The BHS Veterinary Manual

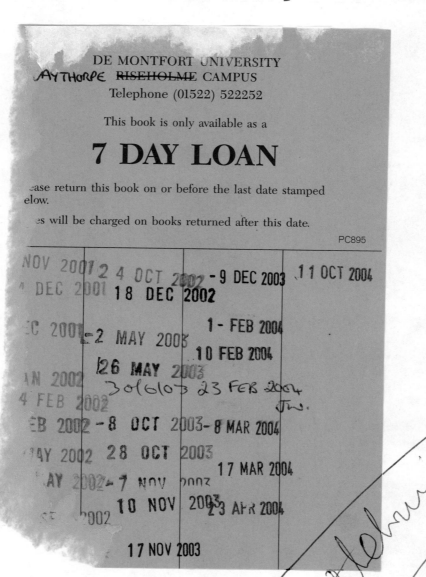

OFFICIAL BHS MANUALS
published by Kenilworth Press

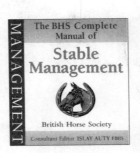

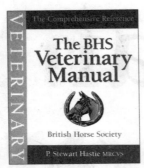

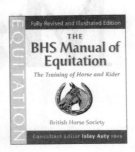

The BHS
Veterinary
Manual

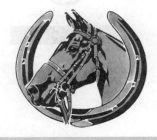

British Horse Society

P. Stewart Hastie MRCVS

KENILWORTH PRESS

DEDICATION

To my wife Jane,
an equine veterinary surgeon, horsewoman and horsemaster
whose loving support kept me 'going forward'
whenever I felt down-hearted.

First published in 2001 by
Kenilworth Press Ltd
Addington
Buckingham
MK18 2JR

Text © The British Horse Society 2001
Illustrations © Kenilworth Press 2001

British Library Cataloguing in Publication Data
A catalogue record for this book is available from the British Library.

ISBN 0-872082-57-2

Layout by Kenilworth Press
Line drawings by Carole Vincer

Printed in Great Britain by Bell & Bain Ltd

DISCLAIMER

This book is not to be used in place of veterinary care and expertise.
The author and publisher shall have neither liability nor responsibility to any person or entity with respect to any loss or damage caused or alleged to be caused directly or indirectly by the information contained in this book. While the book is as accurate as the author can make it, there may be errors, omissions, and inaccuracies.

CONTENTS

PART 3 – LAMENESS: UNDERSTANDING AND DETECTING

PART 4 – VETERINARY ASPECTS OF HORSE MANAGEMENT

PREFACE

My eldest daughter, about to begin primary school, enjoyed being 'mother' at coffee breaks in the Practice. She became privy to the 'shop talk'. The exchange of ideas about 'what animal', 'what was possibly wrong', 'who should see to it', and 'how to treat it', were normal subjects, and the language more vernacular than technical. Carolyn started school. Inquiry as to her progress revealed a heart rending Bible story, about a Mr Saul who had been blinded. Our expressions of dismay were dismissed by her saying, 'Don't worry. God had seen such a case before – so he knew what to do.' There is little fundamental change in veterinary (and medical) practice; there will always be students and teachers, and there will always be patients.

ABOUT THIS BOOK

This is a companion volume to the **BHS Complete Manual of Stable Management** and indirectly to the **BHS Manual of Equitation**. They are intended primarily for examination students but they should also be seen as essential reading for all who care about and care for the horse – as guidelines for horsemastership and horsemanship.

This manual covers health and disease in, I hope, sufficient depth but without unnecessary technical detail, to enable the reader to better understand and therefore to apply the relevant knowledge, essential and background, for the good of the horse.

It is in four Parts. Today's horse is but a genetic extension, altered for good (but sometimes for worse) by man, and an understanding of Part 1, particularly Evolution and Behaviour, is in my opinion essential in order to understand the subsequent Parts. The separation

of disease from health will require the reader to refer back to Part 1 – good revision.

The book is the product both of many years in horse practice and also, importantly, in communicating with those involved with horses – through discussions, demonstrations, lectures and journal articles. The contents are my sole responsibility, as is my interpretation of the vast amount of information gleaned from my own experience and from that of the many other veterinarians, authors, lecturers and specialists, who over the years have been willing to spread their wisdom and to argue their points of view with me. Just as important were the theories and practices of the many experts in horsemastership who were frequently required to put me straight. Collectively they helped make me a better practioner, more able to see more clearly – and hopefully, too, a more succinct writer.

All who have dominion over the horse must 'practice responsibility for it'. I make no claim to do so by original research findings, but like to think that my contribution to this responsibility is in explaining 'the what', 'the why', 'the whom', 'the how', 'the where' and the 'by whom' (Kipling's *Six Honest Servingmen*), for equine veterinary management.

Throughout the book the use of the hyphen in 'dis-ease is', I believe, vital to understanding the concept of 'well' or 'ill', at-ease or dis-eased. The horsemaster must be able to recognise the relevant signs of health and disease which are so important in routine husbandry – if one looks for them – and to so interpret them that correct decisions are made. Veterinary science and practice do not stand still, and so a textbook cannot always be totally up-to-date – but *the basics do not change*.

P. Stewart Hastie

ACKNOWLEDGEMENTS

Where to start, where to finish? There are so many to whom I am indebted, and I shall begin with those no longer with us but whose writings remain, and in particular, among the veterinarians:

Sir Frederick Smith AVC, for his work with navicular disease in the late 19th century, followed some thirty years later by that of my 'boss' Major Oxspring FRCVS, the first (with Col. Pryor) to use radiography for this important 'foot' problem.

Capt. Horace Hayes FRCVS, the original author of *Veterinary Notes for Horse Owners*, such a standard textbook that it has been subsequently edited by three other veterinary surgeons, particularly Peter Rossdale FRCVS who fortunately is still with us, an international authority on diseases of the newborn foal, amongst other subjects, and whose permission to quote is gratefully received.

Professor Linton MRCVS, one time of the Royal Dick Veterinary School, is remembered for his two classic text books, Nutrition and Hygiene, which held much importance for students in the mid-20th century; and Dollar, of surgical textbook fame (and his subsequent editor Professor O'Connor). These books remained in use up to and after the Second World War, as did that of J. Share Jones FRCVS as well as the much earlier encyclopaedias of Professor J. Worthey Axe.

One of my own professors stands out; he taught well, but his emphasis was on 'search': my references to 'Seek, and ye shall find,' come (indirectly) from that. In a similar vein Sam Hignett, a cattleman with more knowledge of the horse than most people, and a personal mentor, advised, 'Treat all research findings cynically – until substantiated.' No-one can forget Professor J. G. Wright, a lecturer and horseman *par excellence*.

Roger Ferguson taught me the necessity of being an efficient stable manager, 'feeder' and tack carer; he revitalised veterinary school riding clubs. Sally Glendinning was one of the first practitioners to establish cardiology, extending the college work of Holmes and Littlewort, both retired and succeeded by Patterson. Lt. Col. Hickman, a doyen of horsemastership and of equine (orthopaedic) surgery and of farriery, was the last to go, but leaving fond memories to many of us.

Thriving veterinarians to whom I am indebted are:

Professor P. M. Dixon MRCVS, Royal Dick Veterinary School (dental disorders); Dr Sue Dyson FRCVS, Animal Health Trust (time after time she has guided and advised on equine orthopaedic disorders); Professor G. B. Edwards FRCVS (colic surgery); Dr Pat Harris MRCVS (nutritionist, exertional rhabdomyolysis); Derek C. Knottenbelt MRCVS (skin and nearly all deeper areas); Professor Leo B. Jeffcott FRCVS (back disease research); Dr J. Geoffrey Lane FRCVS (ear, nose, throat surgery); Dr D. J. Marlin, Animal Health Trust (heat stress); Professor Ian G. Mayhew FRCVS (neurology); James R. Rooney DVM (locomotion); Michael A. P. Simons MRCVS (through his role at the BHS he pushed the need for veterinary representation in training); Ian M. Wright MRCVS (specialist practitioner in orthopaedic problems, particularly of the 'foot'); Sara Wyche MRCVS (locomotion).

Non-veterinary authors whom I have relied upon include:

Xenophon, whose tenets still hold today; E. Muybridge, whose photography was the forerunner of many hi-tech pictorial recordings of the horse in motion; H. Wynmalen, an exquisite horseman; Summerhays, author of a complete book on the horse which is still of value today; John McTimoney, who introduced me to chiropractics; Col. Podhajsky of the Spanish School and a valued friend to the BHS and a patient (very!) instructor to British riders; Moira Williams, an early author on horse behaviour. These have sadly left the horse world, but have passed on the torch.

Dr Debbie Marsden continues ethology at the Royal Dick. Veterinary School. Equitation continues in the hands of authors such as Molly Sievewright FBHS and Charles Harris, a valuable thorn in the BHS's flesh; Noel Jackson, particularly for polo; Sally Swift, USA, on 'centred riding'; Mary Bromiley, who introduced physiotherapy and writes clearly about it.

Other writers are Budiansky, Scruton and of course E. Hartley Edwards, all instructive and of more than passing interest.

I must also mention those who, not in print, still found time to talk, to explain, and to educate. Sherry Scott, electronic therapy exponent; Anneli Drummond-Hay; Christine Dudgeon; David Tatlow; David Gutteridge, osteopath; Paul Belton, master saddler, David Dodwell, a unique horseman; and, last but not least, Mac Head FWCF, this and other practices' hoof balance guru and farrier.

I must also thank Kenilworth Press for their patience and help, especially David Blunt and Fiona Pollard; the artist Carole Vincer; and the staff at Nixon & Marshall Veterinary Clinic.

PART
1

THE HEALTHY HORSE:
ANATOMY AND PHYSIOLOGY

1 EVOLUTION AND BEHAVIOUR

Evolution of the Horse

Some 60 million years ago in the Eocene period there appeared a small, fox-sized, four-toed quadruped, which was a restricted nomad but not particularly gregarious, and which is now recognised by fossil remains as the first or 'Dawn' horse, and given the generic name Hyracotherium (in Europe) and Eohippus (in America). It browsed on soft leaves and flowers and it sought refuge by scurrying, on its short legs, from marshy land into the safety of lush woodland. It was a **scansorial browser**, i.e. able to stand on its hind legs to feed; consequently a long neck was not essential.

Its relatively soft diet required limited mastication, consequently large grinding molars were not yet evident. Plier-like incisors were essential for seizing and snipping off succulent feeds; its skull was therefore relatively small and pointed and the eyes forward-placed. Fibre content was a minor constituent of its food, and its digestion is thought to have been more like that of the simple-stomached animals (e.g. pigs) than that of the later herbivores (e.g. cows and horses).

Over the succeeding fifty million years changing climates, including the ice ages, brought marked changes in vegetation – and during this immense span of evolution Hyracotherium's many descendent branches strove to evolve with the changes.

These changes primarily required an animal to be capable of escape from danger in open country by flight over usually firm ground. Its limbs therefore grew longer relative to body size; and the number of toes reduced to one per limb. Moreover, it stood on tip-toe – which also enhanced its height – with the last bone of the digit encased in a horny hoof. In support of this 'unguligrade' stance, it developed particularly effective stay and suspensory apparatus. All allowed for greater speed.

The sparse coarse grass had to be sought out by continuous walking and eating in the daily search to satisfy appetite; the evolving horse became nomadic, and for safety reasons moved in groups or herds – it became gregarious.

Above all, Equus, as we now name it, had to grasp with its lips before pinching off the stemmy grass with pincer-like incisor teeth, crushing it between large, strong, abrasive molars set in a relatively large head. The bigger head to accommodate the bigger molars created increased weight at the end of a neck itself grown bigger; the neck required stronger muscles; and the weight and leverage of the combined head and neck had to be matched by improved spinal muscles (*see also* Chapter 17, THE LOCOMOTOR SYSTEM).

Horses which evolved in arid lands – e.g. the Arab – lived off the fruit of the palm as well as more succulent young grasses, and retained a narrow head with slightly smaller molars.

A changing feature of the increasing skull size was the position of the eye sockets, which now became more laterally placed. This coincidentally was more advantageous to the nomadic equine's survival requirements. The elongation of the head was not all bone. Rostrally, the nasal bones remained as cartilage. This allowed for a flexible muzzle and upper lip, giving the horse the ability to dilate its nostrils and use the upper lip as a strong and sensitive 'hand' – an important 'feeler' and manipulator.

These were cursorial grazing herbivores, but they retain – to this day – their browsing instincts. All depended on the energy of food from the microbial fermentation of the masticated cellulose-rich fibres in an extra-large caecum and colon, now occupying a larger abdomen and

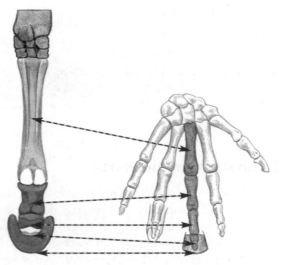

Compare man's hand (and middle finger nail) with the horse's foreleg (and hoof).

round-the-clock pattern of grazing.

The one and, as far as is known, only genus to 'make it' in evolutionary survival terms was Equus. The present-day horse and pony, and other members of the family, all stem from one species progenitor of some five million years ago.

There are six species within the genus **Equus**:

Equus asini – the wild ass, the North African forebear of the donkey

E. *hemionus* – the Asiatic wild ass

E. *grevyi* – Grevy's zebra

E. *zebra* – the Mountain zebra

E. *burchelli* – the plains or common zebra

E. *caballus* – the present-day horse

suspended from a functionally rigid spine. The stomach and the small intestine continued their enzymatic digestion; the stomach itself remained relatively small, being regularly filled, trickle fashion, by a 14–18 hours

E. *caballus* is thought to have appeared in three, possibly four, main types. They first became established in various areas of Siberia and Asia, and migrated to the Middle East and North Africa and westward into Europe, Scandinavia and Great Britain. The early changes produced some variations in structures and related functions suited to

From 'Dawn' horse to the present day.

Hyracotherium (Eohippus) – one of the first creatures that can be considered a true ancestor of the horse. Lived 64-38 million years ago. Height at the shoulder approx. 30cm (3hh). A browsing scansorial 'horse', it walked splay-footed on all 4 toes and its cheek teeth had simple crowns.

Mesohippus – lived 38-26 million years ago. Height at the shoulder 45cm (4½hh). It had only 3 toes. More horse-like molarised tables.

Miohippus – a slightly more advanced form of Mesohippus in respect of feet and dentology. Evolved in the upper Oligocene period, 30 million years ago. Height at the shoulder 60cm or above (6hh). Three-toed, outside toes still remain prominent; incisor teeth becoming more evident.

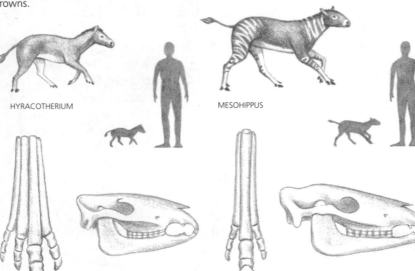

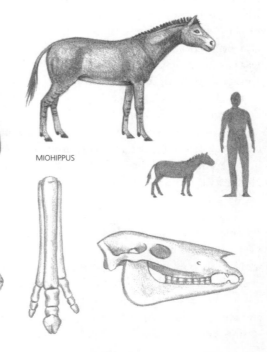

HYRACOTHERIUM

MESOHIPPUS

MIOHIPPUS

local conditions, but fundamentally their major structures and functionings were similar. These were the basis for all successors. No dramatic structural or functional change has occurred during the past million years, except in regard to size, conformation and variety – all the outcome of natural outcrossings and later domesticated breeding.

Today, when man has invested in the characteristics and attributes of *E. caballus*, and especially when he has invested in the athletic potential, he invariably has found that those naturally selected locomotor structures and functionings, which served the genus in survival and had, by careful selection and management, served him in successful and continuing use, were often the weak links – the 'Achilles' heel' when the pressure was on in training and use.

And in addition to exaggerating the horse's physical ability potential, man has also disrupted its gregarious and nomadic instincts. Isolation in stables, confinement in relatively small fields, feeding of different vegetable material in quantities and at times thought correct by man, have all brought many problems, not only of ill-health and disease but also of behaviour.

Simplified Taxonomy

Kingdom	Animalia
Class	Mammalia
Order	Perissodactyla (odd-toed ungulates)
Family	Equidae – the 'Horse', Rhino and Tapir
Genus	Equus
Species	E. caballus

Civilisation and the Horse

Despite or because of domestication the horse has survived and flourished. When first domesticated and ridden or put to chariot, from 6,000BC, it was a small 11–12hh animal – as depicted in cave drawings and early sculpture. Documented evidence, on stone tablets, has been traced to 2,700BC.

Over the centuries, selective crossing of types produced bigger riding horses. Invading armies introduced 'foreign' breeds. Potential progenitors such as the Barb and Arab were purchased to produce the English thoroughbred and, elsewhere, the ancestors of the warmbloods.

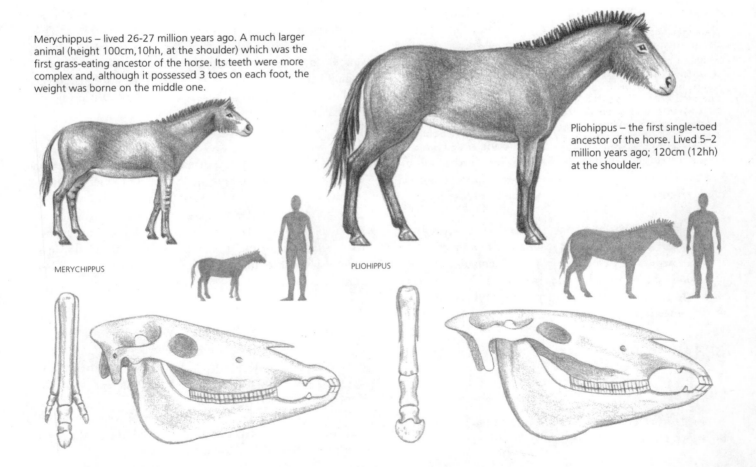

Merychippus – lived 26-27 million years ago. A much larger animal (height 100cm, 10hh, at the shoulder) which was the first grass-eating ancestor of the horse. Its teeth were more complex and, although it possessed 3 toes on each foot, the weight was borne on the middle one.

MERYCHIPPUS

PLIOHIPPUS

Pliohippus – the first single-toed ancestor of the horse. Lived 5–2 million years ago; 120cm (12hh) at the shoulder.

The four types of Equus caballus.

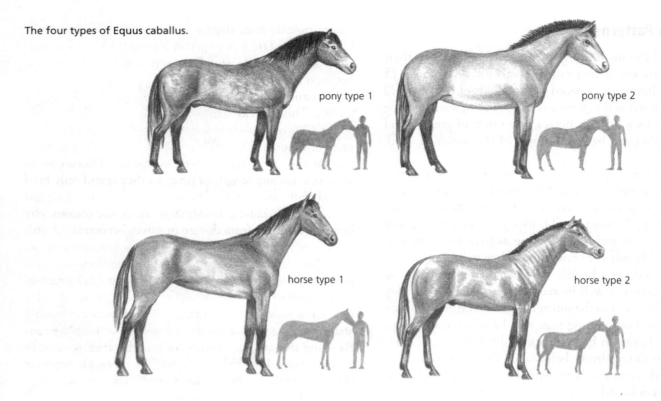

pony type 1

pony type 2

horse type 1

horse type 2

Native British ponies are still relatively unchanged from their origins; and where outcrossed, the progeny have maintained much of the original hardiness and coarse food conversion ability, but have not adapted to the digestion of rich, improved grasses and highly digestible energy concentrates – hence their susceptibility to endotoxaemias such as laminitis, obesity and possibly their intolerance of certain drugs.

Harvested cereals rich in starch, and improved pastures which in their lush growth periods are rich in soluble sugars, are innovations of farming husbandry. Their use dates from late BC for corn and the last 200 years for improved grass pastures.

The larger breeds have not 'changed' sufficiently to be free from the risks of these recent improvements. To a varying degree they can cope with rich concentrate diets and improved pastures, but the change must be introduced slowly to give the digestion microbes time to adapt; *fibre or roughage is still essential*.

BEHAVIOUR

Survival

A horse's instinctive behaviour is that of **fright**, **fight** and **flight**, which enables it to escape by fleeing from danger.

The newborn stays close to its dam and responds almost automatically to her instinctive behaviour patterns. The foal is born with relatively long legs, capable of producing quick turns of speed and its eyes are prominent and capable of great visual acuity, so it can see possible danger and quickly return to the safety of the dam. Within hours of its birth, from the time it has become secure on its limbs, if touched suddenly on its quarters by other than its dam it will instinctively kick out backwards.

Thus it learns from its mother where and what to graze, where to drink and where to shelter and what paths to follow, as well as when to run away. This is all learned from close bonding with the dam, and from an early age the foal has a good sense of survival. This bonding or imprinting, the result of learning added to innate instinct, is early mental programming, and is believed to be more or less completed within the first few days of life.

The horse evolved to survive at grass where, apart from food, it felt free and was programmed to run from danger. It was not an aggressive animal unless cornered. A stabled horse **is** cornered: it will try to escape until it is 'acclimatised' to being shut in but it never forgets its birthright of 'flight rather than fight'.

It is equipped to deal with extremes of weather; it has little need for 'burrowing' for warmth, or hiding. Above all it needs at least 14 hours grazing per day.

Grazing Patterns

Because of the small size of their stomach, horses in their natural state eat at frequent intervals for, on average, 15 out of 24 hours, interspaced with periods of rest. In cold weather, or when the grazing is poor, grazing bouts will be increased. In a herd of horses, the onset of grazing and resting is dictated by the example of the senior or 'lead' mare.

There is no strict pattern to grazing, and it varies according to the season and the weather. Availability of herbage in different seasons will determine the total hours spent grazing. In winter cold, to keep warm, horses will move about day and night, grazing as they do so. In wet, and especially wet cold conditions, they will stand tail to the wind and even huddle together for warmth, day or night; grazing may well be reduced. In summer heat they will seek shelter from the sun at its peak and group together for fly protection; grazing may well be concentrated into the cooler hours. In both situations dry matter intake has priority in determining behaviour; the innate need to trickle feed is constantly present. This feeding programme has certain drawbacks – there is no guideline for how much per day. In poorish grazing, deficiency may occur; so, conversely, will over-eating (especially by ponies) in good grazing or improved pastures.

Stabled horses given ad-lib access to fodder including straw in bedding adopt similar feeding patterns to horses at grass. Behaviour problems may occur if this is not permitted.

Drinking

Horses drink by sucking through partially closed lips, which helps them to filter mud and floating debris. Wild horses do not drink as often as domesticated horses, and herds may roam a long way from a watering hole for grazing, only returning to drink every other day. This is sometimes replicated in stabled horses which may drink only at night or vice versa.

Rest

During rest periods between grazing bouts, horses' behaviour varies according to the time of year. In summer, they usually rest, standing in the shade or in a windy spot to avoid flies, and indulge in mutual grooming or stand head to tail to swish flies away. In winter, a sheltered spot is preferred, and will depend upon the wind direction.

One of the special adaptations which help horses

escape quickly from danger is their stifle joint 'lock' (*see* Chapter 17, THE LOCOMOTOR SYSTEM), which permits sleep or rest while standing and a minimal time lag between awareness and escaping.

In nature, horses spend up to one quarter of the day resting. This is divided into several short periods, but only about 10% of this time is spent actually lying down and most of that is in 'sternal recumbency' (i.e. lying upright, not flat out). The lungs become congested if horses lie on their side for any length of time, so they spend only brief periods fully asleep lying in 'lateral recumbency' (flat out on their side). Lung congestion is one of the reasons why horses recumbent from disease or injury become a difficult nursing problem, and so too with general anaesthesia.

Although horses do not sleep for long, they do need good sleep. By nature they are light sleepers. In domestication, and particularly in training yards, it helps to have a quiet period of up to three hours during the afternoon, in which there are no stable activities going on. By doing this, all the horses have an opportunity to have an undisturbed rest by day as well as by night: whether standing at rest, or lying down with snatches of deep sleep, seems to be a 'personal' decision.

Herding

Horses are herd animals. Herding is a strong instinct and horses are always happier in the company of others. In the wild, a herd normally consists of a stallion, a few mares (usually four or five), their foals and yearlings, and a few two-year-olds. Colts are usually driven away by the stallion when they become mature, at around two years. Herding has many benefits for horses, including mutual grooming and protection from flies and defence against predators. As a group, one or more can be on-guard while the others doze or lie down. In flight, their very numbers can make predators' decisions in isolating individual prey more difficult.

It is difficult for humans to appreciate the importance to horses of the herding instinct. Horses kept in isolation may fret, refuse to eat, or show other abnormal behaviour patterns such as box-walking. These problems can often be overcome by providing companion horses or donkeys, or non-equine companionship such as goats, sheep, rabbits or chickens.

Dominance

Although the stallion will fight for or to retain possession of his mares, he is not dominant over them and, in most instances, follows the herd rather than leads it. Usually, one mare acts as leader. Within a herd, although some animals appear to be more dominant, there does not appear to be a hard and fast 'pecking order' in which each animal is able to pick on those 'junior' to it, as with poultry. Some animals get on well together, others do not; some will not graze together and may show active hostility to one another. Similar relationships also appear to develop under domestic conditions.

Dominance does not appear to be related to age or size, and the relationships between a group of domestic horses are complex. The most important factor seems to be the length of time an animal has been in the group – at least to begin with, any newcomer is 'picked on' by all the established members.

Social Contact

Horses that get on well together are said to show 'positive affectionate behaviour'. This includes nasal contact, mutual grooming, standing head to tail, tail swishing, and grazing near one another. Those that do not 'get on' do not indulge in any of these activities and may even become aggressive. Competition for food will often create aggression between horses which are otherwise normally friendly. This is most frequently seen when hard feed or hay is put out for horses at grass.

Territory

Horses tend to remain in the same extended area (home range), but are not territorial – i.e. they do not defend their area from others. The home ranges of several herds may overlap. The important behaviour is moving away from faeces-contaminated areas to fresh and more abundant grazing, at least for several weeks if not months – an instinctive anti-worm infestation measure. Defaecation in 'domestic' fields is usually restricted to one corner or side, but this produces pasture that tends eventually to become horse sick, with less grazing area than soiled (*see also* Parasitism). Such mis-managed fields lose their effective grazing acreage/hectarage by the subsequent development of unused roughs and over-grazed 'lawns', making worm control doubly difficult.

Growth and Maturity

Colt foals will show precocious behaviour towards their dam by ineffectual, innocent mounting play in the box and in the field.

Both sexes become mature at around 18–24 months; the fillies will display oestrus signs, and colts will respond but are unlikely to be fertile before their second birthday. Exceptions are known.

Separation of the sexes in fully domesticated circumstances follows weaning at about six months of age. This separation is mainly to prevent injuries to male or female, from unwelcome male advances.

In wild or feral situations, the group or herd stallion will drive off two-year-old colts, who then form male groups away from the main herd. Three-year-old and older stallions will eventually break back and attempt to steal mares and fillies by cutting some of them out and drawing these away to form their own harem, rather than fight for the whole herd.

In domestication it is of course essential – by selection or prevention – to control unplanned breeding. Castration of colts not destined for stud work is as a rule carried out in their second spring, as yearlings. In some situations the operation is performed at 6 weeks old. It is arguable that long-term differences between foal and yearling age of operation are significant.

In Thoroughbreds, the young 'go to work' from one to two years old, to race as two-year-olds. Later castration depends on success on the track or lack of it. As in the wild, 2- and 3-year-old future stallions will yard or graze peacefully if not in contact with females, and will practise not only fright, fight and flight action but also sexual attempts at mounting – all youthful games and essential exercise to prepare them for natural adult life. A 2-year-old colt can prove very difficult to manage especially if incorrectly handled at an earlier age.

Breeding Cycle

The mare's breeding cycle is, theoretically, all through the year, but they 'quieten down' from October to March unless encouraged by extra feeding and artificial 'daylight' in January and February.

The cycle is one of approximately 19 to 22 days. The duration of being 'in season' gradually reduces from about 10 days down to 5, and in June and July may even be just 2 to 3 days. The thoroughbred stud world aims for an early foal, and so requires mares to come in season artificially from February onwards. The gestation period is approximately 11 months (336 days), but variations either way are not uncommon; some mares will go 3 weeks overdue with no problems to themselves or to their foals.

BEHAVIOUR AND ITS INTERPRETATION

Horses (foals) learn by **habituation**, **sensitisation**, **association** and **observation**.

Behaviour is the manner in which the horse interacts with its environment – whether living things or inanimate structures. In the mature animal it is a mixture of inherited and acquired components. Inherited behaviour varies from simple reflexes up to complex patterns, while acquired components are conditioned reflexes, general habits and learned habits, i.e. habits both naturally acquired and taught by man.

Many of the natural needs expressed as behaviour in the wild cannot be met in domestication. Some of the taught responses conflict with the innate, and when this occurs the need to escape from control and revert to the behaviour patterns of the wild – with subsequent loss of trained behaviour – becomes psychologically necessary to the horse and sometimes mentally and physically worrying for the owner.

Responsive Behaviour

A horse's behaviour is therefore determined by what its senses tell it.

Take the following example of catching a horse. He will see you moving as you approach the field and will, dependent upon his 'conditioned responses', or training, make up his mind whether to stay out of reach or to approach and be caught. If the latter, he has, in fact, recognised and accepted you. At close range he will sniff proffered feed, check you, and begin to eat. His ears will be 'sweeping' for approaching 'danger', and without leaving the bowl he may pivot on the forehand to gain a better view or to place his hindquarters towards suspected danger. Hearing your voice during this period will reassure him but, unless he really knows you – and your careless habits – he will back off if your hand is inadvisedly raised in front of his face at close range; he cannot accurately see what you are up to, suspects attack from his anterior blind spot, and fears the worst. If, however, your flat hand is placed firmly on his neck, with fairly strong pats, and then tickles up towards mane and withers, contact and reassurance are achieved.

In the loosebox, the noise of your approach – and especially the rattle of buckets – will usually attract the horse to look over the door. Again, your voice will augment what he has already heard and seen. If well trained he will back off on command and, from experience, go to the manger and wait for you to put the feed in.

A horse fully engaged in eating or 'standing asleep' should be attracted by voice, not by immediate direct hand contact. It is then preferable to pat the neck and shoulders before the quarters. A sudden touch on the quarters, which is a blind spot, is likely to cause a reflex kick. Handling should be confident but slow, with firm flat hand contact. Keep talking soothingly, using his name or other constantly used expression – it is not just what you say but also how you say it (the tone, pitch, speed).

New strong-smelling toiletries, bright materials, 'noisy' clothing, or a sudden loud voice, can intimidate the horse. Such breaks in routine handling in the box can upset the

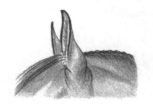

Position of the ears.

pricked – maximum alertness

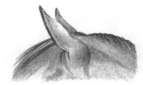

interest to front

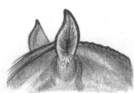

interest to side, or dozing

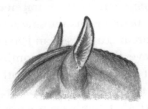

half-back – submission or doziness

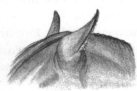

back – interest behind, or submission, or fear

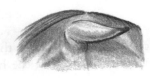

flat back – fear or anger

Body language.

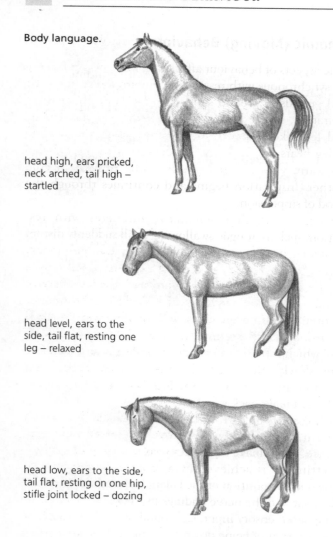

head high, ears pricked, neck arched, tail high – startled

head level, ears to the side, tail flat, resting one leg – relaxed

head low, ears to the side, tail flat, resting on one hip, stifle joint locked – dozing

horse to the extent that he becomes worried and requires room to manoeuvre – or an escape route at your expense.

When adding a new supplement or a powder medicine to a feed try to camouflage the unusual smell or taste by adding a little salt and/or sugar, or chopped succulents, to a small part of his feed, and stir in an equally small part of the unusual addition. Mix well and dampen, which will prevent the horse nuzzling the unknown food away from the known.

When first dealing with a new horse, careful observation should be made of its behaviour when approached in the stable and field. This is especially important in the close confines of a box.

An animal's first line of defence is an innate or unconditioned reflex. Such responses are prompt but brief. In a box, the response is likely to be aggressive; in the field, the horse will look for evasive escape. Attack is by teeth and/or hind and/or fore feet. This may be accompanied by

vocal aggressive noises, laying back the ears, and baring the teeth – a threat.

Some of this response is complicated by conditioned reactions, when a previous painful experience is recalled – the noise of clippers, or the presence of a particular handler associated with something unpleasant in the past. A warning is often given: ears are laid back tightly, eyes are

Aggressive postures.

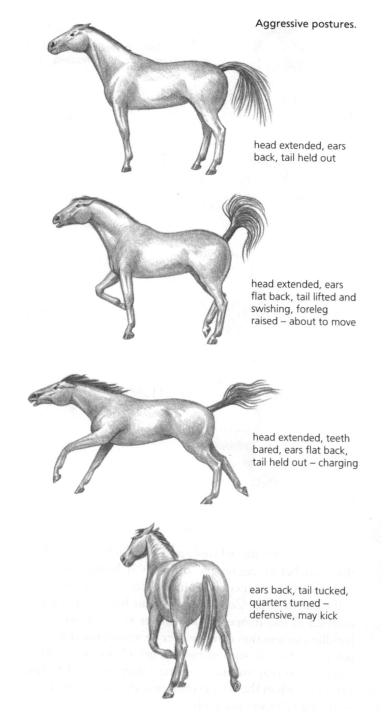

head extended, ears back, tail held out

head extended, ears flat back, tail lifted and swishing, foreleg raised – about to move

head extended, teeth bared, ears flat back, tail held out – charging

ears back, tail tucked, quarters turned – defensive, may kick

Body language – the tail.

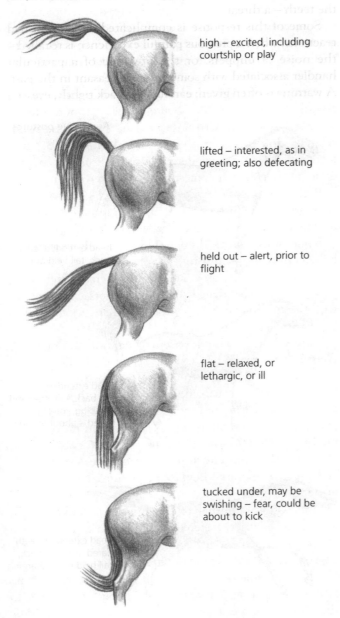

high – excited, including courtship or play

lifted – interested, as in greeting; also defecating

held out – alert, prior to flight

flat – relaxed, or lethargic, or ill

tucked under, may be swishing – fear, could be about to kick

rolled to 'show the whites', and the body is turned to threaten before aggressive reaction is begun. In some animals, their temperament influences these patterns or will come to do so. Consequently, some horses are unfairly branded as bad-tempered, difficult or even dangerous. A handler's assumption can however be wrong; the defensive horse may have to turn its head to get a better view of the suspected threat and in so doing rotate its head to the extreme – when the near eyeball may gyrate to expose the white sclera 'unintentionally'.

Dynamic (Moving) Behaviour

Some aspects of behaviour affect gait; in canter and gallop it is synchronous with respiration. Expiration requires the fixed periods of ground support to facilitate this part of respiration, so the horse begins to exhale as the leading hind leg takes support and finishes when the leading foreleg bears weight – the condensation of the exhaled air's warm vapour can be seen at the nostrils in cold weather. Inspiration begins and continues through the period of suspension.

Anything which momentarily interferes with respiration, such as 'tongue swallowing', will suddenly disrupt the stride. In situations such as obstructive pulmonary disease, the increased duration of expiration will reduce the time for inspiration. This, along with the less effective gaseous exchange, reduces the horse's performance potential and, in severe cases, will interfere with its stride patterns. Such adverse influences are also seen in a tiring horse which is trying to breathe more deeply and therefore more slowly. Repeated changes of lead occur, and thereafter, in an attempt to reduce the need for oxygen, the horse breaks back to trot.

A horse gets up with its head and forehand first, which allows it more quickly to see over a greater and wider distance and to make rapid decisions regarding its safety.

Getting up is achieved by a progressive response to changes in the position of the balancing mechanism in the middle ear and the nerve endings in the neck. A single or a compound sensory input, e.g. sound or smell or touch or proprioception of being down too long, will begin a reflex chain of events beginning with a conscious lifting of the head which is followed by the reflex movement of the neck which then stimulates placement of one foreleg, then the other, with rotation of the trunk and subsequent bilateral push up by the hind legs. It looks clumsy, and once begun cannot easily be stopped – a human, if too close, may be knocked over. The mare takes care of her foal's position before getting up.

The effectiveness of 'sitting on the head' as a means of keeping a horse down depends on having the head/cheek on the floor with the head and neck stretched horizontally. It is the prevention of the initial alteration of the balancing stimuli that stops the 'getting-up' sequence.

Once up, the un-frightened horse will stretch. First, one or other hind leg is fully extended backwards, then the head is flexed at the throat, the neck is arched upwards and the back 'straightened' or 'elongated', and the tail is elevated and swished. Occasionally, the body is leant back so that one or simultaneously both forelegs are extended.

All these movements stretch joints and stimulate muscles. This equates with cat and dog (and some human!) behaviour.

If given the freedom, and reasonable open space, the horse will then proceed to exercise itself. If such kinetic drives or innate behaviours are restricted, anomalous behaviour may follow. Chastising the horse that shows a desire to be natural and do its daily 'stretches', even with a rider up, can be counter-productive. Lungeing a fit horse to 'get the buck out of it' is logical.

To lie down, the horse will circle the chosen resting area, sometimes two or three times and/or in different directions. It will begin to go down, and may change its mind and get up to start again. On going down, it simply folds or flexes all four legs and collapses rather clumsily into the sternal recumbency position, landing fore-end first followed by the hindquarters. This is usually accompanied by a groan and then a sigh. In this resting position the legs are kept flexed; he then leans to one side or other of the centre line. The legs on that side are tucked under the body; the other two remain folded but unencumbered and can be stretched out.

In this upright recumbent position, shallow sleep or drowsing can occur; the horse may prop his head via his chin (his incisor teeth) on the ground, or bend his neck to rest the head on the uppermost side. The horse may also be able to drowse while standing by means of the unique stay apparatus of the equine hind limbs. In safe situations, perhaps with 'guards on duty', he may roll flat over onto his side with head and neck stretched very flat on the ground. Deep sleep (with **REM** – rapid eye movement – or paradoxical sleep) may occur for short periods in this position of lateral recumbency. **SWS** (slow wave sleep) is equated with sleep of the mind, while paradoxical sleep is that of the body. Resting and sleep may occupy a quarter of the 24 hours, usually in several short periods.

Anomalous Behaviour

Stereotypes were previously known as 'stable vices'; 'vice' is an unjustified, unfair, derogatory term.

An affected horse is one behaving in a manner regarded as generally unacceptable **to the owner**. It may seem to be deliberate 'bad' behaviour, but it is not an intentional fault. The adjective 'stable' is, however, most appropriate, as most if not all such behaviour occurs in a stable, i.e. under the restraints of domestication. This fact was first described in 1839. It is a stress response, in some horses, to inappropriate husbandry which blocks their psychological and physiological needs. The consequent mental pressures are apparently alleviated or redirected by the stereotype. It is believed that these horses have a genetic tendency associated with altered thresholds to their neuro-hormonal levels, which reflect their inability to cope 'normally'.

A stereotype is described as a displacement activity of a repetitive nature with no obvious 'goal'. It is not, directly at least, associated with any physical illness. The need-related drives of grazing (natural ingestion) and locomotion (natural wandering or nomadism) are the two basic instincts which domestication interferes with.

If circumstances (such as stabling) block the satisfying of its instinctive behaviour, then a horse may to varying degrees develop stereotypical behaviourisms.

Some horses which do not show clinically may in fact be subclinically 'suffering' in other ways, e.g. lowered performance. In the absence of the recognised stereotype patterns it can be argued that normal horses have coped with the strains of domestication, but there is much yet to be learnt.

Those horses which patently cannot tolerate the stresses will react by refining aspects of the natural repetitive functioning into a parody of them, which they monotonously repeat for no obvious gain other than as a possible escape from unbearable anxiety. That they stop a particular episode, often more quickly than an onlooker might appreciate, without any apparent coincidental change in the overt circumstances, would seem to indicate at least a temporary alleviation, or some more exciting distraction.

Some habits unusual to the human onlooker might appear to be a vice, a stereotype, when in fact they are a temporary expedient necessary for survival. For example **coprophagia**, the eating of dung, by the foal is to populate its bowel microflora with organisms excreted in its dam's faeces. **Soil eating** points to mineral deficiency either in the diet or more probably in the horse's metabolic products, but neither has been proved except where there is a known geographical related problem. **Wood gnawing** and/or tree barking, whilst annoying for the tree owner, is usually instinctive browsing behaviour.

There are some peculiarities such as **hay dipping**, **door banging** and **wood chewing** and **metalwork licking** which are thought to be 'learned' activities for self-satisfaction and, if noisy, for attention-seeking usually at feed time. **Pawing** is one early sign of colic and may be pain relieving, or a frustration act when a decision to lie down is, for one reason or another, not reached. It may also be an inquisitive safety act (or could it be fun?) when water is entered.

Aggressiveness is not a stereotype.

When stereotypes are suspected it is essential to compile a picture of time, place and occasion, and associated events which could be precipitating features. Horses are not mimics.

It is significant that a marked alteration in domesticated circumstances will often lead to the first exhibition of stereotypes even in an adult horse, such as change of ownership or changed work loads – training and/or competing or reversion to a 'life of Riley'! Such, when added to other stresses, can tip the balance. Their occurrence can raise warranty of sale difficulties. Generally they lower an animal's value, not always justifiably.

In general the drawbacks of domestication which are considered of importance are:

- boredom, sees no activity, has no activity
- lack of attention, and handler's ignorance of the horse's natural needs
- failure of companionship
- too little forage, less than 8kg daily, in small repeated amounts
- too little space
- restricted exercise hours – stabled for 22–23 hours
- a total absence of grazing

all of which are accompanied by degrees of anxiety, frustration, fear and – conversely – pleasurable anticipation. The part played by pain is not yet qualified.

Broken expectation of doing things can also be a trigger, for example:

- plaited up but left for several hours before being ridden
- a lorry starts up but drives off without it
- the sound of horn and hounds but it is left behind
- hears feeding activity but is the last stable in the rounds

The first three could well involve box walking and weaving, locomotion-associated 'blocks'; the last, wind sucking.

Similarly, the ending of pleasurable experiences is known to be a cause:

- a hard feed given – and the bucket then taken away
- feeding of tit bits – and then attention to a neighbour
- a good grooming – and the groom then disappears

Two stereotypes are to do with ingestion – wind sucking and crib biting.

- **Wind Sucking**

  It is conceivable that wind sucking is indulged in because of low grade colic pain. The swallowed air is held in the anterior gullet as a bolus, which seems to give 'gratification' or comfort before being returned to the throat for expiration; not a true burp! It is now accepted that this air is not 'deliberately' swallowed into the stomach. Ill effects are rare, so fear of colic and condition-losing indigestion is not justified.

- **Crib Biting**

  The affected animal is thought to practise wind sucking and then finds it helpful to arch its throat against an upper incisor dental hold in order more easily to use its strap muscles, whose contractions create the necessary vacuum in the pharynx to suck in air and then into the oesophagus. The snap opening of the oesophageal entry causes an audible in-rush of air which is the characteristic gurgling grunt. Only occasionally does an inconsequential amount of air leak to the stomach, usually if the act follows closely on a feed or if water or feed is ingested between cribbings.

Recent research in yearlings and 2-year-olds suggests that a deficiency of swallowed saliva and consequent gastric mucosal changes may be involved, but whether this is cause or effect has not yet been established.

Crib biting can be discouraged by keeping the horse at grass entirely, or for as many hours a day as are practicable, and ensuring that it is mentally stimulated:

- double or treble exercise periods
- have long fibre available continuously, but avoid more than three small hay feeds a day as this may increase anticipatory problems
- let it see and hear other horses and exercise with them
- provide tactile exposure to other horses
- increase grooming time and frequency and 'make much' of the horse afterwards
- bed it well

Since mimicry is not a problem, isolating the affected horse is not only unnecessary but also certainly harmful. Neuropharmaceuticals, under veterinary supervision, can be effective.

There are two behaviourisms once thought to be

stereotypes, but not now

- **Head Shaking**

  There is much argument as to the cause of head shaking in the ridden horse. Control through the bit is lost, sufficiently to lose proper collection but rarely to permit bolting. It was said to be self-hypnotic and therefore stress-relieving. The head shaker frequently shows the condition only in months of bright and strong sunlight.

  It is now thought to be a hyper-sensitivity of part of the trigeminal nerve as it enters the base of the skull due to an as yet unidentified allergen or toxic substance. It responds to certain drugs. There is doubt about the photo (light) theory.

- **Sourness**

  The anomalous condition of **sourness** is associated with prolonged fitness and high-performance work, with the horse 'going over the top' so that work ability rapidly fails (*see also* adrenalin exhaustion, in Chapter 38, FITTENING). In chronic form the horse may be seen as a quiet slow-moving 'plug' in a riding school's repetitive work schedule, especially in older horses with low-grade pain. Such horses seem to produce endorphins which 'switch them off' from their environment, and action becomes almost automatic.

In the first type, temperament may change for the worse. Functional ability may also deteriorate. It is important that sub-clinical (i.e. not apparent) disease is considered as an alternative and more serious cause of loss of performance.

Factors Influencing Behaviour

The factors which influence a horse's behaviour are instinct, breed or type, and subsequent experiences.

Instinct

Instincts are behaviour patterns which are common to all horses. They are automatic responses to certain situations or stimuli – the horse does not have to think or learn to be able to carry them out.

Many aspects of a horse's life are instinctive. These include grazing and resting behaviour, reproductive and maternal behaviour, and the very strong herding instinct.

A horse's instinctive reaction to run away from danger, real or imagined, has stood it in good stead in its evolutionary past. This strong instinct for flight, when frightened, is something that must always be borne in mind when handling horses. Likewise, every rider should be aware that any horse can shy, no matter how 'quiet' or controlled it appears.

Shying is usually an instinctive reflex defence mechanism to a sudden movement or to an unfamiliar object, close to the horse – and something which it is not immediately able to see *clearly*. Control of this reflex action is difficult for both horse and rider. It is this which gives the horse the blame for being unpredictable. It may be that it is the rider/handler who cannot sense, and therefore is unable to predict, what a horse may do.

Breed or Type

The horse's breed or type has a considerable influence on its behaviour – mainly because different breeds have been selected by man for certain characteristics. These include not only speed, strength, or stamina, but also the animal's willingness to co-operate and to respond to human instruction. The 'cold-blooded' breeds, which became established first in Northern Europe, tend to be placid and phlegmatic, whereas 'warmblooded' breeds, originating from Southern Asia but settling in Europe, tend to be slightly more spirited – the Arab and the Thoroughbred, as hot-bloods, even more so.

In addition to possessing the general characteristics of its breed or type, each individual horse has inherited characteristics, behaviour patterns from its sire and dam, and to a lesser degree from their progenitors – i.e. familial tendencies. Overall general behaviour is referred to as temperament.

Experience and Learning

Experience and learning influence behaviour because a horse has a very good memory, particularly for unpleasant experiences. These include not only situations in which the animal has been physically hurt, but also when it has had unpleasant experiences with other horses (bullying) or with humans (ill-treatment). Untoward experiences during rearing, weaning, handling and training, can greatly influence a horse's character and its willingness to respond to human instruction. Mishandling of young horses is the commonest cause of trouble.

The temperament is conditioned for the worse by unpleasant experiences, for the better by good handling. Thus, temperament becomes the product of instinct and learning.

It is, of course, essential that the horse learns by schooling in order to perform to the rider's wishes. It is therefore imperative that such learning should as far as possible be a pleasant experience. The definition of pleasure is not always similar for man and for horse, for whom in general it is 'doing what comes naturally' even if under domestication (riding) conditions.

THE PSYCHOLOGY OF THE HORSE

Although the behaviour traits of horses have been closely studied for many hundreds of years, there have been no wide-scale studies of the mechanisms which determine these traits. Opinions are based on the subjective observations of horsemen, or are derived from experiments carried out in other species.

Intelligence in human beings is assessed as the ability to solve problems by reasoning. Intelligence in animals cannot be assessed in this way. Animals are unable to reason – they do not work out the possible solutions to a problem, but choose the most appropriate one. Reasoning's equivalent in animals is based entirely upon past experience. This means that learning plays an essential part in their mental processes. Evaluating so-called 'intelligence' in animals is a matter of assessing their ability to remember, and how they respond to certain stimuli which 'jog' their memory.

Horses appear to be good at learning, i.e. developing instinctive behaviour or satisfying instinctive requirements. They are excellent at 'remembering' their way and can find their way home over long distances. The mechanisms involved in this faculty are not known – it could be sight, or smell, or a combination of sight and smell and other unknown factors. Wild horses can remember, for many years, where food and water are to be found. However, if food is placed on the opposite side of a fence to a horse, it will not usually be able to work out that it can walk around the end of the fence to get to the food. However if, by chance, it does walk round the end of the fence, and discovers the food, it will repeat this behaviour again on subsequent occasions – i.e. it learns rather than reasons.

Training

Training involves getting a horse to respond to instructions. This means persuading it to respond consistently to commands, by voice or by sensory 'aids',

from its rider.

It must be remembered that horses have a limited mental ability – they can only retain and respond satisfactorily to a small total number of instructions (fifteen to twenty in total). If attempts are made to teach any more than this, they become confused and may even forget what they have already learned.

During training, horses learn to associate a given command with a certain reaction or response. This process can be reinforced by reward (positive enhancement) or by punishment (negative enhancement). In time, the horse will learn to know what response is required for a given command. Horses normally respond better to positive enhancement than to negative enhancement. Far more can be achieved by co-operation and reward than by threats and verbal punishment.

Response to any command or aid is mediated via the horse's nervous system. Repeated stimulation leads to nerve fatigue and so to a dulling of the response. This means that over-use of commands or 'aids' may be counter-productive, making a horse less responsive. Training sessions should be kept short and intensive – the horse being made to concentrate for a limited period only. If, after a while, the animal is not responding correctly, it is best to stop and begin again another day, rather than persevere and sour or confuse the horse. To finish on a good note is of course ideal.

Many aspects of horse behaviour other than stereotypes are learned from other horses. Orphan foals reared in isolation may think they are human because of exclusively human contact. This phenomenon is known as human imprinting. Such animals can show normal equine grazing and resting behaviour, but may develop altered characteristics, particularly with other horses. They misinterpret their gregarious instinctive stimuli. Too much unnecessary 'humanising' is very detrimental to future handling, for instance permitting nibbling and pulling on clothing, or developing a persistent expectation of titbits.

Horses are said to be good at learning bad habits from one another, and for years it has been thought that many stereotypes, including crib biting, wind sucking and weaving, are often acquired in this way. However, the imitator may be merely finding out if the other horse is 'on to a good thing'; more probably the copier is equally stressed – *there is no evidence of mimicry*. An exception is the foal of a crib-biting dam, who perhaps because of some as yet unknown inherited tendency, but certainly also from 'doing what mum does', will follow suit at least temporarily.

Handler's Awareness

Instinctively, a horse is suspiciously aware of the possibility of potential predators, even though most are now extinct. Any distant, moving, unrecognised object will stimulate alertness and even apprehension until it is distinguished as friend or foe. A nearby sudden movement will produce instant apprehension, and possible evasion, until its importance is assessed.

Recognition of nearby objects is possible if the horse is free to look; having to reposition its head when encumbered by aids or other restraints may give only partial visual awareness, and evasive behaviour may be the result. New situations require conditioned acceptance behaviour – habituation. Thus the stable cat, yard dog and other farm animals and birds will eventually become part of the horse's environment, especially if they have been close enough to make smell (and touch) contact.

The horse evolved before man 'discovered' fire. In early domestication, horses must have trampled through fire embers, without a burning sensation, because of hoof protection. Had they investigated the hot ashes with their muzzle, a reflex withdrawal would be followed by a conscious acknowledgment of 'that hurts!' A lesson would have been learned.

Grazing animals exposed to torment by flies learn to stand in the smoke of a bonfire for protection, yet the same horses would panic if the stables caught fire. Heat and noise from an active fire, and the sight of flames and the associated inability to escape, would be the stressors for 'fright', leading to either panic or 'freezing' and refusing to be led to safety. It is intriguing to note that some horses will seek the protection of smoke yet have not been 'taught' by others of this anti-fly material.

Assessing Temperament

Temperament means, literally, 'natural disposition'. When applied to horses, this also involves their willingness or otherwise to co-operate. There is no such thing as an overall ideal temperament; an ideal disposition for one type of activity may be unsuitable for another – a placid co-operative temperament, ideal for a child's first pony, may not be ideal for a racehorse.

Temperament is best assessed by someone who is unfamiliar with that horse, as it is the animal's response to humans in general that should be assessed, not its response to the person who normally looks after it. The following factors should be assessed.

1 Gender

Some mares are less co-operative and more difficult to handle when 'in season'. Colts and stallions always need firm handling, but can become even more difficult to handle when they get older. A few become extremely aggressive and can be dangerous, especially when 'at stud' and particularly when running with the mares.

2 Conformation

Horses with small (piggy) eyes set close together are often said to have a less desirable temperament than those with large eyes set wide apart on the side of the head (a 'generous eye').

The type of horse that has a convex nose outline (the Roman nose often seen in cobs) is usually more placid and phlegmatic than those having a concave outline (the dished face of Arabs and some Thoroughbreds).

3 Expressive Action

Alertness

Is the horse keenly interested and taking notice of everything that is going on around it, or does it appear oblivious to its surroundings? Many can 'shut off' and so appear apathetic until engaged in their discipline, especially if that involves fast work.

Movement

Does it stand quietly alert or at rest, or is it continually fidgeting and on the move? This must be interpreted in relation to the amount of exercise and feed the horse is receiving – a fit horse is more likely to be 'on its toes' than an animal at grass.

Ears

Are the ears pricked and alert, a sign of good temperament? Ears continually laid back are usually a sign of a bad-tempered animal. There are variations in the pattern of 'ears laid back'; some indicate abdominal pain.

Exercise

The amount of work a horse is getting can affect its temperament. Horses that are over-fed and under-worked can become difficult to manage; conversely, horses that are over-worked may become sour.

Health

Ill-health, particularly painful conditions such as back and mouth problems, can affect a horse's temperament and make it less willing to co-operate.

Temperament Changes

Factors contributing to the development of altered behaviour are boredom and lack of normal sensory stimuli. In its natural environment a horse is on the move most of the day, in the company of others. It would spend the majority of its time grazing and chewing, and would have an almost continuing food intake (trickle feeding). By confining a horse in a stable, and feeding it a concentrated diet, it is being deprived for much of the time of the stimuli of movement, grazing *and chewing*. Increased exercise, and more fibre in the diet, can help to overcome some of these problems. Periods at grass, whenever possible on a day-to-day basis as well as short breaks out all the time and off work, are of inestimable value.

Handling

This is the most helpful guide to a horse's temperament. A good idea of its temperament can be obtained by watching its behaviour when being approached and caught in a paddock or stable, and how it behaves when being groomed, tacked up, and mounted. Additional guides include the animal's willingness to co-operate when being loaded into a trailer, when being clipped, or when being shod – all relative to how familiar it is with these activities. When going to look at a horse that is for sale it is not usually possible to assess all of these, nor its behaviour in some traffic.

Feeding and Foodstuffs

Feeding can have a considerable effect on behaviour. A horse that is placid when at grass or when fed only on hay can sometimes become 'hot' and difficult to manage when fed large amounts of concentrates or even relatively small quantities of certain cereals, e.g. oats – a complication in metabolism associated with their particular amino acid content. Competition for food can make horses aggressive. Many ponies are spoilt and made 'nappy' by continually being given titbits.

The study of behaviour is known as **Ethology**; practitioners are Animal Behaviourists or Ethologists. It can be seen that all who ride or keep horses should practise the art to some extent – a welfare matter for both man and horse.

2 THE EQUINE SENSES

The five senses of **seeing, hearing, feeling, smelling** and **tasting** have direct communication with the brain via the related cranial sensory nerves. The horse 'feels' with his mobile muzzle; the whiskers, eyelashes and head skin also pick up contact sensations and direct these to the brain. The various body skin, orifice and other external sensations are routed from the source to the spinal cord and then the brain.

Whilst the horse's sense organs are basically the same as those in humans, there are important differences. Of these, the horse's *long-distance visual awareness of moving objects* is the most active and important. **Hearing** comes next; then reaction to **muzzle/whisker sensitivity**. **Smell** and **taste** play a significant role; smell plays a big part in signals related to reproduction. The **skin stimuli** are seen in mutual grooming and sexual foreplay, and is of especial importance in man-to-horse contact as in 'gentling', massaging, grooming and in the aids.

'Proprioception', a sensory input received normally subconsciously from muscle, tendon and joint nerve endings (*see* Chapter 11, THE NERVOUS SYSTEM), plays a big part in the horse's reflex sense of its position in the environment and in its balance and therefore in its safe locomotion. Proprioception is distinct from pain.

The horse apparently does not 'stop to think', but rather responds quickly and reflexly, and then 'asks conscious questions' from a position of safety. It is very debatable how much intelligence a horse possesses and uses. Whatever the sensory inputs or stimuli, the outstanding feature of the horse is its extraordinary memory of 'feedback' information. It is said that horses 'know' from sensations reinforced by subsequent inputs, whereas humans 'know that they know' and can 'consider' such information.

Vision – The Ocular Sense

The horse's visual system has evolved to function in daylight and in dark conditions for both panoramic **monocular horizontal distance vision** to detect the movement of predators, and **binocular vision** for examining items of interest both at long range (a potential predator) or at close range (for recognising grazing).

The equine eye has the largest globe of all land mammals, producing a retinal image 50% greater than that in the human eye. The many structures of the equine eye are more like nocturnal animals' than man's.

The eye, well protected in the bony orbit by skull and facial bones, is in a more or less anterio-lateral position, set relatively far up in the head – and this position, and the eyeball's somewhat bulging contour, permits a wide monocular field of view. The binocular visual field is 65–80°, looking down its nose, but monocular vision is approximately 190° horizontal and 180° vertical. Visual acuity is poor in comparison with man's.

The horse's peak acuity, of approximately 16.5 cycles/degree, lies in a horizontal band just below the equator of the retina at the back of the eye, with poorer acuity above and below this visual streak. In bright light, the normal constricted horizontal pupil maximises horizontal vision, and the horse can effectively obtain almost 350° – *with a blind field immediately ahead of its nose* and another for several metres behind its rump.

Thus when the horse's head is lowered, for instance to graze, the binocular field is directed towards the ground and the horizontal monocular vision is in position to keep the horizon scanned.

For the rider, it is highly significant therefore that when the horse is on the bit, with nose lowered, i.e. the head on

The horse's field of vision.

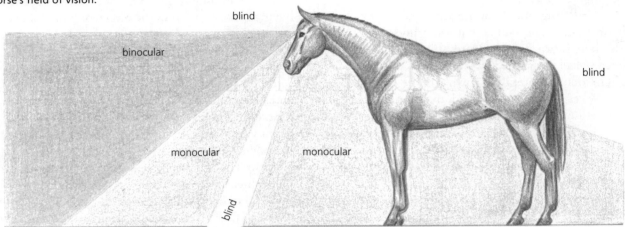

or behind the vertical, *it cannot see directly ahead* and must rely on the rider. If the horse is to see and judge a fence as it approaches, *it must be allowed to raise its nose in order to use its binocular vision*.

The earlier belief that the horse needed to move its head vertically in order to see objects at different distances is not now held; that idea is replaced by one of dynamic accommodation, whereby the horse is able to focus on an object by using monocular 'depth cues'. The distance between the horse's eye level and the ground under natural grazing conditions requires relatively less accommodation ability than man's much shorter distance between eyes and, for example, a page of print.

It is suggested that when a horse pricks both ears forward equally he is using binocular vision. When not drowsing or sleeping, the horse constantly uses **peripheral vision** when on guard. To maintain this visual awareness he behaves like any other look-out. The eyelids periodically blink, momentarily to rest the optic nerves to erase the numbing effect of the fixed stare and the glazed look; the third eyelid may sweep across the eyeball as a 'wiper' to initiate a fresh picture. The eyeballs will be gyrated to the left and to the right and downwards and possibly slightly upwards with minimal head movement. Both eyes move synchronously, one obtaining more of the view than the other as required, as described above for monocular vision. The head may be turned left or right and may be elevated for longer viewing. The body can pivot on either fore or hind quarters to enhance the view, when this is necessary.

When a horse sees an unusual object or movement out of one eye it will turn its head to bring it into binocular vision (not, as was previously thought, in order to bring it into focus). If this is prevented by the rider keeping the

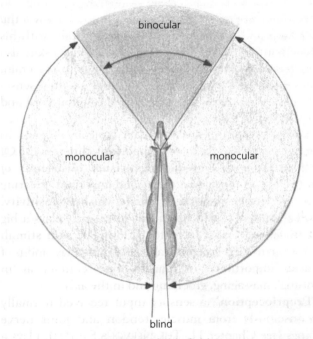

Horizontal field of vision.

horse in a straight line, fear may overcome obedience and the horse will attempt to swing its head and body against the restraints even to the extent of a fast evasion. It is then said to be 'spooking'. It is in fact trying to get away from 'something' seen by one eye but not interpreted by both. In the same context defective vision is often blamed for horses being easily startled and so shying when they become aware of nearby moving objects, but it is possible that when something is 'spotted' but cannot be brought into full view then an 'away from danger' evasion will result even in a normally sighted horse.

When galloping and jumping in company or when driving in traffic or in double harness a horse will try to keep both a forward and a lateral view, and can be distracted or feel threatened by other horses or by traffic to the extent that its lateral vision has to be restricted by blinkers. When trotting up in hand, the runner should for the same reason avoid falling behind the shoulder level, because the horse (particularly if young) may see the runner as a danger or as a 'competitor' and strike out with a hind leg. The same behaviour can also be observed in horses turned out together or as playfulness.

What colour vision 'means' to the horse, and when this skill is used, are still unresolved questions. Colour perception is understood to be good for yellow, green and blue, but red presents difficulty.

The horse's good night vision, reputedly associated with poor colour appreciation, depends mainly on noticing movement and on recognising size, shape and positions rather than detail. Such good vision in a dark environment is said to be due to the presence of an extensive tapetum lucidum at the back of the eye, a light intensifying device which reflects light back on to the retinal nerve endings, and is what makes some animals' eyes 'glow' when lit up in the dark.

Adaption to darkness is slow, but when achieved gives the horse better night vision than man. This slowness may well explain the reluctance of the horse to move quickly from light to dark, and vice versa; cross-country riders must be aware of it, and also handlers when loading into a dark trailer.

Very little information is available on the practical aspects of vision and the evaluation of deficits in vision, let alone on the correction of visual defects; testing for 'sight' in the horse is an inexact science. There is some evidence that domestic horses tend to have short sight, and also that horses generally become longer sighted with age. The altered behaviour of horses with reduced or even absent unilateral vision varies from nil to profoundly different, and is influenced by temperament and environmental familiarity.

Hearing – The Auditory (Acoustic) Sense

As in all species, the ability to hear is very important. Equine 'speech' may not have a large vocabulary but it is an important method of communication, and equine hearing developed in particular to give the horse early warning of predators.

To obtain almost all-round hearing without the horse having to move its body, the **pinna**, or funnel shaped ear, is very mobile, controlled by sixteen independent muscles. Each ear can be operated independently.

The pinna directs the sound waves down into the eardrum, where the sound waves pass through the drum and along a chain of tiny bones. These waves of movement transfer to fluid contained in the inner ear, and its subsequent vibrations are turned into nerve signals which go to the brain's auditory centre.

As well as being highly efficient organs for hearing, the multi-directional ears are also accurate indicators of attention and of body language. When both pinnae are turned to the front there is extreme attention forward. They will be turned to the side when dozing. With the ears half back the horse indicates submission and attention backwards. When the attention is split between different stimuli, or the horse feels anxious or irritated, the ears will move between positions and differently on either side. When the ears are flat back it signifies anger and fear, and this closes the funnel-shaped opening so the horse cannot hear

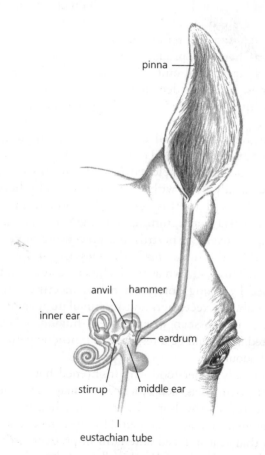

pinna

anvil   hammer

inner ear

eardrum

stirrup   middle ear

eustachian tube

The hearing mechanism of the inner ear.

– 'I am "deaf" to auditory requests or explanations' – and at the same time helps to protect the ears from foreign material particularly water and wind-blown sand or dust.

The horse is able to hear a wide range of frequencies, from very low 'P' waves (as in an imminent earthquake) to a high frequency of 25KHz, compared to the dog's 35 KHz, whereas the human's maximum is approximately 15KHz. Hearing is most sensitive in the range 2–5KHz, which is the level of normal quiet human speech and therefore the ideal communicative pitch for man to 'speak' to a horse.

Horses tend to be 'spooky' when it is windy. This is thought to be partly because the horse cannot hear so clearly, as noises become distorted and therefore unfamiliar.

Smell – The Olfactory Sense

The main function of smell is to receive messages given out by predators, by other horses and by plants.

Herbivores sniff the air to detect the proximity of predators, but do not track a smell as carnivores do. They 'read' messages in faeces and urine. Just as certain chemicals are produced in the body and circulated to other parts as messages requiring action from the receiving organ, so too are certain chemicals produced and secreted from skin glands and via vaginal and other excretions. These are **pheromones**. They are detected and identified by other horses sniffing up the odour of the particular protein molecules.

In addition to the usual olfactory nerve endings, a special area at the rostral end of the nasal passage and the roof of the mouth is developed into **Jacobson's organ**, which specifically deals with pheromones. In the horse, these are directed to this specific location from the external nostrils by an upturning of the upper lip, curling the top lip up over the nostrils and preventing more air entering while the horse 'reads the message' and reacts accordingly. This is known as the **Flehmen gesture**, and it is also used by young horses when first meeting a new smell, to enhance reception and to stimulate memory – learning! It is also seen when a 'new' human is being investigated and could be a response to synthetic perfume or natural odour.

It is not fully understood why frightened handlers or riders are recognised as such by a horse. It may be that it is communicated to the horse by it seeing, hearing and feeling agitated human behaviour. However, recent work indicates that fear-induced adrenalin bi-products in the sweat of the less than confident handler or rider are recog-

nised by the horse – which interprets them as a danger signal, and so takes evasive action. A lack of rapport could be attributed to the horse's dislike of that person's odour, either actual or cosmetic.

When a horse nuzzles something it is first of all sniffing in order to smell, but it does so at close range as it must coordinate with the other senses, including the tactile sense from the whiskers and muzzle skin – one reason why whiskers should not be clipped off – and also taste.

Sharing stables can cause problems with some horses, as they will pick up the previous occupant's excretory scent and so can become agitated. Ripping of rugs can similarly be due to the rugs having a strange smell.

The areas where urine and faeces are deposited serve as territorial markers. The faeces in particular so taint the grass that horses will not graze there for some time. Territory is not too important to herds, but a stallion will quickly recognise the excretion of another encroaching. A mare's marking facilitates herd membership identification and also indicates which dam deposited it, for her foal to recognise.

The foaled mare recognises her foal by smell, and this eases bonding. The foal is attracted to the mother by smell, initially from the udder and nearby sebum glands. The mare spends a long time licking the newborn foal and this allows mare and foal to become familiar with each other's scent. Artificially drying a newborn foal can interfere with this bonding and can even lead to the mare rejecting her foal.

A main function of smell is in sexual awareness. Urine, and to a lesser extent faeces, will carry early warnings of a mare's impending **oestrus**, and alert the stallion. His sniffing where his mares urinate, and where utero-vaginal mucus is ejected, home him in on his next mating appointment; the oestral flow is the ultimate message that she is

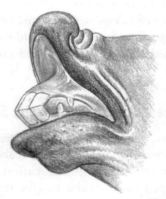

The Flehmen gesture.

receptive and likely to 'stand'.

The smell of food is particularly important. Horses offered a new feed will smell it thoroughly before deciding to eat; it may be because they cannot vomit that horses have to be especially careful about what they eat, unlike dogs (regurgitation of ruminal contents for cudding, as in bovines is not a true vomit and does not serve as a safety valve).

Taste – The Gustatory Sense

As a grazing animal, the horse depends on his sense of taste to determine safe and unsafe materials – for instance, ragwort has a bitter taste as well as a warning smell during its growing and flowering periods, and in situations other than absolute starvation the horse will steer clear. (Most ragwort poisoning follows consumption of baled hay containing ragwort which has wilted and so is not detectable by taste.) Not all potentially poisonous plants have such a warning taste or smell.

The four taste sensations that the human recognises – **sweet**, **bitter**, **acid** and **salt** – are thought to be similar in the horse, and the horse certainly has a highly developed discriminating taste apparatus. The tongue is covered in taste buds, with the highest concentration at the rear.

A salty taste is attractive particularly if the diet is, naturally or otherwise, deficient.

Foals are programmed to recognise their dam's faeces, and they eat some to populate their digestive systems with specific micro-organisms.

It is well recognised that most horses are attracted to the sweet flavours of fruit and vegetables as well as man-made confectionery, but whether this is the sugar content or the peppermint content has yet to be resolved!

Touch – The Tactile Sense

The human can feel, identify, and analyse with his finger tips, toes and lips – an important ability which sets him above the lower animals, because with the information he can then think over the implications. By definition, all that is felt is consciously received, but where safety is at risk then the reflex response is quicker than 'knowing' – e.g. fingers coming near a hot plate. Tactile senses recognise, assess and set in motion reflex actions.

A horse has a true tactile sensory apparatus only in the muzzle skin, whiskers and eyelashes, and these three receivers go direct to the brain, if necessary initiating reflex action before awareness.

Since most of the tactile and other similar sensor nerve endings, including those of pain, are scattered over the skin's sub-surface and on the internal serous surfaces of the body, most such messages are routed through the spinal cord. The specific immediate spinal reflex is then initiated before the message goes on to higher, but not always conscious, centres in the brain. Pain felt by an animal is a clear message to rest the area to avoid further damage – hence lameness. Pain emanating from internal serous surfaces will also interfere with the function of the related organs – hence bowel stasis (ileus), as in colic.

Special nerve endings, proprioceptors, are present in joints, tendons and muscles, which relate information about pressure and stretch, and which, along with the information from the semi-circular canals of the ear, help maintain posture, balance and limits of muscle stretch. This provides horses with a good sense of the terrain they are travelling over and of how to compensate for any changes in it.

Many of these sensory inputs eventually go to specific centres in the brain including some to the 'conscious' cerebrum, where they are recognised. A human might say, *'I like the look of that,' 'Isn't that music delightful,' 'Oh, what a smell,' 'This food tastes sour.'* A horse will, by its behaviour, evince what it has become aware of and what it interprets from the sensation; *'I see grass, so will smell it and taste it and, if satisfied that it is safe, shall eat it,' 'I hear a horn noise – experience tells me that hounds are running – I must be ready to gallop.'*

Only in some situations, for example sexual arousal, defending territory, or warning others, will the horse 'speak' its thoughts and back up this vocabulary with facial expression and postures.

INTRODUCTION TO ANATOMY

Anatomy, from the Greek *ana* (up) and *tome* (to cut), is the study of the structure of the body and the relationship of its parts one to another within the whole. It is one of the oldest of the biological sciences (4th century BC, Aristotle).

All structures have a biological function, a physiological role, and students of horsemastership and equitation benefit from under-the-skin 'inside' information. This should be learnt not just for the sake of remembered knowledge but for a better understanding of what goes on and how the functioning of the parts looks in health and how and why this differs in disease and injury.

Surface anatomy is the visual and tactile appraisal of the skin surface areas and the skeletal promontaries or 'points' which have long been identified by colloquial names, the horseman's terms. The points, and the distances and angles between them, are the basis of 'conformation'.

In the adult horse these parameters are fixed. Although the amount of fat and muscle development also has a genetic basis closely linked to the skeletal map it is an alterable feature reflecting nurture – particularly diet and work – and it is best seen not as conformation but as 'condition'.

The purpose of this chapter is to consider skeletal anatomy and some related ligamental structures, and to do so with reference to the horse's evolved features. Some of these are on the one hand evolutionary survival assets and, on the other hand, potential weaknesses. To the nomadic, herbivorous, unguligrade, free-ranging, gregarious, herd animal which evolved over many millennia, and whose athleticism was restricted to 'fright, flight and fight' actions and whose life routine was a combination of trickle feeding, of being always in the open air and of being unhampered by confinement, these features were not a problem; but, particularly in many 'improved', domesticated breeds, they become 'Achilles' heels'.

Topographic Surface Identification

'Front end' and 'rear end' are explicit terms but do not relate well to other scientifically described features. **Forehand**, referring to head, neck and foreleg, and **hindquarters**, referring to quarters and hind leg, are well recognised descriptions, but the more advanced student requires more scientific terms.

Location of the 'true' points of the horse – the bony prominences (tuberosities – e.g. tuber sacrale = point of croup).

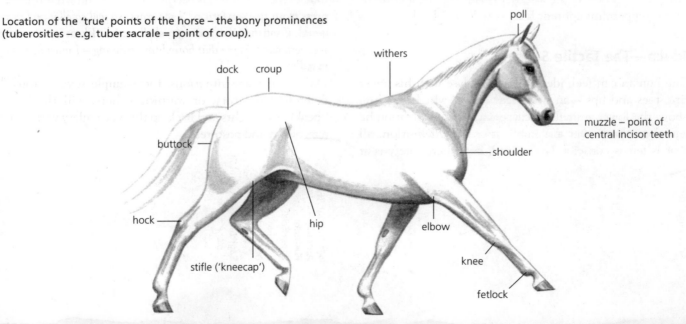

poll

withers

dock   croup

muzzle – point of central incisor teeth

buttock

shoulder

hock

hip

elbow

stifle ('kneecap')

knee

fetlock

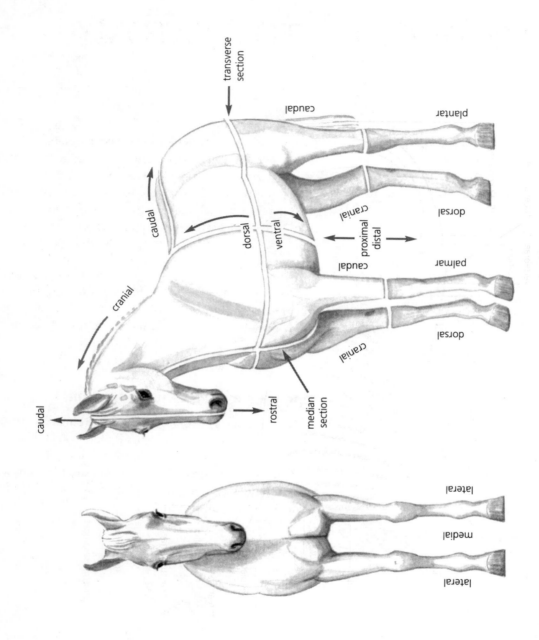

Anatomical directions.

ADDITIONAL TERMS
Anterior – in front
Posterior - behind
Superficial – near the
surface
Deep(er) – furthest
away from the surface
Sagittal – dorso-ventral
plane down the long
axis of the body, any
distance either side of
median

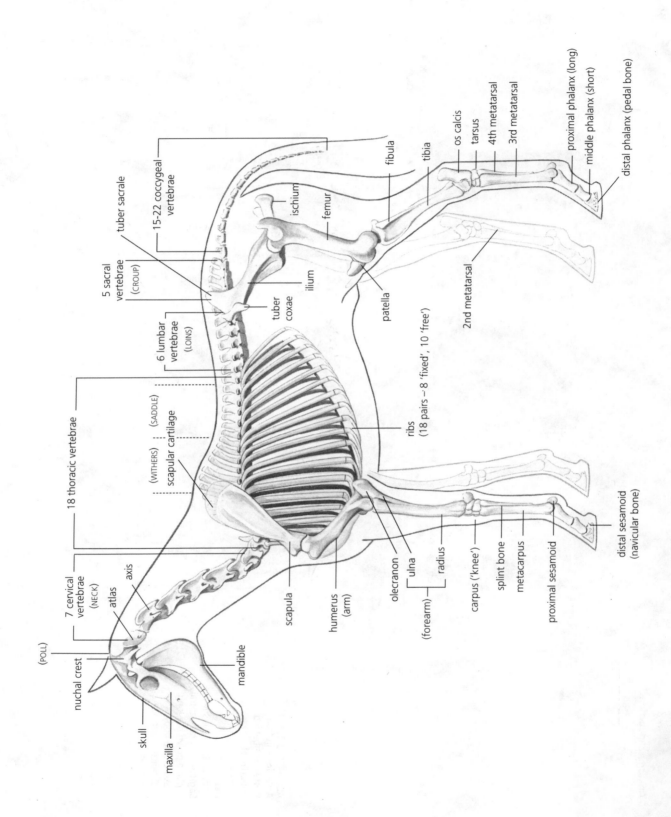

The skeleton.

skull

maxilla

mandible

(POLL)

nuchal crest

7 cervical
vertebrae
(NECK)

atlas

axis

18 thoracic vertebrae

(WITHERS)   (SADDLE)

scapular cartilage

6 lumbar
vertebrae
(LOINS)

5 sacral
vertebrae
(CROUP)

tuber sacrale

15–22 coccygeal
vertebrae

ischium

femur

ilium

tuber
coxae

scapula

humerus
(arm)

olecranon

ulna

radius

(forearm)

carpus ('knee')

splint bone

metacarpus

proximal sesamoid

distal sesamoid
(navicular bone)

ribs
(18 pairs – 8 'fixed', 10 'free')

patella

fibula

tibia

os calcis

tarsus

4th metatarsal

3rd metatarsal

2nd metatarsal

proximal phalanx (long)

middle phalanx (short)

distal phalanx (pedal bone)

The superficial muscles.

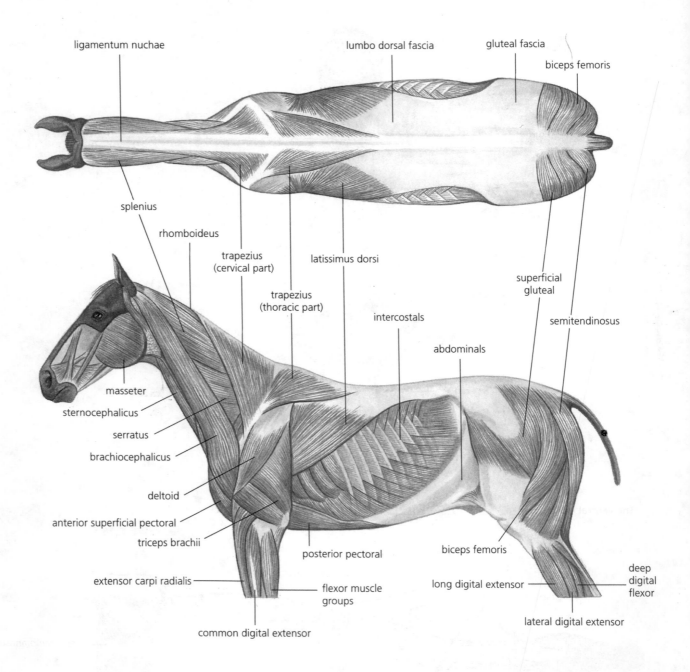

ligamentum nuchae

lumbo dorsal fascia

gluteal fascia

biceps femoris

splenius

rhomboideus

trapezius
(cervical part)

latissimus dorsi

trapezius
(thoracic part)

superficial
gluteal

intercostals

semitendinosus

abdominals

masseter

sternocephalicus

serratus

brachiocephalicus

deltoid

anterior superficial pectoral

triceps brachii

biceps femoris

posterior pectoral

extensor carpi radialis

flexor muscle
groups

long digital extensor

deep
digital
flexor

lateral digital extensor

common digital extensor

Superficial muscles from the front.

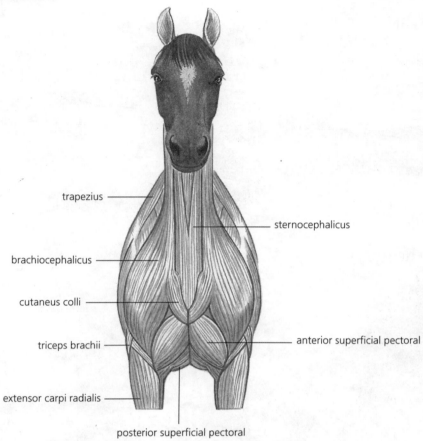

- trapezius
- sternocephalicus
- brachiocephalicus
- cutaneus colli
- triceps brachii
- anterior superficial pectoral
- extensor carpi radialis
- posterior superficial pectoral

The ventral muscles.

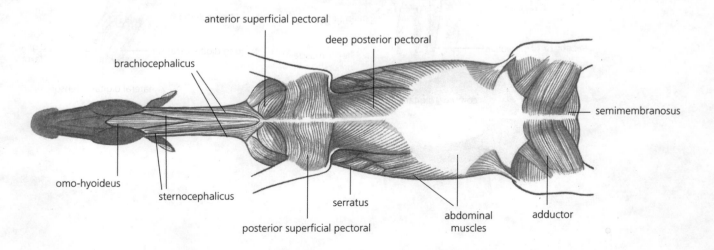

- anterior superficial pectoral
- deep posterior pectoral
- brachiocephalicus
- semimembranosus
- omo-hyoideus
- sternocephalicus
- serratus
- abdominal muscles
- adductor
- posterior superficial pectoral

The deep muscles.

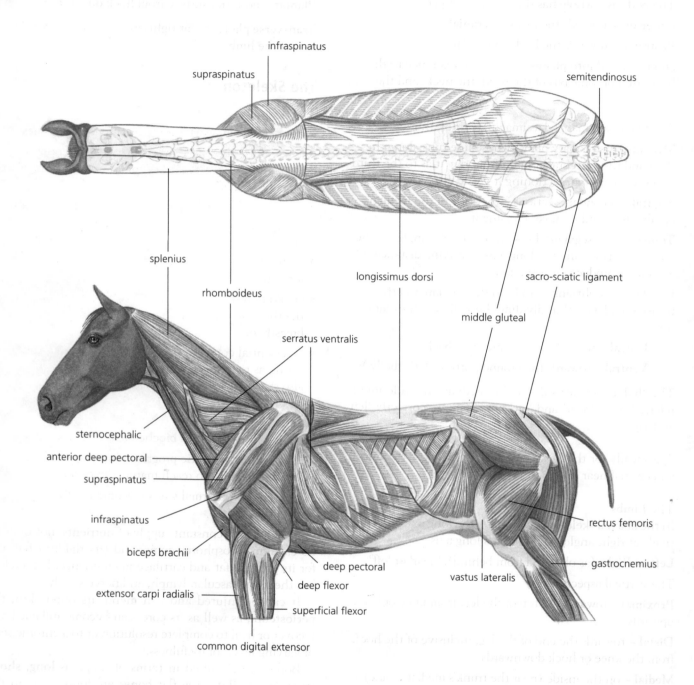

supraspinatus

infraspinatus

semitendinosus

splenius

rhomboideus

longissimus dorsi

sacro-sciatic ligament

serratus ventralis

middle gluteal

sternocephalic

anterior deep pectoral

supraspinatus

infraspinatus

biceps brachii

deep pectoral

rectus femoris

vastus lateralis

gastrocnemius

deep flexor

extensor carpi radialis

superficial flexor

common digital extensor

The body as a whole has the following aspects:

Anterior – towards the head, or **cranial**

Posterior – towards the back, or **caudal**

and is divided into **planes** which have reference to the horizontal or long axis of the head, the neck, and the trunk.

The planes are mapped as imaginary lines, thus:

Median – the primary plane, whose line runs along the skull and the vertebral column from the atlas to the third coccygeal vertebra, sectioning it vertically

Sagittal – secondary sections either side of the median, parallel to it and so never crossing it

Transverse or **segmental** – sections at right angles to the median and crossing the long axis at varying distances of any cut to produce cross sections

Frontal – at right-angles to both the median and the transverse planes, thus dividing the skull and the trunk into:

> **Dorsal** – towards the topline (the 'back')

> **Ventral** – towards the ground portions (the 'belly')

The 'halves' either side of the median are colloquially referred to as 'near' and 'off' but are more correctly 'left' and 'right'.

Specifically for the head, **rostral** refers to near the muzzle and **cranial** near the poll.

The Limbs

In the abaxial skeleton (the limbs), the long axes are effectively at right angles to the body's long axis.

Left or **Right** (as observed from behind), 'near' or 'off'

The vertical aspects are:

Proximal – towards the top of the leg, from knee or hock upwards

Distal – towards the end of the leg, inclusive of the hoof, from the knee or hock downwards

Medial – on the inside (near the trunk's median plane)

Lateral – on the outside (further away from the trunk's median plane)

Anterior – cranial-facing surface down to the knee or hock

Dorsal – anterior surface from the knee inclusive downwards

Palmar – posterior surface from knee downwards

Plantar – posterior surface from hock downwards

Transverse planes are at right-angles to the (vertical) long axis of the limb

The Skeleton

The skeleton provides:

- a general **framework** for the attachment of tissues
- a **beam**, the thoraco-lumbar vertebral column from which is suspended many of the internal organs, as well as being a 'roof'
- a protective **shell**, in particular for the brain (within the skull), for the spinal cord (within the vertebrae), and for the heart and the lungs (within the thorax)
- a site (within long bone marrow) for blood cell formation
- an aid to respiration – the moveable ribcage between the thoracic vertebral column and the sternum or breastbone
- an essential component of locomotion – with the bones acting as rigid levers, especially in the limbs (which are also struts), and the vertebral column

Bone

Bone is a living tissue, a biochemical structure which:

- in response to genetic programming grows in length and in thickness to reach mature dimensions
- in response to normal stresses geometrically adapts inwardly

Bone requires a constant supply of nutrients, not only for its calcium–phosphorus compound (its rigidity) but also for its protein, fat and cartilage maintenance. It therefore has the usual vascular, lymph, and nerve supply.

It can be injured and can mend; its outer skin, the **periosteum**, as well as its core, can become inflamed and recover or heal to complete resolution or to a chronic state of varying levels of usefulness.

Bones are classified in terms of shape as **long, short, irregular,** or **flat**. True flat bones are found only in the skull; these do not develop from cartilage as do all others, but from mineralisation of the facial membranes covering the embryonic brain and other parts of the skull. Some cartilaginous derived bones are flattish in design, but are not true flat bones, e.g. the shoulder blade, parts of the pelvis, and the ribs. Irregular bones are, for example, the vertebrae and parts of the skull

The term 'a horse's bone' is the measurement of the circumference around the fore-cannon just below the knee. This therefore involves not just the cannon bone but also the two splint bones, the ligaments, tendons, blood vessels, nerves and skin. Nevertheless the total circumference is accepted as a measurement of 'bone' – an indication of that horse's weight-carrying ability.

In addition to bone, the skeletal system includes the joints or articulations and the related soft tissues.

Bone Development

All healthy bone is hard. The degree of hardness, the ratio of mineral to the protein complex in which the minerals are deposited, varies. Degrees of hardness can be determined only by scientific techniques, not by manual palpation.

The calcium, phosphorous, other minerals and trace elements are constantly being exchanged with fresh inputs. This flux, and the other living organic constituents, makes bone a remarkably resilient, durable material less likely, in the mature animal, to stress failure than an equivalent mass of inorganic metal.

The architecture of bone consists of the dense cortex of the extremities and periphery of the shaft. Within are less dense areas forming an open framework, cancellous bone – a scaffolding in the spaces of which is the bone marrow.

The long bone's shaft is hollow in the centre – the cavity is filled with fatty material, the **marrow**, of which there are four types, dependent on age:

- in the young horse all bone marrow is **red** and productive and is known as **Type 1**
- in bones other than the ribs, sternum and vertebrae (where red blood cell production is continuous throughout life), production slows with age, and the marrow becomes **yellow** and known as **Type 2**
- production then stops, and the marrow becomes **white** and known as **Type 3**
- in the old horse, where the marrow has become gelatinous, it is known as **Type 4**

Up to the age of ten years, Type 2 can be re-activated in emergencies; reversion is not possible for Types 3 or 4.

The growing animal requires maximum production of red blood cells, but the healthy adult is sufficiently supplied from the red marrow of the thoracic bones.

Immature bone stops growing lengthwise when

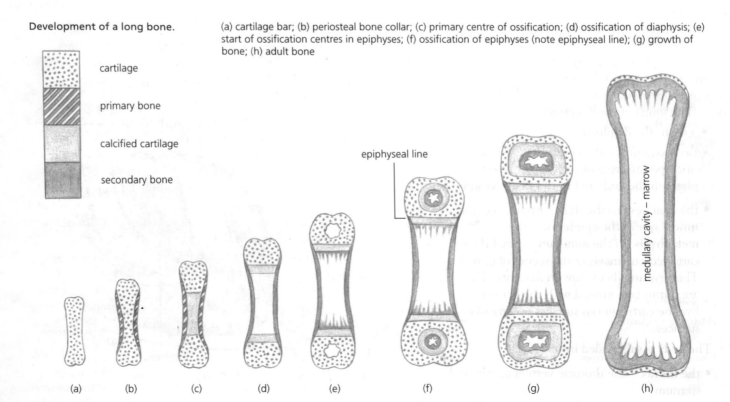

Development of a long bone.

(a) cartilage bar; (b) periosteal bone collar; (c) primary centre of ossification; (d) ossification of diaphysis; (e) start of ossification centres in epiphyses; (f) ossification of epiphyses (note epiphyseal line); (g) growth of bone; (h) adult bone

cartilage

primary bone

calcified cartilage

secondary bone

epiphyseal line

medullary cavity – marrow

(a)   (b)   (c)   (d)   (e)   (f)   (g)   (h)

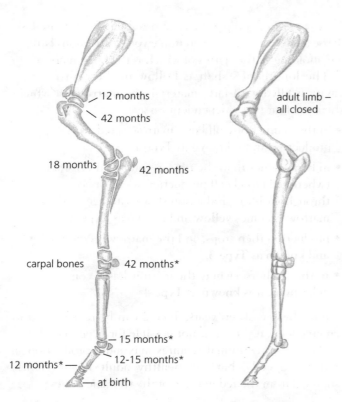

Various bone-closure times between the scapula and the foot – indicators of maturity. (* = important clinically)

cartilaginous growth areas become totally ossified. The limb's long bones stop growing by three-and-a-half years old. The ultimate height of a horse, measured at the highest point of the withers, is a reflection of the ribs' and the vertebral dorsal processes' growth as well as the bulk height of the sternal (fused) and vertebral bodies, and is complete usually at about six to seven years old.

The long bone is structured as:

- a shaft, the **diaphysis**

- two extremities, the **epiphyses**, which incorporate areas of cartilage or growth plates in the ends and in the shaft extremities

- the area next to the shaft cartilage, i.e. the inner layer of the epiphysis, is the **metaphysis**. In the immature animal these cartilaginous areas are the scenes of growth. They eventually close with maturity. They are not to be confused with the periosteal hyaline cartilaginous surfaces on articular surfaces

The body is subdivided into:

- the **thorax** – the thoracic vertebrae, ribs and sternum

- the **abdomen** – the lumbar vertebrae, the abdominal muscles, and the cavities are separated by the muscular diaphragm

The skeleton is in two main parts:

- **axial** – the skull, the vertebral column to the tail bones, and the ribs and the sternum

- the **abaxial** – the limbs, including the pelvis

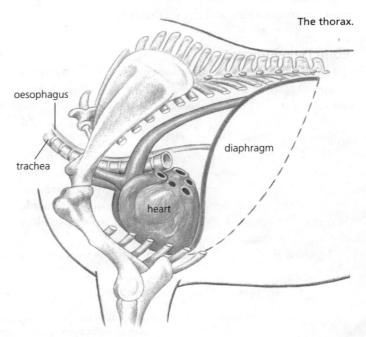

The thorax.

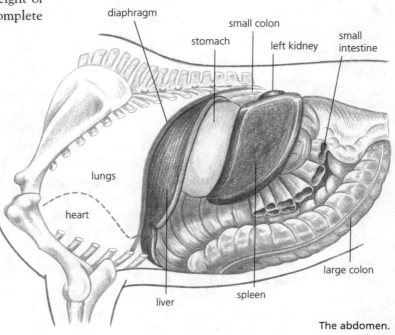

The abdomen.

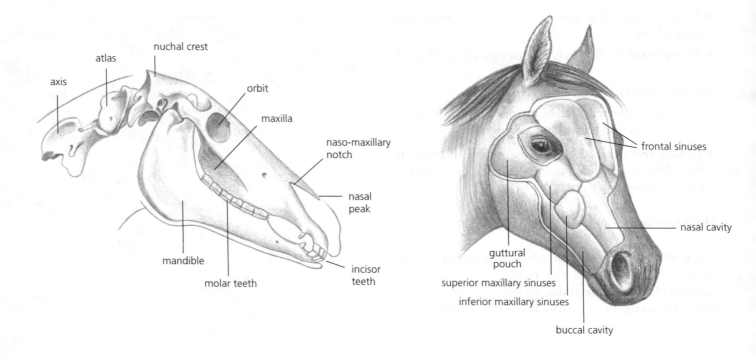

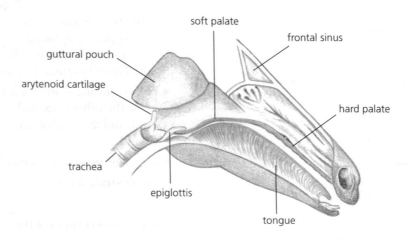

The Skull

The skull, the heaviest bone in the body, gives protection to the brain. The weight of the skull is lessened by the presence of large air-spaces, **sinuses**, within the bony shell.

There are sinuses on each side of the skull. They communicate with each other and with the nasal chamber, but not with the sinuses on the opposite side. The largest is the **frontal** sinus, which lies beneath the bones of the forehead, below and above eye level. Two **maxillary** sinuses lie below the eye and above the teeth; the roots of some of the upper cheek teeth lie within these.

The long upper (**maxilla**) and lower (**mandible**) jaw bones evolved and lengthened to allow room for six large cheek teeth, premolars and molars (*see* Chapter 8, THE TEETH).

Vertebral Column and Ribs

The horse has **54 bones** in its vertebral column (erroneously called its spine, colloquially called its 'backbone'), made up as follows:

- **7 cervical** (neck) vertebrae

- **18 thoracic** (chest) vertebrae

- **6 lumbar** (loins) vertebrae

- **5** vertebrae fused to form a single bone – the **sacrum** (croup bone)
- **18 coccygeal** (tail) vertebrae: this varies from 15 to 25

The horse has **18 ribs** on each side:

- **8 true ribs** attached directly, by individual cartilaginous extensions, to the breast-bone (sternum)
- **10 false ribs** attached by cartilage at their lower end to that of the rib in front, joining the posterior sternum as a 'rope' of cartilage

The Forelimb

The forelimb has no bony attachment (equivalent to the human collar bone) to the thorax. The scapula, or shoulder blade, articulates distally only with the humerus at the shoulder joint; otherwise it is said to be 'free'.

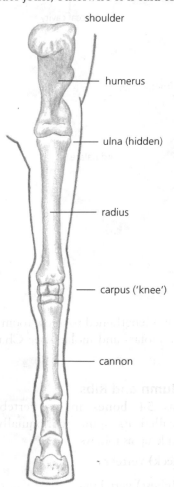

Anterior view of the left forelimb.

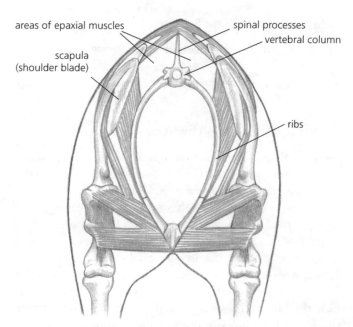

Anterior view showing how trunk is slung between the scapulae and supported by muscles

The trunk is slung between the left and right scapulae, and is supported by muscles. This allows a sweeping, rather than a pivoting, movement of the upper foreleg on the trunk. This gives three benefits:

- ease of **grazing** – one leg is flexed, so becoming 'shorter', while the other is extended and takes support; the trunk and the base of neck can then sink nearer to the ground
- more **agility** – with balanced turning at speed
- longer **stride** length

The forelimb consists of the following bones, down to the knee:

Scapula (The Shoulder Blade)

The two shoulder blades are attached to the chest wall by strong muscles and ligaments. During locomotion, much of the force of concussion is absorbed by these muscles, in which the chest is 'slung'. The angle of the shoulder blades to the horizontal has a considerable influence on the horse's action, and is therefore an important feature of conformation

Humerus (The Arm)

The humerus is the bone running between the shoulder and elbow joints.

Radius and Ulna (The Forearm)

The radius is a large bone which runs the whole length of the forearm. The ulna is attached to the upper end of the radius and forms part of the elbow joint. It does not reach to the 'knee'.

Carpus (Colloquially, The 'Knee')

Its bones are equivalent to the human wrist. There are six of them, arranged in two layers, and a seventh bone (the **accessory carpal bone**) at the back of the knee.

The horse's knee actually contains two joints – one between the lower end of the radius and the upper layer of carpal bones, and the other with a much smaller range of movement between the **upper** and **lower** rows of **carpal bones**. This arrangement allows complete flexion of the knee, allowing the fetlock to come up to touch the forearm near the elbow. There is little if any movement between the lower row and the **metacarpal (cannon) bone**, but both rows do move nominally in a separating fashion to minimise concussion and to dissipate heat.

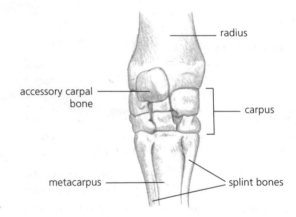

The knee: the carpal bones - left foreleg, posterior view.

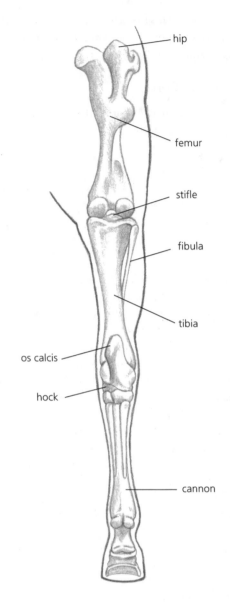

Posterior view of right hind.

The lower limbs of the fore and hind legs have the same structure, and are therefore considered later as one.

The Hind Limb

Down to the hock, the hind limb consists of the following bones:

The Pelvis

The horse's pelvis consists of three parts – the **ilium**, the **pubis** and the **ischium**. It is jointed to the vertebral column bilaterally to the first sacral vertebra, the **sacro-iliac** joints. There is no movement in these, but because of their function as the point where hind leg propulsion force is transmitted to the trunk, the supporting ligaments are exposed to great stress and occasional damage. The two halves of the pelvis come together in a short symphisis to form the floor of the pelvis.

Hip Joint

The coxal articulation is at the junction of the three pelvic bones; the acetabulum ('socket') articulates with the 'ball' of the head of the femur. It has two intrinsic ligaments but depends for security upon the extensive muscular connections which activate it.

Femur (Thigh Bone)

This runs between the hip and stifle joints, and is the longest bone of the body.

Stifle

The stifle joint is the equine equivalent of the human knee. It has two ligaments and two cartilages contained within the joint. The stifle is a strong and stable joint.

Patella

The horse's knee-cap differs from its human equivalent in that it has three ligaments attaching it to the shin bone (**tibia**) below, whereas the human knee-cap has only one such ligament.

In the weight-bearing position the inner and middle of these three ligaments, where they form a loop on the distal antero-medial extremity of the patella, are 'hooked' over the medial 'knuckle' or condyle (a rounded prominence at the medial end of the femur). This helps stabilise the joint and, along with the ligamental structure linking it with the hock joint, forms part of the **reciprocal apparatus**; the horse thereby has security of stance to permit 'sleep', or at least rest, with minimal muscular effort, whilst standing on the weight-bearing hind leg whilst the contralateral (opposite) hind leg rests in a flexed position supported only by the 'toe' of the hoof.

This reciprocal system also comes into play in maximising stability for transmitting propulsion at lift-off.

Tibia and Fibula

The tibia is the main leg bone of the second thigh ('**gaskin**'), and the very thin short fibula is attached to it. As with the ulna, the fibula has no distal articulation, although it is involved in the stifle joint.

Tarsal Bones (Hock)

The hock joint comprises two layers each of three smallish bones, but unlike the equivalent in the fore there is little or no movement in the joints between them and the head of the **metatarsal**. The true joint, that is between the distal end of the **tibia** and the fused upper layer, is capable of considerable hinged flexion and extension.

A dorsal projection of the **fibular tarsal bones**, the

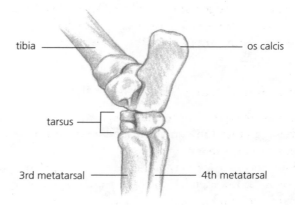

The hock: the tarsal bones – left hind leg, lateral view.

tibia — os calcis

tarsus —

3rd metatarsal — 4th metatarsal

point of the hock, is the point of attachment for the **Achilles' tendon**, formed from the **gastrocnemius** muscle and the **superficial flexor** muscle.

The hock is potentially the hardest-worked joint as, being further down the lever system, it absorbs much of the hind propulsion force. The 'separation' movement of the small non-articular bones of the joint plays a role in anti-concussion and in heat dissipation.

The Lower Limb: Fore and Hind

Below the knee and the hock, the limb anatomy of the fore and hind is the same, except for the differing conformation of the hooves.

- **metacarpal bones** – the **cannon bone** and the two small **splint bones** on either side. The joint with the **long pastern bone (P1)** is called the **fetlock joint**.
- **digital bones** (phalanges) – the **long pastern bone**, and the **shorter pastern bone (P2)** make the pastern joint (the area of these two bones is called the pastern); and the **pedal** or '**coffin' bone (P3)**, which lies entirely within the hoof, forms (with P2) the **coffin joint**.
- **sesamoid bones** – these are the two small inverted pear-shaped bones (the **proximal sesamoids**) at the back of the fetlock joint, and the single **navicular bone** (the **distal sesamoid**) which lies within the hoof capsule, behind the pedal bone and forming that part of the coffin joint known as the **podotrochlea**.

The joints between the distal limb bones are supported by strong ligaments and, when in extension for support and 'take off', their security is enhanced by the stay and suspensory apparatuses.

Anatomically, the foreleg from the 'knee' (carpus)

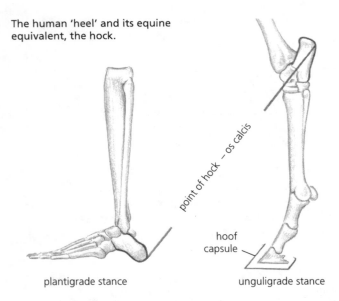

The human 'heel' and its equine equivalent, the hock.

point of hock – os calcis

hoof capsule

plantigrade stance

unguligrade stance

- the sensitive **corium** or laminae
- the pedal or **coffin bone, P3**
- the phalangeal or **coffin joint, P2–P3**
- the navicular bone, the **distal sesamoid**

and the associated

- lateral cartilages
- ligaments
- bursa
- blood and nerve supply

The outer horny capsule is subdivided into:

- the **wall**
- the **sole**
- the **frog**

inclusive to the ground is the 'hand' or '**manus**'. The hind leg from the hock (tarsus) inclusive down is the 'foot' or '**pedis**'.

Failure to appreciate this equine anatomy leads to confusion. We humans talk about 'standing on our feet', without too much concern for what skeletal structures under the skin are involved, and that 'part' on which a horse stands is best seen as a 'foot' even if in reality it is the equivalent to our middle finger or middle toe.

However, in reality the outer structure of the foot is a skin appendage – a very special one, not only in its horn but also in its secure attachment to inner structures. Moreover, this horny skin grows, like our own nails, although in a more complicated way. It is the only aspect of conformation which can be changed during life, by farrier trim and by contact wear. If this does pathologically change, the foot becomes unbalanced and physical forces are involved which have adverse effects on the units of locomotion proximal to it and serious implications for the blood supply to P3, the pedal or 'coffin' bone, and the distal sesamoid (the navicular bone).

The Foot

The equine 'hand' or 'foot' as described above is also known colloquially as the 'hoof'. Anatomically it consists of the foreleg from the carpus down, and the hind leg from the tarsus down, and the hoof.

The actual functioning hoof consists of:

- the **horn**, an insensitive structure which forms a capsule (or hoof) in which is:

The hoof is the focal point of contact with the ground reaction forces. It acts as the fulcrum around which the limb arcs, and rotates or torques against ground surface resistance, with resultant stress forces on the foot and the related joints, tendons and other suspensory/stay ligaments.

The **horn** of the hoof wall is formed exclusively as a specialised layer of skin growing from the coronary band or **coronet**. It is made up of horny tubules bound together by intertubular horn. This gives the hoof wall considerable strength against compressive forces acting along their axis, but it is relatively weak if excessive sheer or torque forces are directed in a manner which separates the tubules or if shear or torque forces are applied horizontally or obliquely across them as in the unbalanced foot. The wall is weight

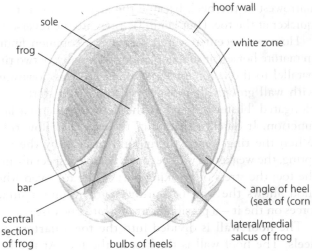

The sole.

sole

hoof wall

frog

white zone

bar

central section of frog

bulbs of heels

angle of heel (seat of (corn

lateral/medial salcus of frog

The structure of the foot.

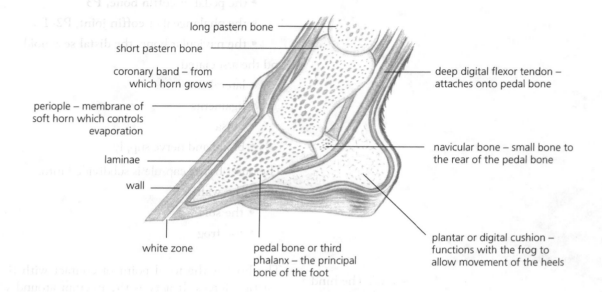

long pastern bone

short pastern bone

coronary band – from which horn grows

periople – membrane of soft horn which controls evaporation

laminae

wall

deep digital flexor tendon – attaches onto pedal bone

navicular bone – small bone to the rear of the pedal bone

plantar or digital cushion – functions with the frog to allow movement of the heels

white zone

pedal bone or third phalanx – the principal bone of the foot

bearing, as are the bars and the buttresses. It grows down at a rate of about 2.5cm (1in) in two to three months. Therefore, on average, it takes from nine to twelve months for horn formed at the coronet to reach the 'bearing' (ground) surface of the wall at the toe (i.e., it takes this length of time to grow a new hoof).

Rings in the surface of the hoof, running parallel to the coronet, indicate variations in the rate of hoof growth. Such nutritionally induced 'stop and go' growth rates are most commonly seen in horses at grass for several months. Fluctuation in grass quality interferes with horn growth; the compression of the horn tubules, especially within the unshod fore feet, produces bulges which encircle the wall. The lines of these rings are widest apart at the toe and narrowest at the heel, because the general growth rate is quicker at the toe. (But laminitic rings are the reverse.)

However, recent research describes a common finding in mature horses, at summer grazing especially, of two rings parallel to the coronary band which progress downwards with wall growth. It is suggested that each starts as an elongated 'blister' formed at the dermal/epidermal layer junction. It quickly 'dries out' to leave a hollow ridge. When the rings reach the ground surface, by the next spring, the weakened wall becomes flexible, especially near the toe; the stress of breaking over at the toe even when shod allows the wall to 'spring', with resultant undue forces on the it – a possible start of white line disease.

The **hoof wall** is divided into the **toe**, **quarters** and **heels**. The hoof wall is thickest at the toe. At the heel

there is less distance from the ground surface to the coronet and the horn is therefore 'newer' and more pliable than at the toe. This enables the heels to expand when the foot is pressed onto the ground, so helping to absorb shock.

The hoof wall turns inwards at the heels, forming the **bars** of the foot. There is a deep groove between the bars and each side of the frog. The corner of the wall and the bar is called the hoof **buttress**. The bar is weight-bearing; the buttress gives added security to the hoof wall and the bars. The bars prevent the heels from collapsing forward.

Bridging the junction between the skin and the hoof wall is a thin layer of soft horn, known as the **periople**. This extends about 2cm (3/4in) down the hoof from the coronet. It has an extra waterproofing function, in both directions.

The hoof wall has three layers – a thin outer waterproof layer, a thick central layer (which contains the pigment cells in pigmented hooves), and an inner layer which is folded into laminae; there are six hundred **primary laminae**, each of which has approximately one hundred **secondary laminae** branching from it – together forming the **insensitive laminae**. None of these three layers of the hoof wall has a nerve supply or blood supply – this is why a farrier can drive nails into the hoof wall without causing the horse any discomfort.

The insensitive laminae of the hoof wall interlock with a second set of highly vascular laminae – the **sensitive laminae** (shown overleaf). These are firmly adherent to the outer medial surface of the **pedal bone**, which lies

Three-dimensional dissection of the coronary region and the hoof wall.

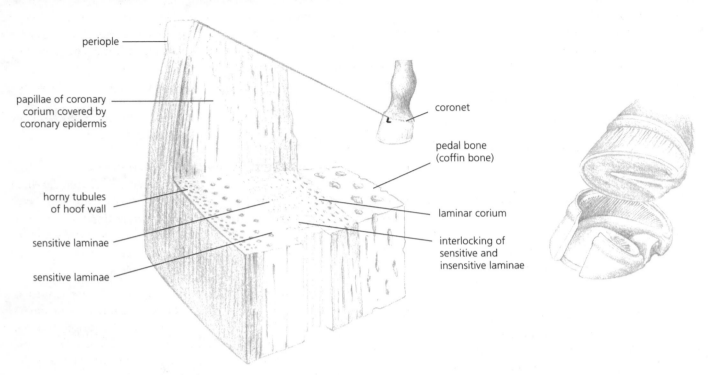

periople

papillae of coronary corium covered by coronary epidermis

coronet

pedal bone (coffin bone)

horny tubules of hoof wall

laminar corium

sensitive laminae

interlocking of sensitive and insensitive laminae

sensitive laminae

entirely within the hoof capsule. The sensitive laminae have both nerve and blood supply, and this is why pain and bleeding can occur if a farrier drives a nail too deep ('pricked foot') or with any other penetrating wound and, to a lesser extent, with bruising of the sole.

This dynamic interlocking of sensitive and insensitive laminae is very important; it is how the pedal bone is attached to the hoof wall, though how the downward growth movement of the horn and its insensitive laminae slide over the fixed sensitive laminae is not fully understood.

The horse takes all its weight secondarily on the pedal bone, not downwards but outwards all round the hoof wall, in effect hanging from the outer wall via the two layers of laminae. It is thus the wall, not the sole or the frog, which is the *primary* weight bearer. The walls of the hoof capsule are physiologically flexible and make an angle of contact with the ground surface. On weight bearing the downward force on the pedal bone is transformed to the upper part of the wall, and because of its angulation the wall spreads outwards as the load is taken. In the anterior two thirds of the foot this spreading is restricted by the attachment to the pedal bone; in the posterior third the wall has no such attachment and the flexible hoof cartilages, bars, and bulbs of the heel allow the heel to spread. The toe conversely

contracts slightly at the coronary band, and the pedal bone rotates downward slightly at the heels, pulling the coronary band back at the anterior aspect and allowing the hoof wall to spread slightly at the quarters. The forward movement of the horse, removing the load, reverses these hoof changes.

These movements help to absorb concussion and assist in the return flow of the hoof's blood supply. If the walls lose their conical design and become more upright, or fail to flex normally, there is often a significant interference with blood flow which can affect stride length and cause lameness. During the gallop, the whole horse's weight (and that of its rider and tack – i.e. upwards of 500kg, or 1,000lbs) is supported on one front foot (the trailing foreleg), the weight being transmitted via the pedal bone and hoof wall onto a shoe of surface area of approximately 60sqcm (9sqin) – a force of over 7kg per sq cm (100lbs per sq in). Appreciating the forces which the hoof attachment to the pedal bone is asked to withstand, makes it easy to understand how painful it is if the laminae become inflamed.

The **sole** occupies much of the ground surface, and protects sensitive structures above. It is concave, particularly in the hind foot. Except in soft ground, the shod foot's sole does not make contact with the ground and does not support the weight of the horse. It flexes with the movement of the hoof.

The junction of the sole and the hoof wall appears white, the so-called **white line** or **white zone**. This line of horn marks the seal between the constantly elongating wall horn and the horn of the sole, and is the junction of the sensitive and insensitive laminae of the hoof wall – which helps the farrier to know where to place his nails to avoid the sensitive layer.

The area of sole between the bars and hoof wall at the buttress is prone to bruising, and is known as the **seat of corn**.

The horn of the sole is produced by a highly vascular layer beneath it, the **sole corium**. It is formed at a faster rate than hoof wall horn, and it flakes off at the ground surface rather than being worn away, somewhat similarly to epidermis – skin – elsewhere on the body.

The rubbery, wedge-shaped **frog** covers the underlying frog cushion and has its apex projecting forward into the sole area. It is composed of softer horn. It has a central cleft. The frog horn is also produced by its own highly vascular layer lying above, the **frog corium**. Recent research indicates that its primary function is to allow controlled expansion of the heels during weight bearing, with reciprocal action which assists in venous blood return. Other suggestions are that it has anti-slip and anti-concussion properties, and is a pump to aid circulation, but these are unproven. It does have ground contact at full weight bearing on soft surfaces, when it protects the underlying tissues.

The three horny structures of the foot all have a different 'water' content: typically, hoof wall 25%, sole 33%, and frog 50%. The water content is not constant.

The **lateral cartilages** are two 'wings' at the edges of the pedal bone. They can be felt just above the coronet at the quarters. Expansion outwards of these cartilages helps absorb concussion. In some horses, especially the heavier breeds, these cartilages become ossified forming **side bones**.

The **digital cushion** is an elastic fibrous pad at the heels, beneath the frog. Pressure from the frog during motion compresses the digital cushion, which is squeezed out to spread the lateral cartilages. Compression and decompression of veins within the hoof helps to 'pump' blood back up the leg (*see* Chapter 6, THE CARDIO-VASCULAR SYSTEM).

The **navicular bone** is a narrow, elongated bone lying across the foot, immediately above the apex of the frog. It lies behind the pedal bone (P3), and beneath the short pastern (P2) at the **corono-pedal joint**. It forms part of the coffin joint, but is so attached that on the support phase it moves slightly apart from the short pastern (P2) and the long pastern (P1) – a heat reducing function. The deep digital flexor tendon (DDFT) runs over a bursa on the lower surface of the navicular bone before inserting into the pedal bone.

The corono-pedal joint, between the short pastern bone and pedal bone, lies entirely within the hoof.

The Stay and Suspensory Mechanisms

The following structures (discussed in greater detail in Chapter 17, THE LOCOMOTOR SYSTEM) are not bony 'skeleton' in anatomical terms but their functioning is described here in relation to the dynamics of the skeleton.

The Stay Apparatus

The **flexor tendons** in the foreleg, the **'deep'** and the **'superficial'**, each have a **check ligament**, the deep's coming from the back of the proximal cannon and the back of the lower knee region, and the superficial's coming from the back of the radius just above the carpus – the **distal** and the **proximal check ligaments** respectively.

These, along with the tendons and other restraining ligaments in the muscles of the chest, of the neck, and of the shoulder and upper arm, form what is known as the horse's **stay apparatus** which links with the suspensory apparatus.

These unique anatomical designs became necessary with the elongation of the limbs which equipped the horse for survival by flight. They are also essential for the horse's ability to rest while standing, since they 'fix' the forelimb in extension – the 'hold' is maintained with minimal muscle action.

The Suspensory Apparatus

The **suspensory apparatus** consists of a ligament (the **suspensory ligament**) arising from the back of the knee and running down the limb immediately behind the cannon bone to its mid point, before dividing into two branches. At the sides at the back of the fetlock joint these branches attach to the two proximal **sesamoid** bones.

From the sesamoids, the two branches of the suspensory ligament run to the front of the **pastern**, meeting with the **extensor tendon** to provide a **suspensory cradle** to the fetlock joint. The back of the fetlock and pastern joints have a trellis of sesamoidian ligaments which help support that area from hyper-flexing.

The suspensory apparatus showing the support of the joints in both the fore and hind leg.

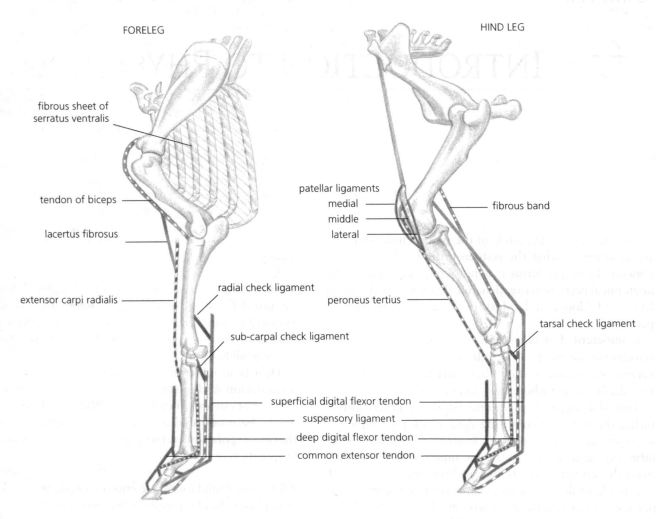

FORELEG

HIND LEG

fibrous sheet of serratus ventralis

tendon of biceps

lacertus fibrosus

extensor carpi radialis

radial check ligament

sub-carpal check ligament

patellar ligaments
medial
middle
lateral

fibrous band

peroneus tertius

tarsal check ligament

superficial digital flexor tendon
suspensory ligament
deep digital flexor tendon
common extensor tendon

In the resting, standing horse, the vertical position and fixation of the limbs is assisted by joint design and ligament alignment and some fixation muscles, as well as by the stay and suspensory structures. These, with the sesamoidean flexible 'trellis' also enable the fetlock joint to 'sink' safely on weight-bearing and, through kinetic energy, then to recoil or 'spring back up again'. The two main systems – stay and suspensory – also help absorb concussion.

In the hind limb more of the 'shock' is absorbed by the ligaments and muscles linking the hock and stifle. This special hind limb arrangement of ligaments makes the hock and stifle joints move together in unison, and is known as the **reciprocal apparatus**. It also produces a more secure hind-leg action, particularly in propulsion.

The equine hock and stifle must always flex and extend in parallel, in contrast with the human knee and ankle which can be moved independently of one another.

4 INTRODUCTION TO PHYSIOLOGY

Physiology means 'the study of the natural functioning of living animals', what the systems do individually and in concert. In simple terms it is how static equipment, the anatomical parts, function dynamically; it is how the horse lives and 'does', and, most importantly, how that is perceived.

Competent horsemastership requires some understanding of the 'working' as well as of the 'structure' of the various organs, and of how they inter-relate, and thus of how the horse as a whole lives and moves.

This skill depends upon understanding practicalities rather than upon memorising data. So, for example, to know the capacity of a horse's stomach and against what other organs it lies is of little use unless *also* it is understood that in nature the horse eats little and often, that it is a trickle feeder whose stomach is never completely full nor completely empty, and therefore that, when stabled, the horse is most at ease when munching fibre, such as hay, whenever it chooses and up to its 'appetite', as when grazing naturally.

The functioning of some of the structures can be improved by man's interference of management and training, or it can be upset by mistakes therein – but the structure of the individual horse cannot be altered during its life, though improved type can be selected and bred for.

Physiology is therefore of more practical importance than anatomy, though less easily understood.

Cellular Physiology

The fundamental or elementary unit of all life is the **cell**. The study of cells is known as **cytology**, from the Latin *cella*, a small compartment or chamber. The term 'cell' tends to be thought of as referring to the cell's wall; correctly speaking, 'cell' refers to the contents within the

cell's wall. Cells vary in size but mainly in morphology (shape). They are diverse in function.

Life is an organic (biological) means of converting one form of energy into another. This means converting chemical (food) energy into, for example, mechanical (muscle contraction) energy and heat. The bio-organic chemical processes are called **vital phenomena** and they occur in all body cells.

Heat is an important by-product of energy conversion, assimilation and storage and it is an even greater by-product of energy expenditure, as in locomotion. Heating has to be monitored and controlled, and this is called **thermo-regulation**; related to it is the production and evaporation of sweat.

All life must fulfil four basic criteria; i.e. all cells, even the individual cells of uni-cellular life, must be able to

- **grow** to a genetically determined size and shape
- **reproduce** themselves, to a variable extent
- **respond** to stimuli from the environment and from within themselves
- effect (bio)chemical **conversions** within themselves for this growth, reproduction, response to stimulation and staying alive

In higher multi-cellular life there is also the need to

- be able directly or indirectly to **pass on stimuli** to other cells, i.e. to communicate
- in embryonic development be able to group cells with others to form **tissues**, **organs** and **systems**
- be able to work with other cells in an ordered way to form a **functioning whole**, i.e.
  - conductivity

- organisation
- integration

The survival of any living tissue depends upon a constant supply of oxygen and essential nutrients into the cells, and unloading of by-products, including waste, from the cells. In a multi-cellular system this requires

- a **transport** system into, through and out of tissues
- a **control** mechanism to maintain **homeostasis** (the maintenance of body fluids at correct pH and chemical composition) to help adherence to a genetically established **lifestyle** which gives
    - a body core **temperature**, within very narrow limits
    - a steady resting **respiratory** rate
    - a steady resting **heart** rate (pulse)
    - an optimal **weight** for height and type
    - **grazing/eating** and **excretory** and other **behavioural** habits essential for the survival of the individual and the reproduction of the species under natural conditions

Domestication should be consistent with the above broad principles as closely as is practicable at all times.

Virtually all cells are composed of

- the **membranous 'wall'** – the cell's flexible and selectively porous, or semi-permeable, framework
- the **cytoplasm** – the protoplasmic jelly-like colloidal intra-cellular fluid which contains
    - the **nucleus** in its **membrane**, which contains a full complement of **DNA**, the genetic plan or blueprint, and the central 'organic batteries'
    - the **nucleolus** – plays a part in ribo-nucleic acid (**RNA**) and protein synthesis
    - the **organelles**, or components
        - **mitochondria** – thought to be the 'power packs' of the cell, from which the cell obtains energy, thus playing a part in the cell's respiratory requirements. The energy is in the form of adenosine tri-phosphate (**ATP**)
        - **ribosomes** – particularly in nerve cells
        - **lysosomes** – the digestive apparatus, working by enzymatic action to produce nutrients small enough for the mitochondria
        - **Golgi** apparatus – involved in producing the products of certain cells' actions, such as mucus, enzymes, and hormones

Structures of the cell.

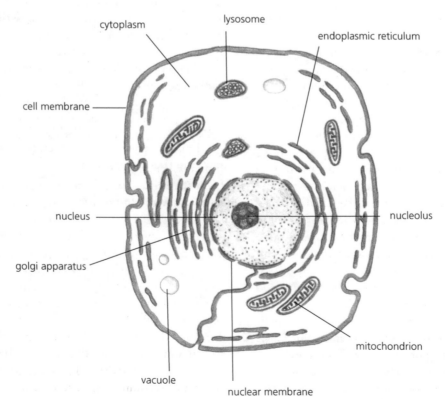

- storage and excretory units
- **vacuoles** – cavities within cells
- **electrolytes**
- **processes**, in some situations

Cells are microscopic, ranging from 10–100µ (1 micron (µ) is 1 millionth of a metre). Their small size ensures efficient functioning, as the rate at which oxygen and other nutrients enter a cell and 'fill' it when transported to it via blood and intercellular fluid is critical. Such substances diffuse through the membrane into (or out from, as in the case of bi-products of their activity) the cytoplasm.

To better comprehend a mammal's many cells it is helpful first to consider a single-cell organism, such as Amoeba proteus, which is 'free living' in a 'sea' of water containing salts in solution which disassociate into separate elements called **ions**. These ions are electrically charged, and in solution are known as **electrolytes**.

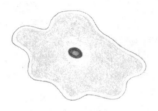

Amoeba proteus, a single-cell organism.

The amoeba cell's membrane is flexible and selectively 'porous', so that soluble substances are absorbed through it. Oxygen diffuses *in*; carbon dioxide, and other waste products, diffuse *out*. The cytoplasmic fluid also contains electrolytes, and microscopic organic material as foodstuff is engulfed through the cell membrane and is metabolised within to liberate energy.

The ratio of electrolytes in the 'sea' is different to that within the cell, and the physical forces of diffusion will tend to equalise the concentration of electrolytes inside and outside. Therefore, the cell must work to pump out unwanted excess ions (typically sodium ions), and to maintain within itself a minimum of such essential ions (typically potassium) which otherwise tend to leak out. This 'electric' difference, which must be maintained within miniscule variations, can be looked upon as the potential 'spark' of life.

Such single-celled organisms carry out work. This work is to keep it alive, allows it to move, and enables it to reproduce by simple division. The energy expended in doing so comes from the foodstuffs metabolised in the

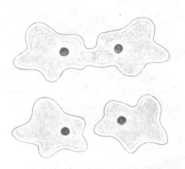

A single-celled organism reproduces by simple division.

presence of oxygen and electrolytes.

This principle applies to very nearly all mammalian cells, though in a much more complex fashion. In higher animal life, the 'sea' is the **interstitial** (intercellular, i.e. between cells) fluid, and the cytoplasmic fluid is the intracellular fluid. There are, of course, many other constituents.

The single-cell organism depends upon a steady-state 'sea', or, within limits, its ability to wriggle to a more suitable concentration of salts, or to adapt its metabolism to change – otherwise it dies.

In multi-cellular animals, each cell is 'fixed' as tissue and organs, and depends upon the correct 'sea' being brought to it via the blood circulation. If their surrounding 'sea' or intercellular fluid does not bathe them consistently in the correct 'mixture' of electrolytes, cells will either absorb too much water and burst, or lose too much water and so shrivel and die. The resultant 'dis-ease' affects not only the cells but also the 'sea' – which in turn will affect other cells in other tissues, organs and systems. Between the lethal extremes, cells become less efficient and so affect local and overall performance of the body. If the cells are those of the **vital organs**, the **brain**, the **heart** and the **kidney**, the upset can be serious. If the dis-ease is of the muscle cells, where their work load can increase forty-five-fold from resting to high performance, a cellular dis-ease, which might be of no clinical significance at rest, can during work involving maximum contraction become an acute and severe illness. Azoturia is an example of this. The higher the athletic performance demands, the greater the need for accurate **homeostasis** (maintenance of the correct balance in body fluid composition).

Animals move about primarily to find food and water, and their nourishment must be taken in by eating and drinking (ingestion). Oxygen enters by the respiratory system and is distributed by the blood. Metabolised nutrients are also so distributed internally and unwanted waste or exhaust substances are excreted to be 'drained away'.

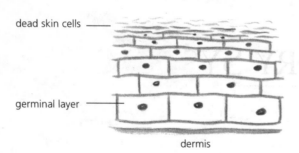

Skin/epithelium.

dead skin cells

germinal layer

dermis

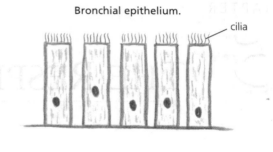

Bronchial epithelium.

cilia

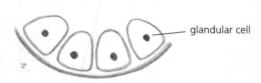

Gland.

glandular cell

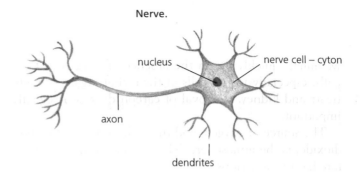

Nerve.

nucleus

nerve cell – cyton

axon

dendrites

Body Cell Organisation

The various types of cell are organised in layers, to become a particular **tissue** (e.g. skin).

Where several tissues are integrated around a transport system, they are called **organs** (e.g. the kidney); organs have specific metabolic functions.

An integration of tissues and organs related by anatomical position and controlled functioning is called a **system**.

The systems collectively work so that the animal **lives**, **moves**, **eats** and **drinks,** and **excretes**, and so **survives** to **reproduce** the species.

CHAPTER 5

THE RESPIRATORY SYSTEM

Mammals quickly die in the absence of oxygen in their cells, especially in the cells of their vital organs – brain, heart and kidney. Removal of carbon dioxide is equally important.

The source of oxygen, and the main disposal of carbon dioxide, is the atmosphere. The respiratory system therefore has two functions

- getting the air *in* and *out*
- exchanging atmospheric **oxygen** for **carbon dioxide** – the **gaseous exchange**

As might be expected in an animal whose survival in the wild depended upon fast galloping, the horse's respiratory system is very efficient and extensive in terms of exchange surfaces. It is estimated that this surface amounts to $2,500m^2$ ($3,000yd^2$). The cow, of somewhat similar size but of different evolutionary type, has but one quarter of this.

The respiratory system is anatomically divided into an **upper** and a **lower airway** or **'respiratory tract'**.

THE UPPER AIRWAY

Upper Respiratory Tract (URT)

The URT, in human terms the ear, nose and throat (ENT), runs from the nostrils through to the end of the windpipe, just inside the chest, although some authorities hold that the trachea (wind pipe) 'belongs' to the lower airway and at autopsy dissections it is removed with the bronchi and the lungs, colloquially known as the 'pluck'.

It is a complicated system designed to allow the various intrinsic and extrinsic anatomical movements.

Defects are invariably induced by man in requiring athletic use beyond the natural, discipline requirements of head carriage, and by conformation 'mistakes' (genetically programmed).

The two nostrils (or **nares**) form the entrances. These are kept permanently open by cartilaginous insertions in the soft tissues under the skin. Muscular attachments to these insertions automatically, reflexly, control the extent of the openings.

When there is a need for maximum inlet and outlet of air, further extension of the opening is possible by the lifting of a fold in the nostrils' structure – the **false nostrils**. This is seen in strong exercise and during recovery from severe exercise, and also occurs when a disease condition interferes with or requires maximal respiratory effort, e.g. in pneumonia, or in occasions of worry bordering on fear. In the latter instance, respiration is usually increased even when the horse is static, 'ready to escape', and the increased intake of air no doubt also enhances the sense of smell.

The airway is continued as the two **nasal passages**, which run the length of the nose and the face, separated by a thin bony **septum**. From both sides of this septum, elongated scrolls of even thinner bone curl outwards – the **turbinates** – thus dividing each passage into several, and so presenting a very large surface area. At the far end of each main passage a small lateral opening leads to two facial bone cavities and one skull cavity. These three cavities intercommunicate, but not across the midline, and are known as the **para-nasal sinuses**.

All these passages and the sinuses are lined by mucous membrane which is rich in blood vessels. The large surface areas collectively present an efficient warming and moistening system for the inspired air, which is thereby presented at the optimal temperature and humidity for

The upper respiratory tract – URT. (Also identified as Areas 1–2 of the respiratory tract.)

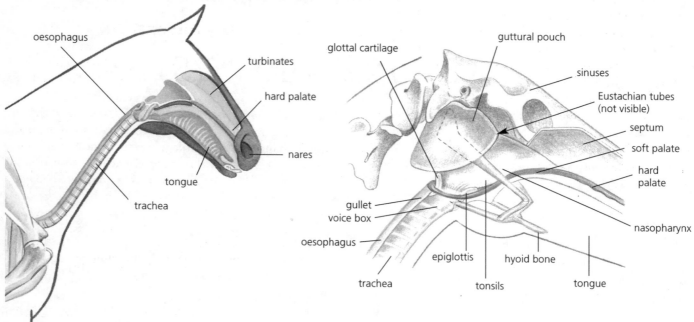

ultimate gaseous exchange.

The nares thus form a double-barrelled airway to open into the **pharynx**, and they are also equipped to act as a surface filter. A secondary but important function is the direction of atmospheric molecules which stimulate the olfactory nerve endings in the organ of **Jacobson**, two small tubes from the nasal cavity floor, for which the air is first trapped by the Flehmen posture of the muzzle.

The **soft palate** lies at the end of the **hard palate**, which is the roof of the mouth and the floor of the nasal passages. It is flexible muscular tissue which, together with the equally muscular pharynx, forms a cuff which encircles the opening to the larynx.

The soft palate is so situated and of such a shape that it prevents a horse breathing in through its mouth, and allows inspired air into the larynx during inspiration. It also plays the important role of directing boluses of food towards the oesophagus during swallowing.

The **pharynx** is the common chamber lying at the far end of the nasal passages and the oral passage, where the respiratory and digestive systems 'cross' one another. The horse's **tonsils** cover a large surface area of the pharynx in small collections of lymphoid tissue and in lymph nodules in the roof.

On either side of the pharynx are two slit-like openings into the **Eustachian** tubes. In the horse, each of these tubes opens into a double-lobed, pouch-like diverticulum

– the **guttural pouch** – before continuing on to end in the middle ear. These pouches, which are in fact cul-de-sacs, lie at the side of the throat about a hand's breadth below the level of the ear. Their function is not fully understood but they act as air pressure modulators. Their disadvantage as part of the horse's respiratory system is that they can act as a trap for inspired fungi and bacteria, which can then colonise on their mucosal lining.

From the opening into the larynx to the end of the URT the airway is a single tube, the **trachea**.

The **larynx**, or voice box, is a system of cartilages which can move under the action of their related muscles, reflexly to increase the diameter of the air-flow as respiratory requirements dictate. Muscle action can completely close the anterior (i.e. cranial) opening of the larynx, also known as the **glottis**, and further seal it off by elevating a triangular-shaped flexible soft cartilage, the **epiglottis**, over the opening, as when the horse swallows. At the glottis, on both sides, is a small diverticulum which incorporates the **vocal cords**.

This mobile anterior end of the larynx, like the nostrils, is capable of significant opening for maximal inspired air flow and for expiration. The flow volume and rate of expiration can be modulated by alteration of the global size and by its vibratory effect on the vocal cords to produce sound, 'phonation'. Such air is usually passed out via the nostrils, whose openings can be so altered as to convert the sound still further.

The **trachea**'s soft tissues are kept open by almost complete rings of cartilage. The trachea runs down the ventral surface of the midline of the neck, and can be palpated (felt) at the anterior end but gradually disappears behind the 'strap' muscles which lie in front of it. These muscles are attached under the jaw and to the **hyoid bones**, which form a cradle for the larynx and the root of the tongue. Their far ends are attached to the breast bone or sternum.

The **trachea** enters the thoracic (chest) cavity between the first two ribs.

The working of the larynx.

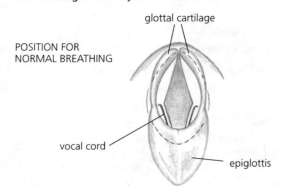

POSITION FOR
NORMAL BREATHING

glottal cartilage

vocal cord

epiglottis

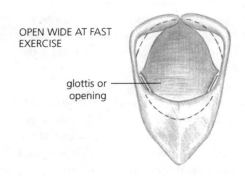

OPEN WIDE AT FAST
EXERCISE

glottis or
opening

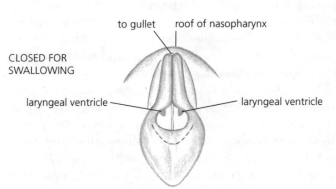

CLOSED FOR
SWALLOWING

to gullet   roof of nasopharynx

laryngeal ventricle   laryngeal ventricle

THE LOWER AIRWAY

Lower Respiratory Tract (LRT)

The **bronchi** are the two airways which branch out from the end of the windpipe to supply air to the left and right lungs. They are kept open by rings of cartilage.

Their subsequent division and sub-divisions within the **lungs** into small bronchi, and eventually into **bronchioles**, sees a change in the cartilage inserts from being semicircular to becoming flat plaques, which continue to maintain some rigidity and so prevent complete collapse.

From the bronchi down to the bronchioles, the lower airways are encircled by smooth muscle which reflexly (autonomically) regulates their diameter.

Beyond that, there is neither cartilage nor muscle, and during breathing these very small bronchioles, which lead ultimately to the **alveoli**, collapse or become inflated by the physical movement of air.

The alveoli are a collection of closed sacs aggregated in very many groups. Each group of alveoli are branching extensions of the end of one bronchiole. Alveoli do not expand or contract. Ultimate pressure changes are allowed for in the non-muscular bronchioles. The whole of the lower airway and the alveoli are held together in **lobules** by very elastic connective tissue. The lobules are grouped as **lobes**, and all are held together by an outer epithelium, an elasticated connective tissue sheet called the **pleura**, to form the left and right lungs.

This lung pleura, is matched by the thoracic pleura, which extends under the base of the vertebrae, down the

Diagrammatic representation of the lower airway – LRT. (Also identified as Areas 3–4 of the respiratory tract) (Not to scale.)

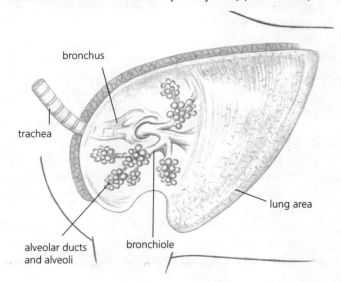

bronchus

trachea

lung area

alveolar ducts
and alveoli

bronchiole

Cross-section of the thorax.

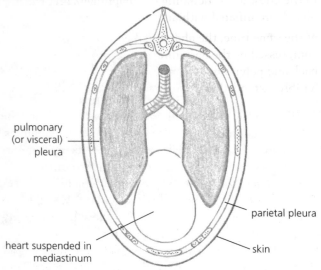

pulmonary
(or visceral)
pleura

parietal pleura

heart suspended in
mediastinum

skin

inside of the ribs, and over the anterior surface of the diaphragm and the inner surface of the breast bone. The space between the thoracic pleura and the lung pleura has a thin film of lubricating fluid which facilitates the expansion and contraction of the lungs within the rib cage.

The area between the two lungs is called the **mediastinum**. Through this channel run the major blood vessels, the oesophagus and certain nerves. The channel is widened anteriorly to enclose the heart, which itself has an outer covering – the **pericardium**. Above and in front of the heart the two walls of the pleura are lace-like in structure, so that the two pleural cavities communicate.

The cells lining the airways from the nostrils to the alveoli are a mucosal epithelium. The outer covering, down to the end of the bronchioles, has a serous epithelium. Only the

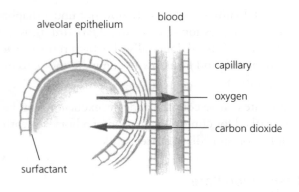

alveolar epithelium

blood

capillary

oxygen

carbon dioxide

surfactant

Gaseous exchange in the capillaries.

mucous membrane of the alveoli is capable of gaseous exchange, although it is thought that a small length of the bronchioles adjacent to an alveolus also has gaseous exchange ability. The remainder of both airways are channels for the flow of air in or out; the mucosae also has defensive functions.

The blood supply to the lungs is from two distinct sources:

- the normal nutrient arterial supply to, and the venous supply from, the tissues. This is the **bronchial system**
- the blood which takes carbon dioxide from the heart and thence to the alveoli, where it is exchanged for the oxygen in the airway, travels by the **pulmonary system**, and the artery (the pulmonary artery) is – in this one special situation – carrying oxygen-poor blood, and the pulmonary vein from the lungs to the left side of the heart is carrying oxygen-rich blood

In the lungs, the capillaries of this pulmonary blood supply form a very close network around each alveolus, so that their single-cell-thick wall is very close to the single-cell wall of the alveolus. This means that oxygen in the lumen of the alveolus is only microns away from the red blood cells in the capillaries, so exchange is assured.

Respiratory Functioning

This system is of the 'to and fro' type – *air in / air out* – oxygen rich air *in* /carbon dioxide exhaust *out*. It is not under conscious voluntary control except when using the sense of smell – sniffing – and even this may be an involuntary instinctive act.

During birth, the supply of maternal blood from the placenta is cut off. The level of oxygen in the foal's systemic circulation begins to fall and, more importantly, the level of carbon dioxide builds up until it causes a marked change in the pH of the blood. This increasing acidity is 'recognised' by the respiratory centre in the brain, which signals a series of reflexes which produce inspiration, and subsequent expiration. From then on, the rate and volume of respiration is controlled mainly from this sensor, through the autonomic nervous system.

Inspiration

Inspiration requires a 'vacuum' to form within the chest cavity:

- the **ribs** are pulled *forward* and, by slight rotation, *outwards*

Inspiration (inflation) – the ribs lift and the diaphragm contracts to draw air into the lungs.

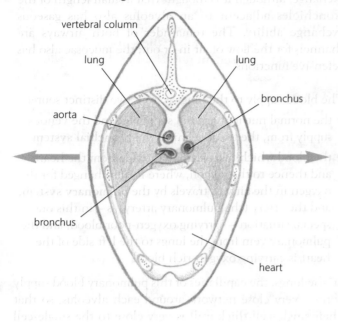

of the chest walls including the diaphragm, and the alveoli are **inflated** with air

- at the same time, the **abdominal contents** are **compressed** by the flattening diaphragm, against the back and pelvis and onto the **abdominal wall**, which is 'visibly' extended *backward*, *upward* and *outward*

In resting respiration, the mechanics are entirely diaphragmatic; further chest expansion by rib movement (costal breathing) comes into play when the air demand is increased.

Inspiration is adversely affected by upper airway resistances, in the nasal passages, the throat and the larynx, all of which are largely a matter of size. Inspiration is energy expensive.

Resistance can be increased by unnatural (imposed) over-flexion of the head at the poll, increasing the obstruction of air flow 2–5 fold. An important element is the relatively long equine neck and so the relatively long trachea. Exercise requires increased effort to accelerate the air from nostrils to bronchi.

Expiration

Expiration is mainly the result of abdominal musculative contraction on the relaxing diaphragm, but elastic recoil of the pleurae and of the lung interstitial and bronchiolar tissues also play a significant part:

- the **diaphragm**, no longer in contraction, is relaxed to fall *forward* into its most anterior position. (Its dome shape still allows for a space either side for the two posterior sides of the lung)

- the lungs deflate by elastic recoil, and *most* of the air is 'squeezed' *out*

- the **ribs** have been pulled *back* and each has been slightly reverse-rotated to further reduce chest volume

- the **abdominal contents** are now not under diaphragmatic compression so can extend *forward*, thus taking pressure off the **abdominal wall** which retracts *inwards*, *downwards* and *forwards* to complete the signs of respiration

- the rate can be counted and the 'excursion' can be described for clinical evaluation of a horse's breathing at rest or immediately after 'work'

Respiration Rate

Breathing rate and flow quantity at rest and at work are related to environmental temperature and humidity and to

Expiration (deflation) – the ribs drop, the diaphragm relaxes and falls forward allowing the elastic lungs to contract and squeeze the air out. Abdominal muscle contraction comes into play when assistance for expiration is required.

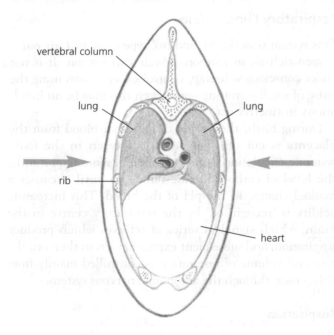

- the **diaphragm** muscle contracts, and the diaphragm 'sheet' is pulled *backwards*

- in the resulting vacuum, external atmospheric pressure causes the elastic lung tissue to 'follow' the movement

Dorsal view of the lungs and diaphragm.

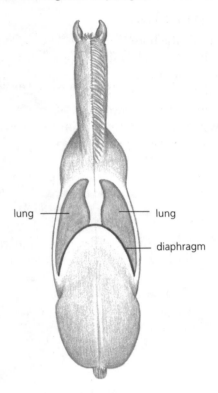

the metabolic demands of living, growing and working.

At rest, there is a momentary halt at the end of inspiration, when no abdominal or other outward signs of breathing are visible. At the slightest increase above the resting rate, this pause is abolished.

The resting rate of an adult horse is 10–15 breaths per minute. When the horse is disturbed, even just by being asked to 'move over', the rate will accelerate to around 25 breaths per minute. It quickly returns to normal when the horse settles. At such rates respiration is usually inaudible.

Any increased demand for oxygen and subsequent need to eliminate carbon dioxide will increase the rate and depth. At maximum exercise the respiration rate will reach 130. Rates above 25 will invariably produce expiratory noise. In the normal horse, no inspiratory noise is audible.

After exercise, to meet the oxygen debt and continue to assist in thermo-regulation, there is a gradual, sometimes 'stepped', return to normal respiration. If the exercise has been extensive, there will be deeper and noisier respirations, and heaving of the abdominal wall for a short period; then over 20–30 minutes there will be a return to normal respiration rate. There may be a nasal drip of clear to cloudy mucus, according to environmental temperature and humidity.

Respiratory Noises

As the respiratory rate increases, the expired air passing through the nostrils produces an expiratory noise. In some horses, the false nostril fold, when not fully dilated, is vibrated and the resultant noise is called **high blowing**. At very fast speeds, expiration can be heard over a long distance.

The anxious horse, whether it be because of an unidentified object or a strange horse, will often force short bursts of air through its nostrils to produce a **snort**. This noise is thought to be a signal to other horses as well as a warning to other animals and man.

If a large volume of air is reflexly expressed forcibly through the nostrils, the resultant noise is a **sneeze**. Its function is to clear the nasal passages of some irritant material.

When an even larger quantity of air is quickly forced out through the mouth, the sound is a **cough**. A cough is not a disease in itself, any more than is a sneeze – it is an indication or a clue that the horse is attempting to rid its respiratory system of unwanted matter or to enhance expiration when it is temporarily more difficult because of some respiratory disease or difficulty.

Factors other than Exercise which will alter the Breathing Rate

- severe **pain**
- Pyrexia (**fever**), with or without other classical signs of inflammation anywhere in the system
- **changes** in the respiratory system, e.g.
  - obstruction to inflow
  - obstruction to outflow
  - interference with gaseous exchange

Pain, fever, toxaemia and other inflammatory reactions, and especially heat stress, will raise the general metabolic rate with consequent further need for more oxygen. All these changes increase the need for more oxygen per minute, to compensate for reduced air-flow and gaseous exchange. The respiratory rate is proportionately increased, although the volume flow may not necessarily equally increase as with 'shallow' breathing.

Breaks in Respiration other than at Rest

Temporary cessation is involuntarily induced – for instance when a horse jumps, its diaphragm is held in the contracted position, and its glottis is closed. It is assumed that this inactivity in respiration permits the explosive impulsion of jumping to be concentrated along the axial skeleton, and not partly dissipated through expiratory deflation.

A horse's breathing may also be held

- during **asymmetric gait** action, when a complete respiration may be 'missed' to allow the horse to swallow saliva without disturbing locomotion

- as an aid to **defaecation** and **urination**, and during **labour** contractions

- on **rising** and occasionally during **post-exercise** recovery, a breath will be 'held' and then released with an audible sigh – this is presumed to be an extra large expiration to clear out carbon dioxide

- a **yawn** is a forced deep respiration, reputedly a reflex action to a temporary reduction in cerebral blood flow

Respiration and the Gaits

The respiratory rate is not synchronised with walking and trotting, but at the asymmetric gaits of canter and gallop expiration begins when the leading hind leg makes support, and ends as the leading foreleg lifts off. Thus it will be seen that **expiration** occurs during the **support phase**, and **inspiration** occurs during the **suspensory phase** – which seems mechanically sensible!

Any defect in respiration which alters the time required – usually expiration against some airway obstruction and the time available for inspiration consequently being shorter – can eventually interfere with gait rhythm.

Supplementary Functions of Respiration

- communication by **voice** production – 'phonation'

- recognition by sense of **smell**

- **heat regulation** – expired air carries heat away from the inner body. When the core temperature is elevated because of strenuous exercise, the horse continues to breathe rapidly after the exercise has finished. The coincidental increase in inspired oxygen helps repay the oxygen debt of anaerobic work, and the expired air dissipates heat by evaporation of respiratory moisture

- **panting** is anatomically impossible for a horse but, in cases of heat stress, very rapid and very shallow breathing is often accompanied by attempts at oral breathing. **This is a serious sign** (*see* Chapter 38, FITTENING)

Defence of the Respiratory System

This is effected as follows:

- when grazing, the horse's head is below the base of the neck, so that the trachea slopes downwards. Any mucus drains down into the throat, from which it can be swallowed; if this mucus is excessive, as following exercise, and particularly if it is of an inflammatory nature, it may run down the nasal passages and exit through the nostrils

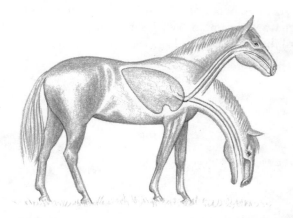

A grazing horse, showing the outflow of fluid and mucus from the lungs.

- the volume and pressure of expired air blows out any unwanted material. The tubes are coated with a mobile but slightly adhesive **mucus**, which has the ability to trap inspired particles, including micro-organisms and spores. Also, lining the airways are epithelial cells from which grow tiny hairs, called **cilia**, which automatically beat in an upward direction and so sweep up the mucus-trapped materials towards the larynx, through which they are wafted into the throat to be swallowed

- large numbers of special white blood cells are present on the airway's surface or in the nearby vascular system, ready to be mobilised in the presence of potentially pathogenic (disease-producing) organisms. The lymphatic system transports lymphocytes from the airway capillaries, with entrapped bacteria, to the regional lymph glands, where they are 'neutralised' and specific antibodies produced as required.

- if any part of the airway is irritated by noxious gases or materials, or inflammatory reactions and exudates, this will stimulate a reflex explosive expiration – a cough or a sneeze

Air hygiene refers to the number of airborne particles small enough (diameter less than 0.005mm) to reach the alveoli.

These are:

- **allergens** – moulds, fungi, forage mite faeces, pollens

- **pathogens** – bacteria, viruses

- **irritants** – plant fragments and other dusts, ammonia and other noxious gasses

Changes in stable management – drainage and bedding and forage – are important, but if ventilation remains poor air hygiene will remain bad. Poor air hygiene increases susceptibility to respiratory disease, increases its severity, and delays recovery from it. Ventilation should bring about 8–10 air changes per hour, mainly by **stack effect** (i.e. heated air rises), otherwise respirable particles rise to three times the acceptable level. Modern stable designs often fail to produce air stack effect, because

- no ridge outlet – hot air rises, cools and falls, and doesn't escape

- the only inlet is the stable door – even with the top half open inadequate air comes in and draughts are more likely

Stabling is a significant drawback of domestication, particularly in relation to respiratory disease and especially chronic obstructive pulmonary disorders (COPD).

6 THE CARDIO-VASCULAR SYSTEM

Blood is the main transporter through the body of essential water, oxygen, nutrients, chemical regulators and waste products. The blood is propelled along the blood vessels by the pumping action of the **heart**

- **arteries** carry the blood away from the heart. They are comparatively thick-walled vessels with a powerful muscular component, the reflexly controlled contractions of which to a great extent determine ultimate blood pressure

- **veins** – carry the blood back to the heart. The veins have thinner walls and less muscular content. They are thus more readily distensible. They are equipped, in the limbs especially, with non-return valves. Venous blood-flow depends on

  - capillary flow **pressure**
  - **movement** of juxta-positioned structures, e.g.
    - skeletal limb muscles
    - abdominal organs
    - thoracic organs

all of which help to massage blood towards and into the heart, and

  - **gravity** flow, from the elevated head and neck
  - **'cardiac suction'** as the right auricle relaxes and opens

In the centre of this circular system are the **capillaries**, a vast network of very thin-walled, microscopic tubes which lie within all body tissues. It is in these tubes and only in these that the transfer of water, oxygen, nutrients, cellular products and waste products occurs.

Apart from this 'exchange' area the system is a closed one. In certain situations, arterial blood may bypass the capil-laries by flowing directly from **arteriole** to **venule**, i.e. from the small arteries just before capillaries to the small veins just after capillaries. This is called the **A-V shunt**. Such by-passing occurs, for example, in the skin during cold weather, to prevent heat loss through the subcutaneous capillaries, and in the distal limbs as part of the physiology of hoof weight-bearing.

The actual transport of the blood fluid is called the **circulation**.

Circulation

Although mainly water – 60% by volume – in the form of plasma, blood is characterised by its red colour, derived from the iron protein content (**haemoglobin**) of the red blood cells.

In health, these red cells cannot diffuse through capillaries. Other blood components which do diffuse to become part of the extra-cellular (interstitial) body fluid, and ultimately intra-cellular (cytoplasm) fluid, are consequently not red.

It should be appreciated that, although the blood circulation is described as a closed loop, it is in fact linked, via the capillary transfers, to the other two extravascular body fluid compartments. Altogether, they form by far the bulk of the total body fluid, which is divided thus

- the **intravascular** fluid – the blood
- the **extravascular** fluid
  - the **intercellular** 'water' – the 'sea'
  - the **intracellular** 'water' – the **cytoplasm**, the largest component by far

It is estimated that a 450kg (1,000lb) horse has a constant circulation of blood, and 'water' derived from it, totalling

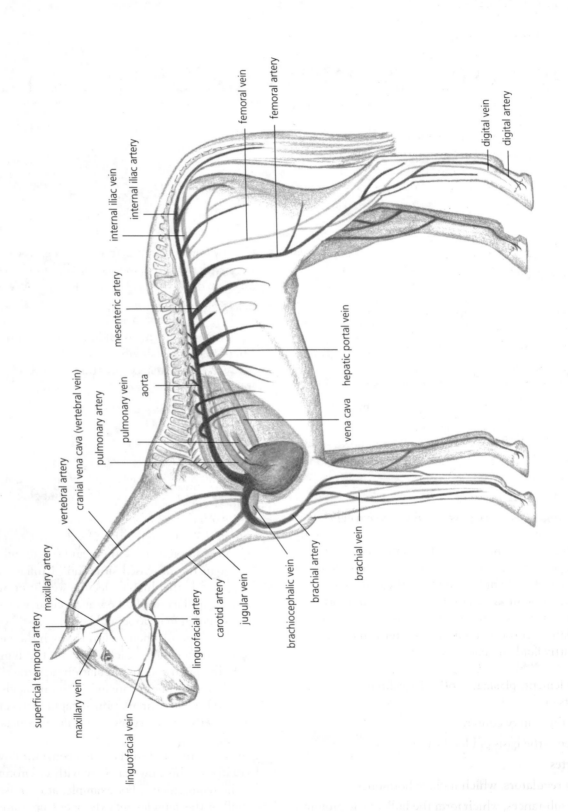

The circulatory system.

femoral vein

femoral artery

digital vein

digital artery

internal iliac vein

internal iliac artery

mesenteric artery

hepatic portal vein

aorta

pulmonary vein

pulmonary artery

vena cava

cranial vena cava (vertebral vein)

vertebral artery

maxillary artery

superficial temporal artery

maxillary vein

linguofacial vein

linguofacial artery

carotid artery

jugular vein

brachiocephalic vein

brachial artery

brachial vein

some *227 litres (50 gallons) per 24 hours*.

As will be described elsewhere, much water is lost in sweat and excretions, but this is replaced by **drinking 36 litres (8 gallons) on average of water daily**, and from metabolism of absorbed nutrients the end point of which is 'energy' and carbon dioxide and water.

Blood, in particular its red blood corpuscles and its plasma carrying antibodies and other essential proteins, cannot afford to be 'lost', as in bleeding. However, a red cell's natural life is measured at some 50 days. There is a replacement mechanism within the blood vascular system to maintain this particularly vital red cell content, whether the loss is natural or from pathological conditions.

The blood vascular system comprises four sections

- the **systemic circulation**, which conveys blood to *all* tissues of the body

- the **pulmonary circulation**, which conveys oxygenated blood from the lungs to the heart and carbon dioxide-rich blood from the heart to the lungs

- the **portal circulation**, which is entirely venous. It carries absorbed nutrients from the stomach and the intestines, antigen elements from the spleen, and hormones from the pancreas, straight to the **liver**

- the **lymphatic system**

Blood

Blood comprises about **10% of the total bodyweight**. It is somewhat sticky (viscous), because of its protein-containing plasma content, which intentionally slows its passage through the narrow capillaries and thus regulates the efficiency of exchange to and from the body tissues. Its constant red colour is brighter in the systemic arteries before most of its oxygen content is handed over, and it becomes darker in the systemic veins after it has done so. Blood is partly fluid and partly cellular.

The fluid element, **plasma**, is **60% by volume** on average and consists of

- **serum** – the watery content

- **fibrinogen** – the basis of blood's ability to clot

- **electrolytes**

- chemical **regulators**, which include hormones

- **immune** substances, which form the bulk of the protein content

The major constituents of blood.

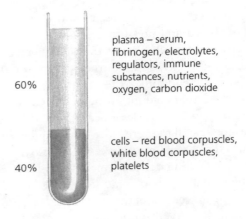

plasma – serum, fibrinogen, electrolytes, regulators, immune substances, nutrients, oxygen, carbon dioxide

60%

40%

cells – red blood corpuscles, white blood corpuscles, platelets

- **nutrients** – sugars, amino-acids (proteins), 'fats', other minerals and vitamins

- **oxygen** and **carbon dioxide**

The **cellular** element is **40% by volume** and consists of

- **red blood corpuscles** – the largest component, approximately 28% of the whole blood by volume

- **white blood corpuscles** (five types) – approximately 7% of the whole blood by volume

- **platelets** – concerned with clotting

Oxygen is transported entirely by the haemoglobin of the red blood cells. Some of the carbon dioxide is likewise carried, but much of it is in solution in the plasma.

Plasma does not leave the blood flow except when the vessels are disrupted, as in injury and severe inflammation.

Except in the dis-eased situation of inflammations, the fibrinogen and other high molecular weight proteins cannot cross the capillary walls. Low molecular weight proteins such as albumen may do so and become 'lost', as there is no local mechanism for their return through the venous capillaries, but they can be 'picked up' by the lymphatics for return to the main venous circulation near the right auricle.

All other constituents, including amino acids and water, can and do leave the circulation at capillary level to nourish the tissue cells and carry away specific products and waste materials.

The fluid content of the body is a **constant flow**. The rate and volume of this flow can vary with environmental and metabolic requirements. For example, at exercise the capillary 'bed' of the muscles reflexly opens up many branches which have remained closed during rest, and so a markedly greater volume of blood flows through the muscles. With increasing exercise, the heart accelerates to send blood more quickly to the muscles and under greater pressure. This speed and pressure is levelled out in the increased network of capillaries, so that muscle cells have 'time' to absorb the oxygen and other essential nutrients for the energy expenditure of their contractions.

The serum content of the blood, carrying with it those substances already described, leaves the system from the arterial capillaries, into the intercellular fluid and thence into the cytoplasm. A reverse flow also occurs and besides, as described under the lymphatic system, returns through the venous capillaries and so to the heart.

The movement of the three fluid compartments – blood, intercellular and intracellular – maintains the vitality of the tissues and the homeostasis of the body generally.

The blood is, of course, also the source and the transport vehicle for the new material of all those fluids excreted and secreted, from specific glands

- **saliva**
- **gastric digestive juices**
- **intestinal digestive juices**
- **transport water** for electrolyte movement into and out of these digestive areas and the caecum and large intestines, with unused water in the faeces
- **sweat**
- **expired moisture** – breath
- **urine**

In addition, the following are also derived from the blood

- **cerebro-spinal** fluid
- the 'waters' in the **eyeball** and in the **tears**
- the **nominal fluid** between the protective coverings of the various body systems, e.g. the peritoneal fluid

Blood Samples

Blood is an easily obtained body fluid, and laboratory analysis of it tells much about the healthy or diseased state of the animal. These tests are basically of two groups

- **haematology**, which counts the numbers of red and white cells, the haemoglobin content, and the relativity of plasma to cells (**PCV** – the **packed cell volume**), and red cells to white cells, and the ratio of the various white cells one to another
- the **metabolic profile**, which measures a vast range of substances such as minerals, proteins, enzymes, and electrolytes in solution, both in the cells but mainly in the plasma or serum. The enzymes and the proteins in particular are indicators of damage to and disorders of the various systems, and pointers to the possible causes

The Heart

The heart is a pump with four compartments, outlet and inlet ducts (arteries and veins, respectively) and its own circulation tract to nourish the constantly contracting and relaxing cardiac musculature. The compartments and

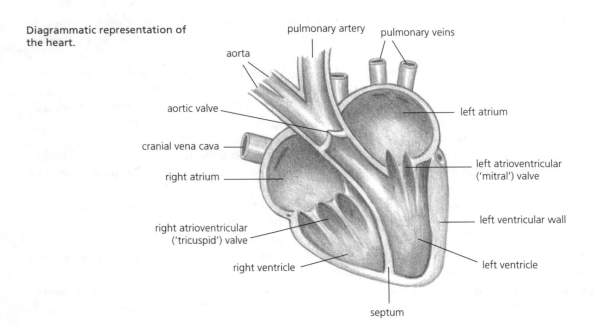

Diagrammatic representation of the heart.

pulmonary artery

pulmonary veins

aorta

aortic valve

cranial vena cava

right atrium

left atrium

left atrioventricular ('mitral') valve

left ventricular wall

right atrioventricular ('tricuspid') valve

right ventricle

left ventricle

septum

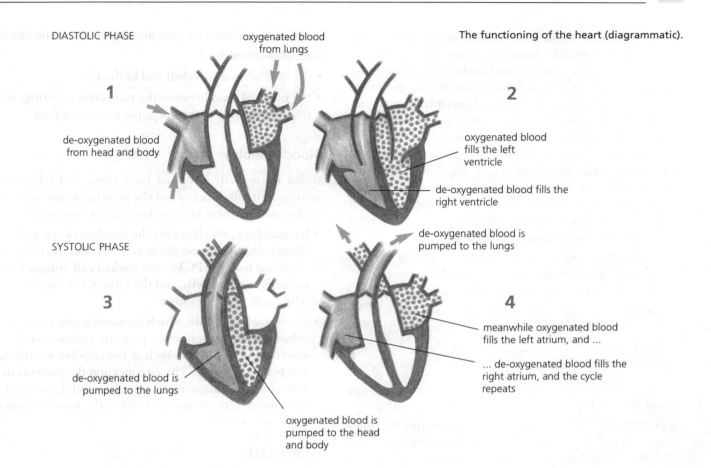

DIASTOLIC PHASE

oxygenated blood from lungs

de-oxygenated blood from head and body

1

2

oxygenated blood fills the left ventricle

de-oxygenated blood fills the right ventricle

de-oxygenated blood is pumped to the lungs

SYSTOLIC PHASE

3

4

de-oxygenated blood is pumped to the lungs

meanwhile oxygenated blood fills the left atrium, and ...

... de-oxygenated blood fills the right atrium, and the cycle repeats

oxygenated blood is pumped to the head and body

The functioning of the heart (diagrammatic).

ducts are fitted with valves which direct the flow of the blood. The cavities are lined with an endothelium, called the **endocardium**, which is continuous with the endothelial lining of the blood vessels.

The walls of the heart are almost entirely 'smooth' muscle, with a variable degree of fat. The outer cover of epithelium is known as the **epicardium**. The whole is encased in another sheet of epithelium called the **pericardium**. The nominal space between this and the epicardium is filled with a lubricating fluid known as the **pericardial fluid**.

Essentially, in terms of its functioning, the heart is a self-contained organ. It has its own intrinsic cardiac nerve-control mechanism, which institutes its contractions in a predetermined sequence and can function without the aid of the voluntary and involuntary nervous systems. These contractions are always complete, i.e. they obey the law of 'all or none'.

The control begins at the sino-atrial node situated at the orifice of the pulmonary vein at the top of the right auricle. It is the primary 'pacemaker' of the rhythm of the heartbeat. This rhythm is conducted to the wall separating the auricles from the ventricles at a second pacemaker node, which is the auricular ventricular, and the subsequent conduction network passes downward and upward along special cardiac 'nerve' fibres (the Purkinje) which then activate the ventricles to contract. The rhythm is determined by the sino-atrial node and is therefore called the sinus rhythm.

The associated electrical changes in the cardiac muscles can be detected and a consequent print-out of them is known as an electro-cardiograph. Changes in the wavelengths enable the cardiologist to detect pathologies within the heart muscle.

The sequence is that the left and right atria (auricles) contract as the left and right ventricles relax, and *vice versa*.

The contractions of the ventricles send the contained blood into the respective arteries, and they occur at regular intervals known as the 'beat'.

Contraction and ***relaxation*** of the ventricles are known as the **systolic** phase and the **diastolic** phase respectively. The associated sounds, as heard through a stethoscope, give information about variations in function in health and disease.

The basic or resting heart rate is fixed genetically and maintained by the intrinsic cardiac nervous system. However, the rate is constantly amended by the other nervous systems, and by certain intra-vascular factors including hormones, to meet the blood demands of the body under different conditions. Sensory nerves go to the central nervous system from sites in the heart wall and the wall of the aorta, and these nerves 'meet' with chemical messengers in the cardiac centre of the brain. This cardiac centre is sensitive not only to the signals mentioned but also to sensory input signals emanating from other body systems. Three main reflex stimuli are involved

- **shock** – over-stress, emotional states, gut and other pain, or severe blows to nerve plexuses outside the heart. These indirect stimuli are **sympathetic accelerators**

- **high blood pressure** – recorded within the right atrium of the heart. This is a direct **parasympathetic decelerator**

- **low blood pressure** – recorded within the aortic arch functions as a direct accelerator via the sympathetics

Autonomous motor nerves reflexly adjust the heart rate according to this information. They are from both of the autonomic nervous system's two divisions (sympathetic and parasympathetic) and work in conjunction with the intrinsic cardiac nervous system as an 'override mechanism'

- *acceleration* of the heart rate is signalled by the messages from the **sympathetic** division

- *deceleration* is signalled from the **parasympathetic** division

The Pulse

As blood is rhythmically pumped down the systemic arterial tree, it flows in short wave formation – beat, pause, beat, pause... The wave distends the elastic muscular wall of the artery. The 'volume' of the wave is determined by the heart strength, and the rate at which the wave passes any given point is determined by the heart's speed. The pulse is taken where the wave can be felt – where a superficial artery passes over a bony underlay, so pushing the wave outwards. The wave is 'smoothed out' by the time it reaches the arterioles, but the pressure continues into the capillaries.

The autonomic system also plays a part in controlling blood pressure through the action of the vasomotor nerves, known as **vaso-constrictors** and **vaso-dilators**, on the smooth muscles of the arterial walls.

The **resting heart rate** of an adult healthy horse varies from horse to horse and also breed to breed, but on average it is *between 36 and 42 beats (pulses) per minute*. At rest, the heart-beat normally runs at the slowest economic speed possible, and some horses will, in addition, regularly miss the odd ventricular contraction.

As an indication of how the whole metabolic system of the athletic horse responds to the demands of strenuous exercise, the pulse will accelerate to *over 250 beats per minute*.

Veins have 'no-return' valves to maintain the blood's flow in the correct direction, and a horse's circulation is generally very efficient, with one exception – in its lower limbs. There is a considerable height difference between the hoof and the heart, and very little muscle tissue in the lower legs to help massage the blood back up the limb veins. To overcome this, the horse has a built-in 'pumping mechanism' in its feet. Veins inside the hoof are compressed by the digital cushion when pressure is exerted on it, especially during weight-bearing, and blood is thereby 'pumped' back up the leg. This remote pump works in conjunction with the arterio-venous 'shunt' mechanism which simultaneously with weight bearing markedly decreases the volume of flow into the hoof.

The cardio-vascular system therefore works best when the horse is able or allowed to move about, as distinct from when it is stabled or in a loose box.

7 THE LYMPHATIC SYSTEM

The lymphatic system is a vital and integral part of the cardio-vascular system.

Structure

The lymphatic system consists of

- **lymphatic vessels**
- **lymph** – the fluid component
- lymph **cells** – lymphocytes
- lymph **nodes** (formerly called **glands**) and related lymphoid tissues
- **organic substances** in solution or in suspension

The Lymphatic Vessels

These begin as microscopic, open-ended, thin-walled tubes. They arise in the interstitial spaces of most tissues and organs and, in joining up, gradually become macro-scopic but still thin-walled tubes, ultimately joining the large veins just before these enter the right auricle of the heart. Throughout the body they parallel the veins.

The lymphatic vessels have no muscle component and, apart from non-return valves along their length, they have no moving parts. The fluid is moved along by other structures' activity, running in close proximity

- skeletal *muscle contraction and relaxation*, a form of pumping action
- *gut movement*, whereby peristaltic activity massages the fluid along the intestinal lymph vessels
- *respiration,* the 'in and out' pressures within the thorax helping to 'pull' the lymph towards the heart
- right heart *'suction'*

The lymphatic vessel system has

- its own **blood supply** to the vessel wall
- **sensory nerves** from the wall and the glands
- no motor nerves, either voluntary or autonomic

The lymph vessels draining the gut, the pancreas, and the spleen connective tissue, are called **lacteals**.

Lymph drainage from the brain and spinal cord via the cerebro-spinal fluid, and from the peri-vertebral neural tissues at the foraminae, is of great importance to neural tissue integrity.

The Lymph Fluid

Derived from the blood stream, lymph is a clear alkaline liquid, equating with serum, yellowish-tinged from any protein content. It is *2–3% of the total body fluid*. In the lacteals, it carries emulsified fat and some vitamins. This is known as **chyle**.

The lymph fluid is the 'siphoned off' excess interstitial fluid which is the 'sea' which bathes the body cells. Lymph flows through the lymphatic vessels and nodes to return to the circulation at the right cardiac auricle.

The Lymph Cells or Lymphocytes

In health, there are no red blood cells in lymph.

Of the white blood cells, the **lymphocytes**, concerned with antibody formation, are able to squeeze out from the capillaries, enter the interstitial fluid, and return to the venous system via the lymph, or regain the lymph nodes and other lymphoid tissues whence they originated. Here, they have an important function in the immunity manufacturing system.

A product of this is **sensitised lymphocytes**, which are 'attracted' to body areas under attack by pathogenic micro-organisms. The ability of lymphocytes to get nearly every-where in a defensive role means that they are often

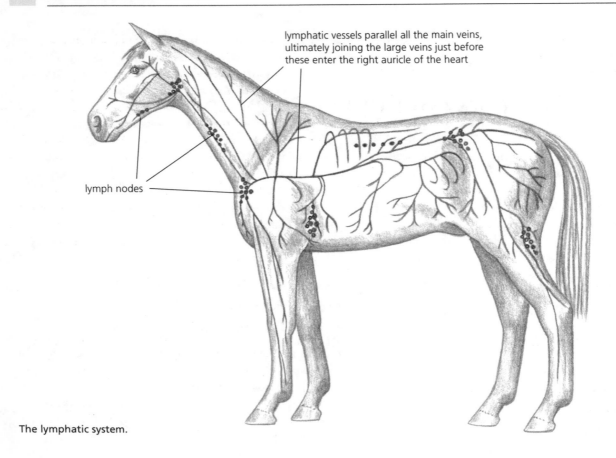

lymphatic vessels parallel all the main veins, ultimately joining the large veins just before these enter the right auricle of the heart

lymph nodes

The lymphatic system.

referred to as one of the 'fluid' components and, as such, act as a 'wandering organ'.

There are also, in times of trauma or infection, **macrophages** and **neutrophils** (which attack bacteria),

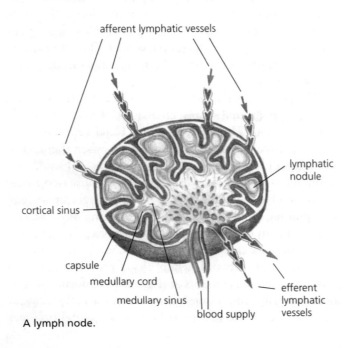

afferent lymphatic vessels

lymphatic nodule

cortical sinus

capsule

medullary cord

medullary sinus

blood supply

efferent lymphatic vessels

A lymph node.

and other white blood cells which are all part of the body's defence mechanism.

The Lymph Nodes, or Glands

Lymph nodes, or glands, are small, ovoid, smooth, pinkish bodies, aggregations of lymphoid cell-containing tissue, positioned in the course of the vessel. Lymph nodes have a soft connective tissue cover, a good blood supply, and sensory nerves.

Those lymph nodes relating to the limbs and the limbs' skin, connective tissue and muscles, are placed some way up the vessel's length; those relating to the mucosal surfaces of the three main body systems – respiratory, digestive and uro-genital – are much closer to their respective organs. Some nodes are on the surface of a system's tract, e.g. the tonsils, on the pharyngeal wall.

Function

The lymphatic system plays a vital role in maintaining general cellular health – through **homeostasis** by the redistribution of body fluid and its contents to prevent either dehydration or over-hydration (waterlogging), and in **transporting** lymphocytes and scavenger white blood cells along with small-sized protein molecules, electrolytes, and waste materials.

In traumatised and infected conditions lymph also carries debris and organisms to the lymph nodes, where germs are destroyed and **antibodies** to them are produced.

In the nodes, micro-organisms 'marked' by lymphocytes stimulate cells such as macrophages and neutrophils to engulf and destroy them. This lymphatic activity involves the intra-glandular reticulo-endothelial system which, with the lymphocytes and other white blood cells is, although not fully understood, found in other sites such as bones, spleen and thymus gland. The lymphatic system's activity has a major role in immune defence stimulation.

In addition to the normal serum contents found in lymph are small-molecule proteins which have 'escaped' from the capillaries but physiologically cannot regain entrance to the venous flow. A build-up of these small-molecule proteins in the intercellular fluid can osmotically retain water and **oedema** develops, with serious effects on tissue activity. The lymph vessels collect this excess protein and return it to the heart for recirculation – an effective conservation as well as a dis-ease preventative!

In Latin, *lympha* means water; in 'poetic' language it suggests 'pure water'. In some disease situations, infected lymph collects in vesicles or blisters such as are seen in cowpox and human smallpox skin lesions, in the vesicles of foot and mouth disease, and in the vesicles of some venereal diseases in the horse – all virus infections. Focal collections of oedematous fluid can appear under the skin where they are known as **weals**. A horse 'marked' by a whip shows a characteristic weal.

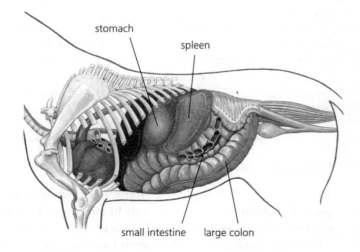

stomach

spleen

small intestine   large colon

Position of the spleen.

It was the cowpox skin vesicle lymph which was used by Jenner (in 1796, long before bacterial and viral infections were even known, let alone the theory of immunity), to stimulate protection against smallpox in humans. He appreciated that this fluid was the vehicle for transmission of the disease to other cows via the milkmaid's hand, and therefore must contain the 'cause'. He had noticed that milkmaids rarely contracted smallpox if, as was usually the case, they had had 'cowpox' on their skin. By scratching the cowpox lymph into the skin of humans at risk from smallpox he obtained protection for them. He called the material 'vaccine' – 'from a cow'. Human smallpox showed as a skin vesicle disease as well as a general illness which was, unlike cowpox, usually fatal.

THE SPLEEN

The spleen is the largest of the lymphoid organs associated with the circulatory system. It destroys old red blood cells, is involved in the formation of lymphocytes, and is concerned with bodily defence.

Although in the abdomen, it is not directly functionally associated with the viscera of the alimentary and urogenital systems in that body cavity.

Structure

The spleen is enclosed in a strong capsule of connective tissue, which extends inwards as a fibrous network for support of the soft functional 'pulp'. In addition to its copious blood supply there is a well developed lymphatic system which, together with the splenic tissue itself, forms the pulp within the fibrous framework. This framework can be compressed by smooth muscle under autonomic nerve control.

The pulp is clearly demarked as red and white, and is fed by a copious arterial supply. Drainage is through the portal venous system. The **red pulp** is for *blood cell storage* – and in particular red blood cell storage – when the horse is resting. In exercise or stress, this reservoir of blood, cells and fluid, is reflexly returned by splenic contraction to the main circulation, where the red blood cells, transported by the plasma, play a vital role in meeting the skeletal muscular activity's increased demand for oxygen.

Recent work confirms that a secondary splenic contraction on reflex demand, when blood pressure falls, will transfer balancing amounts of serum into the main circulation; falling blood pressure concentrates the cell volume at the expense of the plasma volume – the blood becomes 'thicker' and so less capable of perfusion into the vital organs.

In the *foal*, the **white pulp** is where *all blood corpuscles are manufactured*. In the *adult* horse, it is the site for *senile red cell destruction, conservation of the liberated iron* for new haemoglobin, *lymphocyte production*, and *antibody production*.

Paradoxically, the spleen pulp has no lymphatic system, although the connective tissue has.

CHAPTER 8

THE TEETH

In Chapter 1, EVOLUTION AND BEHAVIOUR, attention was drawn to the changes in *Eohippus (Hyracotherium)* as it developed over 50 million years to become *Equus caballus*.

The 'original' small, scansorial, multi-toed, browsing herbivore became a larger, cursorial, single-toed, grazing horse, much as we know it today.

Equus was so structured and functionally programmed that it survived, despite carnivorous predators, in wide open grasslands, as a gregarious, restricted nomad, on **coarse, stemmy herbage**.

This chapter is concerned with its changing dental features, which are essential for the ingestion and, in particular, for the **mastication** of the herbage available to it – in preparation for the subsequent digestion of

- the **soluble starches, proteins, oil** and the minor nutrients of minerals and vitamins liberated by grinding up (masticating) fibrous grass ingesta and by chemical and biochemical (enzymatic) hydrolysis in the stomach and the small intestine

- the **hemi-cellulose**, mainly in lush grasses – an intermediate carbohydrate, similarly digested to produce soluble sugars, important as a potential excess carbohydrate which can lead to endotoxaemia (*see* laminitis) or to upset fermentative digestion if some 'escapes' undigested to pass through to the large intestine

- the **cellulose**, the structural carbohydrate element and the prime source of energy 'released' from the masticated fibres by micro-organism fermentation in the large intestine (*see* Chapter 9, THE DIGESTIVE SYSTEM)

- the **lignin**, a further structural carbohydrate element which is only variably bio-degradable within the gut and, though of limited nutritive value, has to be masticated

Cellulose and lignin form the bulk, or **roughage**, from which comes a grazing horse's (or an entirely hay-fed horse's) main source of energy, the absorbable volatile fatty acids which after absorption are metabolised in the liver into glucose and glycogen. This roughage also plays a vital role during mastication

- in stimulating salivary flow (needed for digestion) by requiring mastication

- in providing 'ballast' to stimulate gut churning and motility – **peristalsis**

- and incidentally in providing silica salts, of no known nutritive value, but whose crystalline nature is abrasive to dental tissue and, within limits, helps to achieve correct enamel self-sharpening

Unlike the human jaw, in which the semicircular arcades of all teeth form a continuous line which limits sideways movement, the articulation between the equine jaws permits considerable lateral movement and some forwards and backward movement of the lower jaw, enabling the molars to grind food very thoroughly.

As a result of the continual friction between opposing teeth in the upper and lower jaws during the grinding of food, the surface (or **table**) is worn down by approximately 3mm ($\frac{1}{5}$ in) each year. And because the lower jaw is narrower from side to side than the upper, the wearing of the **cheek** or **molar** teeth tables is incomplete – the inner aspect of the upper molars, and the outer edge of the lower molars, are worn more, to leave narrow irregular **points** along the less worn edges.

To help withstand the considerable forces placed upon them, adjacent teeth in both the incisor and, more importantly, the molar 'sets', are tightly close to one another, with no gaps between them. For the same reason, horses'

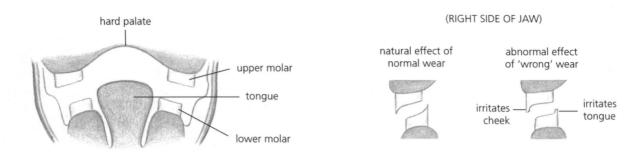

The production of points on molar teeth.

teeth have long roots firmly embedded in their sockets in the bones of the upper and lower jaws.

The part of the tooth that protrudes above the gums is described as its **crown** but, unlike human teeth, in which the crown is distinct from the root, there is no such demarcation in the horse's permanent teeth. Equine teeth have, below the gum level, up to the age of 6 years or sometimes earlier (and by which time it extends 80–90mm (3½ in) beneath the gums), a growing crown, known as **reserve crown**.

At the same time as the table of each tooth is being worn down by friction, the alveolar cavity in which the root of the tooth lies gradually fills with bone, slowly pushing the tooth out of the gum line.

This continuous **eruption**, as distinct from growth, of the horse's teeth occurs throughout its life, compensating for the erosion of the tables of the teeth by friction and so maintaining a more or less constant amount of tooth (crown) protruding above the gums, and a constant molar table area. Such equine teeth are called **hypsodont**, in contrast to the **brachydont** teeth of man.

In old age, upwards of 20 years, molar teeth can 'drop out' – whereas incisors, especially the lowers, tend to be worn down to the gum and held in position by the root and any reserve crown and the cement's 'grip' by the gum. However, at different stages in a horse's life, it will be first the crown, then the 'reserve' crown, and finally (in extreme old age), the by-then inert tooth root itself, that is in wear: it is often a smooth mass of cement. This last is quick to fall out. The rate of wear is not as great in the molars as in the incisors.

The shape and appearance of the tables of the incisor teeth change continuously and considerably with the progress of age, as the teeth wear down.

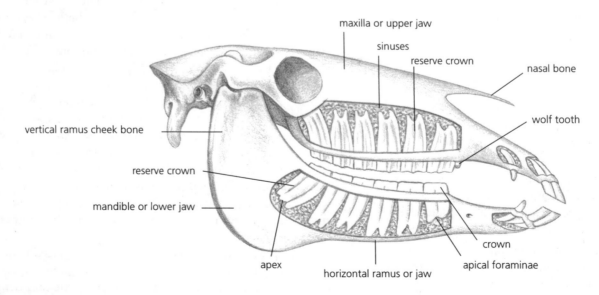

Horses' teeth have long roots embedded in sockets in the bones of the jaws.

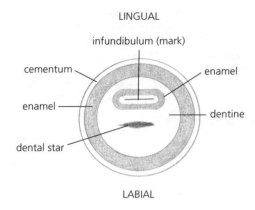

The materials that form the tooth. Shown here diagrammatically is a table of an incisor tooth at age approximately 7 years.

Since this rate of wear is roughly similar as between one horse and another, the outline and appearance of the tables can be used to give an estimate of a horse's age although, depending on the horse's diet, wear can vary by up to about 18 months either side of the expected pattern.

Although the mature horse appears 'long in the (incisor) tooth' as more becomes exposed *above* the gums, its tooth roots and reserve crown become conversely short. The *total length* of the teeth is greatest when a horse is 5 years old; the incisor teeth stop growing once their table is fully in wear, at around 5½ years old, the molars younger.

Teeth are made of four different materials – pulp, dentine, enamel, and cement

- **pulp** is a soft material that occupies the pulp cavity in the root of each tooth, in which are the blood and nerve supply to the tooth

- **dentine** is the yellow-white material that makes up the bulk of the tooth and surrounds the pulp cavity. It is not a 'dead' substance, and in that respect resembles hoof wall. It has no nerve supply. From 7 years on, new dentine becomes thicker and harder

- **enamel** is the very hard shiny blue-white substance covering the exposed parts of the tooth, and which sits on or around the underlying dentine

- **cement** is connective tissue converted into bone-like material, which covers the tooth roots of many animals but, in horses, also forms on the tables and crowns, where it partly fills in the grooves and infundibulae where the enamel ridge-sides and the dentine are exposed. There is little or no cement on the labial surface of the incisors' true crowns

For descriptive purposes, teeth have surfaces that are in contact with the tongue (**lingual**), lips (**labial**), cheeks (**buccal**), and they have a masticatory surface (the **occlusal** surface, or **table**).

Like most mammals, horses have two sets of teeth during their life. They are born with temporary (**deciduous** or 'milk') central incisors; the other, incisors and premolars emerge through the gums in the first few months of life. All the temporary teeth are replaced by permanent ones between the ages of 2 and 5 years. However, there are some teeth (canines and true molars) which have no temporary predecessors, and which only occur as permanent teeth. The ages at which the various temporary and permanent teeth erupt are shown in the table on page 75.

Blood Supply

The vascular system enters via the apical foraminae. It is assumed that there is an accompanying lymph system draining to the submandibular lymph nodes and to those of the deep neck.

Nerve Supply

The trigeminal nerve and its sympathetic fibre components service the mouth and the tooth apices.

In man, the type and duration of pain on noxious stimulation of the sensory receptors distinguishes between heat and cold and 'drilling'; in the horse the situation is unclear. Dentine, sensitive in man, is apparently not so in the horse. There is unproven belief that there may be sensitivity at gum level in the tooth; the gum itself is sensitive.

Dental Formula

Both sides of the jaw contain an identical set of teeth. The adult teeth can thus be represented in a dental formula, as follows:

Incisors	upper and lower x 6 =	**12**
Tush (canine)	upper and lower x 2 =	**4**
Wolf	upper and lower x 2 =	**4**
Premolars	upper and lower x 6 =	**12**
Molars	upper and lower x 6 =	**12**

In practice, the total number of teeth varies. This is because many mares do not have canine teeth; and the wolf tooth is usually absent in the lower jaw and in many horses is absent in both jaws. These wolf teeth are evolutionary remnants of the premolar unit (as PMI); they have no function. The maximum number of teeth possessed by an adult male horse is thus **44**.

The equine teeth are structured as

- **incisors** for cutting growing grass close to the soil, and for defence and attack in the female, grooming self and other horses
- **tushes** or **canines** for attack, by males, after initial incisor aggression
- **molars** or **cheek teeth** for grinding the fibrous constituents and mixing them with saliva with the 'pestling' effect of the tongue

The primary need is for efficient molar teeth, set in the jaws so that their tables form a regular, close-packed arcade or 'battery' of grinding surfaces, and in which the teeth grow from their apices or true roots until 6 years old and thereafter keep erupting more residual 'crown' at a pace of approximately 3mm (1/5 in) a year to meet the attrition loss of the true crowns, so maintaining an occlusal surface against their opposite number.

The molars also need to be able to maintain a self-sharpening enamel, retain (despite diminishing unerupted crown) sufficient hold within the bony alveoli at least until the mid/late 20's, and so function as to keep the formation of enamel points (a natural outcome of mastica-tion) to a minimum size.

Types of Teeth

Incisors or 'Front' Teeth

The middle pairs of the six upper and six lower are the **centrals**. The pair immediately to the outside of these are the **laterals**. The third pairs are called the **corners**.

Temporary incisors are smaller, whiter and more shell like in appearance than the permanents. There is a distinct neck, but this lies beneath the gum.

A feature peculiar to the equine permanent incisor teeth is that the enamel in the centre of the table is infolded to form a large cup or **infundibulum** which with wear gradually becomes smaller and more shallow to show as a dot known as the **mark**.

Wear eventually reveals the tip of the **pulp cavity**, now filled with the yellowish brown dentine; it is called the **dental star**. The star is near the labial (outer) border; the mark is on the lingual (inner) aspect of the table. The star gradually takes a more central position.

The shape of the incisor table changes with wear, from

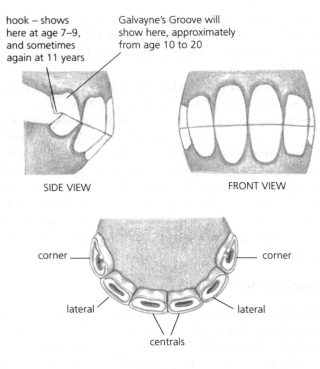

SIDE VIEW FRONT VIEW

The incisors.

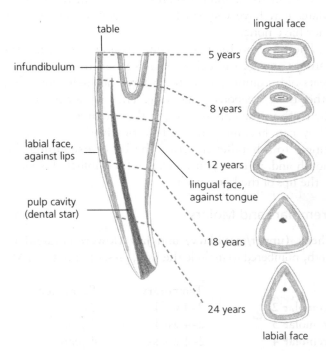

The natural wear of the incisors and the consequent variation in appearances of the table.

elliptical to round to triangular to oval, and it becomes deeper from front to back than it is wide. With age, the angle of the incisors becomes more acute.

The curve of the incisor teeth (viewed from the side)

varies between pony and horse: horses' are more convex, ponies' less so. This is significant for the pony's normal grazing, which is of short-stemmed and leafed herbage requiring close cropping.

An elongated groove (known as **Galvayne's Groove**) may sometimes be seen on the labial surface of the upper corner incisors – first appearing at the gums when the horse is 10 years old, and 'growing' slowly down the tooth crown to reach the occlusal surface by the time the animal is 20 years old. When present, this groove can be a useful guide to the age of older horses, but many ponies, and some horses, do not develop it at all. From 20 years onward this line ceases to appear with the erupting incisor and what is there gradually grows out with tooth wear, by 30 years.

Canine Teeth – Tushes

Male horses normally have two of these teeth in each jaw. They are found in the gum-covered bony ridge – the **bar** – which lies between the front teeth and the cheek teeth and which is the area of bit contact. The lowers are further forward in the mandible than the uppers in the maxilla. Mares may have very small canine teeth or, more often, they have none.

There are no temporary canines, and the permanent canines emerge through the gums when the animal is 4 years old. Equine canine teeth have no useful function, other than 'weapons' in fighting. They do not meet with the teeth in the opposite jaw, so they are not worn down. They can become long and vertically sharp edged, a danger to a handler inserting the bit or examining the mouth and, in later years, a cause of self-inflicted wounds to the lips of the horse itself.

Premolars and Molars

Cheek (upper/maxillary) and **jaw (lower/mandibular)** teeth, numbered to include the wolf, present or not, as PMI

	Temporary	Permanent
Premolar 2	2–4 weeks	2½ years
Premolar 3	2–4 weeks	3 years
Premolar 4	2–4 weeks	4 years

	Permanent only
Molar 5	1 year
Molar 6	2½ years
Molar 7	4–5 years

All adult horses have 6 **cheek** teeth on each side of the

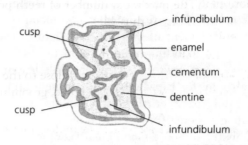

Cross-section of an upper (maxillary) cheek tooth.

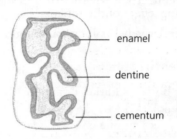

Cross-section of a lower (mandibular) cheek tooth.

mouth and six **jaw** teeth – i.e. a total of twenty-four grinding teeth.

The first three rostral cheek teeth, known as **premolars** (PM), have temporary teeth which are replaced by permanent teeth. The cranial three teeth, known as **molars**, appear only as permanent teeth. The roots of some of the upper cheek teeth lie within the maxillary sinuses, which are covered by a thin layer of bone, below and rostral to the eye.

The **enamel** is laid down as numerous vertical pillars which protrude on the lateral and medial surfaces of the molar crowns as **cusps** and are patterned on the table to form ridges of enamel surrounding the cups or infundibulae, thus forming 'lakes' of dentine covered with cement. This pattern is more complicated in the maxillary tables than in the mandibular but in apposition they form an inter-relating grinding surface.

The molar teeth occlusal surfaces, or tables, with alternating columns of dental material (enamel, cement and dentine) produce self-sharpening ridges of enamel projecting above the other two substances – so that the consequent irregular spaces, top molar to lower molar, produce two effective grinding surfaces. The tables wear down at 2–3mm (⅛ in) per year, to leave an irregular line of tooth, the **points**, on the outside (labial) aspect of the upper and on the inside of the lower (lingual) aspect.

Evolutionally, the accommodation for all these teeth was achieved by elongation of the naso-facial region of the skull, enlargement of the vertical height of the posterior area of the mandible (the vertical ramus), to give the leverage necessary for mastication while leaving sufficient dorsal room for capacious nasal passages and a dilatable oral cavity between the lower molars and the separate mandibular bones (or horizontal rami).

Only the tempora-mandibular (jaw) joint lies caudal to the eye socket; all other components are rostral. Section drawings help to demonstrate that the equine head is mainly concerned with teeth and mastication. It looks even more disproportionate when seen in full lateral plan, with its relatively small cranium housing the brain.

Wolf Teeth

In some horses, additional small teeth which are rudimentary premolars (PMI) are present. These are usually found in the upper jaw, one on each side, immediately in front of the first large cheek teeth. Rarely, wolf teeth may also be found in the same position in the lower jaw.

These teeth normally erupt through the gums by the time the horse is 6 months old. They usually fall out at around 2½ years old, with the temporary first large cheek teeth (second premolar – PM2). However, one or more wolf teeth may fail to erupt through the gums, or may not be lost but remain permanently in position in front of the permanent PM cheek teeth. Thus, an adult horse may have between nil and four wolf teeth.

Unerupted wolf teeth cause gum soreness when pressure from the bit produces a gum ulcer over the tooth. If wolf teeth erupt, which they usually do and remain in place, they can become sharp because they do not come into contact with any opposing teeth to wear them down. Their sharp points can cut the tongue. Wolf teeth are frequently associated with equitation problems (failing to take the bit, hanging to one side, and so on). Wolf teeth do not have deep roots, and so are liable to vibrate onto sensory nerves in the gum, which is thought to explain their irritability. They are removed from many horses, as a precaution.

THE FUNCTIONING OF THE TEETH

The jaw articulations permit the necessary lateral/rotary movement of the mandible against the fixed maxilla, and the chewing action stimulates the flow of saliva. Ingestion

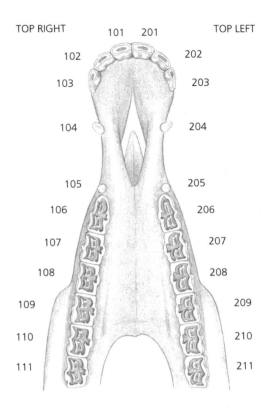

Sequential numbering used in dental records.

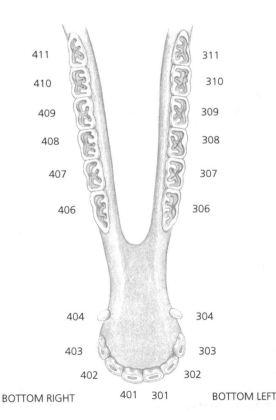

(grazing) continues at intervals over as many as 16 hours in 24. Incising, tongue-directed placing of this feed, and the automatic salivary flow between the molars, and subsequent mastication, is an almost continuous action stopping only for swallowing.

Although line drawings of the dental arcades imply a close match between incisor tables and molar tables it is now postulated that this presumed 'ideal' is maintained *only* when

- the head *and* neck are held *up*, as in reconnoitering, communicating or travelling, and
- the mouth is empty, so not being reflexly stimulated into masticatory action

When the head and neck are *down*, as for grazing and chewing, the mandible is placed so that the lower incisor arcade projects several millimetres, converting the normal 'parrot' mouth into fuller apposition; the molar arcades shift by the same amount, placing their grinding tables into a *maximum surface contact area, with optimal grinding surfaces*.

In the normal mouth

- the *upper* (maxillary) jaw is curved *outward*, caudally
- the *lower* (mandibular) jaw is curved slightly *inwards*, and at no time is its arcade as wide as or wider than the maxillary
- the upper and lower incisors can be manually slightly separated, with the upper and lower molars remaining in contact
- the molar tables face each other, jaw to jaw, at an angle of 10–15°; thus the upper molars slope from the lingual line down and out to the buccal line, and there overhang the lower molars
- during on-the-ground prehension and mastication, the mandible moves forward about 6mm ($\frac{1}{4}$ in), which puts the molar arcades in proper relationship
- the masticatory movement wears the tables across most of their surfaces but not quite all. Consequently the outer and inner enamel columns or cusps are not exposed to full attrition and so remain always a little higher than their table as **points**

The proportion of coarse fibre in the feed has an effect on the lateral excursion of the mandible – greatest with straw, less with hay, variable with grass, least with cereal feeds. This reduced traverse tends to result in more of the table being less ground away and greater formation of points.

The attrition does not leave projections at the occlusal

inter-dental spaces, so the arcades are free to move. The cross action at the end of the lateral and circular sweep by-passes the points. Chapter 25, DENTAL PROBLEMS, discusses abnormalities of this functioning.

What is important to appreciate is that if a horse is fed from a manger and/or a haynet, *rostral or forward displacement of the mandible does not occur* and consequently the molar arcades move against each other out of the optimal occlusion necessary for correct mastication – and wear. *It is these horses which get dental problems!*

The overall dental system has a balance based on three contact areas

- the *'bite'* or occlusion of the incisors
- the *occlusion* of the molar arcades as estimated when the horse is neither eating nor masticating. (The mandible should be easily moveable laterally)
- the tempora-mandibular *articulation* – the jaw joint

Deformation of the contact surfaces will exert undue pressure, causing pain and eventually degeneration of the joint cartilage, thus interfering with good mastication. Osteoarthritis – a permanent condition – may follow.

Horses in the wild must have on occasion lifted their heads to look around – and no doubt continued to chew for a few seconds. If all was well, the head went down to quickly resume eating; domestication interfered with this freedom reflexly to obtain the correct jaw apposition.

One of the important abrasive substances is silica. It is present mainly in herbage – but also in grains (cereals). At one time it was believed that horses constantly at grass did not eat silica whereas horses on hay and cereals – both physically 'hard' feed and requiring relatively more mastication – did have to cope with this insoluble element. Therefore, it was argued, stall-fed horses had for this (erroneous) reason more dental abnormalities than free grazers. It would seem more likely however that the free-grazing head was not only natural, but functioning correctly – whereas 'Johnny Head in Air' was not, with consequent potential for abnormal wear.

So important are equine teeth for survival that they warrant the adage: *'No (correct) dentition, no proper digestion, no healthy horse'*.

Unlike horses, cloven hoofed herbivores get 'two bites at the herbage cherry' – the ingesta is partly masticated and rapidly consumed until 'appetite' is sated or until danger threatens. Thereafter, in a safe place, the cow stands or lies down whilst she ruminates, regurgitates and 'chews the cud'; not for her is there safety in fight and flight.

The horse does 'flee' when required, therefore has no guarantee of a quiet time for regurgitating, even if it was capable of regurgitation. The horse's fermentation vat (as distinct from the bovine's anterior rumen) is in its posterior intestines, so it depends upon on-going fermentation even on the move. The one-time mastication must therefore be efficiently done.

Mastication aims at splitting (opening and breaking up) the stem and the leaf

- to release the solubles
- to expose more surface area for ultimate microbial action
- to stimulate reflexly the copious flow of parotid saliva which softens and lubricates the bolus and supplies buffering electrolytes
- to produce a suitably textured substrate for this activity – a bolus for swallowing

and maintain a variably constant throughput, with a persisting bulk or ballast, as a basis for stimulating peristalsis, making way in turn for the repetitive trickle input.

Dental Check-ups

Regular dental checks should form part of a horse's routine health care. All mature horses should have their teeth examined, by a vet or by a licensed dental technician, *at least once a year*. With youngsters up to 4 years the initial inspection should recognise developmental abnormalities and be carried out twice yearly to deal with excessive points and other projections associated with eruption or 'in wear' attrition.

In the UK any person, subject to the Protection of Animals Act, may

- examine a horse's teeth
- routinely rasp teeth using non-motorised equipment
- remove sharp enamel points and *small* dental overgrowths such as hooks and spurs
- shape 'bit seats'
- remove loose deciduous caps and above-gum-level plaques

(*This is subject to further agreement and regulation.*)

However, there is increasing use of equine dental technicians, trained on validated courses, licensed to do certain procedures which are considered acts of veterinary surgery, such as

- extraction of loose teeth and wolf teeth, via the mouth
- remove dental hooks and large dental overgrowths
- apply techniques requiring dental shears, inertia hammers and powered (motorised) dental instruments
- carry out non surgical orthodontic treatments, e.g. levelling the incisor arcades

Note that **only** a veterinary surgeon may administer any drugs, e.g. local anaesthetics or sedatives, required for these procedures.

Any horse which is not responding properly to the bit, or is having other equitation problems including vertical or lateral evasion should always have its mouth examined by a vet. Dressage horses are frequent subjects. The twice-yearly inspection early on will help to avoid bit evasion later.

Older horses (over 20 years) also require more frequent attention to their teeth. Six-monthly intervals are usually sufficient but some old horses may need to have their teeth rasped every two to three months. Loss of condition in old age is commonly a result of dental problems such as loose, irregular, or missing teeth, or periodontal disease.

AGEING

The appearance of the incisor teeth, their profile and tables, can be used to estimate the age of a horse. This can be done with some accuracy up to the age of 6; beyond this, only an approximate estimate is possible. For this reason, horses over this age are often described as **aged**.

To age a horse, the following must be assessed, usually of the lower incisors

- whether the **incisor** teeth that are present are temporary or permanent. The white shell-like temporary teeth with rounded gum margins must be distinguished from the larger yellow-brown dull-colour, due to the veneer of vegetable juices, and more square-cut appearance of the permanent teeth. It is particularly important to distinguish a 2-year-old (with a full set of temporary incisors fully in wear) from a 6-year-old (with a full set of permanent incisors fully in wear)
- whether the **infundibulum** or **cup** is still present or has worn almost away in some or all of the teeth, leaving just a small **mark**
- whether the brown-stained dental **star** is present in any or all of the teeth, and whether it is elongated or oval in outline

- the 'plan' of the **tables** of the teeth – whether they are round, oval or triangular in outline
- the **angle** (viewed from the side) at which the teeth meet and, in the older horse, the **length** of teeth protruding above the gum
- the appearance of the **upper corner incisors**. These have a 'hook' on their hindmost edge at 7 years until 9 years, and sometimes also again at 11 years remaining thereafter. From 10 years on, they may also have a Galvayne's groove
- whether or not canine teeth (**tushes**) are present; if so, the animal concerned must be over 4 years old

Once all the permanent incisors are fully in wear, *determination of age becomes more difficult, and must be speculative.* No single feature or sign should be considered reliable on its own, and an estimate of age must be based on careful consideration of all the signs noticed. It is now accepted that *individual variations in incisors makes 'ageing' even more difficult than once thought.* Accuracy

lessens rapidly from 5 years on.

There may be small variations in the appearance of the teeth of horses of similar 'age', especially when they are born at different times of the year. There can be variation of up to three months either side of the normally accepted time of eruption of the permanent incisor teeth, and more in the time when they come into wear (normally about six months after eruption).

Evidence derived from eruption and coming into wear should always have more importance attached to it than that relating to the disappearance of infundibulae and the appearance of dental stars. The disappearance of the infundibulum from a tooth is a particularly unreliable sign because it depends on its original depth, which can vary considerably from one tooth or horse to another. Thus, there may be a difference of a year or more between the time of disappearance of the infundibulum from a particular tooth in horses of exactly the same age. The same applies to the dental star's appearance times.

9 THE DIGESTIVE SYSTEM

INTRODUCTION

Ingested vegetation (ingesta) cannot be absorbed from within the alimentary canal until it has undergone digestion. This involves a series of physical, biochemical and biological processes along the system from the mouth to the anus. Food takes typically two to four days to pass through the digestive system.

Foodstuffs or nutrients are organic materials which, when digested and metabolised, liberate energy for cellular activity, especially in striated muscle activity, and also in the building and repair of tissues and to regulate body processes.

In simple terms, the digestive system involves a one-way ongoing flow of **ingesta**, progressively more **digesta**, during which insoluble material in watery suspension and soluble compound organic ingredients in solution are made ready for absorption directly or indirectly into the alimentary venous and lymph circulation, for distribution for other metabolic processes.

The horse is herbivorous; it is genetically programmed to live off vegetable material and, in particular, off 'grass'. Its early ancestors fed on leaves, succulent stems, flowers, and the fruit of low bushes and young trees – all parts of which were rich in soluble nutrients, sugars, starches, proteins, minerals, vitamins and lipids (fats), as well as hemi-cellulose. To obtain these it browsed, often standing on its three-toed hind legs, supporting its forequarters, short neck and small head on the bush with its four-toed forelegs. It was a **scansorial** (standing on its hind legs) **browser**.

It no doubt also grazed the young succulent leaves of the fine-stemmed grasses common to the marshy land it inhabited between forest and river. It did not require a large head with strong jaws and massive teeth, as fibrous food in its diet was relatively soft; nor, for the same reason, did it require such a capacious large-intestinal complex. It is believed that microbial fermentation of cellulose was not called for, at least not as its main source of energy.

Evolution followed the environmental changes imposed by severe climatic fluctuations. Forests disappeared, to be replaced by wide open spaces of coarse stemmy grasses. The horse evolved a longer neck – to let the bigger head reach the ground to **graze** – and to support its extra weight, too. The skull now contained grinding molars, and the jaws required greater muscles to crush this 'new' ingesta, vegetation high in **fibre** (cellulose) and low in solubles.

The thorax enlarged to accommodate an athlete's heart and lungs – for this horse had to flee from predators, and did so on evolved single-toed limbs. More markedly, the digestive organs developed to cope with the now slower microbial fermentation. The enlarged capacity vat-like hind 'gut' required a bigger abdominal cavity.

The modern horse is a **cursorial** (designed for galloping) nomadic **grazer**.

The wild or 'feral' horse had to obtain sufficient **dry matter (DM)** food to supply the average normal requirement of approximately **2.5% of its bodyweight daily** to meet a maintenance diet. In winter this might not supply all the essential nutrients; body condition could become less than ideal, down to the level of starvation.

Both in principle and in practice the horse is a **trickle feeder**. As such, in the wild he grazed in **15–20 minute spells** for up to **18 hours a day** – and still does so, under domestication when turned away to grass or when boxed and with access to sufficient fodder replacement.

The stomach is never completely filled, nor allowed to become completely emptied. The ingested food is held in layers in the stomach, not 'churned up' as in some other herbivore species. It passes down and through gastric acid and other **digestive juices**, which are worked into the layers by a kneading and squeezing action of the stomach wall muscles. This acidic and hydrolising digestion, along with the secreted mucus assisted by a limited amount of micro-organism **fermentation**, gradually converts the ingest into a gruel that is then propelled through the **pyloric valve** – the valve between the stomach and the **duodenum** – to the **small intestine**, while a small amount, digested in the stomach, is absorbed direct. The pyloric valve is stimulated to open by rising acid levels; the opening is consequently intermittent and the gruel trickles through in small amounts at frequent intervals. It is known that a bolus of swallowed food will complete the gastric phase in *one hour*.

In the duodenum, the **acid** gruel is made **alkaline** by the inflow of **bile** and pancreatic **exocrine** digestive juices. This digesta is called **chyme**. It rapidly passes along the small intestine, undergoing further hydrolytic digestion with absorption, before the remainder leaves through the **ileo-caecal** valve into the **caecum**.

It should be appreciated that except in very old, stemmy grasses, there is always some sap in the leaf and stem; in this fluid are the soluble nutrients – sugars, starches, protein, 'fats' and other nutrients such as vitamins and minerals.

In lush grass, these nutrients are present in dramatically greater quantities in comparison to 'old' grass and even to conserved grasses (hay). Concentrates (cereals, etc.) by definition are rich in solubles, especially starch. Equine gastric and small intestinal digestion and absorption had to evolve to become more capable of dealing with these 'unnatural' levels of nutrients; in some situations, especially if over-loaded, they fail, with dis-ease consequences.

The chyme passes through very quickly, possibly in minutes. During this time the digesta – now glucose, amino and nucleic acids, fatty acids and glycerol, plus the minerals and vitamins – are absorbed into the **portal system**, as **chyle**, to the **liver**. Fat, along with some vitamins, is absorbed into the **intestinal lacteals** which, as with other lymphatic vessels, drain into the cardiac inlet of the **venae cavae** of the venous system.

The remaining chyme passes into the **large intestines**, where microbial fermentation of the cellulose constituent of the original herbage takes place. The 'released' volatile fatty acids are the main source of energy in horses other than for those on 'hard work' and related production diets. Even these have a fibre content, both in the grass (if permitted), the hay, and the concentrate's husk. The fibre (cellulose) in food is necessary irrespective of other feeding levels. It requires mastication, with the co-incidental production of essential saliva, and it is the substrate for the eventual microbial fermentation.

The ingesta is moved along the alimentary tract by contraction and relaxation of the smooth muscles in the wall – **peristalsis**. This is involuntary, being under the control of the autonomic and myenteric systems, to produce

- *propulsion*, mainly one-way, from a wave effect

- *churning* or mixing from the muscles' kneading or squeezing through a torque effect, to mix food, water and digestive enzymes and micro-organisms together and ultimately to present the digesta onto intimate contact with the absorption cells of the mucosal lining

- **reverse peristalsis**, as in the caeco-colonic area

- the control of **stop and start** of these, particularly in the stomach

During digestion there is a continuous outflow and re-absorption of water secreted by the intestinal glands. Added to this is the water 'liberated', both physically and by hydrolysis, from the digesta, and the water drunk. Differing and variable proportions of **electrolytes** and **chemical buffers** are transferred in this lateral to-and-fro flow, through the gut wall from intestinal 'waters' to blood plasma and back further down the tract. Vast quantities of this water and electrolytes are ultimately reclaimed via absorption through the distal large colon and the small colon.

The lignous undigested residue of the ingesta, plus other products, mucosal debris and micro-organisms, and variable quantities of water (approximately 40% by weight), is excreted as **faeces**.

The horsemaster must consider these basic physiological facts in his management generally and in his feeding practices specifically. ***This is increasingly important, the further away he gets from a horse's natural lifestyle.*** For example, to satisfy nutritional and digestive needs and the psychological instincts, long fibre on which to chew must be supplied for as much of the 24 hours as is practicable, with due attention to the horse's capacity for dry matter. The horse is left to make the fine adjustments of when and how much.

The horsemaster must be aware that a *concentrate feed should not exceed 2.5kg (5lb) at a time*, and that the estimated 24-hour total should be divided, taking this into account, into the required number of feeds, spaced as equally as possible during the 24 hours, ponies proportion-

The digestive process.

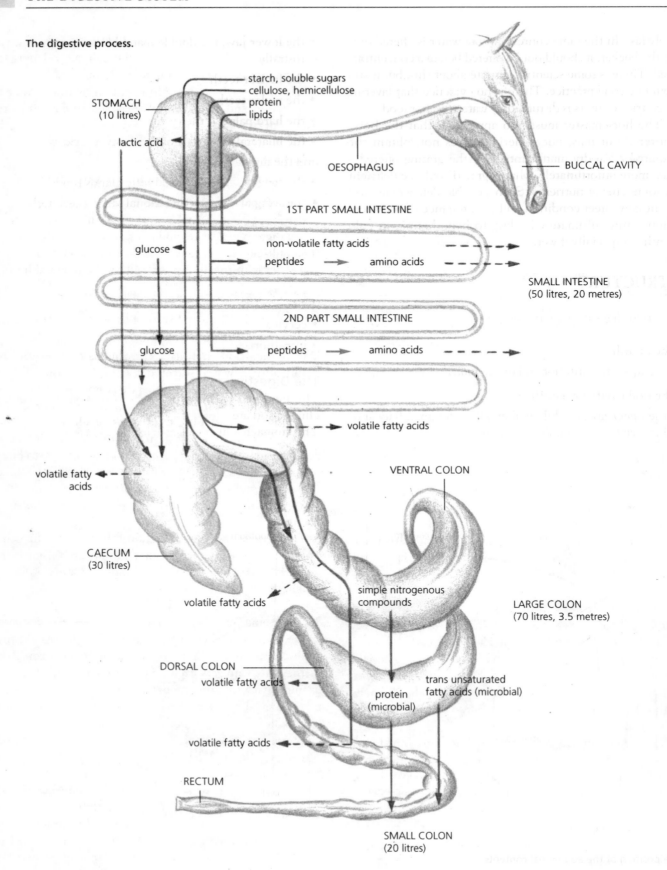

STOMACH
(10 litres)

starch, soluble sugars
cellulose, hemicellulose
protein
lipids

lactic acid

OESOPHAGUS

BUCCAL CAVITY

1ST PART SMALL INTESTINE

glucose

non-volatile fatty acids

peptides → amino acids

SMALL INTESTINE
(50 litres, 20 metres)

2ND PART SMALL INTESTINE

glucose

peptides → amino acids

volatile fatty acids

VENTRAL COLON

volatile fatty
acids

CAECUM
(30 litres)

volatile fatty acids

simple nitrogenous
compounds

LARGE COLON
(70 litres, 3.5 metres)

DORSAL COLON

volatile fatty acids

trans unsaturated
fatty acids (microbial)

protein
(microbial)

volatile fatty acids

RECTUM

SMALL COLON
(20 litres)

ately less. In the same context, where water is offered only by the bucket, it should not be offered before a concentrate feed. There is some scientific dispute about this, but it still could be good practice. There is no evidence that layering of gastric contents is disturbed by watering after food.

The horsemaster must also appreciate that the horse wintered out may, but sometimes does not, obtain the required 2.5% dry matter intake in the grazing offered – and, more unfortunately, what is grazed could be deficient in some energy nutrients. Such possible deficiencies will eventually affect condition and maintenance of body core temperature, ultimately leading to hypothermia in cold weather, especially if wet.

STRUCTURE

The non-digestive regions comprise

The mouth
- the **lips** – the anterior end of the muzzle

The oral cavity or mouth
- the **upper jaw**, the bilateral maxillae, foremaxillary and incisive bones – a unified structure
- the **lower jaw**, the double mandible rami, joined only rostrally
- the **incisor** teeth
- the **molar** teeth
- the **hard palate** – the roof
- the bilateral **salivary glands** – lingual and parotid

and the muscular structures of
- the **tongue** – tip, body and taste glands (buds)
- the **soft palate** – the directional 'door' posteriorly
- the **cheeks** – the walls

The pharynx
- the **throat** (muscular)

The oesophagus length (muscular)
- **cervical**
- **intrathoracic**

The Digestive Areas
The modified and evolved sub-organs of digestion and elimination are
The stomach – average capacity 9–12 litres (2–3 gal)

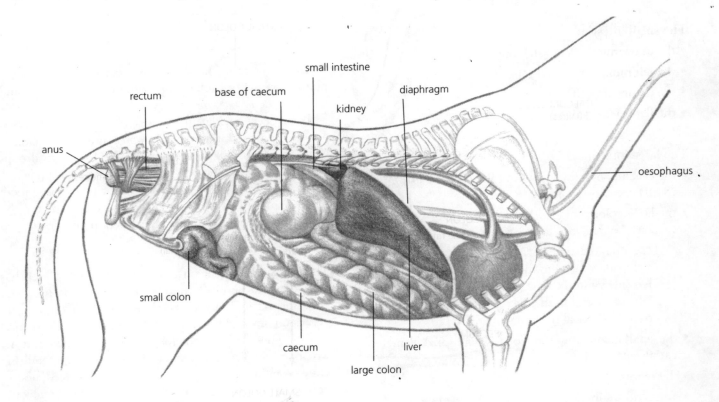

The position of the abdominal contents.

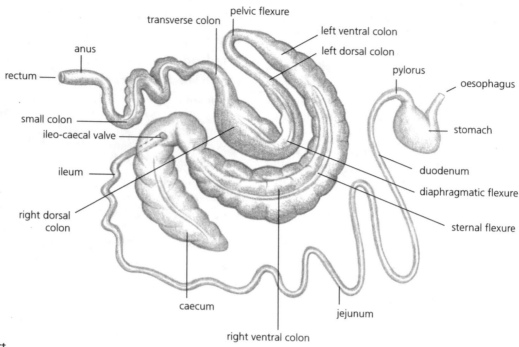

The digestive tract.

The small intestine
- the **duodenum**, 90cm (3ft) long
- the **jejunum**, 18m (60ft) long
- the **ileum**, 2m (7ft) long
- the **ileo-caecal valve**

The large intestine
- the **caecum**, or 'blind' gut, 1m (3ft) long, 35 litre (8 gal) capacity
- the **large colon**, 4m (13ft) long, 108 litre (24 gal) capacity, 'folded' into four sections
    - caeco-colonic valve
    - right side ventral to the sternal flexure
    - left side ventral to the pelvic flexure
    - left side dorsal to the diaphragmatic flexure
    - right side dorsal to the small colon
- the **small colon**, 3m (10ft) long, 7.5cm (3in) diameter, variable capacity
- the **rectum**, a canal, no digestive function
- **anus** and **sphincter**, a valve, no digestive function

FUNCTIONING

The two **lips** form the alimentary orifice. These are very pliable organs of prehension, which have anterior and lateral aspects.

The upper, muzzle lip, is particularly powerful and is able to draw food inwards and to push unwanted material away in a manipulative manner. The lower lip droops beyond the upper, and acts more as a scoop and 'guide'.

The lips are slackly closed when not prehending food; when drinking, they are tightly closed except for the anterior aspect, the water being sucked in and not lapped as in the dog.

The **incisor teeth** cut off growing vegetation, which has been directed between the two arcades by the lips. The curve of the incisor teeth (viewed from the side) varies between pony and horse: horses' are more convex, ponies' less so. This is significant for the pony's normal grazing, which is of short stemmed and leafed herbage requiring close cropping. The incisors also grasp loose feed, and in both situations the prehended material is picked up by the very mobile spatulate tip of the tongue. Jaw and tongue action now distributes it between the molar teeth.

The **tongue** is attached ventrally along most of its length to the soft tissue non-muscular floor of the mouth, and anchored on the framework of the **hyoid** bones. Its whole bulk is extremely muscular, and consequently very vascular. The tip, anterior to the **frenum** (a fold of oral mucosa at the beginning of the attached body), is very mobile. As a whole, the tongue keeps food between the molar tables, and then works it back under the twin columns of ridges of the alternating thicknesses of the palate's epithelial lining, towards the throat where it is moulded into a bolus then guided by the soft palate and passed to the opening of the oesophagus.

The **taste buds** are situated over the dorsal surface of the tip of the tongue, the **dorsum** and the root extremity. It is believed that they 'co-operate' with the olfactory nerves to give a safety awareness of what is being eaten.

Sweet, bitter, acid and salt are the usual stimuli, but it is argued that the horse only seeks out salty ingesta as the result of 'feeling the need for it'. Bitter and acid flavours are usually refused.

Mastication is effected by a side-to-side, slightly circular movement of the mandible (the lower jaw), whilst the maxilla, 'the upper jaw', is held stationary relative to the lower jaw.

The **grinding** of the teeth splits open the stem and leaf to liberate the sap and its soluble nutrients. It also lacerates the fibrous material into small pieces, thus presenting a greater surface area for hydrolytic digestion in the stomach and in the small intestine, but particularly for microbial fermentation of its cellular constituents in the caecum and in the large colon.

The process of prehension and mastication and swallowing is 'on-going'. There is an occasional halt, for deeper respirations and for subsequent swallowing, **deglutition**. On dry concentrates, some horses will spill unchewed feed out of the mouth as they stop prehension momentarily to reposition the feed in the mouth for effective mastication; this is not necessarily an indication of chewing difficulty. Others will pay too much attention to outside activities, and become sloppy eaters with much spillage.

The flow of **parotid saliva** is reflexly stimulated by chewing. This saliva has no digestive enzymes. It is, however, rich in minerals and acid-buffering materials and contains much **mucin** in the secretion which, like all secretions, is water (serum) based. The water, plus this mucin, helps to moisten the food and prepare it for bolus 'packaging', and subsequently lubricates it for swallowing.

About *10–12 litres* (2–2½ gal) of parotid saliva is produced and swallowed each day. It is alkaline in pH; this helps neutralise the acidity of the gastric secretion. 'Working on the bit' will also stimulate salivation, and some of this is swallowed during symmetric gaits. A horse in asymmetric gaits will miss a respiration to swallow; some saliva flows from the mouth, but such loss is not considered significant.

The **lingual saliva** is a steady secretion to maintain moisture on tongue, gums etc, and also acts as a lubricant to the mucosae and lubricates the ingesta. The quantity is not great; it, too, is swallowed. The equine lips and oral cavity are relatively dry when the horse is not eating. The horse does not reflexly salivate at the sight and smell of food, or at the sound of feeding – though it may kick the door if it thinks the feed is late! It will lick its lips, especially when on the meal-type feeds, but not as spectacularly as the canine or bovine.

The **pharynx** is the communal passage for air and food and water. Its muscular activity collects and finally moulds the material directed into it by the soft palate. The resultant bolus enters the **gullet**. Sucked-in gulps of water are likewise individually passed into the gullet or oesophagus.

The soft palate and the pharynx form a muscular cuff which posteriorly encircles the **glottis**. This directs inspired air from the nostrils into the **larynx**. During respiration the **oro-pharynx**, the posterior opening of the mouth into the throat, is shut off by the floor of the soft palate being reflexly kept firmly depressed onto the posterior tongue.

In deglutition (swallowing of water and masticated food) this seal is broken by the reflex lifting of the soft palate, whereby the **cuff** is dislodged. The glottis is closed and the 'swallow' is directed over the posterior top of the larynx into the **oesophagus**.

The **oesophagus** is a musculo-membranous hollow tube, with a diameter varying from nil 'at rest' to several centimetres as a bolus passes down. Down to the mid-thoracic region the musculature is striped. The first few centimetres are under the control of the pharyngeal cranial nerve supply and thereafter of the vagus nerve. The latter part, of smooth muscle, is autonomically controlled by both sensory and motor nerves.

The oesophagus opening is high in the posterior pharynx, above the larynx; it then veers to the left side and downwards, to lie parallel to and just above the **trachea**. It becomes central again as it enters the chest, and traverses that through the **mediastinum** to penetrate the **diaphragm**; 2–5cm (1–2in) within the abdomen it joins the stomach at the **cardiac valve**, just caudally to the liver.

The passage of boluses can be seen going down the full length on the left side of the neck. Eating, chewing and swallowing are possible whether the horse is browsing at a hay net, eating from a manger, or grazing, but 'head on the ground to eat' is the natural and best posture.

Once a bolus 'disappears', the horsemaster knows nothing of what is happening in terms of digestion until defaecation; the alimentary system is out of sight. Careful listening will 'tell of' the movement of digesta, air and fluids being propelled along the tract; the degree will vary. **Borborygmi** is the technical name for the abdominal rumbles.

Eating is such a basic instinct that alterations in the pattern of prehension, ingestion, mastication and deglutition, and especially *the absence of 'eating', even straw if available, for more than four hours, is a strong indication that 'all is not well'*. Even so, defaecation will continue, albeit in reducing quantities, for several days with diminishing abdominal sounds.

Conversely, the absence of droppings, or sudden changes in amount, consistency, colour or smell, and in comparison with that of other horses on the same regime, are significant clues of 'indigestion' of one type or another.

The **cardiac valve** comprises the folds of mucosal-lined muscular-walled flaps which form the junction between the end of the oesophagus and the opening into the stomach at the cardia. It is so constructed that, although there is a sphincter, or valve, it opens for boluses to enter the stomach but not in reverse for regurgitation, let alone for vomiting, except in certain dis-ease states, e.g. grass sickness. Even then, the escape upwards, even of gas, is so impeded that dilation and eventual rupture of the stomach can occur in advanced cases.

The Stomach

The stomach is a muscular, 'J-shaped', hollow organ which lies slightly to the left of the mid-line and in behind the diaphragm and the liver.

It is divided into four areas of different physiological function and size

- the **cardiac** – mucus, non-enzyme, secretion; the expandable container
- the **oesophageal** – no secretory glands at all
- the **fundic** – the principal area
- the **pyloric** – the lesser secretory area with acid gastric juice

The stomach wall is composed of four layers

- the **serosal** – the visceral peritoneum, covers the *outer* surface and is continuous, by reflection, with the parietal (abdominal wall inner surface) peritoneum. The nominal space between, and where they touch other abdominal organs, has a lubricating interface fluid – the **peritoneal fluid**
- the **muscular** – smooth muscles in three sub-layers, so arranged to produce powerful propulsive effect on the contents towards the pyloric valve
- the **submucosal** – with blood vessels, lacteals and nerves
- the **mucosal** – or *inner*, apportioned as above

The **secretory mucosal glands** are primarily in the fundic region. The secretions are of three types, which all produce enzymes, mucus, hydrochloric acid, and an 'intrinsic factor'.

The **pyloric glands** produce lubricant, and small amounts of enzyme for protein hydrolysis.

The Pyloric Sphincter

The pyloric sphincter is the valve between the tubular end of the stomach and the origin of the small intestine. It is responsive to chemical messengers for opening and closing, by local reflex stimulation of the intrinsic myenteric nerve structure.

The Small Intestine

The small intestine is suspended in a mesentery which is a double fold of parietal peritoneum, which surrounds the intestine except at one aspect of the serosal coat; it is through this that vessels, lacteals and nerves traverse to spread within the muscular and mucosal parts of the wall.

Mesenteric lymph nodes are spaced throughout this fold, one for several converged branches of lacteals (*see* Chapter 7, THE LYMPHATIC SYSTEM). The nodes are relatively close to the areas of the intestine being drained.

The **duodenum** is the short portion quite closely

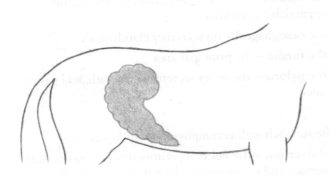

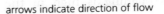

arrows indicate direction of flow

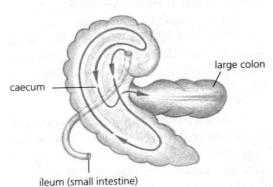

large colon

caecum

ileum (small intestine)

The caecum lies obliquely downwards on the right side.

attached to the stomach by a fold of mesentery, so has little 'freedom'. It is 'S-shaped' and encloses the pancreas in one bend of the serosal wall. The pancreatic and bile ducts disgorge their products through ducts in the wall. The **jejunum** is the major portion; the **ileum** is a much shorter portion.

The jejunum and the ileum are much freer, being suspended on extensive mesentery. Whilst their coils are usually in the left upper anterior abdomen, they are 'free' to move within a considerable area of the abdominal cavity. Apart from the demarcation between duodenum and jejunum, there is no line on the serous coat, or alteration in gut size, to separate the jejunum from the ileum.

There are, however, differences in glandular structure, and function, in the inner mucosal surface. The mucosal surface area is expansive due to its manifold design. In addition to **bile** and pancreatic 'juice', there are the products of three small-intestinal types of secretory cells, each specific to the hydrolytic breakdown – of sugars and starches into **glucose**, protein into **amino acids**, triglycerides into **fatty acid** and **glycerol** – as well as the preparation of minerals and vitamins for transport through the mucosal wall into venous capillaries and lacteals.

The small intestine is not only the site for absorption of its own digesta but also for that from the stomach, together known as chyme. Most of this absorption is through the ileum into the lacteals.

The passage of chyme along the small intestine is very rapid, approximately one hour. On autopsy, it is rare to find the stomach empty but common to find little other than mucoid material in the small intestine, especially the ileum which, in life, empties and contracts between flow trickles. The cubic capacity of the small intestine therefore has little significance. Distension, when it does occur, is due either to short distance impaction, usually with extensive gas production cranially, or to severe marked inflammatory thickening of the wall.

The Large Intestine

In contrast to those of some other herbivores, the equine organs of microbial fermentation of the cellulose content of the diet is not at the fore-end of the digestive system but at the distal part. This necessitates a very marked enlargement of the caecum and colon, in comparison with other single-stomach non-herbivores such as the canine. Not only is the caecum enlarged, but the large colon is enlarged both in circumference and also in length, so much that it has to be 'folded' or 'flexured' at three points.

The **caecum** is a cul-de-sac, somewhat comma-shaped and lying obliquely downwards to the right side. The ileum opens directly into the base, through a muscular valve. Just dorsal to it is the caeco-colonic aperture (from the caecum into the large colon), which has a valvular fold of mucosa.

The four lengths of the **large colon** vary in diameter at the **flexures** (sharp bends), which are sites for the effects of digestive upsets which result in impaction. The large colon is not suspended by mesentery; it depends upon its constant ballast or bulk of slowly fermenting digesta to keep it in place. Consider therefore the need for constant input of fibrous foodstuff and the traumatic effect of any pathologic condition especially if accompanied by displacement, torsion or incarceration.

Within the large intestine, there is much reclamation of water and of electrolytes and metabolic 'balancers', but the main function of the caecum, and of the colon to a lesser extent, is to provide a suitable habitat for the microbial flora to act upon the cellulose to liberate volatile fatty

The large colon, showing flexures.

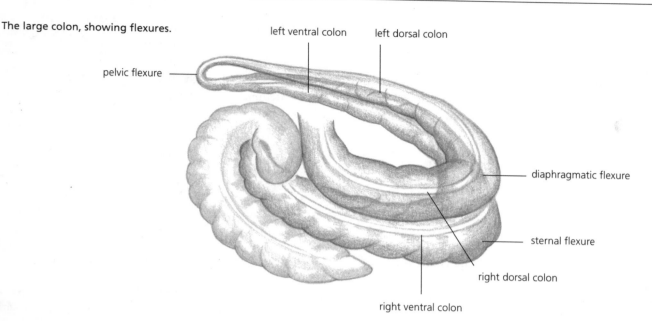

pelvic flexure

left ventral colon

left dorsal colon

diaphragmatic flexure

sternal flexure

right dorsal colon

right ventral colon

acids (which are mainly acetic, butyric and propionic). They are absorbed into the venous capillaries of the mucosa, along with the B vitamins produced in the caecum and amino acids and other vitamins not absorbed from the small intestine.

The millions of protein-material micro-organisms involved in this digestive process have a short life. When dead, they essentially become amino acids, which are thought to be recycled. Other, live ones, are swept out in the faeces.

The **small colon** is a relatively short, tortuous, narrow tube attached to a long mesentery which allows much freedom within the abdominal cavity. Its coils lie in juxtaposition with those of the jejunum; together, their freedom predisposes to **volvulus** and **torsion** – twists. It is in the small colon that the undigested residue is formed into faecal balls by the segmented contractions of its wall, and pushed towards the rectum by peristalsis. It is otherwise active in the final water and electrolyte absorption, and there is some fermentation activity as well.

The **rectum** is a short, straight tube of great elasticity. Its intra-abdominal anterior end has a 'coat' of peritoneum, but the pelvic cavity end has not. It is not held fast in these two sites, and can move horizontally to meet the requirements of receiving colonic faeces and expelling them. This also facilitates careful rectal exploration, as in colic diagnosis and genital ultrasonography.

As well as being unable to regurgitate food from the stomach (unless a neuro-muscular disease of that organ develops) or forcibly to return stomach contents by a form of vomiting, the horse is also prevented from breaking wind orally. Gas produced in the intestines is either absorbed or, mainly, passed as **flatus** through the anus.

Fluid in Digestion

The water content of the faeces or droppings varies considerably. It is a reflection of the amount of water consumed with the food, plus that secreted into the bowel lumen, less that which has been re-absorbed into the blood circulation via the large intestine. It should be remembered that *water is a transport system*.

Fluid movement within the digestive tract plays an important part in equine digestion. Very large volumes of saliva and gastric and intestinal juices are added to the food at the beginning of the digestive tract. This helps to begin the breakdown of fibrous food, and it also helps to present it to the micro-organisms in the large intestine in an ideal form for them to work on. At the end of the large intestine, much of this fluid has been re-absorbed from the contents. There is a vital movement of fluid, varying in type and amount of electrolytes, to and fro through the digestive tract walls, playing a role in homeostasis generally and intestinal content and pH in particular.

Insufficient fluid intake, both direct and from secretion of juices, can thus interfere with digestion. This, in combination with excessive amounts of dry food in the diet, can mean that the passage of food through the large intestine is slowed down – allowing even more time for water to be absorbed. This results in dry intestinal contents, as shown by hard, compacted droppings. Impaction, not really a constipation, can be a problem in stabled horses with access to straw bedding, with insufficient water intake and too much dry food, and/or too little exercise, especially if such management changes have been made too quickly.

In contrast, on lush pasture the faeces may become sloppy and unformed. Another cause may be damage to part of the large intestine, so that re-absorption of fluid may not be complete. This results in loose droppings. In adult horses a common cause of chronic intestinal mucosal damage 'scarring' is from earlier parasitism, but really loose faeces is more likely the result of on-going larval migration.

Diarrhoea is a condition where, due to inflammatory exudates somewhere along the digestive tract, and as a result of the failure of the large intestine to reclaim the water, the excess is excreted mixed with the faeces. Although bowel infections are quite frequently encountered in foals, they are, fortunately, uncommon in adult horses. When they do occur, large volumes of fluid can be lost from the animal's body in just a few hours, with serious consequences for its health, especially in foals. Affected animals appear very sick, and the rapid fluid loss may lead to circulatory problems and signs of shock. Acute diarrhoea is mainly associated with infection causing enteritis. Salmonella germs are an example. Loss of condition varies with the cause and the degree of damage as well as the duration.

The Liver

The largest of all glands, the liver is essential to life. It has several metabolic functions

- the formation and storage of **glycogen** (animal starch) for future breakdown into glucose

- the *de-toxification* of poisons

- the breakdown of **uric acid** from protein metabolism

- the formation of **urea** – part of the bile salts

- the secretion of **bile** from the breakdown of dead red blood cells etc

- the de-saturation of **fatty acids** absorbed from the digesta

The liver lies mainly to the right of the mid-line, just behind the diaphragm and in front of the stomach and parts of the intestine. Its functions are served not only by a normal arterial inflow, but also by the portal vein, which brings absorbed nutrients from the stomach and intestines as well as some of the venous blood from the spleen and the pancreas.

Paralleling the portal vein is the lacteal lymph flow. Together, they form the **portal system**. The lymph brings

fatty solutions direct to the venous system. The portal system also carries foreign material, such as toxins, to the liver. The liver's exocrine function is the production and secretion of bile through the hepatic (or bile) duct, into the duodenum. A horse has no gall bladder; the flow of bile is continuous to support the trickle flow of digesta. Bile assists in the digestion of fats and oils, and helps to alkalise the intestinal contents.

The Pancreas

The pancreas lies within the first loop of the duodenum. It secretes important digestive juices (**enzymes** in water solution) into the duodenum. The secretion is regulated by two hormones, produced by stomach and intestinal glands, to meet the required moisture content; and by the presence of foodstuff requiring digestion, which triggers secretion of the messenger hormones.

The vitally important second feature of the pancreas is its **endocrine** function, the production of **insulin**. This hormone passes directly into the venous capillaries, enroute to the main circulation. Insulin is primarily concerned with glucose metabolism and use. A second endocrine secretion is concerned with the breakdown of glycogen; it is called **glucagon**.

The Peritoneum

The peritoneum is a serous membrane which covers the abdominal viscera, and lines the inner surface of that cavity. It forms lubricating surfaces, enabling one viscus to

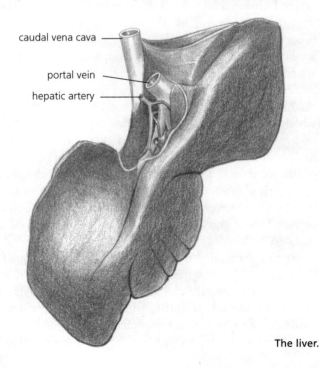

caudal vena cava

portal vein

hepatic artery

The liver.

'slide' over another during peristalsis and other movements.

The abdominal cavity and the peritoneal cavity are not synonymous. The organs actually lie 'outside' the peritoneum. The peritoneal cavity contains, in health, a small amount of fluid.

In addition to the parietal and visceral components, there are also

- the **omentum** – a loose lacey sheet which normally lies on the abdominal floor. It has the property to migrate to plug perforations and seal off acute intestinal inflammations

- the **mesenteries** – the sling of the loose loops of intestines, and a support for blood vessels and nerves to all areas of the gut

- the **ligaments** – thicker lengths which 'anchor' liver, spleen, bladder, kidney and uterus, in place

DIGESTION

Essentially, foodstuffs are composed of four materials: **carbohydrates**, **fats**, **proteins**, **vitamins**. Vitamins, which are either lipid (fat) or water soluble, can pass through the alimentary tract wall once in solution. Carbohydrates, fats and proteins must first be **catabolised** (digested, or reduced) – carbohydrates to glucose (a monosaccharide), fats to fatty acids and glycerol, proteins to amino (nucleic) acids. They then pass through the gastro-intestinal mucosae at appropriate sites. Once absorbed they are **anabolised** or built up into more compound substances for specific use.

The horse, a single-stomach herbivore, is designed to mainly make use of complex carbohydrates, cellulose, for which there are no digestive juices capable of enzymatic hydrolysis; instead they are fermented by micro-organisms, mainly in the caecum and in the large colon. The products of this are **volatile fatty acids** (**VFA**), which are absorbable energy-rich substances. The variable amounts of other nutrients in the typical high-dry matter (DM) fibre content of the coarse grasses for which the horse evolved are digested and mainly absorbed in the small intestine. Any overspill is fermented in the large gut and the caecum. The domesticated horse, often on improved pastures and with supplementary starch-rich but less fibrous grazing, must still be fed substantial quantities of cellulose rich rations to avoid digestive and other system disease.

Gastric emptying is automatically sychronised with ingestion. It ceases when feeding stops. In natural circumstances this is for only short periods coincidental with trickle feeding behaviour.

Fermentation in the caecum and in the large colon requires a constant, if slowly moved on, supply of ingesta prepared by mastication, a primary enzymatic digestion in the stomach and small intestine to minimise the amount of soluble materials (sugars, starch etc.) which would otherwise overflow into the large intestine. The cellulose is macerated to reduce particle size to around 5mm ($\frac{1}{4}$in) in length, which incidentally allows the escape of its sap's solubles into the stomach and small intestine. The rest passes to the caecum and onwards.

Ideally the ingesta should be of constant type – all grass or all hay, or a constant mixture of all foodstuffs in use. If a marked change is likely, as with a change in feeding management, *this should be effected slowly over 10 days or so to allow the large intestine micro-flora time to adjust*.

Micro-organisms in the fermentation process, having produced the volatile acids in the fermentation process, are quickly replaced. A change in this flora takes time to allow sufficient build up. Protozoal micro organisms ingest food particles and carry out ongoing fermentation and liberation of the volatile fatty acids into the intestines over a longer period.

Digestion of some sugars is also by fermentation by micro-organisms in the stomach and the large intestine.

As with all metabolic reactions there are several phases

- **catabolism** – the breakdown of ingested foodstuffs (nutrients) into their basic components, which are
  - stored in the intestinal mucosal area for subsequent release
  - immediately absorbed into the
    - lacteal lymphatic system, as chyle which is mainly emulsified fats
    - portal system, to the liver
    - venous system, to the heart and then into the arterial distribution system

- **intermediate metabolism** – more basic breakdown for primary build up

- **anabolism** – the build up of organic materials in the various systemic organ's cells
  - for their use
  - for ongoing distribution as bio-chemical substances for use elsewhere, e.g. hormones

Movement of the ingesta is, as has been described, mainly under reflex voluntary control as far as the anterior gullet. From there to the posterior thoracic oesophagus, control is by the reflex involuntary system.

Thereafter, to the end of the rectum, control is by the 'minor' nervous system, the myenteric, which controls the visceral smooth muscles. These muscles are circular and longitudinal. They knead and mix the ingesta, producing peristaltic waves which propel the digesta rearwards. Some reverse peristalsis occurs.

The gut has sensory nerves to the central nervous system (CNS), which transmit sensations engendered by distension, constriction, obstruction etc. The sensations pass to the spinal cord, from which reflex corrective action is signalled after subconscious brain assessment and integrated responses. In some cases, especially with pain, the messages pass to the conscious brain, resulting in signs of awareness, as with colic. Any necessary overriding control of the intrinsic (myenteric) nervous system is through the autonomic nervous system, which exerts a physiologically balancing influence. The intrinsic system is sensitive to, and reflexly responds to, various chemical changes in the intestinal wall from the digesta, as well as to specific hormones via the blood supply.

There is no proven evidence that a horse knows what *not* to eat. It is possible that bitterness is sufficiently off-putting to protect it except when grazing is markedly deficient in quantity.

THE ENDOCRINE SYSTEM

The endocrine system is concerned with **hormone** production, distribution and effect.

The Greek derivation, *endo* – 'internal', and *crine* – 'secretion', denotes a system in which special ductless glands within the body manufacture and secrete bio-chemicals directly into one or several of the various channels of communication within the animal.

The channels involved are usually arterial, occasionally venous or lymphatic, and sometimes nerve tracts especially those of the sympathetic (autonomic) nervous system as well as the cardiac (to do with the heart) and myenteric (to do with the digestive system) intrinsic sub-systems.

Secretion directly onto the skin (epidermal) surface does not occur, but some hormones do reach the epithelial mucosal surfaces of the various body systems and will pass to related orifices to be externally active.

An aerosol form is seen in pheromones from the mare's vaginal oestral flow, direct or indirect to the stallion's nasal olfactory nerve endings.

The many endocrine secretions, 'hormones' (derived from the Greek, 'to arouse' or 'to set in motion'), are one form of biochemical messenger. They exert important controlling influences on all body functions except the skeletal muscular system (other than its vascular supply) on a day-to-day and seasonal basis, and they do so by dictating action on *growth*, *reproduction*, *behaviour* and *survival* – the animal's 'way of life' in broad relationship to many extrinsic and intrinsic factors. Except for the adrenalin surge of the 'fright, fight, flight' reaction to emergency situations, they are variably on-going or persis-tent if relatively slow in their action; hormones differ from the control by the central nervous system (CNS) which responds quickly to locomotor needs.

Hormones may act individually, in sequence or in concert. They act on and are intimately connected with organ cellular metabolism and action – one enzyme motivating another. They may accelerate or retard the target organ activity.

The endocrine system is basically one of internal communication, closely involved in **homeostasis**. The secretions are small in amount; a deficiency or excess can readily occur, with consequent metabolic dis-ease.

Hormones have been recognised for some years, but new ones and additional effects within 'old' ones are still being discovered.

The names given to them are not always self-explanatory, for example

- **insulin** is derived from the structural peculiarity of its secreting gland, which is in the form of islets in the pancreas – Latin *insula*, 'island'

- **thyroxin** is secreted from the thyroid gland, which was known of for many years as an anatomical part – shaped like a shield – before its function as the source of this vital iodine compound hormone was discovered

- although **adreno-corticotrophin hormone** does not tell us where it was produced (the anterior pituitary gland), it does say to which organ it is attracted – the cortical part of the adrenal gland, which in response to the message secretes three types of cortico-steroids which themselves are powerful messengers to other systems

Other names tell what message they carry, for example:

- the **follicle stimulating hormone (FSH)** influences the ripening of the graffian follicle in the ovary, to secrete increasing amounts of **oestrogen** which itself feeds back vascularly via the hypothalamus into the anterior pituitary gland, instructing it to reduce the output of FSH and to release **luteinising hormone (LH)** – which stimulates the release of the germ cell into the genital tract

The endocrine system consists essentially of -

- **endocrine glands** – small masses of excretory glandular tissue situated in various parts of the body
- a **blood supply**
- a **nerve supply** – providing sensory *output* to the voluntary and involuntary systems and 'motor' *input* from the autonomic system
- **specific hormones** – the products – either *stimulating* or *inhibiting* in their effect on the target organ(s)

Some endocrine glands are part of a compound production gland, e.g. the pancreas, whose exocrene secretion flows direct into the digestive tract as a digestive enzymatic juice. Some produce several hormones, as in the pituitary. Others, such as the ovary and the testes, responding to incoming hormones not only produce responding feedback hormones but also form and release the reproductive cells.

The Hypothalamus

The neuro-chemical *control centre* for most endocrine secretions is the **hypothalamus**, a small specialised area on the underneath of the brain stem.

The hypothalamus receives sensory information from the brain cortex, e.g. light and touch, as consciously experienced by the horse. Subconscious sensory inputs are also relayed to it via the arterial and venous blood supply (e.g. 'informing' it of body core temperature), and neural connections with the adjacent pituitary gland.

These input messages 'advise' it of the need for control changes in the body. Output messages go to the pituitary gland, via the blood supply, in the form of 'releasing factors' or instructions to actively secrete certain hormones. The hypothalamus itself can also produce certain hormones, which pass along nerve tracts to the posterior-pituitary gland where they are stored until 'released' on demand.

The Pituitary Gland (Hypophysis)

The **pituitary** gland (now more accurately described as the **hypophysis**) is known as the **master gland**, the orchestra leader (perhaps erroneously), as its several hormones function chiefly to regulate the activity of other hormone glands.

The **anterior pituitary gland**, or **adrenohypophysis**, is a major source of wide-ranging hormones for

- *growth* stimulation (**GH** – growth hormone, the somatotrophic hormone)
- *ovarian* activity (**FSH** – follicle stimulating hormone, and **LH** – luteinising hormone)
- **testicular** activity (**SSH** – spermatogenesis stimulating hormone, and **ICSH** – interstitial cell stimulating hormone)
- maintenance of **lactation** (prolactin)
- maintenance of **progesterone** in pregnancy (prolactin)
- **thyroid** gland secretion (**TTH** – thyrotrophic hormone)
- **adrenal** gland (cortical) secretion (**ACTH** – adreno-corticotrophin hormone)

The **posterior pituitary**, or **neurohypophysis** stores hormones produced in the hypothalamus and passed to it

- an **anti-urine** production (**ADH** – anti-diuretic hormone)
- **pitressin**, which acts on the smooth muscles of the blood vessels as and when required
- **oxytocin**, which acts on the udder and on the parturient womb, i.e. at foaling

The Thyroid

The **thyroid** gland is essential for life. It controls
- the **metabolism** generally, by the secretion of **thyroxin**
- the **calcium** metabolism and bone development

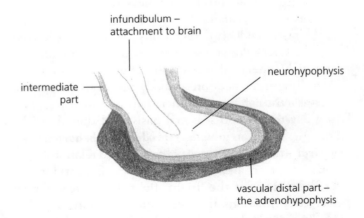

infundibulum – attachment to brain

neurohypophysis

intermediate part

vascular distal part – the adrenohypophysis

The hypophysis.

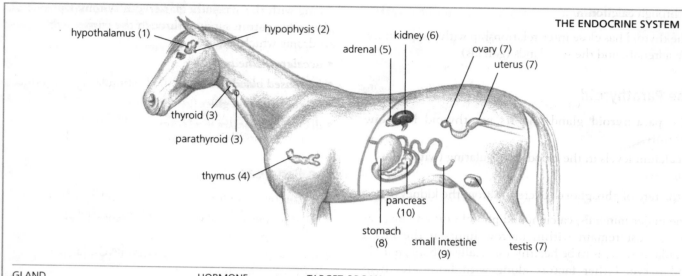

THE ENDOCRINE SYSTEM

hypothalamus (1), hypophysis (2), kidney (6), adrenal (5), ovary (7), uterus (7), thyroid (3), parathyroid (3), thymus (4), pancreas (10), stomach (8), small intestine (9), testis (7)

GLAND	HORMONE	TARGET ORGAN	EFFECT
1. Hypothalamus			
2. Hypophysis (Pituitary)			
adrenohypophysis (anterior)	ACTH	Adrenal cortex	Cortisol secretion
	FSH	Ovary	Follicle development
	LH	Ovary	Ovulation & yellow body formation
	Prolactin	Mammary glands	Milk secretion
	GH	General action on metabolism	Sugar, fat, protein, water in body increased
	TSH	Thyroid	Thyroxine secretion
neurohypophysis (posterior)	ADH	Kidney	Output of urine reduced
	Pitressin	Smooth muscle in arteries	Blood pressure rise
	Oxytocin	Smooth muscle in uterus	Uterine muscle contraction
3. Thyroid	Thyroxine	General	Metabolic rate control
	Calcitonin	General	Blood calcium level lowered
Parathyroid	PTH		Calcium level raised
4. Thymus (temporary – shrinks to become inactive with puberty)	not yet named		Development of lymphocytic immunity
5. Adrenals			
medulla	Adrenalin		Blood flow to muscles increased
cortex	the Cortisones	General	Sugar, water, salt content in blood tissue control
6. Kidney	Prostaglandin		A homeostatic control mechanism and has a neural hormonal function
	Erythropoietin (ESF)		Stimulates formation of red blood cells in bone marrow
7. Genital Organs			
ovary	Oestrogen	Uterus & genital tract	Dioestrus and pregnancy
yellow body follicle	Progesterone	Uterus & genital tract	Oestrous behaviour, lubrication of genital tract
uterus	Prostaglandin	Yellow body of ovary	Progesterone secretion halted in yellow body
testis	Testosterone	Psyche	Libido
8. Stomach's Fundus	Gastrin	Stomach's hydrochloric acid mucosal glands	Stimulates flow of hydrochloric acid
9. Small Intestine	Secretin	Bile & pancreatic juice	Stimulates flow of hydrochloric acid
10. Pancreas (intrinsic)	Insulin	General	Sugar level in blood and tissue control
	Glucogen		Counters the above

through **calcitonin**

The thyroid has close inter-relationship with the pituitary, the adrenals, and the sex glands (gonads).

The Parathyroid

The **parathyroid** gland and its parathyroid hormone controls

- **calcium** levels in the blood, by regulating (with calcitonin)
- the rate of **phosphorus** excretion from the kidneys

The major minerals, calcium and phosphorus and magnesium, must remain within narrow limits if the blood cellular activity is to be healthy, especially in bone, muscle and nerve. Other factors along with hormones help regulate this essential homeostasis.

The Thymus

The **thymus** is active in the very young animal, for which it is essential. It is lymphoid tissue, and is directly concerned with lymph cell production and function. Its hormone, not yet named, is thought to stimulate immunity production.

The Adrenal Gland

The **adrenal** gland has two endocrine producing areas

- the **cortex**, which produces three types of steroids, collectively known as corticorsteroids
  - **glucocorticoids** – promote production of glucose, decrease inflammatory reactions, and generally have other metabolic effects on muscles, nerves and cartilage. It also plays a role in fat and water metabolism
  - **mineralcorticoids** – the principal is aldosterone which regulates electrolyte levels and has an effect on water concentration
  - **androgenic** hormones – similar to the hormone produced by the testes with the same physiological effect, but to a lesser degree
- the **medulla** secretes 'emergency' hormones
  - **adrenalin** – stimulator of the sympathetic nervous system
  - **nor-adrenalin** – produces a similar action, but slightly more slowly

Along with the sympathetic nervous system, the medulla plays a big part in survival through the *fright*, *fight*, *flight* syndrome which requires

- *accelerated heart rate*
- *increased blood pressure*
- *increased blood glucose*
- *decreased intestinal activity*

The Pancreas

The **pancreas** secretes

- **insulin**, which regulates the blood sugar levels and cellular uptake
- **glucagon**, which is involved in the conversion of liver glycogen to glucose

These act as counterbalances.

Regulation of Water and Electrolyte Balance

This important role in the homeostatic control of body water and electrolytes is effected by a system of information feedback.

The concentration of **ions** must be maintained within narrow limits in the blood and in the two extravascular fluids. This depends on the messages from

- the **pituitary**
- the **adrenal cortex**
- the **parathyroids**

all acting on the **kidneys**, and

- the **parathyroid**, which controls the excretion of phosphorus (and so the level of blood calcium)
- the **anterior pituitary**, which controls sodium and potassium levels, and through its secretion of
- **ACTH** (adreno-corticotrophin hormone), which regulates the adrenal cortical hormone, which in turn regulates the excretion of sodium, and thereby water balance

Regulation of Metabolism

The anterior pituitary's **thyrotrophic hormone** stimulates and, by feedback of blood-borne information, regulates the thyroid gland's output of thyroxin – which in turn controls the general level of **metabolism**.

Changes in the rate of metabolism affect heat production, and so body core **temperature**. Variation from the normal temperature for more than several hours affects all cells' enzyme activity, with intermediate systemic dis-ease and with lethal effect in extreme situations.

The control of the **breeding cycle** is essentially hormonal with autonomic and CNS input for secondary behaviourisms in the male and female.

The **digestive system**'s hormonal glands act locally within the wall or on the mucosal surface in the stomach, and in the duodenum, effecting the intrinsic nerves there. Once again the result is to accelerate or to slow gut peristalsis and or to trigger activity in the mucosal juice secretory glands. There is an on-going feedback – **off/on** reaction.

These gut hormones belong to an organ's wide range of protein derivatives or peptides known as **Substance P** or **regulatory peptides**. Examples are **gastrin** which stimulates the release of gastric hydrochloric acid, and **somatostatin** which inhibits the flow.

The renal cortex peptide **renin** (not to be confused with the gastric digestive juice rennin) converts into **angiotensinogen** when renin combines with a liver enzyme produced in the blood.

Angiotensinogen acts on the blood vessel walls as a vasopressor and to stimulate the production of aldosterone in the adrenal cortex.

Some hormones require tactile stimulation to release their flow

- **oxytocin**, to let down milk flow when the calf suckles
- CNS **neuro-hormones** to sedate, as when a twitch is applied

Thermo-regulation

Thermo-regulation is the control of body core temperature, which has a narrow range of normality.

Work generates heat as a by-product; all body cells produce heat from the oxidation of nutrients. At rest, the amount produced is the basic source of heat which maintains the body core temperature.

The animal's normal temperature is maintained by reflex behaviours, and is an example of **homeostasis**. In cold weather, the horse will seek more food and so more heat production. The coat grows longer and more dense with improved insulating properties. Instinct will encourage shelter-seeking, and animals, if more than one, will huddle together to reduce heat loss from wet and wind-chill. The blood flow to body surfaces will be shunted to reduce radiation heat loss. The horse will become muscularly more active to produce extra heat, e.g. by shivering. These changes will, in the absence of extra food, burn off body fat stores – a possible 'catch 22'. In hot weather, it will sweat more, the blood flow being increased to the skin surface, causing dissipation of body heat and increasing water requirements.

Muscle functioning at exercise is more efficient when the core temperature and therefore that of the blood and the muscle cells increases – **hence the importance of 'warming up' before work**.

The metabolic rate will also be raised – at gentle exercise by a factor of 10, and up to 40 times at extreme exercise. Consequently, **a body temperature rise of 2.5°C from 37.9°C (5°F from 100.5°F) is a norm** in fast-exercising animals. Internal controls must not let it get any higher or stay there, however, as there is a risk of heat over-stress through interference with enzyme activity.

Muscle cells use energy for contraction, and – since the conversion of chemical energy into mechanical energy is only about 25% efficient – also produce heat. The rest is excess heat, which must be got rid of not only during work but afterwards as well. The mechanism for heat loss is reflexly instigated and involves a greater volume of blood going to the surface.

The sensors are in the skin, where they record blood temperature increases from the underlying muscles, and in the hypothalamic heat-regulating centre in the brain, which is sensitive to its blood supply's temperature.

As a result, cutaneous blood vessels dilate in order to carry increased volumes, taking core heat to the skin. (There is apparent competition here: the muscles need increasing amounts of oxygen-rich blood; and the horse needs increasing volumes of heated blood to the skin for cooling. This problem is overcome to a great extent by the benefits of training on the muscles.) Skin temperature rises by conduction from the blood vessels, and heat radiates into the atmosphere from the skin. In a cooler environment, or when a wind is blowing over the animal's body surface, there is also greater convection of heat.

Most important of all for cooling, however, is the evaporation of **sweat**; as water evaporates from the skin, the energy necessary to cause the water molecules to turn to water vapour is 'extracted' from the horse as a loss of heat. This is how sweating has a cooling effect. Sweat glands are 'switched on' in response to the adrenalin already released to help the muscles work. But sweating is effective only if evaporation can occur and so is compromised if the ambient humidity is high.

11 THE NERVOUS SYSTEM

The nervous system is the main control of the body and is arguably the most difficult of the systems to understand, especially in detail. Every cell of every tissue, excepting blood cells, is connected to the nervous system in one way or another.

The system is divided into three main parts, functionally and, to a lesser extent, structurally

- the **central nervous system (CNS)** – the brain and the vertebral cord
- the **peripheral nervous system (PNS)**, also known as the **somatic** nervous system, is linked by 42 pairs of nerves to and from the CNS in the vertebral cord (for *reflex* responses) and by 12 pairs of nerves directly to and from the brain (for a '*considered*' response). Each pair comprises an *afferent* nerve from the sensory organs and skin *to* the brain or vertebral cord, and an *efferent* nerve *from* the brain or vertebral cord to the appropriate voluntary muscles
- the **autonomic nervous system (ANS)**, 'that which has autonomy', also known as the **visceral**, is concerned with functions *not* under voluntary control – for example heart rate, airway diameter and respiratory rate, and the functioning of the other internal organs. The ANS is divided into the **sympathetic** and the **para-sympathetic** divisions. These have sensory fibres from the serous coats of the visceral organs, and motor fibres mainly to the smooth (non-striated) muscles. Broadly, the sympathetic nerves, which exit from the thoraco-lumbar area of the cord and run to the viscera, are responsible for *causing* activity; while the parasympa-thetic nerves, from the brain to the viscera, *suppress* activity. Thus, the sympathetic nerves raise heart rate and the para-sympathetic nerves lower it

Neurons

The system consists of large numbers of **neurons**. Neurons are nerve cells; they are the most highly specialised of all body cells but, beyond some re-growth of their processes, they are not able to regenerate, although 're-connections' are possible. A neuron consists of

- a nerve cell body or **cyton** containing jelly-like cytoplasm and, in it, the **nucleus**
- **processes** – fibres known colloquially as **nerves**, along which electrical impulses can be conducted, and which can be very long
  - **axons** transmit impulses *from* the cyton, the nerve cell. Each axon 'ends' at
    - an **effector tissue**, such as a muscle, which responds to the motor message transmitted to it, or
    - links up with a **dendrite** to relay a message from elsewhere within the central or autonomic systems; within the brain and the cord such relays are called **tracts**
  - **dendrites** carry impulses *to* the nerve cell. Each dendrite or receptor 'starts' at
    - a **peripheral sensory receptor**, or
    - a nerve centre or a nucleus within the brain, or is
    - a tract linkage within the cord, or within a **ganglion** (a group of nerve cell bodies)

Since each nerve cell has several dendrites it can receive several 'higher' instructions, but as its axon is a single outlet this information is transmitted to only one effector.

Peripheral dendrite endings have different shapes for

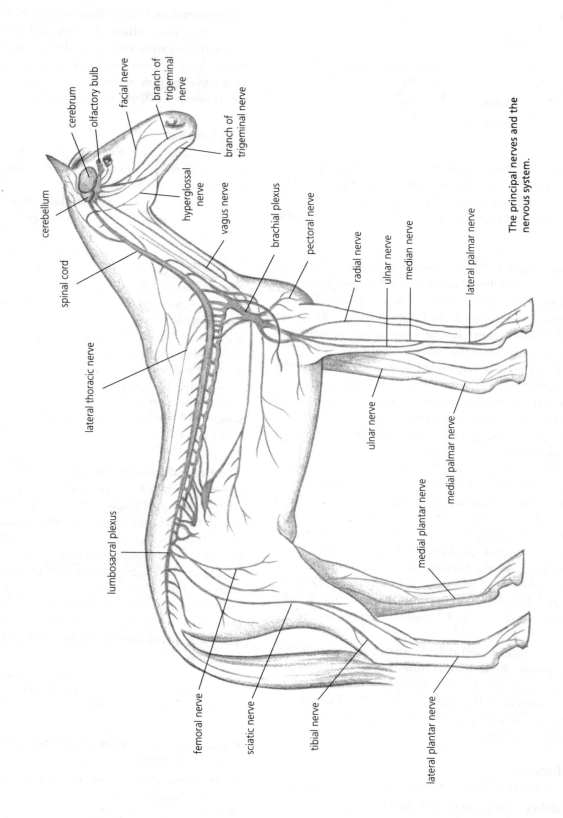

cerebrum

cerebellum

olfactory bulb

facial nerve

branch of trigeminal nerve

branch of trigeminal nerve

spinal cord

hyperglossal nerve

vagus nerve

brachial plexus

pectoral nerve

radial nerve

ulnar nerve

median nerve

lateral palmar nerve

lateral thoracic nerve

ulnar nerve

medial palmar nerve

lumbosacral plexus

medial plantar nerve

femoral nerve

sciatic nerve

tibial nerve

lateral plantar nerve

The principal nerves and the nervous system.

A neuron.

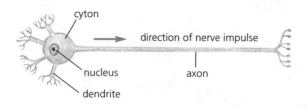

the many different 'sensations' to be picked up, some simple, some very complex as in the retina of the eye. The receptors in the human finger tip can perceive consistency, temperature, and movement – the horse's muzzle is the equivalent.

All sensory input will reach the brain, but not all gets to the conscious cerebral hemispheres. Life would be too complicated and exhausting if each input had to be consciously experienced and 'considered'. Most of everyday living is controlled at lower levels in the brain and, at a reflex level, in the vertebral cord.

The lower cranial centres subconsciously analyse the information, the 'feedback' from many sources. Cranial afferent sensory nerves transmit information gathered *directly* from the eyes, ears, organs of taste and smell, and from the *'feel' receptors* in muzzle, whiskers, and eyelid hairs, and information gathered from the rest of the body *indirectly*, via peripheral sensory nerves, from *exteroceptors* from the body surface, or from *enteroceptors* from the serous lining of internal organs.

A special type of sensory input comes from receptors in the balance mechanism in the ear and in the stretch mechanism in joints and muscles and tendons. These **proprioceptors** are the fundamental source of any animal 'knowing' where it is in stance and movement. They are augmented by visual inputs but are very much sub-conscious messages which stimulate automatic reflex action.

A slower 'receive and reflexly send' function monitors blood pressure, body temperature, hormone levels and carbon dioxide levels, and maintains homeostasis by acting on organs such as heart muscle, blood vessel wall musculature, airway musculature, and endocrine gland secretory functioning.

Nerve Impulses
The main functional characteristics of all nerve fibres are

- **excitability** – they can be stimulated
- **conductivity** – they can conduct impulses

When stimulated, the cell membrane becomes permeable to sodium ions which flow in and change the cell's normally negative electrical charge, of about minus 75 millivolts, to a positive charge. This causes a 'depolarisation wave' to flow along the neuron chain. Nerve fibres can transmit 1,000 electrical impulses a second.

The Synapse
This is the connection which links the systems into an integrated whole, where the axon of one neuron 'meets' the dendrite of another. There is no direct physical connection; a nerve impulse must pass (one-way-only) over the microscopic gap with the aid of transmitting chemicals.

For example, in the *parasympathetic* division of the ANS, one important chemical is **acetylcholine**, and the synapse is said to be **cholenergic**.

In the *sympathetic* division of the ANS, the chemical is **nor-adrenalin**, and the synapse is called **adrenergic**.

A subtle mechanism of enzyme interactions forms the chemical as required, puts it into 'use' position, and takes it 'out of use' when the communication ends.

Any dis-ease in this biochemical area will have a marked effect on neural transmission, with local and even general physiological effects leading to dis-ease or malfunction.

The Cranial and Vertebral Reflex Arcs
All sensory input is sent from a receptor dendrite to a related cyton and then via its axon to the brain, directly, or indirectly along the cord, by inter-connecting neurons. Should the message be that of an unusual sensation, e.g. heat or unlevel footing, this process can be short-circuited to activate an efferent (outgoing) motor axon and so its connected muscle – part of the initial defensive action. Such immediate reflex action is not only involuntary but works without the need to obtain even the lower brain's automatic involvement, let alone the brain's conscious awareness.

The cranial centres are however always (milli-seconds later) made aware of what has been sensed. They can then either

- acquiesce, but store the information as 'memory', another learning input, or

- add to it in whatever way previous programming or instinct 'thinks' best

Good examples of skin (hair) receptors are in the lips,

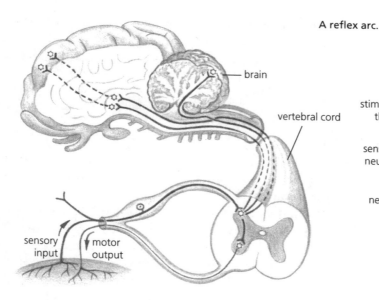

A reflex arc.

whiskers, eyelashes and external ear hairs. Messages from them result in automatic reflex activity – a blink, or a head shake – but are also recorded consciously, so that if the input (from fly irritation, for example) continues then further (conscious) action can follow.

Horses have a high concentration of touch receptors in the skin of the muzzle, and they use this very mobile 'organ' to investigate strange objects and (along with smell and taste) new foodstuffs.

There are no sensory nerve endings in the hoof's keratinised wall, sole or frog. Touch, therefore, is not effective via these insensitive tissues. However, the deeper nerve endings in the sensitive tissues, such as the vascular laminae and the solar corium, will pick up any unusual or changing pressures coming through the ground-bearing surfaces (a form of proprioception). Sub-horn pressures, usually more acute as from pus in the foot, bruise clots and oedema of the sensitive laminae, or space-occupying fluid from horn liquefaction as in a corn's horn necrosis, are pathological inputs producing sensations of pain.

Although all incoming messages evoke a response in one form or another there are examples of 'simple' reflex arcs instigated within the cranial or vertebral arcs which quickly recognise potential danger. A consciously received signal, as when a suspected threat is seen or heard, will arc to central motor nerves and if necessary with interconnection to a vertebral nerve – a **lower motor neuron (LMN)**.

A secondary 'advisory' input is also relayed, slightly more slowly because of the several intercommunications to the higher brain centres, including consciousness, for further action if that is deemed necessary, or to be stored

for 'reference' or learning. This sensation, which is not from stimulation of pain-sensitive nerve endings, is the basis of 'fright, fight and flight' – the simple reflex arc for survival. If however pain is sensed, via the appropriate **nociceptor**, self-preservation activity which has been primarily invoked may well be overridden by the need to respond to the pain – for example, 'don't use a limb that has become lame'.

The reflex arc categories are

- **exteroceptive** – from outside the body
  - via **cutaneous receptors** in the *skin*
  - via **chemoreceptors**, such as *taste* and *smell*
  - via **wave receptors**, as in *sight* and *hearing*
- **enteroceptive** – from inside the body
  - **viscero receptors** in *intestines*, *heart* and *lungs*
  - **proprioceptors**, stimulated by body movements and orientation changes, in *balance organs*, *muscle-tendon junctions* and *joint ligaments*

By definition, pain is a conscious sensation. It can be

- sudden, short acting – a 'stabbing' pain, which will invoke reflex action withdrawal
- longer acting – 'nagging', persistent, varying in intensity, which invokes a protective behaviour such as lameness

Lameness is also a dis-ease extension of proprioceptor reflex activity. Some horses are more sensitive to

- hard going, with the jarring of hoof and abaxial joints – and will alter their stride accordingly, up to the point of unwillingness to perform

- deep soft going, which is more difficult to explain but must incorporate
  - exacerbation of 'stretch' proprioceptors in the limbs – one of the important functions of recording 'stretch' tensions is to minimise the risk of overstretch tearing of the check ligaments in the two flexors and the flexor tendons themselves
  - 'frightening' loss of security in footfall

The 'feedback' warns the muscles that they are at the maximum safe stretch in the relax phase and at the maximum safe tension in the contracted phase, and that the range of activity must be reduced.

The efficiency of the horse's response to all stimuli is refined by training. Thus, improving a horse's co-ordination, balance and response to the 'aids' is ultimately a matter of training its nervous system. Horses have very good memories, but little power of reasoning.

The Central Nervous System (CNS)

The two intra-osseous, skull and vertebral column systems, are collectively known as the Central Nervous System (CNS).

The Brain

Many of the brain's components are structurally bilateral, as left and right sides (or 'hemispheres'). Essentially the brain is a two-layered hollow organ of highly specialised tissue which is almost entirely neural. It is the control centre for all *voluntary* striated muscle activity in

- the locomotor system
- the cranial and caudal extremities of the digestive system and the caudal aspects of the excretory, urinary and reproductive systems
- the other reflex striated muscle action involved in the defensive reactions to cranial sensory inputs

and for *involuntary* 'reflex' smooth muscle activity in the functional body systems, in association with the ANS.

There are distinctions between voluntary, involuntary and autonomic action

- **voluntary** – there is a conscious awareness and control of the activity even though it is eventually triggered and maintained by non-conscious brain areas, as in locomotion. The action can be altered at any time if the conscious brain 'thinks' it advisable to do so
- **involuntary** – movement (muscle activity) triggered by stimulation of a reflex arc involving cranial or vertebral nerves. Here too, conscious overriding can occur, but the reflex activity is spontaneous
- **autonomic** – this is also involuntary but is activity induced by the action of smooth muscles under the control of the autonomic nervous system. The influence of hormones is also involved. By definition there is no conscious input or 'interference', although the ANS is susceptible to feedback messages

The hollow area of the brain is a system of cavities, called **ventricles**, and of **ducts** which 'drain' to the vertebral area. They contain **cerebro-spinal fluid (CSF)**, which is a diffusion product of the blood's serum in the intercellular

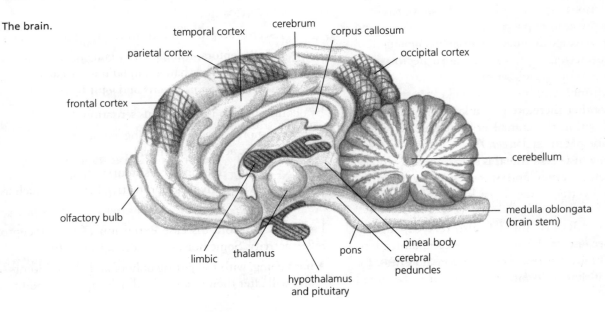

The brain.

temporal cortex

parietal cortex

cerebrum

corpus callosum

occipital cortex

frontal cortex

cerebellum

olfactory bulb

medulla oblongata (brain stem)

pineal body

cerebral peduncles

limbic

thalamus

pons

hypothalamus and pituitary

spaces. The CSF is surrounded by the

- **white matter**, the inner layer of connecting myelinated (sheathed in a white, fatty substance) nerve fibres, and the
- **grey matter**, the outer layer of nerve cells and un-myelinated fibres – the **cortex**

The brain is divided into

- the **anterior** area or **forebrain**, consisting of
  - the cerebral **hemispheres**, with the olfactory bulbs and tracts
  - a group of specialised bodies, the inner brain – the **pituitary** gland, the **pineal** gland, the **optic** chiasma, and the **thalamus** (a major inter-communicating or relay link)
- the **midbrain** area of the cerebral **peduncles**
  - a relay to the cerebral hemispheres
  - contains the nuclei for the cranial motor nerves III oculomotor and IV trochlear (to the eye muscles)
  - carries the neural pathways for ocular reflexes and other reflex tracts
- the **hindbrain** area of the **medulla oblongata** or brain stem, which contains
  - cardiac and respiratory centres
  - nuclei in control of equilibrium and touch sensations
  - the origin of the cranial nerves
    IX glossopharyngeal (to the tongue)
    X vagus (to the heart, larynx, lungs, stomach)
    XI spinal accessory (to the neck muscles)
    XII hypoglossal (to the tongue muscles)
- the **pons**, part of the brain stem which contains
  - nuclei for postural reflexes, and is
  - the outlet area for the cranial nerves
    IV trochlear (to the muscles of the eyes)
    V trigeminal (to the skin of the face)
    VI abducent (to the muscles of the eyes)
    VII facial (to the muscles of the face)
- the **cerebellum**, which functions primarily to
  - maintain **muscle tone** via feedback links from the 'stretch' proprioceptors
  - respond to reflex stimuli concerned with **posture** and **equilibrium** or **balance**

The brain is enclosed in 'skins' called **meninges**. There are three fascial layers

- the inner, the **pia mater**, a Latin name derived from the Arabic for 'tender mother', presumably 'protective'
- the middle, the **arachnoid**, a spider web-like structure which carries the vascular supply, the source of the lymph-like cerebral fluid, which bathes it and the other two fascias
- the outer, the **dura mater**, the tougher protector, firmly adherent to the bones

Within the cerebral cortex, the grey matter, the cytons are arranged into specific organ- or function-related groups called **nerve centres** or control nuclei, which with their axons are called **upper motor neurons** (UMN) and lead directly (or via interconnecting neurons) to peripheral motor nerves, both cranial and vertebral. Recent research suggests a greater divergence into subgroups of these nuclei, with more diverse interconnections.

The Spinal Cord

The cord is the tract for the neurons to and from all parts of the body, other than the head, to the brain

- **afferent** – sensory neurons *from* the periphery to the cord
- **efferent** – motor neurons from the cord *to* the periphery

Except for cervical nerve I (Cn1), which enters and leaves the cord through foraminae in the sides of the first cervical vertebra (the atlas), and cervical nerve II (Cn2) which enters and leaves the cord through foraminae in the sides of the second cervical vertebra (the axis), these bilateral paired nerves leave or enter the cord via the spaces *between* each vertebral body – Cn3 between C2 and C3, Cn4 between C3 and C4, and so on along the cervical, thoracic and lumbar vertebrae. The spaces between the cervical vertebrae thus have 8 paired nerves leaving and entering, the thoracic vertebrae 18, and the lumbar vertebrae 6. The sacral vertebrae accommodate five notwithstanding that the cord itself does not extend the full length of the sacral vertebrae.

In the cord the **grey matter**, consisting of relay cytons and their processes, forms an H-shaped column. The arms of this H at the level of each paired intervertebral foramina are the dorsal and the ventral nerve **root horns**; the dorsal are the entry roots for the afferent sensory elements of that nerve, the ventral the exit routes for the efferent motor elements. The **white matter** is on the outside – the reverse of the cerebral design.

The spinal cord.

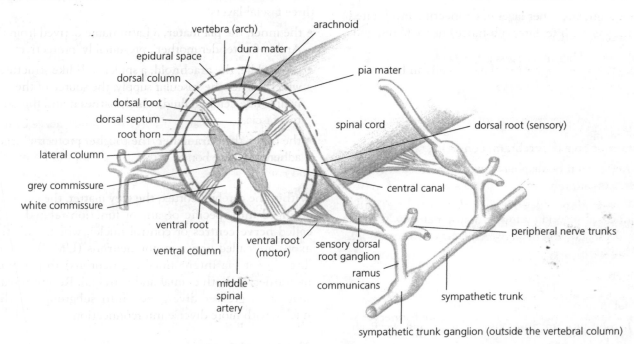

The cord is also covered by the meninges, but the duramater is but loosely attached to the inside of the vertebral column's individual body arches. The resultant area is called the **epidural space**.

The cerebro-spinal fluid (CSF) continues along either side of the arachnoid layer to the end of the column, where it enters the venous return system.

The vascular supply is functionally similar to that for the other body systems.

There is no lymphatic system as such within the brain and the cord.

The Peripheral Nervous System (PNS)

Each cranial and spinal nerve trunk ('nerve') is derived from the dorsal or ventral root horns which part (or come together) outside the brain and the cord (but inside the cranium and the vertebral column), and they are still within an extension of the dura mater.

The sensory nerve, the afferent, after the separation has a ganglion, the **sensory root ganglion**, an aggregate of cytons.

The motor element has a **lower motor neuron (LMN)** within the ventral horn, in the vertebral cord.

Each peripheral nerve trunk has two main branches

- the dorsal to the somatic muscles
- the ventral to the viscera and glands

Each trunk carries both sensory and motor fibres as in cord nerves and also in some cranials, but the cranial nerves (e.g. the cranial sensory inputs of smell, taste, sight and sound) are usually directionally single.

The afferent sensory fibres carry information from

- peripheral nerve endings, as with the above mentioned organs of sense
- skin and other epithelial surfaces – touch, pressure/stretch, pain from inflammatory dis-ease or serous coat distensions (as in some colics)
- the locomotor system via
    - proprioception with feedback information loops involved in monitoring that all is or is not 'well'
        - stretch, as in
            - tendons
            - muscles – voluntary and involuntary (cardiac and myenteric)
        - pressure (a form of stretch) in
            - joint synovia
            - vascular walls, and bronchio-alveolar walls
- ANS feedback from smooth muscled organs (the viscera)

Such information is carried to

• the brain, direct via cranial nerves

• the vertebral cord, and thence to

> • the brain, but not necessarily to conscious level, or into

> • the spinal arcs

In the brain they are: assessed, integrated, relayed, and/or stored as memory.

From the brain and the cord, 'decisions', either conscious, or sub-conscious, are transmitted outwards through the efferent motor nerves via **upper motor neurons** (UMNs), and indirectly through the cord via interconnected secondary **lower motor neurons** (LMNs) as well. As a subsequent peripheral nerve they will also carry ANS fibres.

Such instruction can be

> • voluntary, conscious, to striated

> • involuntary, unconscious compound reflexes from the lower areas of the brain stem

> • simple cord reflexes, and

> • autonomic nervous system (ANS) responses.

In man it is for example easy *consciously* to speed up or slow down respiratory rate and to change from diaphragmatic to costal breathing 'at a whim', but in doing so conscious, striated muscles are involved, e.g. intercostal and abdominal muscles; there is no evidence of animals having any wish or ability to do so – in other words, such visceral organs, in this case the lungs, are under involuntary control

It should be appreciated that the cranial sensory afferent nerves to the brain all go to the conscious brain and are dealt with there as above. The horse may, for instance, look and see, then act, to 'look more closely' or 'jump out of the visualised object's way', or 'weigh up what it sees and decide to ignore it', and similarly with sound, smell and taste.

Many such on-going sensory inputs seem to be ignored even when awake; they are 'recognised' as non-threatening, accustomed-to, inputs. When asleep, if the inputs are 'strong enough' – such as a loud unusual sound or a burning smell – they will arouse consciousness.

These and other 'usual' proprioceptor input feedback loops become more efficient and better defined with practice – hence the need for training.

The Autonomic Nervous System (ANS)

It is not possible to separate anatomically the ANS from the CNS and the PNS. Autonomic nerve fibres are frequently carried in nerve trunks along with peripheral fibres. There is a physiological division in as much as the ANS is concerned with the control of viscera and secretory glands and performs by means of reflex, feedback arcs which do not necessarily involve the higher nerve centres.

Man can hear the abdominal rumbles of a horse's digestive system, or the noise when it exhales during exercise and can see a horse sweat. Who knows, so too might the horse. What it cannot do is voluntarily control these bodily functions. The adrenalin responses, however, might be susceptible to training; for instance, the event horse can be taught to switch off the athletic adrenergic excitability which is appropriate for the gallop but not for the relaxed steady trot or canter required in phases one and three, so avoiding the unwanted and unbalancing energy-waste which may be induced by distracting aural and optical inputs – people and other horses!

Sympathetic Division

This is also known as the **thoraco-lumbar ANS**, because its fibres connect to the spinal cord in only these two lengths of the vertebral unit.

The exiting, afferent fibres leave the cord along with the paired segmental peripheral 'nerves'. Outside the vertebral foramen, or opening, most of them leave the main trunk to link onto the sympathetic trunk ganglia which run bilaterally along the external latero-ventral border of the vertebrae. At each ganglion the sympathetic fibres form synapses and then go in several directions

> • along the trunk, to interconnect with other ganglionic fibres

> • directly into visceral ganglia or direct to visceral effectors including the heart (but doubtfully to the lungs, as distinct from the bronchial walls)

> • to somatic glands – sweat, sebum and mammary – and to the muscles which erect the body hairs (or which are allowed to fall back, when the message is switched off)

A group of fibres returns via the spinal nerve and so back to the CNS – a feedback loop.

Sympathetic nerves also travel to the head, but do not reach the effector ganglia until the anterior cervical vertebrae level, and from there go to salivary and lacrimal glands and to intrinsic muscles of the eye such as the dilators of the pupil.

Similarly, extended fibres pass from the last lumbar ganglia to service the udder, the urogenital apparatus and the glands of the terminal colon, rectum and anus.

Parasympathetic

Also known as the **cranio-sacral ANS**, since the nerve fibres arise from the cranial nerves III, VII, IX and X, and from the sacral portion of the spinal cord. They parallel the sympathetic fibres, but unlike those the para-sympathetic cyton lies in the brain and the sacral cord, and the respective ganglia are located at the organ supplied. Those from cranial nerves III, VII, and IX are distributed only to the head – along with the sympathetic fibres from the anterior cervical ganglia.

Cranial nerve X, the vagus, carries parasympathetic nerve supply to the gullet, stomach, small intestine and anterior large intestine, as well as to the heart and the bronchi. The sacral portion follows the sympathetics, except that there is none to the udder and skin and only doubtfully to the gonads.

The cardiac and myenteric ANS sub-systems are referred to in Chapter 6, THE CARDIO-VASCULAR SYSTEM and Chapter 9, THE DIGESTIVE SYSTEM.

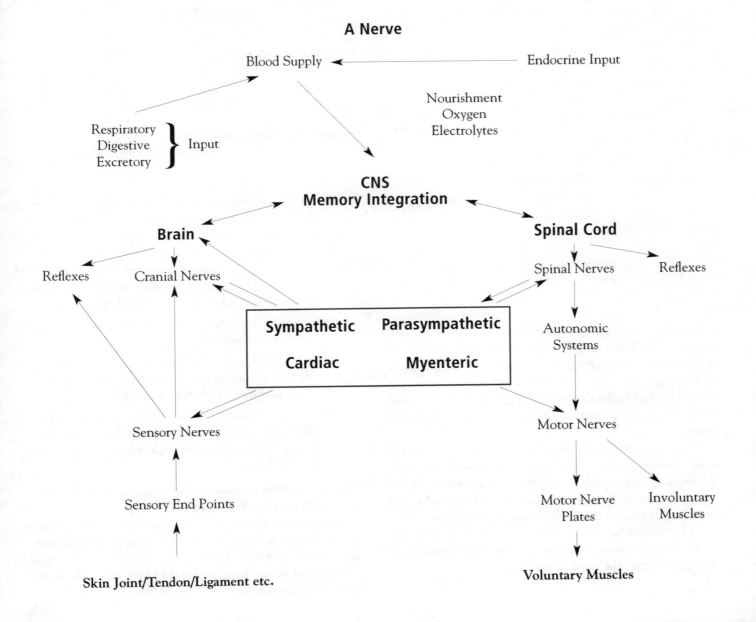

A Nerve

The Nervous System

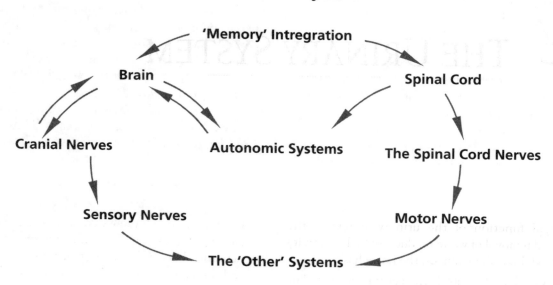

'Memory' Intregration

Brain   Spinal Cord

Cranial Nerves   Autonomic Systems   The Spinal Cord Nerves

Sensory Nerves   Motor Nerves

The 'Other' Systems

Endocrine System

Blood Vascular

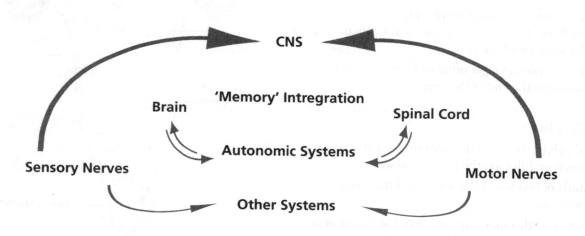

CNS

'Memory' Intregration

Brain   Spinal Cord

Autonomic Systems

Sensory Nerves   Motor Nerves

Other Systems

12 THE URINARY SYSTEM

The principal function of the urinary system is the extraction and removal of waste products of bodily activity from the blood. Like all mammals, the horse has

- two **kidneys**, which lie outside the peritoneal cavity but within the abdominal cavity, just under the lumbar vertebrae. The kidneys are closely attached within their own capsule to the surrounding fascia. The right kidney is slightly larger, slightly more anterior, and more firmly in place than the left

- drainage tubes, or **ureters**, one for each kidney, which travel backwards and downwards to enter the bladder

- a **bladder**, which lies within the abdomen just anterior to the brim of the pubis, connected to the outside by a single tube, the urethra

- a **urethra**
  - in the female, a short, urine-only carrier exiting on the floor of the genital passage at the junction of the vagina and the vulva
  - in the male, a longer urine and semen carrier, exiting at the end of the penis

Each kidney has

- a **renal pelvis**, the collecting area situated at a depression or 'hilus' on the medial surface

- a **medulla** of two zones, the water- and the electrolyte-regulating areas

- a **cortex**, a single outer zone, the major secreting area, all within the capsule, which is surrounded by peri-renal fat

- a **nephron** which, with its **tubule**, is the unit of kidney function. There are many nephrons in each kidney and each is a continuous convoluted tube. The blood supply is copious. Urine production begins with serum (water) passing from the capillaries into the proximal end of the nephron. There follows a complex movement along and through the various loops of the tube. Urine is excreted at the distal end, into the renal pelvis. The roles of secretion, conservation and excretion are within the renal zones

The urinary system.

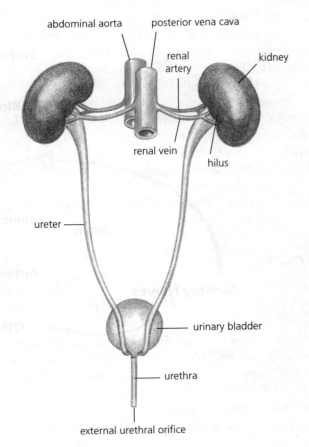

- abdominal aorta
- posterior vena cava
- renal artery
- kidney
- renal vein
- hilus
- ureter
- urinary bladder
- urethra
- external urethral orifice

The kidney.

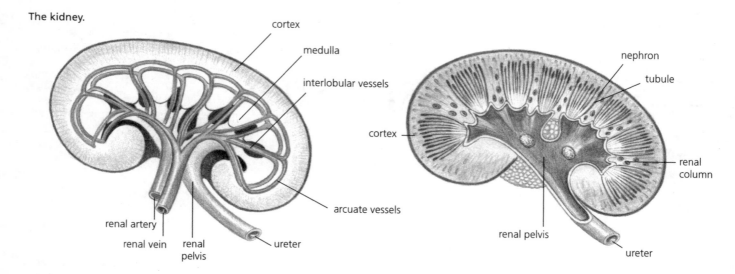

• **peri-renal fat**, the last body fat to 'go' in starvation. It is shock-absorbing and insulating

The **kidneys** play a vital role in regulating much of the body's internal environment, i.e. **homeostasis**. They conserve water, and regulate the acidity and alkalinity (pH), fluid balance, and osmotic pressure, and the composition and levels of many electrolytes, within the body's fluid compartments. They also play a vital role in excreting unwanted waste materials from the body. The ability to endure exercise stress and to benefit from it is dependent on healthy kidney function.

Hormonal action *reduces* urine flow to conserve water; enzymatic action *increases* urine flow to maintain fluid balances.

Up to 10 litres (2½ gal) of urine are produced daily, the colour and consistency of which vary in normal situations.

Urine samples are important laboratory aids to clinical diagnosis and are often examined in conjunction with blood samples.

Physiology

The amount of blood passing through the kidney determines the amount of urine excreted. It is subject to three controls

• **neural control** regulates the amount of blood flow. *In 5 minutes, the total blood volume will pass through the kidney circulation*, and within *15 minutes the extra-cellular body fluid will have been cleansed and returned* – natural dialysis

• **hormonal control** – the **anti-diuretic hormone**

(ADH), in response to blood concentration and increased osmotic pressure. **Aldosterone** from the adrenal cortex promotes **sodium** retention

• **enzymatic control** – responding to an increase in arterial blood pressure from inefficient kidney function. A substance called **renin** triggers a chain reaction

The kidneys themselves produce hormones, the principal one being **erythropoietin** which stimulates the production of red blood cells in the bone marrow (and increases their iron content).

Body Water

Water is the basis for most body fluids. It is the major portion by weight of the body, averaging around **65%** in the adult resting horse, some 40 litres per 100kg (9 gal per 100lb). It is derived in a replacement form, from what is

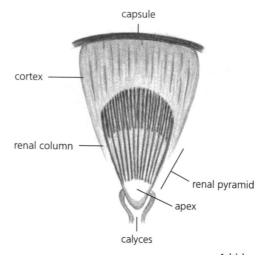

A kidney tubule.

- *drunk*, or absorbed from the gastro-intestinal tract
- *eaten* on wet feedstuffs or in the sap or juices of succulent feedstuff (all food has some fluid, water, content)
- the end-product of terminal **catabolism** along with carbon dioxide, as the 'water of metabolism', absorbed directly into intercellular fluid and so to the blood plasma

It is augmented by the secretions involved in digestion, most of which are re-absorbed further down the digestive tract as the transport for a different 'cargo'. As straight water it is not a nutrient: in itself it cannot be metabolised. It is vitally importan,t as

- the fluid part of all **cytoplasm**, the intercellular fluid component of total body water
- liquid blood, the **serum** (or intravascular part)
- the **intercellular fluid**, with a small protein content
- **transcellular fluid**, e.g. fluids of the eye, peritoneal cavity, joint fluid, cerebro-spinal fluid etc
- the liquid component of the **gastro-intestinal** tract

These five are collectively the **extracellular** components.

Water acts as

- a **transport** medium
- a **lubricant**
- the basis for sweat and other **secretions**

These are apportioned

extracellular	30%
intercellular	20%
gastro-intestinal	12%
intracellular	10%
intravascular	5%
lymph	2%
transcellular	1%

Intracellular fluid and intravascular serum are kept within narrow limits of variation, this being important in maintaining blood pressure as part of homeostasis. There is a constant interchange of their solutions – a persistent throughput of electrolytes and in the gastro-intestinal tract. It is said that the fluids therein are exchanged with that of the blood serum at a rate equal to total body weight every 24 hours.

Natural fluid loss is physiological, as in

- sweat and other **secretions**
- **expired** air
- **urine**
- **faeces**

and is reflexly 'made good' by increased drinking 'to meet need'.

Pathological loss, of varying degrees and severity, occurs in

- **diarrhoea**
- failure to concentrate urine – **polyuria**
- inflammatory **discharges**
- **haemorrhage**
- **heat stress**

The horse will reflexly attempt to counteract unacceptable loss by increased thirst, but in some situations appropriate therapy will be necessaary.

Effect of Fluid Loss

The body can lose a significant percentage of its water content through **haemorrhage**, through profuse **diarrhoea** (especially in the very young), and through excessive **sweating**, particularly in long distance work.

Clinical records show that when the water loss is

- *between 6% and 10%* – the animal exhibits *thirst*, *muscular inco-ordination* and *laboured breathing*. The blood has become concentrated, with an effect on the perfusion of tissues, particularly the vital heart musculature, kidneys and brain
- *between 10% and 20%* water loss, there will be *functional dehydration*, shown by *shrivelling of the skin* with persistent folding, *delirium* and *coma*
- *over 20%* water loss, the metabolic heat removal system fails, leading to a *fatal* rise in body temperature

CHAPTER 13

THE REPRODUCTIVE SYSTEM

BREEDING – CONSIDERATIONS

Punch (magazine) reputedly answered a young man who was seeking advice on marriage, with a cynical 'No'! Similar advice to a mare owner not to breed from her is less likely to be heeded, but at least considerable thought is advisable before deciding. Consider the following

Costs – cost-cutting is a bad policy

- stud fee
    - special care, e.g. if left at stud or 'walked in'
- foaling expenses
    - special care, e.g. if taken back to the stud for foaling, or if foaling at home with suitable pasture before and after and special lay skills and close watching during expected foaling period
- extra costs involved in
    - veterinary fees, especially at foaling
    - supplementary feeding of the mare and foal
    - rearing costs, plus breaking and training
- sale price potential

The mare

- suitability – age, any breeding history, value (**not** just because you have a mare available)
- pure bred or not – maternal influence
- athletic conformation
- showing and/or performance history
- temperament (temporary alteration with oestrus and/or suckling may change this)
- engage a veterinary practice for further advice regarding the mare's suitability with a special respect to
- athletic importance of locomotor deficits, which might be hereditary
- her past and present health – or specific lack of it – which could debilitate her during heavy pregnancy and foaling, as for example the risk of laminitic flare-up and COPD especially if stabled and on dry feed
- maintenance of breeding health before service
- attention to vulva seal deficits
- recommended swabbing
- any other debilitating factors
- during pregnancy
- pre- and post-foaling (teeth, worming, vaccination, hoof care)
- when to call the vet
- facilities and help required
- breed of stallion to be used (a stallion will not always improve the mare's suitability)
- which particular horse
- discussion with relevant Breed Society is worthwhile
- and also with recommended stud owner

THE MARE

The mare's genital and reproduction system functions very much 'behind closed doors', with only periodic surfacing to enable the observer to recognise that all is going well and, with training, to perceive the behavioural and other clues that point to something possibly being wrong.

The visible or external structure is limited to the **vulva** orifice and the intermittently exposed **clitoris**. The internal structures can be palpated by a veterinary surgeon

- *per vaginam* – forward to the **cervix**, the external neck of the womb

- *per rectum* – down onto all the structures and more anteriorly around them, as with the **ovaries**, the **horns** and the body of the **womb**

The innovation of ultrasonography has dramatically increased the ability of the veterinary surgeon to monitor the organ changes during the reproductive cycle, and the presence and development of the foetus during early pregnancy. Disorders can also be discerned (thus increasing the opportunity for treatment and re-service where applicable).

In the Thoroughbred a significant disorder is the relatively high incidence of twin pregnancies which usually leads to abortion or death of both embryos. Ultrasonography has not only enabled early and accurate diagnosis to be made but also has facilitated manipulative removal of one foetus to the benefit of the other. Twin abortion loss is now a rarity.

The hormonal (physiological) functioning controls of reproduction are now well understood in the mare, so much so that blood analysis for 'sex' hormone level abnormalities can be related to cyclical structural changes. In some cases this permits timely therapeutic intervention for further covering in the same breeding season.

Most research and development has been carried out in Thoroughbred breeding, and the benefits have been readily transferred to other breeds, thus allowing better understanding and subsequent management of the Warmbloods and crosses. In particular it helps the amateur mare owner to better appreciate what little information a brood mare gives him as to the significant behaviour of being 'ready for service', not returning to service and therefore probably pregnant, and eventually entering into Stage I labour.

The owner can therefore relate the obvious physiological (functioning) happenings to the many unseen structural changes necessary for

- fertilisation

- pregnancy

- parturition (foaling and passing of the **placenta)**

- lactation

Man, when he interferes with natural, herd reproduction must 'go along with nature' as much as possible within the limits of domestication; that is, the breeding season and within that the repetitive oestral cycles. He must therefore correctly interpret the mare's biological behaviour and also correctly present the stallion who, as a rule, is always ready and willing!

In the wild, the horse lives in groups (small herds) with one stallion who guards his mares jealously for many years until 'sacked' by a younger, stronger replacement. The incumbent can manage to cover up to 15 mares during a normal breeding season with 4–5 coverings of that mare during one heat period. The overall number of services required for the herd as a whole varies primarily with his own fertility and, to a lesser extent, that of his mares. Repeat coverings because of his low fertility will weaken him physically, making him more liable to be fought off by a newcomer. In this way the herd fertility is maintained.

In domesticated situations, man

- selects the stallion

- in a closed stud, the mare is also determined by the management

- in a public stud, mare selection is usually effected by financial constraints. Non-Thoroughbreds may be accepted, but the 'nomination' (stud fee) is relative to the potential value of the mare. In some situations the management cannot be too choosy

Whatever the politics and commercial considerations, it is essential that prevention of contagious disease is of paramount consideration for both parties, so the latest Codes of Practice must be followed.

Anatomy of the Mare's Genital Tract

Vulva

- **lips**
  - vertical
  - a seal, except at **micturition**, or when **winking**, as during oestrus behaviour, to disclose the (normally hidden)

- **clitoris**, the sexual function of which is not fully known, but its smegma coating retains olfactory and gustatory pheromones cyclically secreted into
  - the body with a central sinus, and two small sinuses laterally, all in a surrounding fossa

- cavity or **vestibule**
  - a short mucus-lined passage
  - the anterior end has the opening of the **uretha** on its floor

- anterio-dorsal to that is a constriction, a second seal, a defence against aspirated air and faecal matter

Vagina

- during **anoestrus** and **dioestrus** (see later) the vagina is a flexible 'collapsed' tubular passage leading to the **cervix**

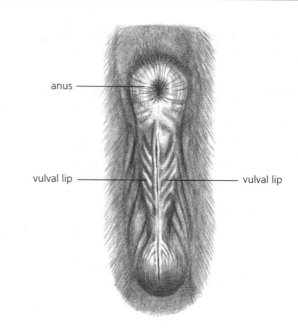

Cervix

- a protrusion backwards into the vagina from the uterus, its potential opening is the **'os' cervix**
- acts as the third and final seal between the womb and the vagina
- its tone and size varies with the physiological changes in the oestrus cycle, as does that of the vulva and vagina

External appearance of normal vulva, showing how close the dorsal aspect of the lips are to the anus.

Uterus

- T- or Y-shaped, a body running forwards and downwards on the anterior floor of the pelvis, in contact with the bladder
- about 20cm (¾in) in length when not pregnant
- divides cranially into two horns, which run laterally, each
  - 20–25cm (¾–1in) long
  - narrowing towards the cranial tips
  - each a potential cavity during oestrus and pregnancy

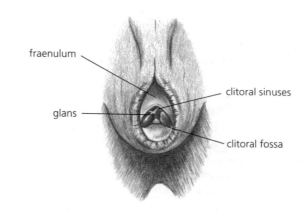

Exposed clitoris, visible by parting lower end of vulva.

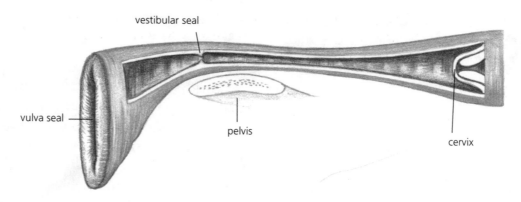

The position of the vulva in relation to the pelvic floor and the seals which prevent air being sucked into the tract.

- the **broad ligaments** suspend the uterus and ovaries; they contain contractile smooth muscle

Ovaries

- two bean-shaped structures
- main contents are an essentially embryologically determined number of dormant **follicles** in highly vascular tissue, one of which ripens and ovulates in each oestrus cycle
- ligament attachment, which carries the
- **fallopian tubes**, the narrow continuation of the uterine horns; they end in
- **fimbria**, open-ended fringes into which the liberated ripe ova passes at ovulation

Physiology of Reproduction – The Oestrous Cycle

Each species of mammal has a specific gestation period for the foetus to develop. In some, the neonate requires a further period in the security of a nest to mature sufficiently to become ambulatory. Others, such as the cursorial grazing ungulate's neonate, have to quickly be capable of running with the herd for safety and for the dam's nutritional intake as a trickle feeder.

In the mare, the gestation duration is approximately 11 months. In temperate zones the optimal grazing is spring to summer, consequently conception has to occur almost a year earlier. The ideal equine breeding time is, therefore, late spring to mid-summer. The mare is seasonally **polyoestral** and is programmed to begin the breeding cycle from mid-April to the end of July. Before and after the breeding season she is **anoestrus** (in the northern hemisphere, October to March). There are transitional periods before and after these dates when she will present abnormal cycles, usually with prolonged oestrus.

The actual date of foaling is said to be strategically controlled by the embryo through its developing endocrine system's circulation back through the mare's. (The foaling *time* is controlled by the mare to occur in the early hours of dusk and dawn.) This leaves a post-foaling interval for recovery of the genital tract before conception is required again, if annual foaling is hoped for. There is

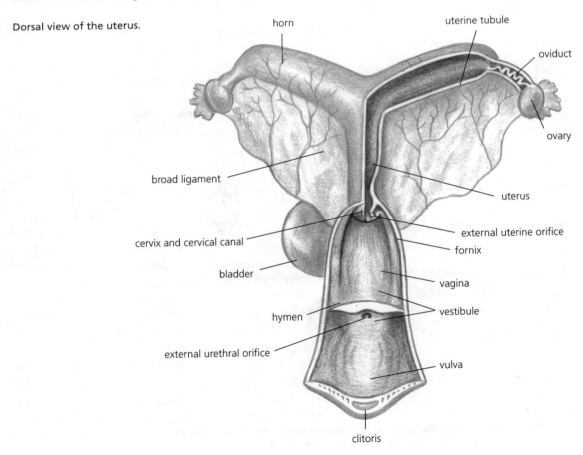

Dorsal view of the uterus.

horn

uterine tubule

oviduct

ovary

broad ligament

uterus

cervix and cervical canal

external uterine orifice

fornix

bladder

vagina

hymen

vestibule

external urethral orifice

vulva

clitoris

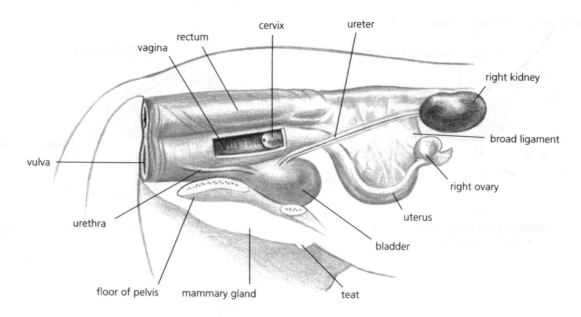

The genital organs of the mare.

often a foaling heat some 9 days post-foaling which, if all is well, is fertile.

The length of the true oestrous cycle of the mare is **20 to 22 days**. It is separated into **oestrus**, lasting 3 to 6 days, and **dioestrus**, the period between the end and the start of each oestrus, lasting 16 days.

A mare will show that she is 'in oestrus' by her behaviour, e.g.

* passing frequent small amounts of pheromone-rich urine
* being attracted and eventually receptive to a stallion or gelding
* raising her tail and contracting and expanding the vulva to evert the clitoris – winking
* a placid mare may become irritable; a difficult one may quieten

These changes are produced by the effect of hormones on the reproductive organs. The **follicle stimulating hormone (FSH)** is secreted by the pituitary gland under the influence of the **hypothalamus**, which responds to increasing hours of daylight and better nutrition in the mare and acts on the ovaries stimulating the growth of undeveloped follicles. Each follicle contains an ovum, and as the follicles develop they secrete another hormone, **oestrogen**. It is this which effects the physical signs of being 'in season' and the changes (increased **vascularity**, a congestion) in the reproductive tract, e.g. relaxing of the cervix and lubrication of the walls of the vagina and vulva from the increased mucoid secretions.

Once a certain level of oestrogen is reached in the blood, the pituitary gland releases an increasing amount of the other gonadarophous hormone, **luteinising hormone (LH)**. This has the effect of reducing the production of FSH and finalising the development of one follicle in the ovary, which eventually ruptures and releases the ovum – **ovulation**. This occurs about 24 hours before the end of oestrus.

After ovulation the level of oestrogen falls, the mare 'goes out of season' and is no longer receptive to the stallion. The empty follicle develops into the **corpus luteum**, which secretes a hormone called **progesterone**. This prepares the uterus for the implantation of the fertilised ovum, ensuring that the lining is ready to maintain early pregnancy. It also reduces the amount of FSH, thereby slowing down the development of further new follicles.

If fertilisation has not occurred, the 'empty' uterus produces a hormone called **prostaglandin**, which neutralises the corpus luteum in the ovary, thereby causing the level of progesterone to fall. The **pituitary gland** reacts to this drop by stimulating an increase in the amount of FSH to repeat the cycle. A feature of this hormonal control is the interplay of negative and positive feedbacks.

Oestrous cycle – hormonal stages in adult mare

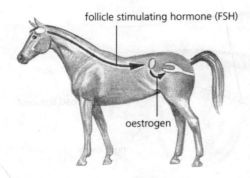

OESTRUS (0–5th day) – tail up, winking, cervix relaxed, tract moist

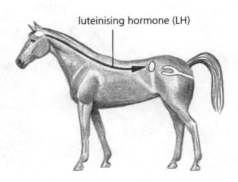

OVULATION (5th day) – tail up, winking, cervix relaxed, tract moist

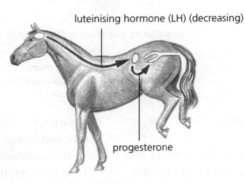

DIOESTRUS (7th day) – ears back, kicking, cervix closed, tract dry, progesterone dominant

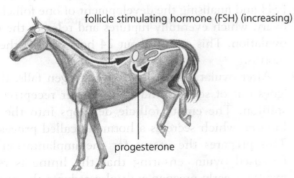

DIOESTRUS (13th day) – mid-cycle surge of follicle stimulating hormone, progesterone dominant

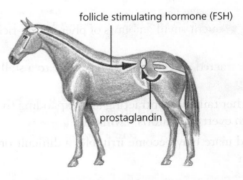

NEW OESTRUS starts (20th day) – follicle stimulating hormone and prostaglandin dominant

Pregnancy

A physiological state from conception to birth

- **conceptus**, the developing embryo and yolk sac (from 1st day to 5th)
- **embryo**, so-called when the fertilised ovum, the original conceptus, moves from the **fallopian** tube to a

uterine horn (5th–6th day)

- is implanted (attached) to the horn wall (16th day)
- the embryonic cells remain just cells. i.e. undifferentiated into tissues (until after 21st day)
- is now known as a **foetus** (at 40th day) complete with

The oestrous cycle.

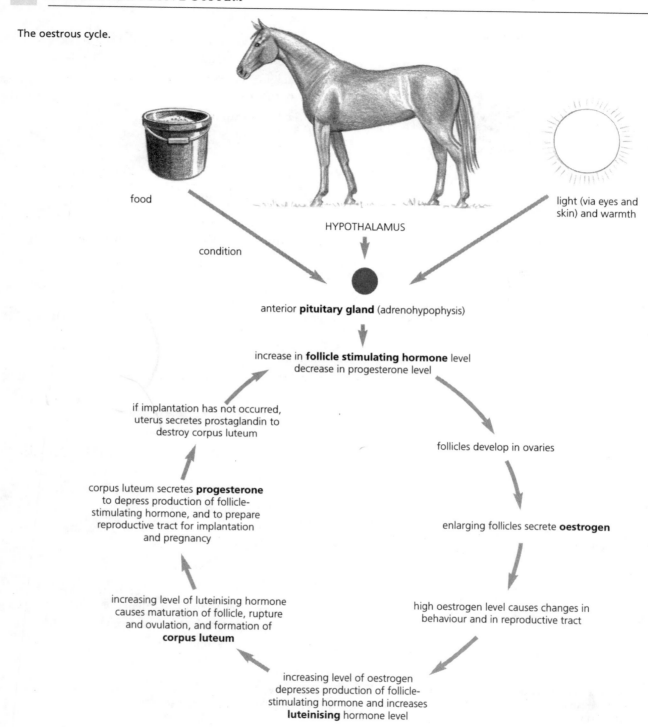

food

condition

HYPOTHALAMUS

light (via eyes and skin) and warmth

anterior **pituitary gland** (adrenohypophysis)

increase in **follicle stimulating hormone** level
decrease in progesterone level

if implantation has not occurred, uterus secretes prostaglandin to destroy corpus luteum

follicles develop in ovaries

corpus luteum secretes **progesterone** to depress production of follicle-stimulating hormone, and to prepare reproductive tract for implantation and pregnancy

enlarging follicles secrete **oestrogen**

increasing level of luteinising hormone causes maturation of follicle, rupture and ovulation, and formation of **corpus luteum**

high oestrogen level causes changes in behaviour and in reproductive tract

increasing level of oestrogen depresses production of follicle-stimulating hormone and increases **luteinising** hormone level

placental membranes and **foetal fluids**

- the **endometrial cups**, a specific area of the placenta, produce **chorionic gonadotrophin** – a temporary source of this endocrine secretion which helps maintain early to mid-pregnancy (36th day). They degenerate (from 100th–150th day)

- the foetus and its membrane extend into the uterine body (60th day)

- the increasing foetal fluids distend the whole uterus (90th day)

- the foetus takes up a long-axis gestational rotation, either head to mare's pelvis, or (less commonly) tail to mare's pelvis (180th day)

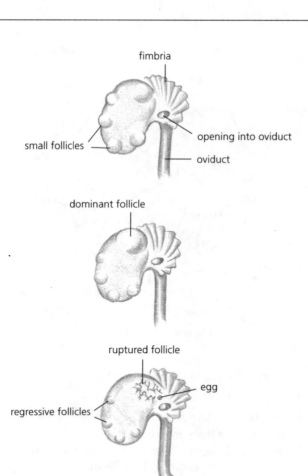

Stages of ovary development.

labels: fimbria, small follicles, opening into oviduct, oviduct, dominant follicle, ruptured follicle, regressive follicles, egg, yellow body, egg descending oviduct, sperm swimming up oviduct

visual changes of the external *os* of the cervix and lower genital tract, indicative (18th–21st days)

- further changes in size of uterus, and increasing tone (21st–60th days)
- uterus falls forward into abdominal cavity, leaving base and cervix palpable. Lessening accuracy (60th–120th days)
- uterus enlarges and partially re-enters the pelvic area. Now more accurate except in older mares where it is still forward (from 120th day to full term)
- visible from outside, foal's exercising movement – 'quickening' – limb thrusts onto left flank (from 180th day)

eventually

- enlarging lips of the vulva
- slackening of pelvic sacro-sciatic ligaments and the tail head
- enlarging udder (near foaling)

all associated with increasing hormonally controlled vascularity

- blood samples, both variably accurate, for
    - progesterone level (18th–20th day)
    - equine chorionic gonadotrophin (80th–120th day)

    (there is a recently introduced test of plasma by a safer chemical. The originally used reagent for the urine test is now known to be carcinogenic for the lab technicians!)
- urine sample for
    - placental oestrogens (150th–300th+ day)
- ultrasonography
- *per rectum*, highly accurate, particularly valuable for twin diagnosis at time of routine pregnancy evaluation (arbitrarily from 10th to 40th day)

STALLION

The Genitalia

Both anatomically and physiologically there are a similarities in the male and the female.

The male **gonads** (**testes** or **testicles**) are, like the female organs, the source of the male **gametes**, or the **sperm**, the ova in the female. Like the ovaries they are

Pregnancy Diagnosis

- presumptive if no return to service after 21 days. Low accuracy, for example the mare can go from dioestrus into anoestrus
- rectal examination

    palpable changes in the uterus
- *per vaginam*

'paired' but, unlike them, each foetal testis descends from the abdomen through the **inguinal ring** in a double peritoneal sac, to lie externally in the scrotal area of skin through which they are discernible and palpable. This extra-abdominal position is due to the physiological need for a lower but controllable temperature for spermatogenesis, development and early maturation.

The testes have a two-fold purpose from two distinct glandular structures within each

- **spermatogenesis** – the production of spermatozoa. This takes 50 days within the testis and **epididymis**

- production of **testosterone** and other androgen male sex hormones in the **leydig cells**. These are responsible for the development of puberty and subsequent maintenance of the secondary male sexual characteristics

  - growth of the penis and testicles
  - stimulation of sperm production under the influence of the **spermatogenesis stimulating hormone (SSH)**, the equivalent of the ovarian FSH
  - conformation, as with stallion crest
  - muscularity, possibly athleticism
  - 'voice'
  - libido or sex drive
  - knowing 'what to do, when (and when not to!)'

The androgens are thought to play a role in the sexual rhythm by shutting down the level of gonadal **interstitial cell stimulating hormone (ICSH)**, which is the primary trigger for androgen formation – a positive feed-back – the chemical equivalent of LH of the ovary.

The testicular products are steadily passed to the **epididymus** or dorsal cap of the testis in which spermatazoa finally mature before entering the **ductus (vas) deferens** of the spermatic cord for eventual transport to the intra-pelvic urethra.

The **spermatic cord** is originally 'let down' with the descending testis, and maintains a connection with it. Its constituent parts are

- the **cremaster muscle** which reflexly tenses or slackens the scrotum, and so regulates its and the testes' exposure to external temperature
- somatic nerves to the peritoneal tunics, the muscle and the skin
- artery
- veins – the **pampiniform plexus**
- lymphatics

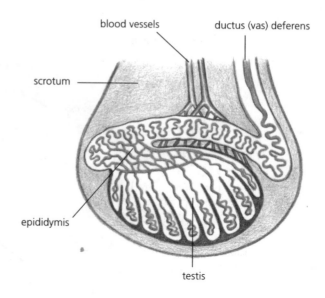

Detail of the testis in the scrotum.

- autonomic nerves of the testis
- smooth muscle fibres
- **ductus deferens** in a separate inner pouch – the passage-way for the concentrated sperms to get to the urethra via the inguinal canal; it enlarges within the abdomen as a storage area, the **ampulla**

All these are held together in the visceral layer of the descended peritoneum, now called the **inner vaginal tunic**, within the scrotum. Attached to this and to the outer lining is the cremaster muscle. The two scrotal sacs, although they can drop, are mainly held variably taut and therefore close to the abdominal wall area. They are separated by an inner septum of abdominal peritoneum, which divides proximally around the penis before entering their respective canals.

The **penis** is held close to the abdominal external wall within a fold of skin. It ends just posterior to the naval scar where the skin fold opens at the orifice of the sheath. It is the common terminal route for

- **urinary** excretion
- **semen** outflow, and by copulation into the female

These respectively require that

- the urine should be passed clear of the body surface and, as a rule, of the lining of the **prepuce** and the **sheath**. For this the penis is autonomically dropped flaccidly down. The **distal urethra** ends in a process or tip enclosed in a **urethral fossa**

- the semen has to be directed to the external os of the

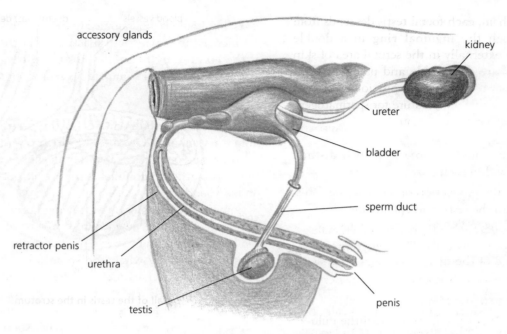

The genital organs of the stallion.

female's uterine cervix through the vulva and the vagina. This necessitates a marked protrusion and stiffening, an 'erection' as well as an active effort. The erection is brought about by autonomic closing off of the return blood-flow from the erectile tissues of the penis, whereby a hydrostatic pressure is quickly increased to give the required rigidity. When erect, and intromission occurs, the urethral tip flares into a **cup** which is said to form a seal onto the external os of the mare's cervix

- after **coitus**, **detumescence** occurs and the now flaccid penis is withdrawn backwards and into the sheath by the contractions of the **retractor penis** muscle which originates at the base of the penis within the pelvic

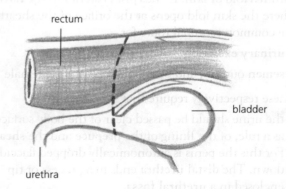

Sagittal section through the male pelvis showing how the rectum and bladder are held together within the peritoneum.

cavity and is inserted onto the ventral surface of the length of the penis

Parts of the penis become periodically visible
- at the dropped down flaccid state, when **urinating**
- the erect, or **tumescent** state, at copulation

In both situations the external orifice of the urethra and the exposed penis can be examined: in the former it can also be brought down manually, as for swabbing and for cleansing, along with the sheath. The internal tissues can be palpated *per rectum,* but the intra-pelvic accessory glands rarely require examination and nor does the out of sight urethra, certainly not as part of a genital problem.

The **sheath** is an invagination of the skin which, as the name implies, forms a sheath in which the penis is concealed and protected after it leaves the pelvic cavity to run forward along the ventral abdominal wall from the perineum to just short of the umbilical scar.

Posterior to the inguinal region the sheath is not distinct from the overlying skin although its area is delineated. It enlarges cranial to the inguinal region to become the sheath proper, in which a secondary invagination occurs called the **prepuce**. The outer skin is more or less hairless as far back as the scrotal level. The sheath contains an oily, waxy material, **smegma**. It is this area which can become infected contagiously during coitus

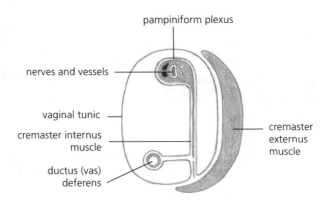

Cross-section of spermatic cord and vaginal tunic.

(compare the clitoris of the mare). The outer surface is rich in sweat glands.

The **mechanics of reproduction** involve, specifically

- the male's penis, for gaining **intromission** of the female and **ejaculation** of seminal fluid carrying (transporting) his sperm, to be deposited into the uterus. There, the sperm mobility carries it to the oviducts or fallopian tube(s) – for one sperm to meet and fertilise one ovum

- the female's tubular tract, to allow the penis to penetrate as far as the cervix, where the ejaculate is received into the external os to be temporarily sealed therein. In oestrus the tract is lubricated and the valves relaxed

Male Reproductive Behaviour

Male reproductive behaviour complements that of the female except that the stallion does not 'cycle' as such. Maximal reproductive capacity of the male is from 4–20

years. His libido is programmed to increase in keeping with the increase in female oestral activity, but the actual flow of the controlling hormones has to be triggered by the mare's signals, which stimulate his sensory organs.

Olfactory

To detect female pheromones in the oestrogen exuded from the vaginal mucus, some of which is washed out with her urine and onto faecal pats. This begins early in oestrus. In the wild, the stallion makes routine inspection of these on his 'rounds'.

Some of the pheromone becomes airborne and is attractive from a distance downwind to his incidental sniffing. On homing-in to an in-season mare, her initial readiness is confirmed visually when she spreads her hindlegs and partially lowers her buttocks, carries her tail to the side, then rhythmically everts her clitoris to perform the 'winking' act, which not only gives a visual sign but also exudes scented smegma. The male then adopts the **Flehmen** head posture, whereby scent molecules in solution in the female genital vestibule are inhaled into a separate nasal area – the **vomero-nasal organ** – which is said to have a direct afferent nerve route to a specific cerebral centre.

In some instances the horse will muzzle the clitoris and add the gustatory sense of taste to that of olfaction. This contact may have a reflex feedback to the mare's anterior pituitary's secretion of sex hormones. The mare, as already described, if she is 'fully on heat', i.e. near ovulation, responds by acceptance.

In controlled mating, as in stud work, the stallion signals his belief of a mare being near ready or actually so by

- vocalisation
- behaviour
- rearing

The penis.

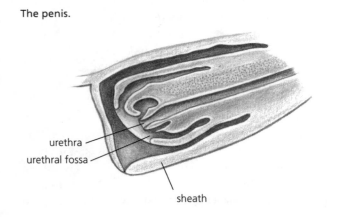

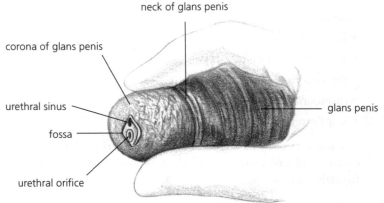

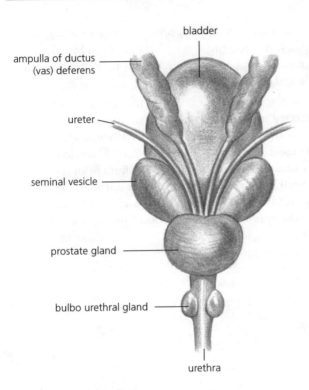

The intrapelvic genital organs of the stallion.

Labels:
- bladder
- ampulla of ductus (vas) deferens
- ureter
- seminal vesicle
- prostate gland
- bulbo urethral gland
- urethra

endocrine systems. In the male

- **puberty**, when sperm count rises in association with gonadotrophus, around 18 months of age

increasing **daylight** hours stimulates the secretion of

- **gonadotrophin releasing hormone** in the hypothalamus, which is neurotransmitted to the
- pituitary gland, which in a pulsed mode secretes the male equivalent of the two gonadotrophins
  - **luteinising hormone** (LH) is the first to be increased; its effect is immediate but transitory to give a periodic effect on the leydig cells of the testes to produce testosterone and other androgens
  - this is followed by follicle stimulating hormone

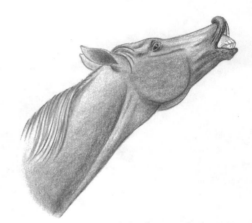

The Flehmen posture.

- pawing
- erecting
- further vocalisation
- Flehmen posture
- holding the mare's tail in his teeth
- nuzzling her perineal area
- and then her neck by
- mounting
- intromission with thrusting
- ejaculation (with pulsation, which can be palpated by the stud groom)

when complete he

- ceases thrusting
- rests on the mare
- flags his tail laterally
- dismounts
- loses interest

On some occasions the first thrusting period does not result in ejaculation; he will then remount to try again (usually successfully).

There is a basic similarity in the male and female

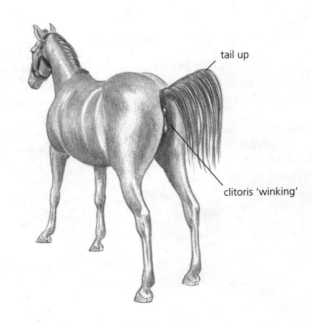

Mare indicating oestrus.

Labels:
- tail up
- clitoris 'winking'

(FSH) equivalent, but stimulates the testes; this is slow but progressive in the amount secreted from the leydig cells in the testes

- **testosterone**, some of which enters the main circulation where it controls the formation of the male secondary sexual characteristics
  - 'manliness', aggression, crest formation, libido. That which is secreted directly into the sperm-producing area of the testes initiates and maintains spermatogenesis
  - levels vary, but there is an on-going spermatogenesis to keep storage levels up after coital use
- **oestrogens** are also formed in the testes (compare ovarian follicular oestrogenesis). When a stallion is exposed to a receptive mare his oestrogen blood levels increase within 10 minutes. He has to be 'teased', it is believed, for maximum output
- the accessory sex glands within the pelvic cavity around the penis and draining into the urethra all produce a varied amount of **seminal fluid** which acts as a transport mechanism for the spermatozoa. They do not have any sexual hormone function; the fluid from the seminal vesicles is thought to have antiseptic properties and its viscosity is believed to act as a cervical plug to seal the cervix after ejaculation of semen into the uterus

CHAPTER

14

THE SKIN

INTRODUCTION

The skin, or **common integument**, is the largest organ of the body.

Skin is much more than an efficient cover to the internal tissues and other organs. It is a tough, resilient and highly elastic **multi-function system**.

It is made up of tissue known as **epithelium**. It consists of two distinct layers

- the **epidermis**, an avascular, **keratin-rich** layer of outer

protective covering, divided into two sub-layers, the outer called the **stratum corneum** and the inner, the germinal replication area, called the **stratum germinativum**

- the deeper layer is the **dermis**, or **corium**, an intricately woven 'underfelt' of collagen strands, elastic fibres, and fat. It includes hair follicles, sweat and sebaceous glands, and the udder in the female. Blood and lymph vessels, muscles and nerves are embedded at various levels. The dermis is the flexible nourishing source of the epidermis. It is attached to the underlying structures

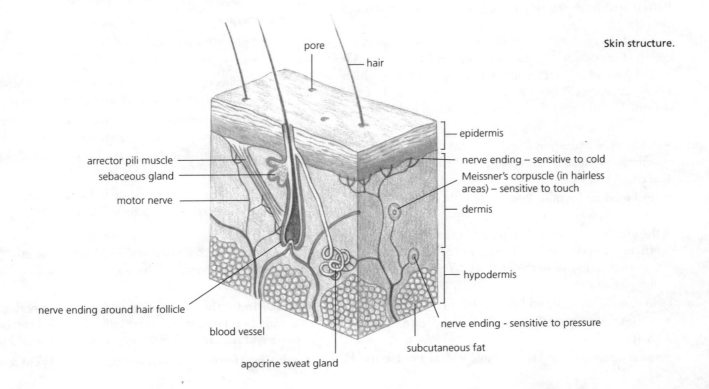

Skin structure.

pore

hair

epidermis

nerve ending – sensitive to cold

Meissner's corpuscle (in hairless areas) – sensitive to touch

arrector pili muscle

sebaceous gland

motor nerve

dermis

hypodermis

nerve ending around hair follicle

nerve ending - sensitive to pressure

blood vessel

subcutaneous fat

apocrine sweat gland

by the subcutaneous tissue or **subcutis**

The variable thickness of the skin – 1–5mm (0.04–0.2in) in general – can be felt through the hairs and assessed. It is greatest at the roots of the mane and the dorsal surface of the tail root (the dock). In both areas grow the coarser, more slowly cast, weather-protective and rain-shedding hairs.

Skin is thinner on the dorsal trunk, thinner still on the ventral neck and throat. It is thicker again on the dorsal aspects of the limbs but thinner on their palmar and plantar aspects. It is minimal on the lips and on the eyelids.

The variable looseness can be judged by picking up a fold between finger and thumb; its moveability is in keeping with the more mobile articulations such as

- the lateral surface of the neck
- the front of the shoulders
- the trunk (as judged by range of reflex 'twitch' reactions)
- palmar and plantar aspects of limbs

In the 'tied-down' areas it is less moveable – over the limb joints (for stability) and the loins and quarters (where it is involved to some extent in muscle attachment).

The 'pinch test' is applied by picking up a fold of skin, for example of the eyelid or over the eyebrow, or the lateral aspect of neck, and when it is let go **the 'tent' will flatten within 3 seconds to indicate healthy, hydrated skin.**

This looseness and mobility reflects the amount of fat cells and elastic fibres in the subcutaneum (subcutis) and is an indicator of general health and bodily condition, which when 'satisfactory' gives a springiness to the feel of the dermis. The intrinsic elasticity of the dermis is determined by

- the level of **hydration** (fluid content) of its dermal cells and intercellular spaces and those of the germinal layer of the epidermis
- the **blood and lymph flow** in the subcutis (hypodermis)
- the **vitality** (nutritional state) and the **metabolic efficiency** of the germinal layer, which has a direct influence in regard to the production of hair, keratin, and pigment

as well as the quantity and the quality of

- **sebum** coming into the follicles and onto the hair shafts
- **sweat** coming onto the epidermal surface (and so its pH

and micro-climate)

The skin must be seen as much more than superficially 'dead' or 'inert'. It is a flexible physical shield against external factors – wind, water, trauma (physical, chemical, and thermal), and the sun's actinic and UV rays – and a useful 'map' of the individual horse's characteristic colour, markings, and hair flow pattern.

It is also, physiologically

- an extensive diffuse surface for sensory nerve endings for **'contact' awareness**:
  - tactile hairs of muzzle and eyelids
  - 'ordinary' coat hairs
  - pressure changes on the skin
  - temperature variations in the micro- and macro-climate being a guide to heat radiated from subcutaneous and deeper tissues

all with protective reflex ability and a potential for transmitting, via hair follicle and skin nerves, warning input, and (in the skin only), pain

- **thermo-regulatory**
  - a radiant surface for heat loss
  - an evaporative surface for sweat
  - variable through the reflex modulation of the hair's insulating ability (standing or flattened)
  - deeper insulation through
    - epidermal and dermal thickness
    - hypodermal fat content
    - reflex opening and closing of the blood flow volume, especially in the smaller vessels
- **communicative** through special sweat gland secretions – one source of **pheromones** (e.g. female to male)
- **biochemically active** – e.g. the site of the synthesis of vitamin D
- **biologically active** in its response to local cellular antigenic stimulation and dermal inflammatory responses

The appreciation of dermal and hypodermal health and, through that, the health of the animal as a whole, is based on

- **visualising** of the outer surface, for the lay (smooth or 'staring') of the coat and its variable shine and for the shine and smoothness of the skin where that is visible
- **palpating** (feeling) for its resilience (elasticity) in terms

of epidermal softness, thickness, and mobility (relative to the area), and

* assessing the hair's cleanliness from scurf and oiliness

It must be remembered that what are actually seen and felt are the physiologically 'dead' or 'inert' tissues of **'hard' keratin** of the hoof (see later), **'firm' keratin** of the hair, and **'soft' keratin** of the superficial epidermis, with the impregnating sebum and apocrine sweat and the deeper sensation of the underlying more active germinal layer of the epidermis. Together these constitute the 'practical' surface forming the protective physico-chemical cover and barrier for the underlying tissues.

The inert layers of the epidermis and of the hairs are the end result of the reproduction of the **stratum germinativum** basement cells in the epidermis and the ingrown follicles respectively.

As a new layer of epidermal cells are formed, they elevate the previous layer away from the germinal and vascular tissues. Successive layers become so distanced that they dehydrate and die, becoming flattened eventually into **squames** (scales) and relatively more keratinised.

In the follicles, as a new hair bud forms, it pushes the old and now inert hair shaft upwards and eventually out, to be 'cast' at a much slower rate than the skin loses its squames. The shaft is enveloped in its squames and the follicle opening is plugged by them. Both sets of squames are coated with sebum which protects the interspaces.

The normal abrasive effect of daily 'wear and tear' removes the oldest squames and 'ageing' hairs as 'dander', the skin cells falling as scurf (not to be confused with dandruff which is a 'dis-ease' exfoliation) and the hair as 'cast hairs'.

FUNCTION

Skin, as an organ and system, has many functions

* **barrier**
  * it is a barrier to the many micro-organisms which are on its surface and on the hairs. These cannot damage healthy, intact epidermis, nor penetrate it to the subcutaneous tissues

* **protection**
  * it is a pliable, tough protection against reasonable everyday conditions, with hair over much of its surface which grows and lies in 'streams' to encourage rain and sweat to run or drip off. The skin of a horse also contains many **sebaceous** glands which produce an oily material (**sebum**) which 'waterproofs it'
  * it is a base for the production of **vitamin D** in response to the **summer** sun's rays on the **intra-dermal calciferol**
  * pigment in the dermis protects against solar radiation

* **sensory**
  * the hair bulbs have special sensory nerve endings which, on stimulation, 'trigger' the early warning system to activate avoidance procedures such as skin twitch, 'scratch' reflexes, tail swishing and ear, eyelid, and muscle twitch to ward off potentially dangerous insects, and to get rid of inanimate annoyance
  * its nerve endings, cutaneous sensory receptors, can detect varying **pressures**, **heat/cold** and **pain** sensations
  * specialised hairs are the long sensory whiskers, eyelashes and ear hairs, and the coarser, rain protection hairs of the mane and of the tail (it is the presence of hair which identifies the bearer as being a mammal; no other classes of animals have hair)
  * the thin **panniculus muscles**, lying as sheets in the subcutis of the thorax and forequarters, react to that hair's sensitivity to flies' contact. The relevant receptor sensory nerve endings are in the hair follicles. The rapid contraction of these muscles 'twitches' the skin to displace insects

* **thermo-regulation**
  * **reflex dilation** of skin blood vessels permits heat loss by radiation and, conversely, constriction of them reduces body heat loss
  * hairs can be erected by a small muscle at their roots. The resultant 'deeper' coat traps air, which together with the hairs forms a more insulating layer. This **erector muscle action** is a reflex response to low skin temperature. (In modern man, where body hair is too sparse and fine to be effective as an insulating feature, the skin is still responsive to cold; the follicles rise up as 'goose pimples')
  * the **sweat** secreted onto its surface and evaporated

from there also acts as the main thermal regulator

The thickness of a horse's skin, and the amount of coat it will grow in winter, varies from breed to breed. While many native pony breeds and coarser-bred horses are well-protected from winter conditions, thin-skinned horses, such as Thoroughbreds, Arabs, and their crosses, do not develop such thick coats and so are much less well protected, and cannot be expected to winter out without being affected adversely unless rugged.

Pigments, such as **melanin**, help to protect the skin. They are manufactured in the epidermis and in the hair follicles, where they become incorporated in the hair to give the eventual colouring. Thus, flesh-marks and areas of white hair (in which there is no pigment) are more prone to sunburn and possibly to problems caused by skin irritation associated with 'cracked heels'.

Skin Glands

Sweat glands develop from those epidermal ingrowths which also form hair follicles. The gland's secretory coils are situated deep in the dermis and its ducts penetrate the base of the follicle to emerge near the surface onto which it secretes, as and when required. Sweat glands are most common on the nostril, the flank and other hairless areas, but they appear over most parts of the body.

Sebaceous glands are also associated with hair follicles, and they open into them. Their product, sebum, of high fat or lipid content, adds to the skin's water propellant property. The sebum is the 'shine' of coat and hair, and its odour is an identity signal. Larger sebaceous glands, independent of hair follicles, occur in various parts of the body such as the lips, the vulvar lips, the prepuce and the anus.

Ceruminous glands are found in the **ear flap**; their secretion is a heavy, waxy material.

Other Derivatives of Skin

Hair, hoof and other horny appendages are derivatives of skin. For example:

- the **chestnuts** are a horny plaque on the inner surface of the forelimbs, above the knees, and on the hind legs just below the hock. They are believed to be the remains of pads which, in shorter-legged prehistoric ancestors of the horse, protected the knee and hock joints from ground contact, or remnants of the now absent first digits. Their exact position, and especially their outline, are thought to be identifying features for each horse

- the **ergot** is a horny plaque embedded in the skin at the back of the horse's fetlock. It is the remains of a pad that protected this part of the body from ground contact in the horse's evolutionary past (similar to the large pads under dogs' feet). In some horses, particularly the coarse breeds, it projects through the skin as a horny outgrowth. In heavy horse breeds, the ergots can be quite large, but in many finer-bred horses they do not protrude at all

- the **feather**, a rain- and mud-shedding clump of hair growing from the skin at the back of the fetlocks, can be very plentiful in 'heavy horses' (and 'encouraged' for show purposes) but is absent in hot-bloods and their crosses, an indication of their arid, desert origins which is still inherited

- the **horn** of a horse's hoof wall is a highly specialised skin which is formed by a special layer of skin cells at the coronet, known as the **coronary band**. The keratin content is much greater, and so harder, to form the protective 'hoof capsule'

THE SKIN'S EXTERNAL ORIFICES

Mammals take in air, water and nutrients essential for the metabolic processes of living, and void the waste products of these biological processes back into the environment.

The systems primarily involved are the respiratory, the digestive and the urinary. Input and output requires orifices in the external surface of the body: openings in the skin.

It is logical that air, food and water enter at the anterior aspect (the front) and that waste leaves at the posterior (the rear). Thus, the nostrils and the mouth are in the head; the anus and the urinary exit are at the hindquarters. The male urinary outlet is directed forward and downwards as part of the combined uro-genital system's positional requirement. The female's uro-genital outlet is also situated 'conveniently' for mating and foaling as well as for urinary excretion. A temporary orifice is the new born's umbilicus which closes soon after birth.

Two further pairs of twinned orifices in the head are the appendages of the external auditory canal, the ears, and the eye orbits. The variable positions and shapes of the lips, nostrils and adjacent cheek tissues and ears are communication signals – the 'looks' a horse can give!

At these natural orifices the skin 'changes' to the **mucous membrane** type of epithelium which lines the passages of the 'internal' systems. The skin is invariably devoid of hair, or has only very fine hair, for several centimetres before the change-over, especially where the opening leads directly into or out from the system.

Where the orifice is 'occupied', as with the orbit, the mobile lids are fringed with special protective hairs, the eyelashes. The external ear, the flap or pinna, also has a hair fringe to help prevent entrance of coarse material and insects. These are also sensory organs of touch. The inner surface of the pinna is still skin, 'becoming' smooth as it approaches the base of the external ear at the 'drum'; it is kept flexible and protected by the presence of ear wax secreted from its glands.

The Ears

As described in Chapter 2, THE EQUINE SENSES, the equine pinnae are cartilaginous structures activated by muscles at their base, very mobile and independently so. The outer surface carries short coat hairs, which lengthen at the edges into fringes and act as partial filters to dust, sand and water, enhanced by the re-positioned ears as well as having tactile sensibility.

When laid back and down, as in the anger/fear position, the canal is virtually closed to material or sensory impact. This is a very important signal to others, as well as a guard to the delicate ear drum at the distal end of the outer canal. **The horse becomes 'deaf' to the human voice** in such circumstances and no doubt to other horses!

The inner skin is soft, thin and slightly shiny from the oily wax which further protects the passage; in health, this rarely exudes from the pinna. Apart from their use in signalling mood, the ears are only for sensory input. Any metabolic waste products of the middle and inner ears are dealt with via the circulatory and cerebro-spinal fluid systems and do not escape externally unless in exceptional circumstances (dis-ease), e.g. a ruptured ear drum with pus formation, or bleeding following cranial trauma.

The Eyes

The skin over the skull bones is continuous with that which forms the integument covering the cartilaginous framework of the outer eyelids, or **palpebra**, of which the upper is the more extensive. When closed, the edges form an oblique slit of some 5cm (2in) long; when open, the edges are concave, the upper more so especially nearer the inner corner. In this inner corner, commissure (joining), or **nasal canthus**, there is a small rounded nodule, the **caruncle lacrimalis**, covered by skin and bearing a few hairs and sebaceous glands.

The edges of the lids are stiffer than the surfaces, especially on the inner part of the edge, where there are some 45–50 special glands in the upper and 30–35 in the lower lid; these are **tarsal glands** which secrete the **palpebral sebum**, a lubricating and protective fatty material; and on the outer part of the edge, from which project the eyelashes. These are long and numerous on the upper lid, except in mid line. They are either very short or absent on the lower lid, although whisker-like tactile hairs project from it.

The inner surface of the lids is lined with mucous membrane, the **palpebral conjunctiva**. This is reflected over the eyeball, first as the tough, white, blood vessel-lined **sclera**, and then, in the centre, as the thin, avascular, transparent **cornea**. The lids have a neuro-muscular system of control.

Near the nasal end of each lid is a small opening into a tube which join together to become the **lacrimal sac** or pouch, from which the lacrimal, or tear duct, traverses down within the nasal bones to open near the internal aspect of the respective nostril. As the name implies, these drain the tears from the eyeball surface, the tears having been secreted by special lacrimal glands between the posterior, temporal commissure or canthus of the upper part of the eyeball and the bony orbit. Tear is a clear, serous fluid which moistens, lubricates and flushes the conjunctivae of the eyeball and lids. It is this fluid over the cornea which reflects light to give 'bright eyes'.

In the medial angle, or **nasal canthus**, of the eye is a half-moon shaped fold of **conjunctiva** which covers a small plate of thin cartilage. The outer surface is variably pigmented. This is the **third eyelid**, or **membrana nictitans**. In the quiescent state its outer edge is just visible.

The Nostrils

The nostrils are necessary for the intake of air and its oxygen, and they also serve as the outlet for the expired air waste – heat and carbon dioxide. They must remain open at all times, yet have extra opening ability at times of increased oxygen demand. The rims are partly cartilaginous and flexible with an additional fold, the false nostril. The aperture is determined by muscle action which is under automatic reflex control, to open this fold into a circular dilation.

The overlying skin is thin, carrying many nerve endings and specialist long tactile hairs. The skin continues a short distance inside the mobile area of the nostrils, where the hairs are very fine and short. The nostrils' partial closure can be augmented by upturning the upper lip, as when exhibiting the **Flehmen** sign, and when the horse is swimming or in dust or sandstorms.

The Lips

The lips are the external boundaries of the mouth, and as such are the digestive system's anterior orifice. Both can be moved independently. The upper is the more mobile; it is the manipulative organ of the horse, highly sensitive and strong. Externally, the lips are covered with thin skin over very dense subcutaneous tissue; there are tactile whiskers present. Internally, they are covered by the **oral mucous membrane**.

The prehensile facility of the lips is the first stage in prehension of food. By the very nature of the use of the lips, there is no survival need to have them 'tight shut', so from that point of view they do not act as a seal. However, a horse drinks by sucking water through nearly closed lips, thereby preventing extraneous, possibly dangerous material, as found in ponds, streams and watering holes, from being ingested.

The Anus

This is a sphincter seal, produced by muscular action on the thick ring of the thin, hairless, skin-covered, terminal portion of the alimentary tract. It is in the shape of a short cylindrical projection, ventral to the root of the tail. There is a central depression when closed.

There are, obviously, good functional reasons why faeces is not allowed to trickle out of the tract as it arrives at the end. It is not a social necessity as in humans, but nonetheless it must be included in disease-prevention; (parasitic), along with the taint of grass which prevents horses grazing too close to where worm larvae have been deposited in a concentrated fashion; the domesticated horse has a defaecatory territory and the donkey more so. Moreover, the softish faeces of a grazing horse have to be excreted well clear of the buttock and thigh skin, so the expulsion will be improved by a build up of bulk output.

The mucous membrane of the distal rectum is everted through the widely opened anal sphincter at the end of defaecation, but is quickly withdrawn before the seal closes.

The closed anal sphincter and its protrusion move backwards and forwards in rhythm with non-resting respiratory rates and is a feature, in advanced obstructive pulmonary disease cases, of the exaggerated expirations when it is compressed well out between the buttocks and conversely drawn well back in, even in the resting horse.

The Orifices of the Reproductive System

The reproductive system also requires access and outlet.

The female's urethra brings urine from the bladder to just inside the genital tract, the nominal junction of the vagina and the vulva. It is hidden by the lips of the vulva, which form the actual orifice.

The male's urethra, conversely, runs to the extremity of the dual purpose penis, and the genital ducts enter the urethra at its bladder origin. The penis, except at mating and at urination, is kept withdrawn in a fold of mucosal-lined skin, the **prepuce** or **sheath**, the external perimeter of which is the actual and visible epidermal orifice.

The Vulva

This does act as a seal. Situated as it is, just below the anus, it must prevent any faecal or other extraneous material from entering the uro-genital tract. Vertically, it is bounded by the lips, which are narrower at the top end and wider at the lower end, where they enclose a fossa, the inner wall of which houses the clitoris. The lips are kept together and opened by opposing muscles, some of which mould the shape of this external orifice. The skin is hairless but, like the rest of the perineal skin, it is richly supplied by sweat and sebaceous glands.

The vulva opens at urination; the mare's posture, and the fact that the floor of the pelvis is much nearer the top than the bottom of the vulva lips, means that the urine, forcibly expressed, culminates in being passed clear of the buttocks and upper hind legs. Most importantly, the final contractions drain the urethra, and the spout-like lower end prevents any urine tracking back to pool in the floor of the vagina. These final contractions also result in a rhythmic exposure of the clitoris, a function which also occurs during oestrus display – 'winking'.

The urinary tract is a one-way-out system. The opening from the urethra is covered by a flap of mucosa, sheltering it from any contamination at mating.

The Prepuce

The outer skin is soft, elastic and thin, and extends from the scrotum to within 5–8cm (2–3 in) of the umbilicus on the underneath surface of the abdomen – where it turns back inside as the sheath. Invariably dark and black in colour, it is smooth and slightly oily to the touch. Hairs are few and short, but it has copious sweat and sebaceous glands. The inside skin is hairless. Special glands inside the sheath produce a fatty secretion, **smegma**, which collects deep inside.

The external orifice of the prepuce tends to fall in, thus

forming a skin fold and partial seal.

Orifices and Organs as Indicators of Health

Some appreciation of the systemic 'regional' and 'local' health of the horse can be made by visual appraisal of these orifices and of their structure and functioning as 'outside' features of the systems.

The Ear

- the inquisitive and 'semaphoring' movement of the ear flaps, and the flick response to fly irritation

The Eye

- the closed lids of the sleeping horse and the partial closure, principally by the upper lid, in the drowsing animal

- the irregular blinking of the outer lids to help push the tears over the two conjunctivae and out through the ducts

- the closure, blink, reflex in response to sudden threats or to periodically break a stare which becomes unfocussed

- the appearance of the third eyelid as the head, and within it the eyeball, gyrates to accommodate vision away from straight ahead, and when the horse yawns. (This can be partially elicited by 'chucking' it under the jaw. The extrusion is rapid and the position momentarily held if this sensory input, the knock on the chin, is inflicted on a horse with tetanus – it is almost a diagnostic test)

- the small slick of overspill tears down the face at the inner corner of the eye, and an increase in this and a thickening of it during the fly season (a white blood cell reflex extravasation in response to a low-grade local infectious and mildly toxic irritation)

- the 'bright eye' in natural and artificial light

The Nostrils

- a thin, serous flow is seen at the lower corner, which is part nasal mucus which increases in cold weather (nose drip) and following exercise, and part outflow of tears

- the inner aspect of the still skin-covered nostril often has dust and food particles sticking to it. (Unlike the cow, the horse cannot wipe its nostrils with its tongue!)

- in cold weather, the expired air condenses to produce vapour 'clouds' – this is best seen in asymmetric gaits, just as the leading foreleg takes support.

- the nostrils dilate with increasing oxygen demands, whether from exercise or from abnormal respiratory functioning and marked fever

The Lips

- unlike other species, the horse salivates only in response to mastication or, similarly, when working on the bit. In mastication, the saliva is swallowed; when working on the bit, the mouth fills, most is swallowed and the excess froths at the lips. The lips are otherwise dry. The lips will alter their tension in communicating the horse's attitude to others. The lips will search the proffered hand for recognition smells and for possible food – if (erroneously) trained to do so

- the lower lip, with the chin, will droop in the drowsing horse

The Anus

- the sphincter and valve are tight, except at defaecation

- the hairless skin has a mild glisten

- there is no on-going mucus flow

The Vulva

- the vertical valve is firmly, but not tightly, closed, except during urination and oestral display, when it relaxes open and may be held open as in 'winking'

- the hairless skin has a mild glisten

- there is mucus flow at oestrus, but little or none at other times in health

The Prepuce

- the orifice is moist with glandular secretion

- the penis, at urination, should 'drop' down easily to fall clear of the prepuce

- the penis is usually retracted out of sight, except when the horse urinates or is sexually aroused – even geldings. Conversely, in hot weather when drowsing, the penis is often pendulous and 'down'

CHAPTER

15

THE EYE

See also Chapter 2, THE EQUINE SENSES.

The eye is a fibrous walled sphere, the 'eyeball', only a small part of which is visible. The greater part is contained within the prominent bony orbit of the skull, which gives protection. Its shape is maintained by internal fluid pressure.

The outer surface of the sphere is the tough white fibrous **sclera**, a small area of which is visible as a surround (the 'white of the eye') to the bulging highly touch-sensitive transparent **cornea** or 'window' through which light rays enter the eye. The hidden surface of the sclera has a fascial outer layer which forms insertion areas for the muscles which move the eyeball in its socket.

Inside the sclera lies the **uvea**, comprising

- the **choroid**, or vascular coat, a layer of sensory peripheral nerves
- the **ciliary body**
- the **iris**

The **choroid** is divided into two sections

- a pigmented area called the **tapetum nigrum**
- a smaller unpigmented area, the **tapetum lucidum,** at the **fundus** or back of the eye. The tapetum lucidum is crucial to 'night vision', acting as a light enhancer particularly in very low light conditions by reflecting *back through the retina* light which has already passed through it. It is what causes the eyes of horses and many other animals to glow brightly in the dark as when illuminated by car headlights

The **ciliary body** is a ring of specialised tissue at the junction of the sclera and the cornea. It is divided into three parts

- the ligaments of the lens – the **ciliary ring**
- the **ciliary processes** – the ligaments which suspend the lens
- the **ciliary muscle** – the smooth autonomic muscles of 'accommodation' or focussing

The outer surface of the **iris** is visible through the cornea. It is a smooth-muscled oval diaphragm, with a variable central aperture, the **pupil**, the size of which controls the amount of light falling on the retina. Projecting into the aperture from the upper and lower margins are irregular small black bodies, the **corpora nigra** or **iridic granules**, whose function is believed to be to reduce glare. The iris's pigment is the 'colour' of the eye. Lack of pigment produces the 'wall-eyed' horse; total lack produces an **albino**.

The light-sensitive **retina**, or **nervous coat**, a 'neuro-epithelium', is an extension of the brain. It extends from the border of the ciliary ring to the optic disc, at which all the retinal neuronal dendrites converge to pass through the sclera to become the optic nerve.

The neural receptor cells are known as **rods** and **cones**. The rods differentiate black and white and are particularly for night vision; the cones differentiate brighter light and colours; they can interpret blue, yellow and green but are believed to have difficulty in distinguishing reds and tones of red. The cells are in ten layers and convert light into neural volleys of electrical impulses which are transmitted by the optic nerve to the brain, where they are interpreted as composite pictures. If responding action is necessary, the cortex then transmits efferent motor messages via the CNS to the body's musculature and to the autonomic nervous system.

Paradoxically the **optic disc** itself is not covered by retinal cells, and is the 'blind spot'. It lies, within the

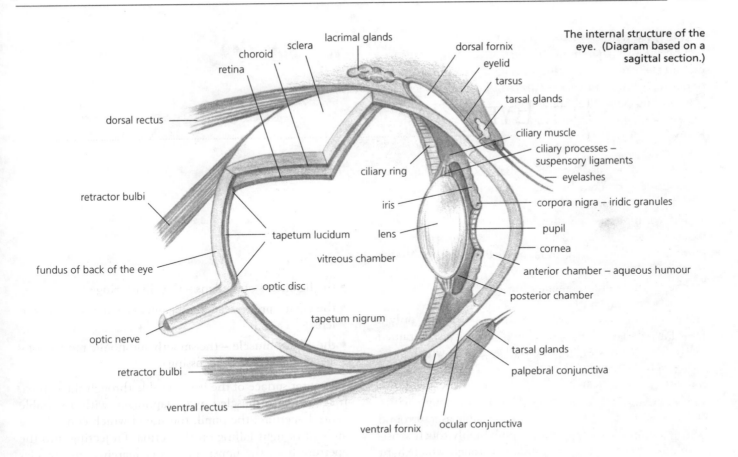

The internal structure of the eye. (Diagram based on a sagittal section.)

Labels: lacrimal glands, sclera, choroid, retina, dorsal rectus, retractor bulbi, fundus of back of the eye, optic disc, optic nerve, retractor bulbi, ventral rectus, tapetum lucidum, ciliary ring, iris, lens, vitreous chamber, tapetum nigrum, ventral fornix, ocular conjunctiva, dorsal fornix, eyelid, tarsus, tarsal glands, ciliary muscle, ciliary processes – suspensory ligaments, eyelashes, corpora nigra – iridic granules, pupil, cornea, anterior chamber – aqueous humour, posterior chamber, tarsal glands, palpebral conjunctiva

retinal layer, at the posterior of the vitreous chamber and is the exit point for the single optic nerve and a foramen for blood vessels supplying the choroid.

Before reaching the brain, the optic nerve from each eye sends branches to join its opposite nerve, a partial cross-over which is believed to help cerebral interpretation of incoming messages.

Only a small part of nature's radiant energy waves, the light waves between 4,000 and 7,200 Angstroms, from thermal infra red to ultra violet, produce effective and safe retinal stimulation.

The eye has two **bulbar chambers**

- the posterior, the more voluminous **vitreous chamber**, contains a jelly-like transparent material, the **vitreous fluid**, or **body**. It bathes the retinal and the choroidal mucosae

- the anterior or **aqueous chamber** contains a watery fluid, the **aqueous humour**. It has a small posterior portion lying behind the iris and in front of the ciliary body and the lens, and a larger anterior portion whose anterior surface is the transparent bulbar epithelium – the cornea

The **cornea** is a special, non-vascular, several layers thick continuation of the non-transparent fibrous **sclera**. The latter has a profuse, mostly microscopic vascular supply. The size and therefore the appearance of the arteries can vary significantly between health and local disease.

The cornea and the aqueous and vitreous fluids and the lens all refract light rays to sharpen the image projected onto the retina.

The crystalline **lens** is round and disc-shaped, with a thin transparent fibrous capsule retaining its jelly-like contents.

The lens is suspended by ligaments and intrinsic muscles arising from the ciliary body. Autonomic ennervation of the muscles determines the shape and so the refraction of the lens and its focussing; the horse is not thought to require much lens alteration.

The Adjacent Structures (The Adnexa)

The eyeball rests within the orbit on a pad of **periorbital fat**. This forms a cushion onto which the globe can be quickly and safely retracted reflexly during the 'blink' reaction, and it also acts as a shock absorber to a globe under pressure in disease or if accidentally struck.

The fat fills the supra orbital fossa, the 'open' area behind the rim of the orbit. With age or malnourishment or during debilitating illness this fat is burnt up to leave an obvious and palpable hollow above the eye. In Cushings disease a diagnostic clue is an infilling of this geriatric hollow.

The protruding area of the globe, the sclera and the cornea, are protected by the conjunctiva and the third eyelid.

The **conjunctiva** is a thin transparent epithelial sheet, vascular over the sclera and avascular where it forms the outer layer of the cornea, and is a reflected continuation of that which lines the eyelids.

The **third eyelid**, or **membrana nictitans**, is lodged in the inner or nasal canthus of the socket. It is part cartilage and part fibrous tissue within a semi-lunar fold of conjunctiva. Periodically it sweeps over the eyeball as a wiper. Under threat, it is quickly extruded as part of the blink reflex. This movement is passively activated by strong retraction of the eyeball, so allowing the third eyelid to slide out over the eyeball.

The uppermost of each pair of **eyelids** has a complement of eyelashes which are long except in the mid area; the lower, smaller eyelids have very sparse eyelashes. The eyelids contain mucus secreting cells, the **conjunctival epithelium**, which lubricate the movement of the main lids and the third eyelid over the eyeball.

The outer surface of the upper and lower eyelids is formed of skin similar to that of the face but thin, pliable and hairless. Between this outer skin and the conjunctival epithelium lie two further layers – a subcutaneous layer, and a fibrous layer called the **tarsus** (from the Greek for 'flat surface') along the edge of which are embedded the **tarsal glands** (30–35 on the lower lid).

The **lacrimal (tear) glands** are located beneath the scleral conjunctiva, just above the temporal canthus of the orbit. These secrete a clear serous fluid which persistently washes over the eyeball to exit through dorsal and ventral openings in the nasal canthus into a communal **lacrimal sac** which drains down through the facial and nasal bones to exit visibly just inside the nares.

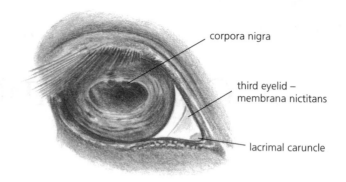

The external structure of the eye.

Excess tears can be induced by irritation of the ocular and palpebral (eyelid) conjunctivae, as by an 'oat flight' on the cornea or by flies feeding on the tears. There is often an overflow spilling down the face.

In the commissure of the lids at the medial canthus there is a small, rounded, pigmented prominence called the **lacrimal caruncle**. It carries sebaceous glands to moisturise the lids, and from it project several hairs. Other glands are in the borders of the lids. Some of the fluids secreted have antiseptic properties.

The eye's **nerve supply** is complex, involving the primary afferent sensory optic nerve to the brain and the efferent motor nerves to the many intrinsic muscles which move the eyeball.

Neural activity is mainly concerned with cranial reflexes engendered by 'requires a closer look' or a threatened blow when the eyeball is rapidly retracted. Ordinary motor decisions occur when the horse moves his line of vision voluntarily.

The eyelids have their own muscles which are both reflexly (especially) and voluntarily controlled.

Autonomic control brings about changes in focussing by stimulation of the ciliary muscles on the lens, and changes in the diameter of the pupil engendered by alterations in the intensity of light falling on the retina. Dilation and restriction of the pupil in response to variations between darkness and light are brought about by two groups of opposing smooth sphincter and circular muscles activated by (for dilation) the parasympathetic and (for restriction) the sympathetic autonomic nervous systems.

CHAPTER

16 CONFORMATION

A horse's 'conformation' is its 'make and shape' as determined by its skeletal outline, which is an inherited immutable feature. Conformation is a reflection of the dynamic skeleton, and influences the horse's manner of going, its 'action'. This in turn is a major factor in a horse's ability and in its durability.

Within each gait there is an accepted 'ideal' movement of the whole body and in particular of the limbs. The gaits should present an overall appearance of

- **balance** – 'self carriage'
- **straight flight paths** of each limb
- **symmetry** of the left with the right
- **security of foot fall** and support

all maintained by

- controlled **elasticity**, reflecting an
- **economy** of effort

The horsemaster will emphasise the benefits of 'straightness' of a horse's action, referring to the appearance of the forelegs as seen approaching and of the hind legs as seen going away, at both walk and trot. Variations from this fore-and-aft flight – deviations from 'straightness' of action – are usually the result of

- **conformation abnormalities**, whereby the flight paths describe a circuitous direction, either outwards or inwards, after and before foot fall

- the **foot fall** being unlevel from side to side as the foot makes contact with the ground – the foot lands 'outside in' or 'inside out'

- the **lift off** being completed too soon or too late and/or not correctly relative to the 'column of support' line of the limb above it

In the unshod horse, foot fall, support and lift off will be amended by ground forces on the hoof wall which, as a skin derivative, is constantly growing and being worn down by ground contact. Hoof horn conformation *faults* are therefore usually *acquired* from such limb faults and/or by faulty trimming and shoeing.

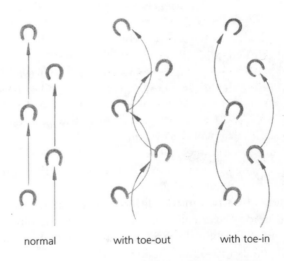

normal   with toe-out   with toe-in

The effect of toe-out and toe-in on foot fall.

Conformation defects may be

- **congenital** – foetal growth defects present at birth
    - hereditable
    - not known to be hereditable
- **acquired** – neonatal and young horse defects not present at birth
    - **hereditable**, but with a variably delayed onset
    - **limb growth defects**, possibly resulting from a lack of synchronisation in development and/or

influenced by defects in limb action with subsequent mal-effects through upward ground force reactions

The immature horse, with growth plates still open, i.e. not fully mineralised, can have its skeleton altered by 'nurture' inputs affecting footfall support

- **nutritional**
  - mineral and trace element imbalances
  - excess body weight
- **hoof trimming** faults altering the direction of ground surface forces
- incidental **injuries** or **defects** in the locomotor system, causing limb weight-bearing inequality

The effect of these actions may, in later life

- interfere with performance
- predispose to injury and so to reduced durability
- be displeasing aesthetically

The outline has been changed pathologically and this must be distinguished from congenital conditions.

Although conformation has the greatest influence on equine biodynamics of locomotion, other management factors play a part, such as fitness, training and using, by undermining the benefits of the inherited conformation.

Some inherited conformation faults predispose to lameness

- 'cow hocked' and **spavin**
- 'sickle hocked' and **curbs**
- 'back at the knees' and **tendinitis**

These three disease examples can also occur in horses with 'normal' conformation as the result of other forms of over stress.

Conversely, newborn animals with angular limb deformities (which are primarily faults of the developing knee and to a lesser extent the hock joint) which improve so as not to alter action so seriously as to cause interference or incorrect footfall, will 'grow to live with them'. The column of support has adjusted to, or accommodated for, the defect.

Until all limb-bone growth plates are 'closed', at approximately 3½ years, some corrective adjustments can be made by upward leverage through manual alterations in the hoof wall by corrective trimming, wedges, 'insoles', and redesigned shoes, and the subsequent contact with hard surfaces. Some require surgical intervention.

Overall conformation is the key to a horse's manner of progression. As a working animal its value is primarily determined by this: 'it looks the part'. The related appearance is determined by the numerous promontories of a horse's skeleton at the extremities of bones at

- an **end point**, or
- where **two bones meet** at a joint's most prominent knuckle, to form a protruding **angle point**

Such visible and palpable landmarks are known as the **points of the horse**. Their relationship one with another can be measured as

- the **distance between**
- the **angle** they form with one another and the horizontal
- the **distance from the ground** to the highest point, etc

Common conformation faults.

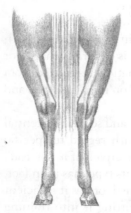
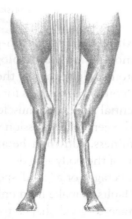
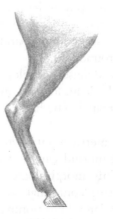
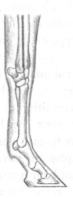
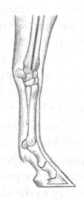

normal   cow hocks   sickle hock   normal   back at the knee

The shoulder joint.

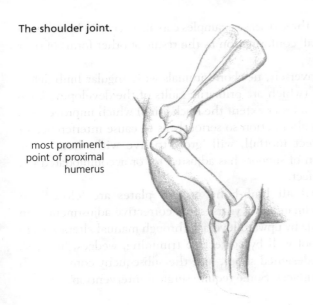

most prominent point of proximal humerus

The skeletal 'shape' when seen 'in the flesh' produces an outline which can guide the onlooker in identifying the breed/type of horse.

This appearance overall is permanent but can be visually altered by infilling differences in muscle development and fat deposition, to give '**condition**', which can vary from very thin or emaciated (which respectively, by definition, imply no subcutaneous fat, limited body fat, and symmetrically wasted musculature – the animal has, through starvation, burnt up fat reserves and has catabolised the protein of muscles, the flesh) to over-fat or **obese**, when fat stores are excessively full. The muscle development may be fair to good, but the horse cannot be fit – it is carrying excess 'dead' weight of fat.

A **fit condition** implies that the ratio of fat to trained muscle is correct for a particular discipline. The show horse is so managed that muscle fitness is sufficient for the limited athleticism of the show ring and the fat deposits sufficient to give an unreal, sometimes dangerous, level of 'good condition'. Such animals are often too heavy for their limbs, especially in the growing show animal and when asked to go repeatedly on hard ground.

Elite athletic fitness is exercise-induced muscle development with a minimal amount of fat: the lean, fit look, in which muscle groups are clearly demarcated. The horse is said to be in **hard condition**.

Muscle development can be asymmetric relative to unbalanced action from a variety of morbid causes, to produce hypertrophy or atrophy. This morphological appearance must not be interpreted as true 'conformation'. Injury to the skeleton can amend the bilateral positioning of the points as in a healed pelvic fracture: the horse's

appearance is altered, the basic conformation is not. A common example is the knocked down hip.

The skeletal topline is an assessment of the outline of the tops of the dorsal processes of the thoraco-lumbar-sacral column, the vertebral column, commonly called the 'spine'. The cervical vertebrae, the neck, do not immediately enter into this picture. The dynamic topline reflects the development of the epaxial muscles from the poll to the dock, and includes the relatively large expanse of cervical muscle infilling the space below the ligamentum nuchae and the cervical vertebrae. The fit athletic horse is primarily judged on this top musculature and especially on the muscles of the neck. The horsemaster views this topline with the horse at halt and the subtle movements of the abaxial muscles play a big part in the rhythm of dynamic movement as seen in the horse in its various gaits.

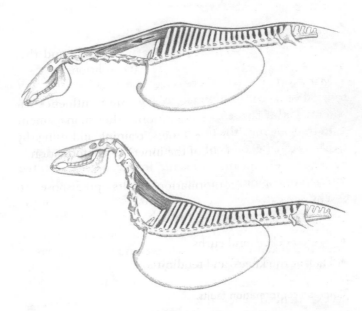

The skeletal topline.

Altogether, skeleton-plus-condition equates with phenotype or morphology, that is overall shape or contours. Nevertheless the conformation, as judged from the 'points', is the basis for a 'correct' or 'ideal' skeleton and potential associated muscle power.

The general impression as to type, and so to its potential usefulness, can then be analysed with regard to specific areas of the body – to determine subjectively if it is a 'bad', an 'average', or a 'good' specimen of its type: has it, in fact, bad faults to make it an unlikely animal, or has it sufficient average-to-good shapes to justify putting it into training and work?

'Ideal' conformation.

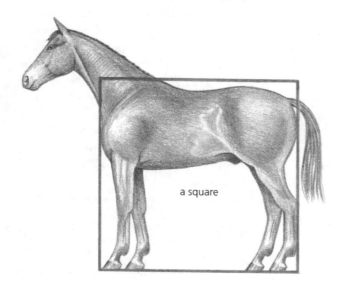

a square

symmetry, viewed from above

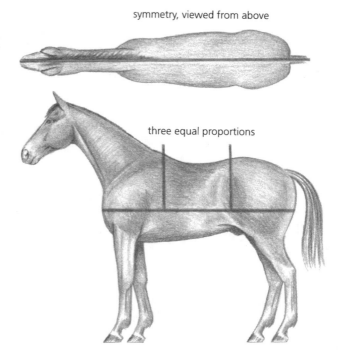

three equal proportions

Many formulae have been suggested as guides not only to good or to bad conformation, but also as indicators of potential athletic use.

In the long run, 'the proof of the pudding…'. An objectively assessed good conformation can be confirmed only by objectively measured results in the horse's selected activity: the opinion is confirmed or refuted by facts!

The subjective view is taken from both sides, from the front, from the rear, and sighting above and along the back to judge this aspect and to compare the left and right top sides. It is taken when the horse is standing four-square at the halt on a flat, level surface and also, most importantly, from the action and balance observed in the various gaits or 'experienced' when ridden. On these observations an assessment is made of the horse being able to do certain work, and subjective opinion is made of it being able to do and to stand up to this work.

Ability and durability are

- **bred** for, on the basis of parental appearance and past performance – the **genotype**
- **selected** for, on conformation – the **phenotype**
- and **confirmed** by **performance**

Different breeds have different conformation standards or specifications, whereby all members conform to an acknowledged appearance. Within a breed, the expert judge will recognise features which are 'ideal' and which should be bred for. Not all of these are working attributes; some are in the 'beauty competition' class, and are often more fashionable than useful.

Over many centuries, breeds have been bred to meet specific work requirements – for instance, racing, endurance, or haulage. Within a breed, a particular horse can be judged more suitable for a specific discipline – dressage rather than show jumping, for instance. By selective breeding, this strain can be more or less established but temperament will always play a significant role.

A type, the result of interbreed crossing, no matter how suitable it proves to be, is more difficult to establish or fix. To attempt to do so invariably means breeding back and forth, but eventually the offspring becomes nearly purebred for one or other of the original breeds. Some good points will vanish, and some bad points will become more prominent.

When speed and cross-country jumping ability are required, an input of Thoroughbred or Hot blood is necessary to 'upgrade' warm and cold blood types, no matter how good they were in the originally established purebred role. Some of this input relates to a determination to 'go'. It is also related to the air flow tract with minimal dynamic interference.

As a type, whether a purebred or a cross, it will be assessed by experienced users in whatever discipline required, for potential ability and durability.

Within a particular use, there is always an accepted way

Three genotypes.

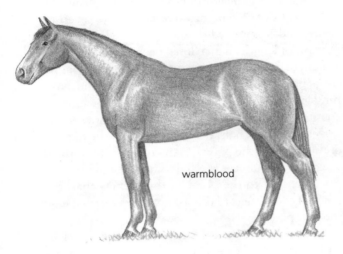

warmblood

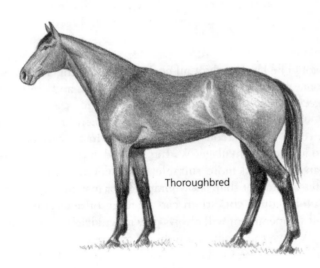

Thoroughbred

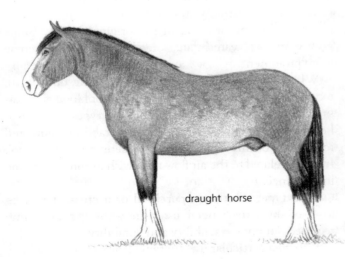

draught horse

of going which usually, but not always, is associated with the 'ideal' conformation for that use.

Whatever is hoped for, it is essential to breed from stock which

- looks the part
- acts the part
- moves well, and has
- stayed sound, whilst
- competing (or working) successfully

Conformation therefore can be seen as being a factor in the locomotor system – abaxially and axially. A good average conformation promises a balanced bio-mechanical structure. A poor average conformation warns of the likelihood of sub-optimal performance, injury risk and reduced durability – all of which influence the animal's value.

Conformation assessment is based on the relationship of form to function; body type is the inherited characteristics of a horse that best fit it for a specific function.

Most horses 'learn to live with' their defects in conformation. Some perform remarkably well despite them, to the surprise of the pundits and to the delight of the breeder or owner. 'Handsome is as handsome does' is often quoted. There is always the 'one-off' exception to any rule; significantly, it does not refer to *'for how long will such a horse keep doing so…'* A profitable but short flat racing career, before being retired to stud, is one thing; early retirement of a winner from racing especially is usually due to injury. It is important to consider this as possibly being the result of poor conformation and 'constitution', and **not** just accidental. Retirement to stud can therefore be the perpetuation of poor durability type. A short-lived success in other disciplines, no matter what the transient glory, is quite another from an economic point of view.

A good conformation which produces a balanced, 'straight moving' athlete from age 5 to 15 years should not be an unrealistic hope, provided the management factors of feeding, training and using are good.

The almost unmeasurable 'will to win' – the temperament or 'heart' – is a vital component for success, as is the ability to obtain maximum airflow and gaseous exchange. Airflow is a feature of respiratory tract airflow capacity, e.g. laryngeal specifications, which in turn relates to the skeletal width between the mandibular rami. Gaseous exchange, however, is more a reflection of system health. These can only be subjectively assumed during training, and objectively measured by actual performance in competition over the years.

It must not be forgotten that potentially elite athletes can become their own worst enemies who will persevere when overfaced, tired or over-stressed – states which are overlooked by the trainer or rider at the horse's peril. The horse with anatomical defects which predispose to injury, a less than good conformation, 'driven' by excellent temperament, can be a dangerous combination.

The guidance given here is concerned with conformation, good and not-so-good, as related to present function.

Head Conformation

Parrot mouth (overshot), **sow mouth** (undershot), rare and related mal-alignment of the molar arcades, and the presence of **wolf teeth**, require veterinary opinion. (*See* Chapter 8, THE TEETH.) They can affect prehension, mastication and **bitting**.

Intermandibular space, in the 15–17hh adult horse, a good guide is a minimum 10mm (4in) space – a closed knuckle's width, approximately – as judged at the angle of the jaw. This will 'permit' a good airflow diameter in a well-conformed larynx.

Neck Conformation

The neck, with the head, is the 'fifth appendage' of the horse. Anatomically, it is the front or cranial end of the vertebral (axial) column. It is the most flexible area of the

spine and, in comparison with the limbs, has greater potential for movement in more than one plane.

No matter the length, there are always seven cervical bones, and it is argued that a 'short' neck has more range per unit of length than a 'long' neck.

Length does, however, have an influence, in as much as the appendage acts as a counter-balance to the mass of the hind legs and of the trunk, pivoting over the forelegs. This counter-balancing is functionally important. As a guide, with the horse at halt, the distances from the highest point of the withers (the point) to the muzzle and to the start of the dock should be equal, but a neck should be no longer from the poll to the point of the withers than from the point of the withers to the start of the dock (as measured at the halt posture).

From the side view, the neck vertebrae describe an 'S' curvature. The correct 'development' of this, through trained muscle action, influences not only the head carriage on the bit but also the extension or telescoping, and the flexion of the neck as a whole. Together, these maximise potential hindquarter engagement and self-balance through 'lifting of the back' above the forehand by the pull of the ligamentum nuchae on the withers and seat area of the thoracic vertebrae. The closer to correct proportions, the less fatiguing it will be for the horse to obtain and to maintain balance.

It is suggested that geldings over 16.2hh with a neck which is relatively too long are prone to **laryngeal hemiplegia**, but many such horses do not suffer from this. There is scientific evidence that laryngeal hemiplegia is an inheritable condition, but whether a direct neurological or an indirect one through conformation is not yet clear.

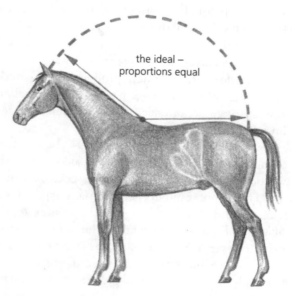

the ideal –
proportions equal

Assessing neck length. (There are breed variations from this.)

Back Conformation

It must be emphasised that symmetry of bilateral points, and bilateral muscle development and tone, are pre-requisites of good back functioning. This can be judged accurately only in the square-standing animal, so that, as viewed from *above*, there is a straight medial line from the dock to the poll and symmetric bilateral conformation and condition.

Absolute symmetry of musculature may not be obtained. 'Left-' or 'right-handedness' will have some influence; and unbalanced riding, in its many aspects, will produce compensatory muscle over-development and converse atrophy from lack of use.

Such affected horses invariably compound and prolong

the problem by 'throwing' the rider on to the 'easier' side, by going on three tracks, or by leading with the less uncomfortable side, as well as having a displacing effect on the saddle.

The basic skeletal symmetry must be there, otherwise symmetric muscle development is compromised. Action can be effected within any such deficit, usually by contra-lateral development – and so further apparent asymmetry of 'condition' will follow.

The four main features along the 'topline' are

- neck and withers – conformation and condition
- loins and croup
- 'back' length relative to whole horse, i.e. length from wither point to lumbo-sacral joint, compared with length from point of shoulder to point of buttock
- relative lengths within the topline as a whole
  - T7 to T18 – the seat
  - T18 to L6
  - tuber coxae to tuber sacrale

In general, one is looking for

- a *short loin*
- a *smooth curve* from dock, along croup and over its points onto the loins, effected by good muscle development
- a *forward position of the lumbo-sacral joint*, as judged from the position of the tubera sacrales (points of croup) – the nearer to the line transversely 'joining' the tubera coxae (points of the hip), the better; the loin is thereby 'shorter' and the quarters relatively 'longer'

An overall short back (loins plus 'saddle') is more likely if the horse is 'close-coupled' – has a space of four knuckles' width, 10cm (4in), or slightly less, between the last rib and the point of the hip, and its withers are well developed.

A long loin weakens the back, irrespective of the overall back length; it is usually **loose-coupled**, i.e. more than 10cm (4in) as measured above.

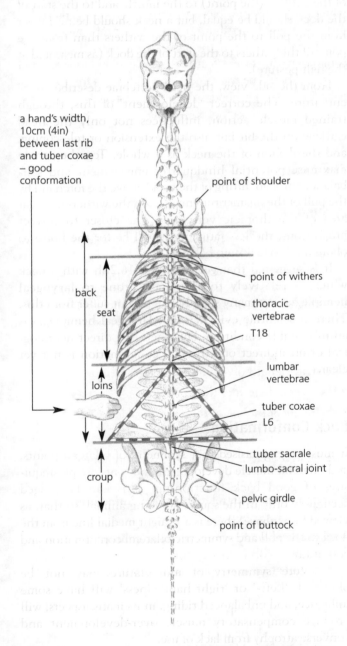

a hand's width, 10cm (4in) between last rib and tuber coxae – good conformation

point of shoulder
point of withers
back
seat
thoracic vertebrae
T18
lumbar vertebrae
loins
tuber coxae
L6
tuber sacrale
lumbo-sacral joint
croup
pelvic girdle
point of buttock

Measurements in assessment of back length – dorso-ventral view.

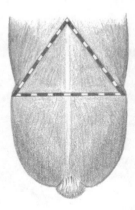

A long back.

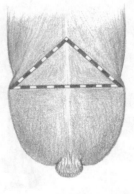

A short back.

A good (relatively long, slightly sloping, broad) croup, for power to extend the lumbo-sacral joint and the hip joint, thus reciprocating the flexion induced by strong ventral musculature under short loins and in the abdomen wall – will augur well for

- good lumbo-sacral **flexion**, and subsequent

- forward **engagement** of the hind legs, as induced by fit ventral muscles with

- good propulsive **power**

The withers should be prominent, to provide a large attachment area for the ligaments and muscles which support the head and thorax and 'lift' the seat as well as playing a significant part in 'slinging' the thorax between the forelegs. The conformation of the withers, including their dorsal process height, the muscle/fat development between them, and the cartilaginous extension of the scapulae on both sides, as well as the symmetry of muscle under the 'saddle' area (and even along the loins), all determine the required 'fit' of the saddle. An ill-fit will affect performance.

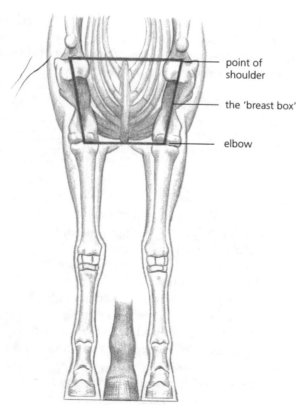

The column of support.

point of shoulder

the 'breast box'

elbow

feet 'one foot-width' apart

Chest Conformation

The 18 thoracic vertebrae and paired ribs give the horse a large chest cavity as well as protection for the vital organs within. Athleticism requires a well developed cardiac musculature; it also requires voluminous lungs. For comparison, cattle and sheep only have 13 ribs.

The external appearance of the chest should be both broad and deep, to provide ample room for the heart especially and the lungs. The breadth of the chest (viewed from in front) affects the distance between the forelegs which, if placed too close together or too far apart, can produce weight-distribution-associated problems. Ideally, the distance between the front feet, when the horse is standing with its front feet level (square) and viewed from in front, should be the same as the width of a forefoot; this is an indicator for good chest room. A narrow chest may also influence security of the saddle.

The Limbs

Foreleg

To a varying degree related to the gait, the foreleg carries 10–20% more body weight than the hind leg. It is at its maximum in the asymmetric gaits when, for a short time in each stride, the leading foreleg momentarily carries all the weight. A conformation defect which compromises the security of support of the foreleg can become important.

The **stride length** of a foreleg is determined by

- the overall *length of the limb*
- the *angle of incline of the shoulder blade*, which enhances its 'gliding' action

The **relative length** of forearm to cannon bone determines

- *long forearms* with relatively *short cannons* gives increased lever **power** potential
- relatively *short forearms* and *long cannons* promise **speed**, but with increased risk of tendon and ligament over-stress (strain) – speed is always the enemy

Durability is a reflection of

- the **angle** made by the hoof wall at the toe with the ground – it should be **45–50°** in the foreleg

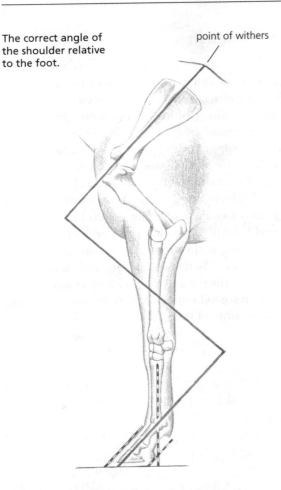

The correct angle of the shoulder relative to the foot.

point of withers

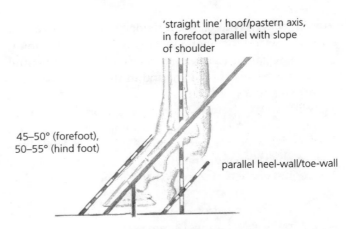

'straight line' hoof/pastern axis, in forefoot parallel with slope of shoulder

45–50° (forefoot), 50–55° (hind foot)

parallel heel-wall/toe-wall

Good foot conformation.

- a '**straight line**' hoof/pastern axis
- a **parallel** heel-wall/toe-wall profile
- heel-wall/toe-wall **parallel** with the slope of the shoulder blade on a line from the highest point of the withers to point of shoulder
- a good **column of support** from the hoof to elbow
- a **balanced** foot fall

The customary description of an 'ideal' conformation is

- *sloping shoulders* give a comfortable ride with **long sweeping strides**; this conformation is desirable for **speed** and **cross-country jumping**
- *upright shoulders* are biomechanically more powerful and are desirable in **draught horses** and possibly in **show jumpers**; the volume of proximal limb musculature and therefore of potential power is determined by this uprightness or otherwise, particularly in the posterior groups

When viewed from in front, in an 'ideal' foreleg conformation an imaginary line from the point of the shoulder should pass through the centre of the knee, fetlock and foot. When parts of the limb deviate inside or outside this imaginary line, extra strain is put on the leg, and there can be uneven weight distribution on the foot.

When a horse is viewed from the side, the forearm and cannon bone should be in a straight line. The length and slope of the pasterns influence the horse's action, and can affect the amount of strain on the foreleg tendons and fetlock joints. Short, especially upright pasterns with an upright shoulder give a shortened 'choppy' stride, making for an uncomfortable ride, and predispose to concussion. Long, sloping pasterns give a longer 'springing' stride, but if the length of slope is excessive it predisposes to tendon strain. Whatever the slopes, they should be parallel throughout, for pastern and shoulder blade.

Hind limb

When viewed from behind, in a horse with so called 'ideal' hind-leg conformation, an imaginary line dropped from the point of the buttock should directly pass through the centre of the hock, fetlock and foot.

If the hock is outside this line, the horse is said to be **bow legged**, and this puts extra strain on the outside of the hock, which can lead to such problems as **thoroughpin**. It is also biomechanically inefficient.

The opposite conformation, in which the hocks are inside this line, **cow hocks**, is usually accompanied by hind feet that turn out. This is quite a common hind-limb fault and can, if pronounced, predispose to strain of the inner aspect of the hock joint, leading to **bone spavin**. This must be distinguished from the correct conformation described below.

Few horses have hind-leg conformation to match man's ideal. The toed-out type, if excessive, is more prone to brushing, as one hoof passes very close to the other fetlock and, in heavy going or when tired, such interference can occur.

A short gaskin and a relatively long cannon promises speed; a long gaskin and a relatively short cannon gives increased power potential.

When viewed from the side, an imaginary line from the point of the buttock should pass through the point of the hock and down the length of the back of the cannon.

If the hind legs are 'straight', the horse is likely to give a jarring and uncomfortable ride but may be better suited for speed.

Excessively angled or curved hocks, **sickle hocks**, are weak, and place additional strain on the back of the hock joint. This conformation is likely to cause strain of the plantar ligament at the back of the hock, a condition known as **curb**, and is described as **curby hocks** when the os calcis (the point of the hock bone) is angled forward, which can be present on its own.

Of necessity, the hind limb when protracted should not move in a true 'fore and aft' plane, but rather in an 'out-in-out' flight; essentially, so that the front of the stifle does not strike the lower posterior abdomen. This preferred movement is determined by

- hip sockets set wide apart
- outward deviation of the femurs as they descend from the hip joint, with outwardly inclined stifles
- hocks that are directed forward

- vertical cannons
- hooves parallelling the stifles, and so standing toe-ed out below the fetlock

The planes of the stifle and true hock articular surfaces determine much of this out-in-out flight. The overall appearance is that of 'straight' action, i.e. without distal curving action such as winging or dishing. The levelness of hoof fall and support is, as always, vital.

Foot Conformation

The old horseman's adage, *'No foot – no horse'*, is as relevant today as it has been in the past. Although some defects can be present at birth, in most instances important defects develop during life. Many can be corrected by judicious trimming. They are not true conformation deficits: they are better seen as acquired faults of shape which invariably alter the ground reaction force effect and thereby the biokinetics of the horse's dynamics.

A horse's feet should be two identical pairs, fore and hind. A foot that differs from its opposite should be viewed with suspicion unless it is a known confirmable congenital fault. Even then, the smaller foot may give less supporting surface and/or be more upright, and predispose to one cause of tripping. The fore feet are rather more circular than the hind, reflecting the shape of P3, the pedal bone. The fore is more engaged in landing and in support; the

Correct hind limb conformation.

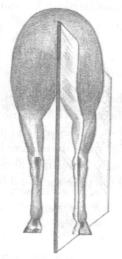 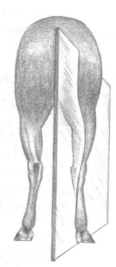 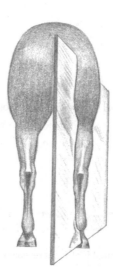

correct – plane bisects hoof, fetlock, hock and stifle

cow hocked – hoof and fetlock lie outside plane, hock is inside

bow legged – all or most of hoof lies inside plane, all of hock lies outside

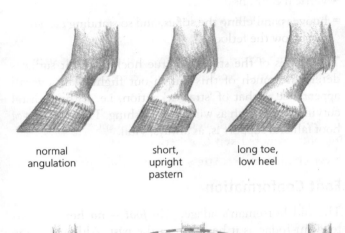

normal
angulation

short,
upright
pastern

long toe,
low heel

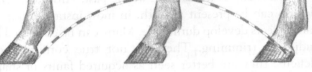

normal angulation – foot flight as previously thought

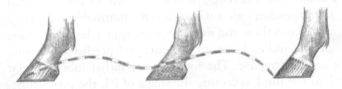

normal angulation – actual foot flight revealed by recent research

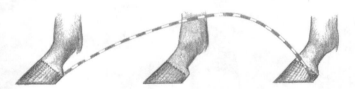

long toe, low heel – foot flight as previously thought

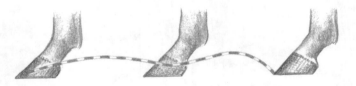

long toe, low heel – actual foot flight revealed by recent research

The effect of pastern conformation and foot flight arc.

oval hind foot is primarily for 'digging in, to kick off'.

It is an over-generalisation that the side walls of the fore and of the hind foot should, in antero-posterior profile, always be of equal length and fall from coronet to ground at the quarters at the same angle, i.e. that there should be the same distance from the coronet to the bearing (ground) surface on both sides of the foot at any given point. A non-horizontal coronet, with associated differences in inside and outside wall lengths and angles of ground contact, is acceptable if the column of support is correct.

The **hoof/pastern axis** can have a considerable effect on the length and character of the flight of the foot, and the length of the stride during motion. When a horse has a normal hoof/pastern axis, the foot flight should, when viewed from the side, make a smooth arc whose apex occurs as the foot passes over the vertical line of the opposite (supporting) foot.

With a sloping hoof/pastern axis, especially if broken back is acquired, the break-over is delayed – so that the foot has already reached the apex of its flight *before* it passes the opposite one. The horse has a longer stride, and keeps its foot closer to the ground. If the hoof/pastern axis is upright, and especially if broken forward, the foot reaches the apex of its flight *after* it has passed the opposite one. The horse has a short stride, and brings its foot to the ground quickly. True conformation deficits are less likely to alter flight patterns, even though they may predispose to eventual morbidity from stresses imposed during work.

The recent research involving slow-motion photography indicates that the varying flight arcs described above are not so readily associated with broken hoof/pastern axis as once thought.

Front Feet

Broken **pastern/hoof axes** as mentioned above inflict compounding influences on distal limb function and structure. A number of such cases respond in time to corrective hoof balancing, i.e. they are acquired and not inherited defects. Some such inherited abnormalities can be improved up until the time the distal bones are ossified, at around 1½ years.

Hind Feet

The **angle** of the front of the hoof wall and the pastern should again be the same but, in the hind limbs, the angle is about 5° steeper than in the forelegs – i.e. about 52°. A range of **50–55°** is normal.

A congenital broken back axis in the hind limbs creates a significant weakness and causes overstress of the plantar suspensory ligaments and the superficial flexor tendon.

There is no doubt that unbalanced feet, especially in a latero-medial (acquired) conformation, are the greater fault, both contemporarily and even more so from a long-term point of view.

The Horse in Motion

See also Chapter 17, THE LOCOMOTOR SYSTEM.

There are colloquial names for alterations in action due to conformation defects, which affect flight paths and foot fall

- **dishing** or **paddling** – both fore and hind
- **winging** – both fore and hind
- **plaiting** – both fore and hind

Body Proportions

The **long-backed** horse can, if not properly fit, and especially if not ridden in collection, develop a lateral swing at the trot and at faster gaits. This can

- put *stress on the thoracic lumbar-sacral* musculature and ligaments
- *affect limb action*, predisposing to interferences such as **speedy cutting, cross firing** and **vertebral soft tissue trauma**

A **short-backed**, close-coupled horse, especially in show jumping, is more likely to suffer

- vertebral joint over-stress – **arthritis, spondylosis**
- vertebral **bone injury**
- **over-reaching**
- **forging**
- **scalping**

Such altered balance may be compounded by

- too long a neck
- upright shoulders
- limbs relatively too long
- short pelvis, weak quarters
- too heavy a head
- tiredness

THE LOCOMOTOR SYSTEM

The aesthetic appearance of the ridden horse, the pleasure of the rider, and the ability and durability of the horse all depend on the balanced functioning of the 'locomotor system'.

A major requirement for this balance is that the moving horse attempts to keep its dynamic centre of gravity as close as possible to where it would be when it is standing at the halt; hence the expression **in self-balance**.

The co-ordination of the rider's centre of gravity with that of the horse is an essence of equitation, and is vital to the ideal movement within any gait.

The locomotor system subserves the two primary functions for an animal's 'being'– that is 'existing' (staying alive) and 'reproducing the species'. To these ends, the locomotor system is integrated with the other vital systems, to fulfil the roles of

- **mobility** – to food and to water

- **posturing** – for grazing and drinking and for excretory and reproductive acts

- **resting** – standing at ease, sternal recumbency and lateral recumbency

- **alertness** and awareness

- **defence**

- **flight**

The necessary 'machinery' is provided by the many units of the locomotor system. A 'unit' is an articulation which, as the 'centre' of a particular movement within the whole, consists of

- two **bones**

- their **cartilage** with its **synovial capsule**

- the supporting **ligaments**

- the **muscles** and their **tendons**

- the **blood** supply and drainage, including the **lymphatic** system

- the **nerves**

The **limbs**, as organs of locomotion, have three functions

- to maintain a particular position for the body, i.e. posture – stationary, albeit if only for a short time

- to propel, or 'move', the body by overcoming inertia

- to reduce the movement, eventually to a standstill

The limbs are also organs of defence and attack.

All these functions are 'against' the force of gravity, which is centred at the **centre of gravity**. In the horse at standing rest, on the horizontal plane this is between the top two thirds and the bottom third of the trunk, and in the

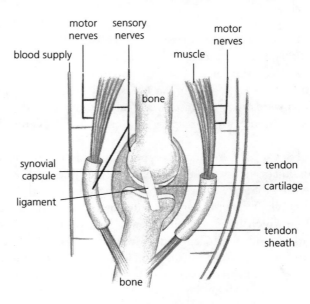

A typical joint.

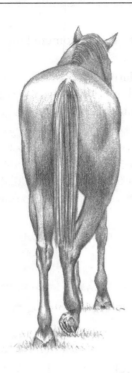

A resting stance.

the 'engagement' of the hindquarters, both of which actions move the centre of gravity backwards and so lighten the forehand. The musculature of the vertebral column plays an essential role in augmenting and directing the forward movement induced by hind quarter propulsion.

A number of technical terms are used

Biomechanics
This deals with facts and figures which relate to the *forces* working on the horse, and the resultant changes in its component parts. Such changes are called

- **accelerations** – which may be 'up' or 'down'. For continuing well being, such accelerations should be elegant, i.e. accomplished smoothly, through the range of the articulations' flexion and extension. A jerking change – third degree acceleration – inflicts 'dis-ease' stress on the involved units of locomotion. In the horse at standstill biomechanics are also involved in maintaining this posture

Kinesiology
This is the science and study of *movement*, and in the living animal is divided into:

- **biokinetics** – concerns the forces required for start, alter, stop, and 'hold', whose accelerations are used in balancing and re-balancing

- **biokinematics** – analyses movement, and so the geometry which characterises particular motion in an animal type or species. As such it is two-dimensional

- **biostatics** – relates to the resting animal, or to one moving in a straight line at a steady velocity, both of which situations require an input of force to balance the output of gravity's force

- **biodynamics** – relates to moving and the involved accelerations (changing velocities). Thus, dependent on gait and terrain, the position of the centre of gravity changes and so requires complementary re-balancing – a 3-dimensional input and output
  - **gravity** – 'output', influenced by mass-x-speed
  - **muscle forces** – 'input', subject to
  - **environmental changes**
    - internal – appropriate gaits
    - external – terrain, fear, etc.

In technical language, as in recording on paper or on screen

vertical plane it is towards the cranial, fore-end, of the trunk; looked at from the side it is typically on the line of the rider's calf. ***The forehand therefore carries approximately 60% of the body mass*** of the horse standing at ease and slightly less at the halt.

This force of gravity is equal to the mass of the body at any one time. 'Weight', scientifically, is the product of 'mass x velocity'. Thus, at rest, speed is zero; so, at rest, weight = mass.

In practice, mass is measured on a weighbridge or from formulae based on certain body linear measurements.

At rest, the force of gravity pulls the mass downwards and, because of its forward position, it tends to pull downwards in a forward arc. The locomotor forces, i.e. work input, are (in part at least) to prevent this happening.

Forward locomotion is propelled mainly by the horse's hindquarters. In consequence, in forward locomotion the centre of gravity is directed both downwards (by the force of gravity) and further forwards (by propulsion), with a force which increases with speed. This 'on the forehand, with a tendency to pitch downwards' situation requires a constant opposing force in order for an upright equilibrium to be maintained – and the forelegs' primary propping action, as well as their secondary propulsive role, is augmented by the elevation of the head and neck and by

- the movement of the horse from one place to another is called **displacement** – from A to B
- the measurement of any displacement distance is a **scalar** – e.g. 100m is of necessity shown as a scale, such as 1cm = 100m
- the direction, or orientation, of displacement is shown on paper as a **vector** – e.g. '100m northwards'
- the combined displacement distance and direction is a **scaled vector** – e.g. a twisting road drawn on a map
- the time taken in scalar terms for a displacement is **speed** – expressed, for example, in kph or mph
- the term that describes speed in a given direction is **velocity** – which describes kph or mph. It can be written as $V = {}^{d}/_{t}$ where V is velocity, d is displacement and t is time, but these figures provide only a gross overall view of direction and speed; they do not record minute-by-minute changes in velocity brought about by gradients and alterations in surfaces etc. These require differential calculus!
- **acceleration** (+) and **deceleration** (–) occur with a change in velocity

Many other words are used to expand on these and to describe the methods of measuring and recording them. They are required knowledge for students at degree level in biomechanics with special regard to athletic performance.

There is argument about nomenclature within **bio-kinematics**, but

- **stride** is the cumulative effect of those movements of all four limbs required to bring a designated part of one limb back to the same position a second time round. Within this, there is 'cycle' and 'step'
    - **cycle** is the series of movements of a limb which return it to its original position. In practice, a stride involves four cycles; the actual distance is not cumulative – footfall overlap must be taken into account
    - **step** is the movement of a limb away from or towards the other limb, either on the same side (that is, in the same plane) or contralaterally on the same plane or laterally (that is, to the opposite side)

Stride has four parameters

- **length** – the linear distance which a hoof moves between two successive imprints of that hoof
- **duration** – the time taken to do so
- **frequency** – the number of strides per unit of time
- **pattern** – the variable sequence of repetitive limb movements; a particular sequence is described as a **gait**

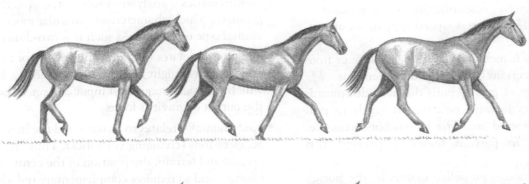
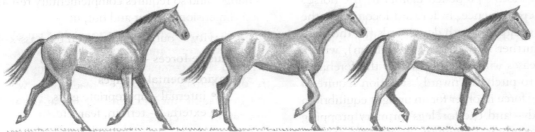

A sequence of movement – as an example, the trot.

Gaits are

- the **walk** – symmetric
- the **trot** – symmetric
- the **gallop** and, with altered hind footfall, the **canter** – asymmetric

Within each gait's stride, a limb has two positional elements, **stance** and **swing**.

Stance

Stance describes the position of the limb and its joint angles in relation to the trunk when it is weight bearing. It has three components

- **initial contact** with the ground – 'landing'
- **support** – on the foreleg, when the cannon is vertical; and on the hind leg, when the hoof is right under the hip joint
- **final contact** with the ground before going into flight – 'lift-off'

Stance has three 'effects'

- **initial deceleration** on landing
- **support** and stability throughout
- final acceleration, i.e. **propulsion** on lift-off

and it has

- **duration**, especially during support
- **pressure** – all forces are equal and opposite, so during stance the ground exerts an equal and upwards pressure on the limb as that exerted downwards by the 'pull' of gravity

The stability of the limb when in the stance element of a gait depends on

- the **antero-posterior** hoof capsule balance, and
- the **medio-lateral** hoof capsule balance

as they affect foot-fall, support and lift-off, and as they influence the column of support and subsequently the distal limb joints. Reduced stability induces torque stresses, e.g. landing on the outside wall and then rolling onto full contact

There are two facets of this torque

- the initial hoof-wall ground-surface contact which receives the upward force input up, for example, the lateral wall if the footfall is 'outside in', and on up the

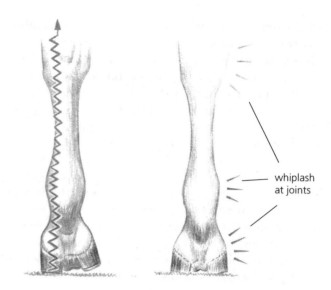

(In the same leg) the torque stresses of landing on the outside wall (left) and then rolling onto full contact (right).

lateral aspect of that distal limb. This is quickly dissipated as eventually the medial wall takes its share of the load and the ligaments come into total support, and therefore the pathological effects will be on this aspect

- the secondary action when the medial hoof wall whiplashes down onto support. This is said to cause third order acceleration, a jerk action, on the distal components of the hoof and the limb

Dis-ease severity is a reflection of the integrity of the stay and suspensory apparatus and of the related intrinsic muscle fibres and tendons.

Swing

Swing is a dynamic repositioning of the limb's parts. It has

- **duration**
- vertical and horizontal **ranges**
- **phases**: the **posterior** and the **anterior**, in relation to the flight path past the opposite leg's stance

Swing and stance have functional and time relationships to the other three limbs and to the trunk, neck and head. Left and right comparisons (remembering the 'action' on the other rein or lead) are best made at the walk and at the trot in straight lines and circles, and at the walk and trot and canter on a circle.

The **dynamics** or 'in motion' of support and flight of a stride correctly begins with one hind leg. The subsequent limb movements, as well as trunk, neck and head related activity vary with gait and the speeds at that gait.

It is easier to understand this in a horse that is already moving; when this hind limb is fully lifted off it has played its part in propulsion, the trunk will have been propelled in advance of the limb which, momentarily, will have been left behind (extended caudally) only to be then carried forward by its proximal attachment at the hip.

This initial extension is smoothly translated into flexion of all the joints to lift the limb clear of the ground, and then into protraction to take it level with the opposite limb which, in symmetric gaits, will now be weight-bearing. This is the **posterior phase**. As it passes in front of the supporting limb it now extends to move into the protraction of the **anterior phase**, before being retracted and a final extension towards foot fall. These take it onto ground contact and support once more.

The flexion also effectively minimises the limb's weight and so its resistance for ease of protraction and, to a lesser extent, retraction. Extension, i.e. lengthening, in the return phase, allows it to 'reach' the ground relative to the same part of the body as before. Ideally, the two phases should be equidistant. The contra-lateral limb's parameters should mirror these.

The stride is said to have a period of suspension when no limb is in support.

The co-ordination of all parts of limbs, trunk, neck and head is essential for rhythm, balance and security in locomotion, whatever the gait.

A horse 'goes' according to the path described by the **limb flight path**, and by the **foot-fall** pattern irrespective of the limb flight path, both of them as judged *head on* (for forelegs), *going away* (for hind legs) and *from the side*. (*See also* Chapter 16, CONFORMATION)

THE APPENDICULAR SKELETON – THE LIMBS

The limbs have a two-fold function:

- as 'inclined' **struts**, for support both at rest and in the support phase of motion
- as **levers**, imposing forces at lift-off and again at foot-fall, through the hoof acting as a fulcrum

The series of struts and levers are the structural and functioning components of the locomotor system. They

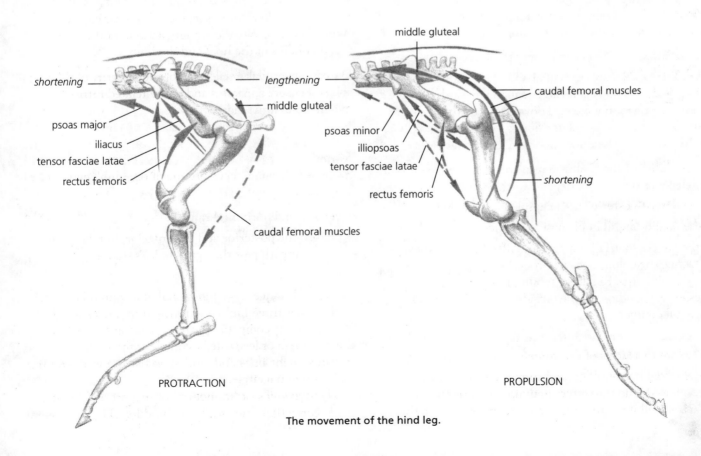

The movement of the hind leg.

are guided and supported by their ligaments, and motivated by their related muscles under the control of the nervous system.

It is primarily the action of the limbs that supports the horse or moves it from the static position. The horse's body is 'suspended' from these four columns; the fore end is 'slung' between the forelegs and the hind is attached by bony articulations to the pelvis.

The hindquarters *carry only approximately 40%* of the horse's effective weight at rest, *but they provide approximately 85% of the propulsive force* required for locomotion at maximum levels. They have

- a bilateral 'fixed' articulation through the pelvis onto the first of the fused sacral vertebrae, thus establishing a bony direct line for a horizontal forward thrust along the axial vertebral column, from the propulsive forces generated by

  - the extensor muscles of the hip
  - the kinetic energy developed in the stay/suspensory apparatus from the stifle distally

- a locking reciprocal structure and functioning between the stifle and the hock joints, thus involving the femur proximally and the cannon distally, sufficient to form an *almost* rigid lever over the major length of the limb to more effectively transmit the propulsive force, as well as a degree of stability in the support phase, yet maintain

  - a degree of 'give', a stress absorber, to minimise the risk of strain, augmented by
  - the distal stay/suspensory apparatus of the fetlock region and the related 'let down' potential of that joint which action induces a kinetic rebound for lift off

The hind leg does not depend to the same extent as the fore upon its proximal musculature, for shock absorption. Moreover, in the hind leg, ground reaction forces on footfall are significantly less; most of the time the emphasis is more on lift off than on support.

Conversely, the horse is equipped to land on extended fore limbs with no restriction from a collar bone, the force of landing being absorbed by the thoracic muscular sling as well as the distal joints.

This all-important difference has evolved a hind foot which concentrates its functioning requirements into a solar surface area which is

- narrower from quarter to quarter and at the bulb of the heels, and

- longer from toe to heels

both giving an ovoid ground plan, and

- has a sole which is more concave
- has a more upright wall at the toe, and
- is longer in the heel wall

all of which make the hind feet better suited for a 'digging in' propulsive lift-off than for a 'safe landing'. At foot fall there is often a slight horizontal twisting of the hind hoof.

At the walk the foot is set down flat, or the toe may just land first. The heel always leaves the ground first, in all limbs and at all paces. At faster paces, the toes of the front feet are flipped forwards and upwards at the end of their forward flight (protraction); it is not until the leg has been fully retracted that the foot makes contact with the ground – the heel landing slightly before the quarters and toe.

Although it is normal for the front feet to land slightly heel-first at paces faster than the walk, if this is excessive it can predispose to injury from whip lash to the distal joints. At a fast gallop, the heels of the hind feet hardly come into contact with the ground at all.

It must be remembered that trimming can, at any age, alter hoof wall growth and its final geometry – unfortunately, if not done well, for the worse.

THE AXIAL SKELETON

The quadrupedal horse's body functions on a horizontal plane. Bipedal man's functions on the vertical plane, whereby his 'hind legs' appear to carry the body.

The long axis of the body of the quadruped's vertebral column is called the **axial skeleton**. It consists of the various regions of vertebrae: **cervical (C), thoracic (T), lumbar (L), sacral (S),** and the first three **coccygeal (Cy)**. The head is attached to the C1 (atlas), and the last lumbar (L6) articulates with the anterior sacrum (S1) to which the pelvis is also attached (though in Eastern breeds there are often only 5 lumbar vertebrae, and this is 'made up' by a 19th thoracic and an extra pair of floating ribs). In addition, there are

- 18 pairs of **ribs** – the last pair are free or 'floating', i.e. have no distal cartilage connection to the sternum

- the **sternum** or breast-bone

In more general terms the axial skeleton has **neck, back, loin** and **pelvic** divisions, collectively known as the **vertebral column** (known colloquially as the 'spine').

The area behind the withers to the 18th thoracic is

colloquially known as the **seat** or 'saddle'. The lumbar area is the **loins** or the 'link' to the sacrum and so to the hind limb. To the horseman the 'seat' is seen as a logical place to sit comfortably, safely and in balance between the fore and the hindquarters. To the biomechanic, the back is seen as a bridge from which is suspended the mass of the internal organs and an incidental, if fortuitous, area for a rider.

The pull of gravity, the 'gravitational force', acts on all parts of the body; perhaps most of all, it acts on the vertebral column – supporting, as that does, the relatively greater 'pull' of the digestive system mass, compared to other parts, and 'carrying' the rest of the trunk and the limbs when in suspension.

In movement, with acceleration, this mass is increased by a factor of speed. The product is the effective weight, or gravitational force active at any one moment. In changing accelerating motion, therefore, the equine vertebral column is exposed to varying gravitational forces; it must be able to exert an immediate opposite and equal force – a resistant stability to withstand the stress, especially in suspension, an increasing rigidity.

The inter-vertebral discs are much firmer than in man and much less liable to 'slip'. A horse's vertebral column is *anatomically flexible* but, of necessity, *functionally rigid*.

In the quiet (relaxed) standing animal, the flexibility can be induced and the reflex movements seen. Such flexibility is more readily assessed by watching the horse move at walk and trot, either free or led or lunged or ridden.

- the swing of the head and the quarters, with marked flexibility between them through the back, at the walk's three-foot support gait

- general horizontal stability at the trot, as the stride length increases

- the horizontal undulations through the head with the neck and the quarters, over an increasingly rigid back at the canter. *As gait speed increases, the back (withers to croup) becomes more rigid*

Similarly, the imbalance of the immature or unfit or tiring horse, whose muscles are unable, or no longer able, to keep the vertebral column 'rigid', can be appreciated both from the saddle – **kinaesthesia** – and when viewing from the ground. This imbalance is felt and seen especially during the canter.

In an amenable horse, at the halt, it is possible reflexly to stimulate vertebral column movement – to a degree. A pressure on the midline drawn from behind the withers and again towards the point of the croup induces a 'hollowing' of the back and actual extension – to some extent along the thoraco-lumbar region, but mainly between T1 and T2 with the neck being elevated and between L6 and S1 whereby the croup to the dock is elevated to become more horizontal The overall visual 'picture' is that of hollowing of the back. If the linear stimulus is taken midline from mid-croup to the dock, a reverse movement immediately occurs – **flexion** – with the back apparently 'humping up'. Here, again, most of the movement is from the two ends, although the impression is of total arching. A play of rising and falling can be obtained until the horse voluntarily overrides this involuntary reflex activity and says 'Leave me alone!' Lateral movements can also be induced.

In post mortem examination with the vertebral column stripped of ribs and muscles, movement can be manually effected between

- the skull and the atlas (C1) – flexion, extension and some lateral movement

- the atlas (C1) and the axis (C2) – rotation

- C2 and C3 and, with decreasing range, to T1 –

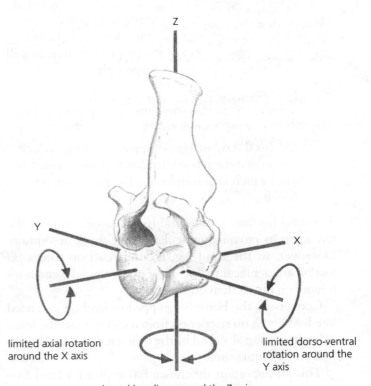

limited axial rotation around the X axis

limited dorso-ventral rotation around the Y axis

lateral bending around the Z axis always results also in X axis rotation

The vertebral column – movement around the three planes is possible but very limited.

rotation, flexion and extension

- T1 and T2 – marked flexion and extension
- T1–T14 – cumulative lateral flexion to give a horizontal range of movement in arc shape at T1
- T14–T18 – none
- T18 and L1 – limited flexion and extension
- L1–L6 – limited flexion and extension
- L1–S – torque effect, diminishingly from sacrum to L1, i.e. 'screwed' round to left or to right along the long axis
- L6 and S1 – marked flexion and extension
- the fused five sacral bones and the first three coccygeal (Cy) bones – flexion, extension and lateral movements
- from the fourth Cy backwards – tail swishing

The first three of these movements (i.e. those involving the skull to T1) are functionally active in life.

Two are vitally important – L6–S1 which is the source of 'engaging the hindquarters', and T1–T2 which is involved in the flexing of the neck. The remainder are blocked in live faster movement. The lumbo-sacral torque does occur at rest and at the walk, though not at the faster gaits. At rest, with one hind leg flexed, the pelvis rotates down on that side, and the lumbars follow to a decreasing extent – they rotate over. The swing of the hips at the walk is a somewhat similar movement.

The Biomechanics of the Vertebral Column

The theory of the **bow and string** axial column is applied to all quadrupeds. In the horse, as has been emphasised, vertebral column rigidity increases with speed. Where there is no suspensory phase, as in the stance and the walk, balance is not at great risk, so rigidity is less vital. The trot, a two-time movement in a symmetrical gait, has a balancing effect even at the extended pace, but at the gallop (and the canter) the asymmetry of the action is fundamentally unstable and must therefore have vertebral column rigidity to compensate.

In nature, when a horse gets up, the slight increase in gravitational pull mechanically causes a hollowing. The proprioceptor sensations in the vertebral column joints immediately and reflexly trigger an opposite and equal 'humping', and then a quick repositioning into intrinsic weight-bearing – and the ideal neutral position is attained. In equitation, a similar situation occurs when the horse is mounted; leg and seat aids 'send' messages to amend the central balances, and so signal transitions and changes in direction, but all these require development of the vertebral and other related musculature – appropriate fittening, and 'training' of the related nerves by practice.

Vertebral column rigidity is dependent on

- the natural vertebral column articulations and overall linear shape being stabilised by the horizontal ligaments, assisted by the action of the epaxial cybernetic muscles, to make this line of vertebrae from T2 to Cy3 (the tail bone) the potentially **rigid bow**
- the variable tensions, counter forces, of two groups of muscular **'strings'**
  - the **dorsal** string

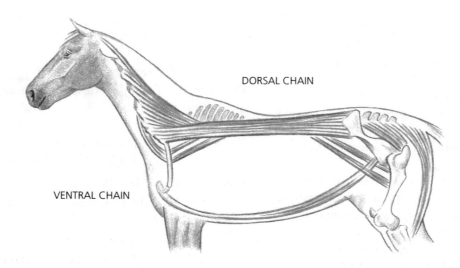

DORSAL CHAIN

VENTRAL CHAIN

The dorsal and ventral muscular chains.

- **uninterrupted** epaxial gymnastic muscles along the top and sides of the vertebrae from quarters to neck and head – which act by straightening (extending) and compacting the line of vertebrae: they stiffen the bow horizontally

- **interrupted** (the hypaxial)– two series of muscles along the base of the vertebrae, one in the cervical and anterior thoracic region, then a gap before other muscles in the posterior thoracic and the lumbar to sacral region and proximal femur

  - the **ventral** string

    - the abdominal muscles running from the sternum to the pubis and via these to the anterior and posterior regions of the vertebral column respectively

The dorsal and other muscles extend the vertebral column at their respective ends, but the hypaxials also assist in this stabilising but can flex the pelvis on the lumbar vertebrae as required. The ventral muscles act by flexing the bow more extrinsically through their contractile pull from sternum to pelvis, and so indirectly onto the vertebral column. Proximal limb muscles and others from the rib cage to the ventral mid-neck complete a coil of muscle activity to augment the action of the bow string complex.

Flexing, when required, occurs only at T1–T2 and at L6–S1; otherwise, the dorsal muscles are compacters and stabilisers. When bowing is induced, the major effect is the building up of kinetic energy in the vertebral column's dorsal 'string'. Conversely, when the bow is released, more kinetic energy is built up in the 'opposing' structures. In consequence, there is a two-way elasticity of 'hold', or rigidity, and 'pull'. The ventral string has, as well, an important role in limb movement at the shoulder and at the quarter. In natural or in induced reflex vertebral column movement at rest, there is variable flexion and extension along the 'back' especially at T18–L1.

The galloping and jumping horse certainly requires fit abdominal muscles. These play a significant part in getting the sacrum/pelvis flexed on the backbone for forward engagement for better propulsion into a longer stride or into a jump.

In the wild, the horse's evasive actions and ultimate flight for survival required agility, speed and endurance. Balance had to be achieved through a functionally rigid 'backbone'. If this failed, propulsive forces lost their input and balance became compromised, with potentially fatal effect – from unacceptable stress and strain on the vertebral column and, indirectly, upon other locomotive structures. The horse became a very easy prey as it lagged behind the herd in flight.

As has been described, the 'bow and string' principle of locomotion involves not only the vertebral column, the 'bow', but also the other skeletal structures, the ribs and sternum, interposed between the bow proper and the ventral muscles for attachment of these muscles. The associated movement is primarily in the one plane of flexion and extension.

The skull on C1 and the other cervical vertebral joints permit a varying degree of three plane movements, with the addition of lateral and rotational 'bending'.

The specific functional requirements of the horse, especially in the asymmetric gaits, are

- counter-balancing by the head and neck, through three plane movements

- flexion at L6 and S1 to permit 'engagement' of the hindquarters

- maintaining extension of the back, the 'bridge', to give it rigidity to

  - accept the propulsive power of the hind legs

  - maintain stability for carrying the weight (mass x speed) of the internal organs – and of the rider

  - yet allow a degree of shock absorbing, and

  - facilitate balance

and so minimise the risk of

- overstress to the

  - bridge's units of locomotion, the thoracolumbar vertebrae, ligaments and muscles

  - subsequent overstress to the limbs and to the neck

This intrinsic flexibility of the whole axial region is a summation of the 'give' between the vertebrae and is determined by the

- compressibility and resilience of the species' relatively thin intervertebral discs, the connecting 'washers'

- 'give' (and recoil) of the

  - dorsal vertebral ligament (the supra spinous ligament)

  - inter-dorsal process ligaments

  - ventral spinal canal ligament (attached to a disc as it passes over it)

- ventral vertebral ligament (attached to a disc as it passes under it)

These have limited 'stretchability'.

The total possible vertebral movement is reduced by the

- lateral vertebral articulations
- attachments of the ribs, each one onto two adjacent thoracic vertebrae on both sides
- articulations between the caudal lumbar transverse processes

The muscles which 'service' the vertebral column can act on the 'flexible' column

- unilaterally, to turn it laterally
- bilaterally, which aims to compress the vertebrae, i.e. by extending the column into compaction

Thus, within limits, these muscles can obtain a three-plane movement, but it is limited. Their main work is to stabilise the vertebral column and to flex the lumbo-sacral joint.

Each inter-vertebral joint has six possible movements. However, when the limiting factors, as described above, are overstressed there can be trauma to the soft tissue, muscles, tendons and ligaments, and to the bones to which they are attached. These become the points of ultimate overstress into injury and even fracture with displacement.

The normal movements are around the three planes of

- *flexion and extension* – dorso-ventral bending (rotation) around the Y or **horizontal axis**
- *rotation (sideways)* – around the **X axis** along the axial plane
- *lateral bending* – around the **Z axis**

The first two can occur independently. The third can do so only if there is a coupling with the second, that is a combined twist and a lateral bend – a torque. Such movements are functionally possible in the standing horse when they are maximal, declining to rigidity as required with locomotion. The twist and lateral bend can be seen, and on riding, felt when the horse walks.

In rigidity the ligaments and discs still retain a compressed resilience to allow 'give' to a degree; this absorbs the stresses imposed on the maximally impacted vertebrae. The muscles which motivated this can, of course, release their hold if and when required. To do so suddenly could court disaster – accelerating forces' trauma – and a serious imbalancing.

The **epaxial** muscles (upper group, above level of the vertebrae) of the back run segmentally (i.e. in a series of origins and insertions) from the pelvis to the skull attaching, en route, to the

- vertebral processes and bodies of lumbars and thoracics
- ribs
- cervical processes and bodies
- skull
- subcutaneous fascias
- other adjacent muscles

The **hypaxial** muscles (lower group of dorsals) run in support, from the ventral aspects of the

- cranial thoracic vertebrae back to the ribs and the forehand fascia
- caudal lumbar vertebrae back to the pelvis and its fascia with the hind limb

The **ventral** muscles, the 'antagonists' run

- from the first rib and the cranial sternum to the caudal cervical vertebrae, with the
- abdominal muscles from the caudal sternum inserting onto the pelvic brim
- giving stability to the back
- helping balance the impulsive forces of the limbs by the
  - engagement of them and their force through the sacro iliac joints and along the spine

This unified system, the mainspring of all the gaits, especially the asymmetrics is

- an elastic, variable rigidity of the dorsal trunk
- a regulated, rhythmic muscle action of contraction, hold; relaxation, 'give' and repeat

which has to be under a refined neurological control

The co-ordination depends upon

- sensory proprioceptor inputs
- cranial, conscious sensory inputs
- conscious voluntary motor outputs (decisions if change is needed)
- involuntary upper motor neuron (UMN) outputs and spinal reflexes

The Thorax

As in other areas of the body, the skeletal structures play more than one part in the overall functioning of the animal. The **thorax**, the chest or 'ribcage', protects the heart, lungs and other vital structures, assists respiration, and affords attachment areas for the extrinsic muscles of foreleg locomotion. It consists of

- the **sternum** or breast bone – the base or 'floor' of the cage – **8 bony segments** united by discs of ossifying cartilage to give a resilient but fundamentally rigid structure. It maintains a functional 'give' which absorbs stress, and thus assures durability. In front, it is a narrow, flat vertical extension or keel. At the rear, it extends horizontally as a flat 'tail'. Both these are firm but flexible cartilages: the fore-end is the **cariniform** and the hind the **zyphoid**. The overall appearance of the wall is that of a high-prowed canoe

- the **ribs**, the walls – the **8 pairs of 'fixed' bony ribs** are individually attached to the sternum by short, flexible extensions of cartilage which act as non-articular hinges. The **10 pairs of 'free' ribs** also have distal extensions of cartilage which unite to attach to the sternum on either side by a single 'rope' of cartilage which is quite flexible. Together, the sternum and the ribs afford extensive areas for muscle attachment. The first pair of ribs, hinged by true joints, two each side, to the last cervical vertebra and the first thoracic, describe a relatively small ovoid space which is the entrance to the chest. Successive rib pairs are longer and more outwardly convex to form the capacious chest cavity wall, and are mobile in respiratory movement

- the **roof of the thorax** is formed by the **18 thoracic vertebrae**

- the caudal or **gable wall** is the **muscular/fibrous diaphragm**. Its main function is in inspiration. It is attached to the caudal inner surface of the sternum, to the last ribs, and to the last thoracic vertebrae. In locomotion it 'holds' at the end of inspiration, especially during explosive hind leg action, to maximise that propulsive effort and not dissipate it by relaxing into expiration thereby loosening the contractile force of abdominal musculature

- the **zyphoid cartilage** and the posterior ribs and their cartilages are sites for the origin of the abdominal muscles, and especially those which insert at the brim of the pelvis. These muscles form the ventral uninterrupted 'string'

The Pelvis and the Pelvic Cavity

This consists of three pairs of fused bones, which diverge cranially to form part of the walls, come together ventrally to form a short floor, and then diverge once more caudally. The rest of the walls are the tough sacro-pelvic ligaments. This infilling lessens the weight of an all-bone cavity, and although giving firm foundations for muscle origin, they impart an essential resilience and elasticity. The roof is the fused sacral bones and first three coccygeal vertebrae – the croup. The extremities of the pelvis are

- the close-together **tuberi sacralae** – the *points of the croup*
- the wide-apart **tuberi coxae** – the *points of the hip*
- the posterior mid-spaced **tuberi ischii** – the *points of the buttock*

The pelvis is the origin foundation of the proximal extrinsic muscles of the hind legs. It is the all-important linkage between the hind limbs and the axial skeleton. The 'joints' are the **sacro-iliacs** – anatomically true articulations, though functionally fixed from a very early age.

The pelvis's cranial brim, the insertion point of the abdominal string and the outer surface of the ilia and the femur of the caudal, interrupted string, are the areas on which these muscles exert their ventral flexion effect on the lumbo-sacral joint. As such, this special articulation, particularly in faster gaits, is the primary joint of hind limb extension and flexion. The pelvic cavity is a passage for the rectum and posterior urogenital organs. It is not lined by peritoneum.

The 'bow's' purpose is not to project an arrow; paradoxically, a sudden forceful 'bending' or flexion will project a rider out of the saddle, but this is not a primary function! However, when 'well drawn' at its extremities, the tension in the vertebral column, its discs, ligaments and dorsal muscular strings will have built up a considerable kinetic potential. The 'draw' will have been assisted by protraction of the hind legs and retraction of the fore.

Their prime function is to elevate and propel; this occurs at 'lift-off'. The subsequent converse action relaxes the bow, and its recoiling extension results in further propulsion into a forward period of suspension, or a jump, as required.

Not only throughout the 'bow and string' complex, but also throughout the skeleton, muscles must work in harmony, so that the horse, free or ridden, goes in self-balance. Such a state is important in dressage and show jumping. In racing and cross-country work, the aim of equitation is significantly different; such balance therefore is compromised for the demands of speed and agility **but must not be ignored**. An unbalanced horse is bordering on instability; instability leads to injury.

Balanced locomotion allows fit muscles to obtain their optimal effect; balance implies co-ordinated 'give' and 'hold'. 'Give' does not necessarily mean action, but excessive 'give' against 'hold' can be unwanted movement leading to lack of rigidity, as in the vertebral column, when, especially in asymmetric gaits, it permits instability – and so possible injury. Total relaxation means physical collapse. This balance is in essence the basis of athleticism and durability – a controlled gradation within the demands of the gaits and jumping to the limits imposed by the anatomically designed range of the units of locomotion (joints).

Before present-day understanding of these dynamics, certain equitation beliefs, now seen to have been wrong, were sincerely held. The reasoning behind them was from an interpretation of what even the experts **thought** they saw when the horse was in action

- **'Lateral Bend Around the Inside Leg'**
  The **impression**, especially with a rider up, is certainly one of a curve from poll to tail. To have the horse on such a 'circle' it must reduce the forward reach of the inside shoulder, and step forwards **and** under with the inside hind.

  Even in a well-schooled and fit horse which can keep upright, the quarters must engage further forward on the inside. The posterior or lumbar vertebral column cannot laterally bend on the horizontal plane, only tip down or rotate to the inside and so 'screw the lumbars'. This gives a forward displacement as well. The effective distance between the inside shoulder and the inside point of the hip is now less; and that between the outside points relatively greater.

  The 'leg' aid inside reflexly stimulates a greater forward reach, and engagement of the inside hind leg. The neck, 'hand-led' into the appropriate lateral bend, restricts the protraction of the inside fore shoulder. Riding, conversely must prevent the outside shoulder falling out under the rider's weight

- **'The Horse Must Bascule Over a Fence'** – and in doing so must describe, at any point in flight, a symmetrical curve or parabola from poll to dock.

  No way! What does describe a perfect parabola is the top line of the swinging centre of gravity or, in this situation, the identical 'centre of rotation' of the body. The horse lifts off his forehand into an elevation to start a trajectory which will 'clear' the obstacle. The hind legs kick off together to propel the trunk along the projected incline. The fore limbs are tucked up, and the head and the neck flexed down on T1 and T2 after the head has passed maximum height. The hind feet move from extension into flexion and then protraction, with the croup well flexed at L6 and S1. The horse can and must keep its head and neck down until the quarters have passed maximum height, when the neck begins to elevate ready for a secure landing.

When take off, elevation and landing are reasonably spaced and equidistant, the centre of gravity or rotation moves in a perfect arc. No flexion occurs along the thoraco-lumbar vertebral line. The straight line from posterior withers to point of croup is maintained; in any ideal and correct jumping the back is held rigid

Certain requirements are feasible

- **The Vertical Carriage**
  The desired curve, from base of neck to the poll without a break or bend around C3–C4, is anatomically and functionally possible, but it requires expert schooling not so much to attain this ideal within 'self carriage' but more to prevent the wrong bend occurring

- **Lateral Bend of the Neck from Withers to Poll**
  This is similar

- **Head Carriage From the Occiput/Atlas Joint**
  This is also a matter of schooling. A natural head carriage of 30–40° in front of the vertical (depending on individual conformation) is naturally possible. The dressage 'on the bit with muzzle just ahead of the vertical' is, however, a schooling requirement

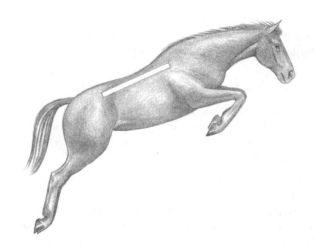

No flexion occurs along the thoraco-lumbar vertebral line – it remains straight.

There is much sense in the need to *'more fully engage the hindquarters'*.

The lumbo-sacral flexion, just below the point of croup, is an essential movement whereby the femero-pelvic joint or hip is brought forward and lower; the hind leg therefore can reach further forward.

The horse moves within the limitations of its conformation and its state of health. The rider may be an added handicap to perfect locomotion if his centre of gravity does not relate to that of the horse.

The dynamics of movement require the interaction of rigidity and elasticity in the limbs as well as in the spine and trunk.

When the horse leaves the ground by pushing and lifting his mass up and along, he will return to a new point on the ground at a force which reflects the speed at which he is moving *and* the elevation he attained. The ground if firm and too hard will offer an opposite and equal force to this dynamic weight: the ground force reaction. It is therefore important to be aware of the nature of the surface. 'Give' in the ground absorbs the impact of the downward force and the upward force. In 'soft going' this minimising of concussion can go so far as be 'holding'.

All the tissues involved in the structure of the horse and, in particular, the connective tissues of hoof, bone, cartilage, ligament, tendon and muscle, have to be conditioned and the muscles trained or fittened. Within them all, even the bone, there has to be an element of 'give' or elasticity. Working the horse to an extent to which it has not been conditioned or fittened places over-stress on these tissues.

At any given level of stress, there are four possible responses: competence, adaptation, fatigue, and failure

- **competence** is where the stress level is within the horse's capacity and does not produce any increased biological activity; there has been no training benefit

- **adaptation** is where the higher level of stress is sufficient to develop more capacity without damage

- in **fatigue**, stress has been sufficient to weaken the involved tissues temporarily. However, these can still adapt if the over-stressed system is given time to regain integrity. Most adaptation levels induce some degree of fatigue; the trainer's skill is to be aware that he has reached this but has not yet 'over-fatigued' a particular system or part therein, and then to judge how far to go back in the training programme before stressing the system again

- **failure** indicates that the integrity of the system or

tissues has broken down. It may be the result of a single severe overloading or, more commonly, a succession of lesser overloadings which lead to excessive fatiguing over-stresses and so to failure

Adaptation stresses are said to have imposed a desired, reversible, **elastic deformity** on the tissues; whereas any fatigue – from which the system recovers only after a long delay or, in fact, never – is said to produce a **plastic deformity**. In the young, immature horse the careful monitoring of these stresses is particularly important. Even in the older animal it is important that the training rate is no greater than that which allows rapid and uneventful recovery from fatigue.

It is those structures and functioning which have been advantageous to the horse in his evolution which are often its weakest links in these domesticated athletic circumstances.

MUSCLES

Muscles are units of force production: they perform 'work'. They expend (spend) energy.

All animals have three types of muscles: **cardiac**, **visceral** and **skeletal**. The cardiac and visceral types' smooth muscle fibres, known as involuntary muscles, are described in their respective chapters.

In the horse, as in many other animals and man, two sub-types of skeletal, striated, voluntary muscles are recognised, according to their microscopic appearance, their biochemical characteristics and their potential biomechanical effects.

When the flesh of an animal which depends for its survival on quick bursts of speed (a rabbit, for example), is examined, the *pale* colour of all the flesh is noticeable. In a hare, on the other hand, whose survival depends on twisting and turning during a long period of escape, the appropriate group of muscles is *redder*, more capable of endurance work.

The difference in muscle 'colour' is due to the amount of myoglobin and other energy-producing pigments, the greater capillary blood circulation, and the greater number of the mitochondria in those muscle cells which work aerobically, i.e. are able to use maximum oxygen. These are known as **slow twitch** muscle fibres.

Physiologically they respond to training for increasing fitness in slow to medium work. Theoretically they can work for ever!

Conversely, the speed fibres, the **fast twitch** type, are

metabolically anaerobic and as such are much less dependent on oxygen. These fibres are greater in cross section to store more muscle sugar; they are paler.

This colour difference is blended in the horse and the difference is not macroscopically obvious. Histological and biochemical examinations of muscles can reveal this metabolic difference.

Individual muscles have both sub-types; it is the ratio which is significant. Basically, the fibres are

- **slow twitch** (ST), which function *aerobically*
- **fast twitch** (FT), which function *anaerobically*, have a limited action time – up to about four minutes. As they work in the absence of oxygen, they produce a larger amount of lactic acid and hydrogen ions. When the levels of these build up in the muscle cells, surrounding fluid, and in the capillaries, they have a limiting effect which can terminate the fast twitch muscle action. Such muscle fibres do not respond to training in speed and duration but 'practising' their use, as by galloping, increases their strength and 'skills'. A sub-group

  - **fast twitch high oxidative** (FTH) form a variable proportion of all horse muscle fibres, from one third to one half. They are capable of being trained to work aerobically. Their usefulness is at a maximum when their oxidative aerobic potential is developed by training. They are athletic essentials

The proportion of muscle fibre types in any one group of muscles is genetically determined, but the investigative work done several years ago from muscle biopsy, either in the adult competition horse or in the foal for its potential, has not proved as predictive as was originally thought. Recent research shows that relative fibre composition is similar in pattern within a breed, but variable in an individual in as much as different biopsy sites in any major muscle group reveal variable proportions – making predictions of potential performance unreliable. Athletic potential does, however, seem to be reflected by mean fibre area, capillary density, biochemistry characteristics and enzyme activity.

The aerobic fibres are the primary focus of **muscle tone**, which is a persisting force active even in apparently resting muscle and/or in muscles involved indirectly in posture and stance support. Such **tonus** is a healthy state of readiness for immediate full contraction when required for action. Anaerobic fibres build up to peak contractions, and thus generate stronger force in a short phase before relaxing; muscles with a predominance of these are engaged in propulsive effect.

The training of muscles, and the fundamental nourishment of them, is dealt with in Part 3.

Muscular Action in Locomotion

During evolution the horse 'became' a solipedal unguligrade which improved its chances of survival from predators through flight over wide open spaces. It had to become a galloper but with three basic gaits for nomadic purposes, with ease of transition between them, and in the asymmetric gaits an ability to change the lead to maintain balance as it twisted and turned and to delay total fatigue by alternating unilateral action.

The ungulate's horny hoof gave protection to the pedal bone, the third phalanx, on which tiptoe he had the benefits of an enlongated stride and an increase in relative height for better vision.

The solipedal structure of such an elongated limb required fewer limb muscles, and these came no lower than three-quarters of the way down the radius and the tibia, in which the respective ulna and fibula bones did not have a distal extremity let alone an articulation there. Resistance of elongated muscle bulk to wind while galloping, and the reduction of distal weight for ease of flexion, were both important further coincidental benefits. Other, propulsion muscles, of necessity of considerable bulk, were concentrated high on the shoulder and pelvic girdles. The disadvantages of the subsequently required elongated tendons and distal ligaments is considered under Lameness.

Motion is produced by the **contraction** and **relaxation** of alternating, opposing groups of muscles acting reciprocally on the skeletal levers and eventually on the hooves as fulcrums on the ground surface.

Each muscle bundle is made up of many, many fibres, cells of an elongated design. Each bundle of fibres can contract and then must relax. The contraction of all individual bundles to their maximum extent, that is when they have been fully shortened, will have exerted a maximum effort on the related bones over one or more articulations.

Conversely, as explained above, no muscle ever relaxes completely; a degree of tone is always retained.

Full effect is gained when all bundles in a particular muscle are stimulated. Gradation of power relates to how many fibres in any one muscle bundle are recruited. The more forceful the movement, the greater number of fibres that come into play.

The converse of tonus is **spasm** following fatigue, injury or dis-ease of the neuro-muscular skeletal unit. Spasm reduces muscle ability and may even prevent any action at all from the muscle.

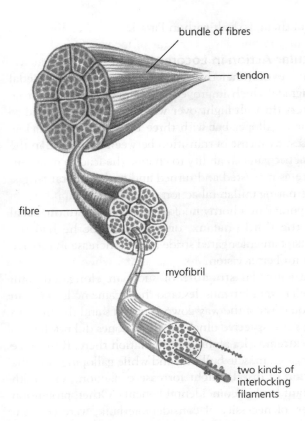

A muscle bundle.

In action, one muscle or group of muscles will contract to a predetermined extent, and the opposing muscles will relax at the same tempo and to the required extent. Thereby, the movement of the joints and bones are controlled and free of any inelegant, jerky action – a smooth excursion from a predetermined range of the joint; totally, or to a degree between. The aim is to avoid inflicting third order acceleration forces on the joint with resultant overheating, or to avoid loss of control of the extent of the movement which would impose an overstress on the supporting ligaments.

The only way a muscle can perform 'work' is by contracting and, therefore, shortening, so that the result is a pull. It cannot 'push'. It can be stretched to its original relaxed tonic length by the action of the opposing muscle, and its degree of tone or readiness to 'take the strain' prevents an overstretching and subsequent tearing of its fibres and the fibres of its tendon. A tired muscle can fail in these functions, especially with regard to the tendon which is 'left' to take the over-stress or strain.

Once locomotion has started, subsequent steps are automatic but always under lower cerebral central nervous system control based on feedback information through the proprioceptor system from sensory nerves in joints, tendons and ligaments relayed via the vertebral cord to the lower centres of the brain. If there is no adverse information, that centre continues to send the reflex messages to move the next leg in the sequence, and so on until the first and subsequent strides are completed to effect the desired movement.

Many influences will determine changes in speed, and transitions up or down through the gaits to accommodate these. The horse makes voluntary decisions based on information received via the external sense organs, or involuntary ones if, for example, the going dramatically alters and, of course, when tiredness and fatigue set in. Training not only delays the onset of fatigue but also teaches skills which enable the horse to move more efficiently and safely.

The motor nerves to muscles come from one to several cervical, thoraco-lumbar and sacral segments of the vertebral cord. Those to the limbs are from nerve roots in the forequarter area C5–T4 and in the hindquarter L3–S5. Sensory nerves travel back to the vertebral column within the anatomically related nerve trunk along with the outgoing or efferent motor nerves.

Horse and human muscles are arranged differently, as far as locomotion is concerned. In the human, the muscles are relatively long and lie parallel to the bones which they move; in horses, the key propulsive muscles are in the quarters, the thigh and in the shoulder and the neck; generally speaking, they tend to meet the bone at a greater angle.

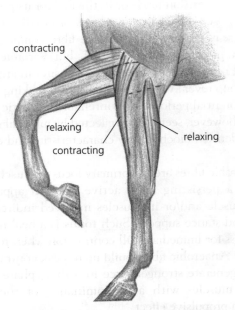

Muscles in contraction and relaxation.

This gives them greater power in a slower and so shorter stroke. The positioning of such muscles on the level of the trunk not only minimises the weight which the limb would have to overcome when in motion, but also gives a better overall biomechanical effect on the action of the legs. In biomechanical terms, a 'mechanical advantage' is said to exist if strategic design has the fulcrum so placed that a small force can move a heavy load a short distance; this is rare in equine locomotion – the more common 'mechanical *dis*advantage' obtains, in which the light load is moved a long distance by a larger force, e.g. the stride length of a lightened limb.

Motion depends on the limbs being moved through radii, with the feet being the fulcrums which, because they are furthest away from the muscle mass, makes the effects of muscle contraction more effective. This power is enhanced by the functional rigidity of the vertebral column, the lumbo-sacral capability, and through the 'gliding' potential of the shoulder blade. It also depends upon a secure foothold or stance.

Joints

The limb joints of the horse are nearly all hinged joints subject to flexion and extension and so moving in one plane. The joint with its cartilage, bone, ligaments, tendons and muscles is the unit of locomotion; the articular surfaces are the part of the limb which takes much of the concussion and compression involved in weight-bearing and lift off.

A joint consists of two bones which are said to **articulate** with one another, and the articular surfaces are moulded to fit into each other as a single or double 'ball and socket'.

Each surface is covered by **hyaline cartilage** which, whilst it has neither blood supply nor nerve supply, is the focal point of joint action. Forming a cuff round the articular heads is a double layer of connective tissue called the **joint capsule**. The outer forms a primary support and also an area of attachment for ligaments, when these blend with the periosteum of the bone. The inner layer, the **synovial membrane**, secretes a lubricating oil, the **synovial fluid** and, on weight-bearing, the water content of this is squeezed into the cartilages for an added hydraulic shock-absorbing effect as well as nourishing this subtly designed tissue. The capsule layers are well supplied with nerves but only the outer layer of the synovium has the blood vessels, a self-preservation of the synovial mucous membrane which is biomechanically exposed to various stresses which could traumatise superficial blood vessels with the risk of haemorrhages into the joint cavity.

The limb as a lever system.

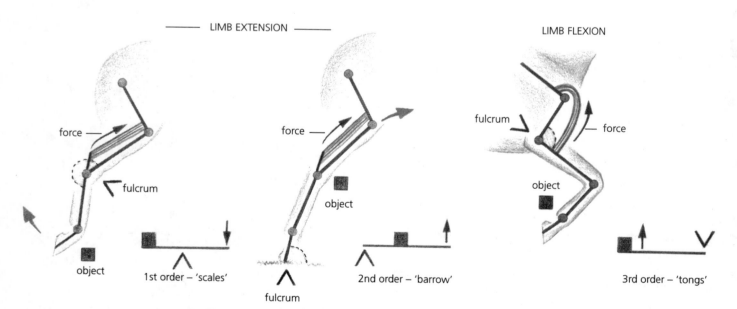

LIMB EXTENSION

force

fulcrum

object

1st order – 'scales'

hind leg extends to kick out backwards

force

object

fulcrum

2nd order – 'barrow'

hind leg extends on a fixed fulcrum and so propels the proximal limb forward

LIMB FLEXION

fulcrum

force

object

3rd order – 'tongs'

the leg flexes on the joints and so shortens to lift the free leg off the ground

The joint is further stabilised by ligaments running from bone to bone, and their positioning not only supports the joint but frequently directs and limits its range of movement. The nerve supply is of sensory proprioceptors which feed positional information back to the central nervous system and sensory nociceptors for pain information.

Almost all joints of the limb function on the principle of the lever, of which there are three 'orders' in all mechanics. In the horse, the first order is involved in free limb extension backwards – a kick. The second order is involved in the hind leg on a fixed hoof fulcrum extending; the third order is that of flexion, as in the elbow and 'knee' and in the stifle and hock and the three distal joints of both fore and hind limbs. Each joint or 'linkage between levers' has its own order, but in the unified limb movement within a cycle it is the hoof which is the primary point.

The joints are activated by the opposing action of flexor and extensor muscles augmented, in certain joints, by other muscles, *synergists* or *agonists*, which have a stabilising and in some cases alternative directional property. The muscle contraction power is passed to the bone through an intervening **tendon**, and where that tendon passes over a joint surface it is encased in a synovial sheath; all the sheaths in a particular joint area are held close to the bones by surrounding anular ligaments and fascia.

The Role of Non-Articular Ligaments

An important feature both of the forelegs and of the hind legs is the quantity and distribution of the non-articular ligaments. These play a part in supporting the limbs on landing, on weight-bearing, and at take off, as well as having an important role in permitting the horse to rest whilst standing – the **stay apparatus** and the **suspensory apparatus**.

PROPULSION

Forward propulsion requires the hoof (or hooves) to have a ground friction resistance, against which the limb forces work.

Before the advent of slow-motion photography, it had been assumed that the forelegs played little part in propulsion but were mainly concerned with 'catching' the weight of the body when it finished a cycle and holding it upright against the force of gravity. Although most of the propulsive power does come from the hind legs, it is now seen that the forelegs contribute a significant percentage of the overall power, in the asymmetric gaits particularly, in the lift-off from weight-bearing and in forward movement, as well as adding to the overall asymmetric stride length.

All muscles play a part in locomotion, including the ring of vertebrals and others involved in the control of 'back' movement. In the foreleg, the major muscle involved in the forward motion of the shoulder region is the **brachiocephalicus**. This muscle is indirectly attached to the scapula via fascia and runs on over the point of the shoulder, attaching at one end to the head and the atlas, and at the other end to the mid-front portion of the humerus. It thereby serves to rotate the scapula forward, and to very slightly straighten the angle between the scapula and the humerus. When the horse is stationary or on turning, contraction of either one of the muscles will pull the head and neck round to that side. When the brachiocephalicus muscles contract simultaneously, they not only elevate the forehand well off the ground but also bring the points of the shoulders forward: the horse elevates into forward movement. It is by no means the only one so involved.

In addition, when the support phase of the forelegs is finished, the potential energy stored in the tendons relating to the fetlock/pastern region is translated into kinetic energy and, with the help of the digital flexor muscles, adds to the lifting of the horse off the ground.

The various neck and shoulder muscles and the **latissimus dorsi** all play their part, the latter forming a linkage from the pelvis via fascia and the humerus via insertions thereon to effect retraction of the forelimb.

In the hind limb, there is a direct bony connection to the axial skeleton, since in the adult horse the pelvic girdle with the sacrum and the first three coccygeal vertebrae are effectively fused together; the sacro-iliac joints are non-functional. This required fusion is to benefit the transfer of the power created by the hind limbs onto the spine, as well as to form a stable area for the origin of the hindquarters' extrinsic locomotor muscles. It should be noted that the hips, stifle and hock joints must move synchronously, which also helps stabilise the propulsive power from the hindquarters.

The bilateral **longissimus dorsi** and other muscles compress the vertebrae of the thoraco-lumbar vertebral column to add to its stability by the associated extension of the column from wither to dock.

The lumbo-sacral joint is the most movable in the axial column; its flexion, most noticeable in asymmetric gaits, permits the pelvis to move downward and forward, thereby giving the hind legs more forward stride range. At support and at lift off, the leg has to be 'held' in order not to dissipate the forward propulsion – hence the functional advantage of patellar lock and subsequent synchronised hip/stifle/hock action.

The limbs are held in extension at the appropriate times of support and take off, and then are folded up to reduce the drag effect of their relative long length. Finally, they are extended into the protracted position of flight so that, on subsequent retraction, the feet are brought to the ground in a correct position for maximum security of landing and maximum support. Holding in extension for this stance phase does not necessarily mean a completely straight limb; in the foreleg there is flexion between scapula and humerus, and in the hind leg the angulation begins between the pelvis and the femur. In both legs, further angulation occurs distally: the fetlock is 'let down'.

The elbow joint angulation at support is in the 'extended' position for that joint. The same applies to the stifle and to the true hock joint. All these merely 'look bent' – anatomically angulated to varying degrees relative to type and to individual conformation.

FLEXION AND EXTENSION

The anatomical design of the joints determines the direction of movement of the limbs. In the majority of cases in the limb, it is flexion and extension in a forward and backward direction, and this is related to the construction of the limb with a single toe protected by horn. The horse cannot rotate a limb from the elbow or hock (ankle) as can man. It can **abduct** (carry it out from the mid line) and can **adduct** (carry it over and beyond the mid line) from the proximal aspect of the limb, but the hoof still points forward relative to the whole column of support.

The two rows of small bones in the carpal and tarsal joints, whilst of limited flexion and extension range, have a sliding action which produces a minor separating one from the other in a plane which is oblique to the horizontal. This has heat reducing and anti-shock faculties. The main joint in these two areas is above the small carpal and tarsal bones: the radio-carpal and the tibio-tarsal joints respectively.

As previously described, the forelegs 'carry' about 60% of the total body weight at rest. This is due to the anatomical and functional design of the horse where it can stand, at rest, with minimal muscular effort provided

- both forelegs are at halt position, i.e. in maximal weight-bearing position

- the neck is 'let down' to about the horizontal position
- the head is so suspended from the neck that it is approximately at right-angles to the neck, and therefore, at right-angles to the ground

In this position the head and neck counter-balance the rest of the body, pivoting over the forelegs with the thorax 'slung' between the scapula. One hind leg takes around 40% of the body weight in the reciprocally locked position – which requires little muscular supporting action. The other hind leg, alternating at 3 to 5 minute intervals and with no postural muscular effort, 'rests' on the toe part of the hoof wall with all joints in the relaxed position.

Moving off from Standstill

Displacing the centre of gravity back from the position at rest comprises two obvious movements (lifting the neck and head, using both hind legs to support), and one subtle movement (a slight flexion of the stifles/hocks to fractionally lower the croup and pelvis usually more on one side than the other).

Most 'moving off' begins with a hind leg. Although it may be remarked that a horse, said to be heavy on its forehand, is pulling or 'clawing' its weight forward with its forelegs, this is not so; propulsion has to be initiated from behind. A foreleg at standstill can be protracted and the hoof made to make ground contact ahead of the original position, but the subsequent retraction produces a 'pawing' action only. Before a foreleg influences forward movement the forequarter must be propelled beyond the foreleg's vertical; then lift off, then protraction with subsequent retraction to footfall and backward effect will have 'propulsion effect'.

When the 'selected' gait requires an explosive start-off, as in starting stalls or for flight, the hindquarters perceptibly sink; the flexion of the hip, stifle, hock and fetlock induce a store of kinetic energy in the associated ligaments and tendons which, with appropriate extrinsic muscle action, is released to give a powerful lift-off from both hind feet. The forehand is then elevated for protraction into the next stride.

At slower gaits a single hind leg begins the action, propelling the body mass forward. An opposite foreleg lifts off to protract forward, and then retracts to 'take the weight' to maintain balance – and so on.

The young, untutored horse is not so elegant in these starting movements and will elevate its forequarters to clear the forelegs for protraction.

The muscles involved can be named individually,

especially the synchronised give-and-take, by agonist/antagonist, flexor/extensor – both in the intrinsic, which motivate the limbs alternately as struts and levers, and in the extrinsic in the shoulder and hindquarters which elevate and propel.

What is important is the ability to recognise the development of them with increasing fitness (and co-incidental loss of fat), to appreciate from palpation that such fitness is not a hard tissue but, in relaxed mode, has a soft elastic palpable tone and, in contraction, a firmness with greater rebound to digital pressure. Above all, it is important to appreciate that such development is *bilaterally symmetrical*.

The good rider must be able to 'ask' for such activity so that symmetry can be regained by work (provided any underlying functional defect has been rectified or ruled out), and to know how to 'engage' all parts of the body to this end. Such an ability requires good perception as well as 'good feel' through the breeches – kinaesthesia – and, of course, a detailed understanding of the horse's action in all the gaits.

Balance

At the free **walk** a free moving horse will

- swing his head and neck in rhythm with the foreleg stride's protraction phase
- swing his quarters alternately forwards, in rhythm with related hind leg stride – the appearance as seen from behind is that of laterally swinging hips
- give a feel of rhythmic movement to the rider (much exaggerated in a steep descent, for the required braking effort), with the tail swinging laterally in opposing rhythm

At **trot**

- the head is held comparatively still
- the foreleg action, in time with the diagonal hind leg, will give a vertical (and horizontal) lift and fall through the back
- the quarters will show little lateral sway; the hind leg action is mainly that of flexion and extension of the stifle and lower joints, with hip involvement related to the required stride length. As seen from behind, the

promontories of the entire vertical limb will alternately rise at footfall and fall with support, before rising again into the swing phase

At the **asymmetric gaits**

- the head and the neck will rise and fall relative to foreleg suspension and support
- the quarters will elevate at hind leg lift off
- the hind legs, aided by increased lumbo-sacral flexion, will 'engage' further forwards under the abdomen. The hind limb engagement depends on
    - the initial flexion at the lumbo-sacral joint
    - the synchronised stability of support and lift-off of the extension of this joint *and* the other distal articulations
- the overall motion is that of a controlled up-and-down swing, with appropriate functional rigidity in the thoraco-lumbar vertebral column. The faster this gait, as in racehorse 'gallop', the less the switchback; the good horse is said to move *level and close to the ground* – all the effort is in forward movement

The elevation into suspension comes with the leading foreleg lift-off, but the propulsion comes through from the leading hind leg thrust, which ultimately lifts the forehand at the withers. Here there is greater need for vertebral column stability or rigidity, but this should not interfere with neck and quarter flexion and extension, but rather give a sensation of elasticity as well as balanced power.

The young, inexperienced horse being broken to faster gaits will develop 'balance' when it exercises freely in a field or in a large indoor school: this is a self-preservation requirement. When first ridden this balance will be upset, hence the need for a balanced rider. It will have to re-learn self carriage, gradually, progressively up through the gaits and, if necessary, into jumping. An assessment of a 'new' horse's self carriage is best determined when it is viewed 'loose' in a school and then, when reasonably fit, correctly ridden.

Recent biomechanical slow-motion photography and upward ground force analyses show that the trailing foreleg at 'let down' and at lift-off experiences the major stress, thus explaining the greater incidence of superficial flexor tendon over-stress (strain) in that leg.

CHAPTER 18

FUNCTIONAL CONTROLS

Chapter 1, EVOLUTION AND BEHAVIOUR, describes the behaviour patterns induced and ultimately built into the horse's genetic make-up by the demands of evolutionary development. Eating, drinking, locomotion and reproductive activity all patently occurred day by day, season by season. All became *instinctive*, some refined by mimicry and others by 'experience'.

Some of the behaviour and its instigation, and the resulting sensory feedback input which influenced subsequent action or reaction, was *subconsciously* determined – 'intuitive', not reasoned – under the control of the **lower cerebral nervous system** and therefore *involuntary*, and any outward signs such as breathing and eating were the result of 'inward instruction' which was not consciously appreciated by the horse. The vital functions of living – breathing, circulating the blood, digesting food, and nerve activity – were too important to be left to the animal, and too 'delicate' to risk being exposed to the individual whim of man or horse.

How these body systems function is described under the related chapters, and much mention is made of the integration of one system with another, all to subserve a horse's life as a **nomadic**, **gregarious**, **herbivorous**, **solipedal quadruped**. Such controls are genetically imprinted to 'regulate the regulators', so that the rhythm of living and reproducing is maintained.

The living animal does not function 'like clockwork' with an unalterable output from its many working parts, but it does have a 'biological clock'.

The horse is programmed to have a *resting heart beat of average 36–42 beats per minute (bpm)*, to have a *resting respiratory rate of average 10–15 per minute* with the related systems immediately responsive to altered demands for oxygen, in order to *move quickly* as required

to safety, to use *appropriate gaits*, to *trickle feed* in short but frequent periods in response to 'hunger' and to meet a bulk input requirement, to *rest and sleep* in small but frequent periods, and to *reproduce.*

It is also programmed to recognise day from night, though only in so far as changes in ambient temperature (and so the presence of flies) influences comfort to eat, move and rest. In the horse's evolution, predator habits must also have had an effect; predators usually hunted in daylight but not in the 'heat of the day'.

Diurnal Rhythm

The body core temperature is maintained within very narrow limits. However there is a recognised **diurnal rhythm** which particularly influences body core temperature – *the evening temperature is 0.5°C (1°F) higher than the morning's*. Such an increase is significant in an elite equine athlete, so it is essential that a trainer is aware of this possible individual idiosyncrasy and is not surprised into thinking it a significant rise (a mild fever), sufficient to cancel a race or competition or training

Resting heart rate and resting respiratory rate may also vary, but not as significantly as to require bi-daily recording.

Seasonal Rhythm

In response to longer hours of daylight (*not* environment temperature), sensory input via the eyes and subsequent neuro/hormonal integration

- the winter coat is **cast**, and a summer coat grows
- mares begin to show **oestral behaviour**
- stallions become more **sexually active**
- **helminth** (worm) populations within the gut become more prolific – the Spring rise of egg laying to 'meet' ideal external conditions for hatching

Oestral Rhythm

In response to the seasonal rhythms' influence on **pituitary hormone secretion**, the sexual rhythm within the 'breeding season' becomes patent in *cycles of 20 days*. The rhythm 'shuts down' completely if pregnancy supervenes, and wanes if not ceases as daylight hours diminish in the autumn.

These three rhythms – diurnal, seasonal and oestral – are reflex activities begun by

- sensory inputs to the brain, via cranial nerves
- other inputs to the brain, direct or via the cord and the autonomic system, which 'trigger' motor messages from them to larger organs – in many cases through hormonal stimulation but often with the possibility of sub-conscious motor correction (of, for example, posture when that is the end result)
- conscious motor activity, to meet one-off contingencies

Body Systems Co-ordination

As humans, we take our breathing and our heart beating for granted; we are rarely aware of their activity until we exercise beyond our normal limits – and our breathing becomes 'laboured' and we feel our heart 'thumping'.

We can be aware of hunger; but once food is put before us, eating is almost automatic. We give no thought as a rule to our digestion; we give a little more thought, for social reasons and comfort, to our excretions. Similarly, our daily work can with practice become routine, unless our skills alert us to a problem – admittedly, we have to decide where to go, know what to do and recognise our equipment, but we give little if any attention to how the energy for our muscles gets to them and how they actually work. Likewise, we may feel hot from our exertions, and be aware of 'sweat on the brow', but how our body knows when to sweat, and where it comes from, raises but little interest. There is no reason to believe that a horse is different.

As we ride, we do not think about our horse's muscle cell contraction, carbon dioxide excretion and electrolyte loss in sweat. After all, the horse does it all involuntarily, without 'inside' concern! It recovers, ready to go the next time.

Body Systems Controls

All animals function in a manner natural to their evolved, specific requirements. Fundamentally these functionings are to facilitate *living*, *moving* and *eating*, for *survival*, in order to *reproduce* – the criteria of all life, whether uni- or multi-cellular. To function effectively, the animal's systems must be co-ordinated and under control. Much of all this takes place unseen and is taken for granted by the horse-master.

Whilst the nervous system control plays a major role, it is not the only one. Thus

- the foal's behaviour is **imprinted** at an early age. Its gaits are genetically determined, so that it 'goes like a horse', and its dam sees to it that it practises these, so that
- its locomotion, either as an individual or as one within the herd running as a group, is in a safe, balanced manner. The posture necessary for grazing is copied – *'What's mother doing with her head down there?'*, and *'What is this 'smell' and 'feel' she is eating?'*
- the posture of defaecation reflexly follows the sensation of 'something close under the tail', which reflexly stimulates straining by the rectal musculature, which in turn is augmented by abdominal musculature – a combined voluntary and involuntary activity

The foal uses sensory interpretations from the cranial sensory centres to 'advise' it. The brain's cerebral cortex, now aware of suitability and safety for moving and where to go (the foal sees grass, and the ground between seems all right), and it knows what to do when it gets there (eat), all of them conscious decisions (*'Hurry, before others get there'*), leaves the setting of the decided gait pattern and its repetition 'canter on, keep cantering left lead' to the sub-conscious centres in the lower brain.

A fixed pattern of movement is more efficient without constant, conscious, sometimes contradictory and often confusing decisions. It certainly is more economic in energy expenditure and in stress on the suspensory apparatus. Consider the balanced, steady control of the cross-country rider, especially on roads and tracks – the horse canters at a set rate (seemingly 'asleep!') and pays no attention to extraneous distracting information.

But changes may be required: the rider foresees the need for them, or the horse sees something in his path or feels something through his proprioceptor sensory input. The rider 'wakes' the horse up, and the horse changes his speed or his gait just as he did when he moved free in a herd – *'Look out, there's a ditch ahead,'* *'Beware that aggressive horse,'* *'I don't like the smell of this grass.'* All this new sensory information must be analysed consciously but quickly, and action for safety and survival follows.

Proprioception information may require little thought; righting or rebalancing of ongoing action is often automatically reflexed through lower brain centres, and the horse successfully copes with undulating or changing 'going'.

Fear of what is seen, heard or felt (e.g. the whip), 'mind over matter' inputs, can over-rule these, so that the horse 'keeps going at all costs'.

Many conscious-led decisions are intuitive in the horse; they are based on instinct and experience, not on reasoning or intelligence.

All nerve (sensory) inputs and (motor) outputs describe 'arcs'. Some arcs are a series of relays through several brain centres, others along the vertebral cord and 'out' further down via a relay; but the most quickly effected are into, and immediately out of, the central system, whether brain or cord. Hence

- wave a hand in front of a horse's face, and he will blink, or perhaps even jerk his head away, before his brain had 'time' to weigh-up the situation

- prick the skin of the coronary band, and there will be an immediate withdrawal of the limb. Do the same to a hind leg, and the reflex withdrawal may be quickly followed by a reflex survival fending-off kick, which also does not depend upon a conscious 'decision' unless input persists, when the horse will more consciously attempt to evade or get rid of the perceived cause

- but tap its hoof sole, no response; he has been 'conditioned' to such by the farrier. However, if there is pain already present, the tap will cause increased pain and evoke a withdrawal followed by a conscious attempt to stop you doing it again – because it has, and will again, hurt

All these are in-built self-preservation features.

Reflexes may have to pass via relays through brain centres. These involve the re-balancing requirements – and some are useful in restraint. Lift a foreleg, and the horse will be reflexly reluctant to lift the hind leg on the same side; to ease the lifting of a foreleg, have his head and neck moved over to transfer weight to the *other* foreleg. A farrier's trick on his new apprentice is to move the head and neck over, and then ask his pupil to lift the leg on the same side: *'Can't do it!'* Surreptitiously, the farrier has the apprentice move the head and neck the other way, and – *'Look. Easy!'*

The horse in the wild depended upon learning and practising different activities, not only for defence and for escape, including how to rise fore-end first for early visual activity, but also for daily living, including getting to and eating his grass. He has been instinctively programmed

- to look for, sniff at, and decide where to graze and to drink, and where not to

- to graze frequently, in short spells, over most of the 24 hours
- to consume, daily, an amount of dry matter approximating to 2.5% of his body weight
- to drink

All these involve sensory input and **controllable** decisions, albeit to a built-in programme. He 'decides' that he would eat and, once started, the process of prehension, mastication and first part swallowing continues automatically by voluntary muscle action. He can stop if it seems necessary to do so.

The flow of saliva is, however, **autonomically** stimulated by mastication, and is not under voluntary control. Swallowing is also an **involuntary** activity – by reflex arcs from the sensory nerves in the throat and the gullet, which activate peristaltic muscle contraction for two thirds of the way. Eating and swallowing are activities indirectly visible to the onlooker as far down as the caudal end of the neck, but not from there on. Thereafter, the nerve control is fully autonomic and is eventually under the **myenteric system**. The horse has no conscious awareness of post-swallowing movement through the digestive tract unless pain sensations develop, as in choke, gastric bloat, enteritis, colic, etc. His awareness of these abnormal sensations stimulates abnormal reactions and behaviour, partly autonomically and partly voluntarily.

Defaecation is the next and last visible digestive activity. It can be voluntarily, tactically determined, to comply with species requirements of where to do it – sufficiently controlled for the horse to get to the 'correct' part of a field. It can be done 'on the move', but it is easier to do in a standstill posture.

This **myenteric nervous system** specific to the digestive system acts without central nerve involvement except for sensory awareness of upsets in the digestive function. It is one of the minor branches of the autonomic nervous system, and as such removes the major part of the digestive system from the horse's conscious concern. Conversely, and perhaps more importantly, it keeps the horse from interfering, except for deciding when to eat and what to eat, as determined by instinct and modulated by conscious sight. Conscious control of digestion associated with voluntary interference with 'what' and 'when', would be too much for safety.

The digestive system does not invoke wide ranging control changes. Its blood supply is reflexly 'shut down' during periods of strenuous exercise, to 'free' more blood for the skeletal muscle activity. But there is a constant movement of water and electrolytes (a large part of the total body fluid) through-and-through and in-and-out of the vascular system. The body fluids and their electrolyte constituents are under the control of the autonomic nervous and endocrine systems, and ultimately active through kidney function. A subsidiary is thermo-regulation, as it relates to body core temperature control following exercise and in disease, and water and electrolyte loss through sweating.

The major components of the **autonomic nervous system** (ANS) can also function independently of the central nervous system. The ANS is concerned with transmitting motor stimuli to the muscles of the heart, to the smooth muscles of the gut and other viscera, to the muscles of the blood vessels, and to those of the respiratory airways and of the secretory hormone and other glands. There is also a sensory input, from these 'active' tissues and related areas, to the central nervous system.

Another neurological control of living is the **cardiac**, the second 'minor' autonomic system. It is not, strictly speaking, entirely or actually nerve tissue, but it does have an autonomic reflex capability. It is fundamentally independent of all the other nerve systems; it is vital that the heart should continue to beat, irrespective of all other factors.

However, to meet the hour-by-hour (or more frequent) – variations in blood flow requirements, there are overriding control systems. Thus the 10-fold increase of oxygen requirements of the muscles in work necessitates

- reflex stimuli of the **sympathetic nerves** to accelerate the heart for work
- the auxiliary effect of **adrenalin** on the sympathetic system, then

- when the 'pressure is off', a reflex stimulus of the **parasympathetic** to slow the heart to its resting normal rate

These reflexes and the hormonal influence are via the cardiac centre in the brain, which is receptive to blood chemical changes, for example the hydrogen/ion level. There are further barometric (pressure) centres in the atrium (auricle) and in the aortic arch. There are sensory nerves from the heart to the voluntary nervous system but this has no converse direct motor input. The horse cannot consciously dictate the blood's flow, speed and volume.

In summary, all parts of the nervous system are involved in the control of life. For effective overall control, opposing systems can be seen to be at work (though not always simultaneously or as direct opponents)

- the *sympathetic* – and the *parasympathetic* nerve systems
- *adrenalin* – and *insulin* (controlling blood sugar levels)
- *oestrogen* – and *progesterone* (in reproduction)

'Information' is fed to a control source, 'telling it' about events in the body. Delays in feedback produce rhythms, as in the sexual cycle.

If, in response to a hormone, a targeted organ does its work, the output of the target is coincidentally fed back to the source endocrine gland – and says either 'No more' (a negative feed-back), or 'More, please' (a positive feedback). Most feedback information asks for 'No reaction – all is well' (a negative feedback).

19 SIGNS OF HEALTH

When all the structures and the functionings in all the horse's systems are normal, they produce certain signs or indicators perceivable by the trained horsemaster.

Such a normal horse will have a collection of signs which will produce a general picture of

- **A**ppearance
- **B**ehaviour
- **C**ondition

which imply that it is *healthy* and *at ease* with its environment.

This **A** **B** **C** will be broadly similar for all horses, more so for those of the same breed or type, and relative to age and use.

Individuals within such a group will have slight variations peculiar to their living and action and idiosyncrasy. It is therefore accepted that, for example

- **feeding patterns**, likes and dislikes, can vary

but

- **heart rate at rest**, and
- **respiratory rate at rest**, and
- **temperature at rest**

will all fall within a very narrow range, and that these (especially the temperature, as with some other functioning patterns) may well vary between morning and evening – the **diurnal rhythm**.

The **seasonal changes** also have an influence on the **A** **B** **C**.

Temperament as it affects response to training, and the 'will to win', are all **individual traits** within the general pattern of equine behaviour; they too must be taken into account, as must

- the more mundane **excretory habits**

- the rhythmic effects of the **sexual cycle** – especially in the mare
- the **metabolic response to feed input**, the so-called 'good and bad doers', with or without the secondary influences of **work**, can vary quite widely within the limits of normality for that horse

It is the often slow but recognisable variation from these limits which becomes important; it is difficult to define the limits, and common sense and experience both play a part in the horsemaster's skill.

Locomotion, especially the individual horse's action, its 'way of going', is an important feature of the healthy horse which has to be distinguished from a 'new' abnormal limb action as in lameness.

The qualification of 'sound' is often misleading. Legally, unless in its negative form of 'unsound', it is not acceptable. 'Sound' means free from all aspects of disease, illness and defects. In practice, no one can be legally certain that such a Utopian situation exists, and a veterinary surgeon cannot and must not give such a statement, especially when advising a prospective purchaser. The long-accepted description *'Sound in eyes, heart, wind and action'* is now frowned upon as not being a legally worthwhile guide to future usefulness. The vet at a pre-purchase examination can only say that under certain conditions, present on the day of examination – and using only a thermometer, a stethoscope, hoof testers and, of course, his expected powers of perception – he could find no clinical signs of defects in the eyes, the heart, the wind and the action, and elsewhere as judged from the 'outside', before and following exerting exercise. Such an opinion implies that it has been reached by comparing a study of that horse with the yardstick of many similar horses 'known' to be all right.

In routine daily assessment of the health of a known horse, or the immediate assessment of an unknown one for acceptance into a livery yard, for example, the horsemaster is looking for signs that 'all is well', but he is constantly on guard that something may be wrong. In that event, recognising that 'something is not right' is more important than knowing **what** it is that is 'wrong' and the implications of that unsoundness or unwellness.

All physiological functions are carried out as economically as possible. Thus, at rest, a normal adult horse's heart rate is just as fast and as powerful as is required to circulate sufficient oxygen-containing blood and other nutrients to the tissues, to maintain life. Similarly, in respiration, slow shallow inspiration is followed by a momentary pause before expiration and immediate inspiration again. An occasional deep respiration – a sigh – may be interspersed. At rest, except in very hot and humid weather, the excess heat produced merely by living is easily dissipated, and there is no visible sweating. Even moderate light work and its associated muscular effort will not produce extra heat beyond the capacity of latent thermo-regulation, and so the body core temperature is kept normal.

Harder exercise will call for greater effort from circulation, respiration and the associated heat-losing sweating which will become obvious. These can be monitored. Conversely, the increased metabolism of fever, an illness, will also produce increased heart and respiratory rates as well as sweating dependent on the degree or severity and also degree of pain. *The immediate history is thus seen to be important.*

Daily Routine

A daily routine carried out by the horsemaster, to check on normality in **A** **B** **C**, could typically be

On Entering the Yard
Is the horse's greeting *as usual*?

- watching?
- listening?
- calling?
- impatiently kicking the door, or *whatever is usual for this horse*?

In the Box
Does the horse look *as usual*?

- is he dozing in the far corner, as is his custom? or

- alert – pricked ears, bright eyes?
- interested?
- has the usual amount of feed and water been consumed?
- is the bedding as usual?
- droppings – same number, same place, same consitency, colour and smell?
- is he standing as usual?
- does he move over as usual?
- is the rug tidy – no excess bedding on it?
- with rug off, are there any signs of sweating?
- does he go eagerly to the feed bowl, then turn back to a fresh haynet, perhaps drinking in between?
- has he urinated as usual, as far as you can ascertain?
- is there any variation in wetness of the bedding?
- when settled, is respiratory rate normal?

On Grooming
Is all as one would expect in respect of, or felt through, the skin?

- especially on tack areas?
- in mud-fever areas?
- mouth and nose on spongeing?
- are the corners of the eyes and nostrils free of discharge?
- feel of tendons and other locomotor stress points?
- back reactions, under the saddle and the girth areas?

When Led Out in Hand and When Ridden
Are there any perceivable alterations in his way of going?

Changes from Normal

Note *any* change from normal – notice, for instance, if the horse is usually

- uninterested
- not welcoming or
- won't (can't) get up
- gets up awkwardly
- moves stiffly
- hasn't and doesn't eat and/or drink
- has dirty eyes and/or nostrils, and coughs or sneezes
- is or has been sweating
- has produced less and/or altered faeces and urine

- has sores on skin
- has heat or pain in limbs on palpation
- when standing, rests a foreleg or a hind unusually
- has disturbed bedding and rugs
- has made scuff marks on walls, or on hooves, etc.

If such changes are noticed, then it will be necessary in most of these situations to

- take pulse rate
- take respiration rate, and assess depth and rhythm
- take temperature
- listen for unusual sounds in the breathing and in the abdominal area

If any of these are abnormal, stop work, get advice and help; the same applies to defects in walking or trotting.

Taking the Three Basic Parameters

The three basic parameters of: **heart rate** (pulse), **respiratory rate** and **temperature** are used, usually with the horse in his box

- to confirm an alteration away from resting normal – usually upwards
- in association with other known facts, to determine if the changes
    - are as expected in a healthy horse, e.g. after hard work; and if so, do they return towards normal within the expected time after work
    - are *not* as normally expected – in which case, how significant are they?

Generally, a non-normal rise is significant but its interpretation may well require skilled (veterinary) help.

Whether taking the measurements at rest or after exercise, the horse must be approached and handled in a manner that will not confuse the issue by exciting or alarming it. Most horses will react to unusual situations by accelerating both heart and respiratory rates – *fright*, preparing for *fight* and subsequent *flight* – so time must be given either to prevent these or to allow them to settle. The athletic horse will have had these parameter readings made so frequently as to make it accustomed to the procedure, but even so – and especially since it is tuned up for fitness – such an action will accelerate the heart and lungs albeit momentarily. The horse not used to it will require

greater care, not only to obtain more accurate readings but also to avoid violent and therefore potentially dangerous reaction.

Respiratory Rate

Respiratory rate is taken first, from outside the box

- let the horse become aware of your presence outside his box, but away from sniffing distance
- let him settle, and eat if he wishes
- look at his abdomen; preferably with him standing tail towards you
- watch the abdominal wall move
- look for the short pause
- watch the wall move again
- now count the number of times of 'in, pause, out' in sixty seconds or, preferably, in 4 separate periods each of 15 seconds
- gauge the range of 'in and out' (but it is the rate which is more important)

The resting normal is typically 10–15 respirations per minute.

Heart Rate

Now enter the box, and attach the head collar and rope preparatory to taking heart rate.

- gentle the horse; talk softly, firmly but kindly, and stroke his neck
- when quiet, take his pulse. Ensure that helpers are quiet and out of sight, and that no other horses walk past

The heart rate is typically 25–40 beats per minute.

If at any stage in the counts of respiratory and heart rate recordings there is a sudden marked rise, ignore and restart, unless the rate is persistently higher than normal from the start.

Temperature

You will require a helper, and a thermometer – a stumpy bulb one. (When not in use, it should be kept always in the same safe place.)

- remove the thermometer from its case and (if it is a mercury type) shake down until the mercury is below 37°C (98°F) . The shaking should be done over straw –

The three points at which the pulse can most easily be felt.

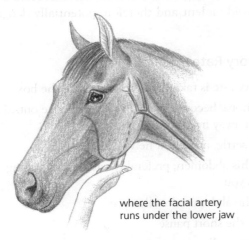

where the facial artery runs under the lower jaw

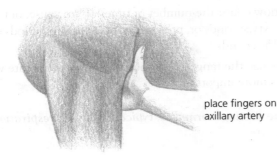

place fingers on axillary artery

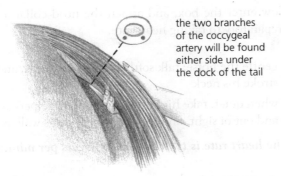

the two branches of the coccygeal artery will be found either side under the dock of the tail

you might drop it – but out of range of the horse's tail!

- carefully lubricate bulb end and a short way up the stem with a little liquid soap or similar
- have the helper hold the horse close to the wall most suitable for you, with the horse's head near the corner, and lift the outside foreleg
- stand on the 'up' foreleg side, close to the quarters and just behind
- grip the tail, and pull well to the side of the quarters
- speak soothingly to the horse

- gently insert bulb into the anal sphincter
- insert three-quarters of the thermometer
- angle the stem to one side, in order to have the bulb rest against mucous membrane and not in a ball of (colder) faeces
- holding thermometer, leave for at least half a minute
- withdraw, and move out of range of the horse's tail swish
- have helper release leg, but continue to hold head
- read thermometer – *if the reading has not risen at all, repeat the above procedure, pushing bulb well to one side*
- if satisfied, have the horse released. Outside the box, shake thermometer down, clean it with cotton wool moistened with luke warm water with a little antiseptic diluted as for wound dressing, and replace it in its cover and store safely
- write down all readings, along with other relevant information

Temperature is typically 37.8–38.3°C (100–101°F).

It is always advisable to know a horse's normal readings. They should be taken each morning and evening for several days, after it has been got up and stabled for about one week. The readings will give an average and enable the horsemaster to recognise any diurnal rhythm, especially of the temperature. Thus a base line for that horse can go on a record sheet. *Do not wait until the horse is suspected of being ill.*

Quick Method

Experienced workers will be able to take all three measurements together, more or less simultaneously

- with horse held, leg up if deemed necessary, and allowed to settle
- stand behind and to one side
- lift tail
- count breathing
- take tail pulse
- insert thermometer and take reading

Know your horse. Be constantly aware of <u>A</u> <u>B</u> <u>C</u> changes. Take no chances by ignoring them. *Be particularly observant the evening and morning after strenuous work.*

DISEASES OF THE HORSE

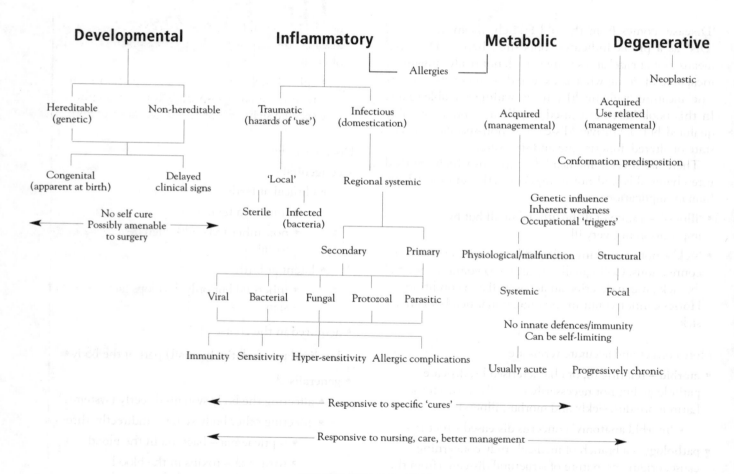

Developmental

Hereditable (genetic)   Non-hereditable

Congenital (apparent at birth)   Delayed clinical signs

← No self cure Possibly amenable to surgery →

Inflammatory

Allergies

Traumatic (hazards of 'use')   Infectious (domestication)

'Local'   Regional systemic

Sterile   Infected (bacteria)

Secondary   Primary

Viral   Bacterial   Fungal   Protozoal   Parasitic

Immunity   Sensitivity   Hyper-sensitivity   Allergic complications

Metabolic

Acquired (managemental)

Physiological/malfunction

Systemic

No innate defences/immunity Can be self-limiting

Usually acute

Degenerative

Neoplastic

Acquired Use related (managemental)

Conformation predisposition

Genetic influence Inherent weakness Occupational 'triggers'

Structural

Focal

Progressively chronic

← Responsive to specific 'cures' →

← Responsive to nursing, care, better management →

TYPES OF DIS-EASE

CHAPTER

20 DISEASE

'**Disease**' comes from the old French, meaning 'sickly'. '**Dis**' as a prefix indicates 'opposite'; hence **'Dis-ease'** means 'not at ease' and so 'unwell, ill, not ready, unwilling, incapable of doing what is expected' – in contrast to 'at-ease' meaning 'well, healthy, ready, willing and able to do'. In this book 'disease' is used usually as a noun, suitably qualified but definitive; 'dis-ease' is non-specific and is a state of altered functioning and structure.

There are several 'medical' descriptions which are used interchangeably and not always correctly, and most have human implications, e.g.

- 'illness' – a state of ill-health, being ill but by implication not very ill
- 'sick' – not in working order, in humans in a variety of connections. Colloquially, meaning to vomit, hence to 'be sick', it can describe an act as well as a condition. Horses cannot vomit in the human manner, but can 'be sick'

More correct and accurate terms are

- **morbid** – relating to, or characterised by, dis-ease: pathologic but not necessarily mortally so (from the Latin morbidus, sickly and morbus, illness)
  - **'morbid anatomy'** concerns dis-eased structures
- **pathology** – a branch of medical study concerning cause, origin and nature of structural dis-ease (from the Greek partheia, suffering)
  - **pathophysiology** specifically refers to the associated functional (physiological) disorders with or without cell structure morbidity
  - **pathologic** (pathological) – relating to, involving or caused by, dis-ease
- **clinical** – pathologic signs which are 'patent' (evident),

usually functional, changes. In some cases, as in skin diseases, the structural changes are macroscopically obvious as well

- **sub-clinical** – not obvious except by special techniques, and suspected from indirect non-specific signs of altered behaviour or performance

Disease can be

- **congenital**
  - clinical at birth
    - inherited (genetic)
    - non-inherited – although developed in the womb
  - latent at birth
    - inherited but only develops later into clinical signs
- **acquired** in the course of life
- **localised** to a (relatively small) part of the body
- **generalised**
  - affecting the body systems directly (systemic)
  - affecting other body systems indirectly, through
    - septicaemia – bacteria in the blood
    - toxaemia – toxins in the blood
    - abnormal glandular secretions into the circulation
      - hormonal and/or
      - nutritional deficits
  - interference with homeostasis

The dis-eased state is influenced by the *age* of the horse, its sex, its **condition**, its **environment**, the **feeding** practices, **use** and associated '**contacts**', and (in the injury type) by **athletic use**, **temperament**, and **fitness**.

'Diseased' is the state or condition in which signs or clues may 'surface' from an underlying morbidity of the horse's tissues. Such pathologic information is there to be **perceived**.

Functional disorder clues are more readily available than structural ones, unless these originate in or on the skin and orifices. Internal lesions can be observed by

• biopsy through the skin or via system tract endoscopy

• autopsy (a post-mortem examination)

The findings of both of these can be related to earlier clinical signs.

Pathologic findings and their interpretation are

• **indicative** of something wrong

• **suggestive** of the type of disease in most but not all cases

• **diagnostic**, in some cases

thereby possibly permitting a 'name' to be applied or, at least, directing the veterinary surgeon to further diagnostic aids.

The conclusion may be related to the

• system, organ or tissue involved – e.g. pneumonia (of the lungs)

• type of disease – e.g. inflammation, possibly an infection

• sub-type – e.g. a viral infection

Some pathological changes produce reasonably specific, characteristic signs which, short of being fully diagnostic, can be perceived and described as a syndrome suggestive of which anatomical site is involved and what general type of disease is present. It is often sufficient to institute initial treatment and, where relevant, suitable management pending a specific diagnosis, e.g. from laboratory findings.

Trauma, especially if presented with external signs of 'injury' (from the Latin meaning 'injustice') or surface distortion, is easier to perceive. The physical forces involved are

• external onto the skin and possibly to deeper tissues

   • the skin may be penetrated

• 'internal' (subcutaneous) as the result of 'over-stress' from

   • concussion

   • compression

   • 'stretch'

Many such traumas involve the locomotor system, where limb lesions are frequently clinical, but vary according to the stages of the disorder; the functional deficits also vary, but not necessarily in parallel. The tissue contour and consistency changes are often patent in both acute and chronic.

Nerve tissue pathology is mainly clinical through functional deficits.

External signs of structural changes and functioning are reflections of morbid lesions present in dis-eased tissues. These can be

• gross, i.e. macroscopically visible and palpable through the skin

• invisible, subcutaneous or 'deeper' and not palpable, requiring

   • biopsy samples, for

      • gross changes in tissues

      • histopathology of cells (microscopic)

      • biochemical evaluation of cellular by-products and their altered effectiveness

         • direct

         • on target organs

The cell is the primary focus of all pathologic conditions – the smallest unit of life, the basis of all structure, albeit in many forms and of many functions.

Cells have a genetically determined life span and many wear out and can be replaced within hours. They degenerate and are regenerated in sequences which do not compromise the effective functioning of the tissue. Note, however, that cardiac cells and neural cells (cytones) cannot divide and therefore cannot regenerate.

Blood cells in particular, but also those of the epithelia and especially of the dermis, have a short life. The effete cells are taken out, in the case of blood cells, and scavenged into the reticulo-endothelial system; 'surface' cells are shed unnoticed into the system tract 'exits'.

In dis-ease situations, greater proportions of such cells can not only indicate histo-pathology but can be *en masse* clinical signs, as in dermatitic disease, in lower respiratory disorders or with blood disorders and inflammation. Pathologic cell death, a necrosis, is distinct from physiologic degenerative loss.

Pathological cell change is due to

- Disturbances in nutrient supply, from
    - mal-nutrition, or starvation generally
    - impaired local blood supply, in specific instances

 giving rise to degenerative changes

- inflammatory reactions and their sequelae, from
    - sterile trauma
    - infections (primary and secondary)
    - allergic reactions
- neoplastic invasion
- toxic factors
    - chemical
    - thermal
    - nuclear radiation
    - from microbial-multiplication bi-products (toxins and inflammatory enzymes)

Signs of 'Dis-ease'

These are related to the type of dis-ease and to the various causes within the type; they are **clinical**, perceivable by routine horsemastership, and may be

- **sudden**, as in injury and acute illness, such as azoturia, 'choke', allergic reactions

- **marked**, as in severe trauma, acute systemic illness, some colics, acute laminitis, fractures of long bones

- **indistinct** – vague, non-specific, as in low grade lameness (especially bilateral), capricious appetite, dullness

- **slow in development**, as in lameness-inducing degenerative joint conditions

The important skill in horsemastership is to know that 'something is wrong' – that a functioning upset has occurred; and that until the implication of it and its severity have been determined

- the horse should not be worked

- its concentrate feed intake should be reduced accordingly, and

- further and more experienced help should be sought

A human can answer a doctor's questions as to '*what seems to be wrong?*' The answers describe what are called **symptoms**. Animals can only evince signs; they may vocalise their 'feelings' as in some acute colics, or quantify pain when the affected area is pressurised on palpation by withdrawal of the leg or other more forceful evasive factors, a form of talk-back. These signs are perceived and interpreted using all the senses – plus 'common sense'

- seeing
- hearing
- touching – contour, consistency, heat
- smelling
- tasting (often only inadvertently!)
- kinaesthetically – the sensation of movement

The acuity and accuracy of such perceptions are reflections of knowledge and practice, i.e. experience.

Some morbidities can be insidious in onset, producing no immediate or primary discernible structural changes and consequently no mal-functioning clues – but yet are present, albeit in sub-clinical form. In many such instances careful evaluation of the horse's overall behaviour – the side effects – will raise questions in the observer's mind as to possible ill-health. Such indecisive signs are frequently interpreted as

- 'one degree under'
- not looking or acting as it should
- losing fitness and/or condition

Some dis-ease is discovered fortuitously during

- a pre-purchase examination – a vendor's unawareness!

- an assessment for insurance cover – by the veterinary surgeon who, by definition, is clinically 'more astute'

The normal '**A B C**', **A**ppearance, **B**ehaviour, **C**ondition (*see* Chapter 18, SIGNS OF HEALTH), of a horse is a reflection of the healthy functioning of all its systems. It is essential that the normalities for horses in general are known and, in particular, that the normalities for the horse(s) in the horsemaster's care are known and checked for as a daily routine, when any alteration is quickly recognised.

'Something wrong' is suspected when *one or more* of these regular signs is missing or *changed*. This must be looked for – in the widest sense.

For example, if the at-rest respiration is different from that horse's resting normal (**typically 10–15** respirations per minute), the first thought is *Why is the horse not 'at ease'*? Has it been unusually stimulated or frightened, so that it is reflexly preparing for fight and flight? If not

- are the nostrils more dilated than normal?
- do the respirations remain accelerated and more obvious over several minutes' inspection?
- is it dull, and *not* interested in one's presence?

If the answers are affirmative, it is sensible to monitor

- **heart rate** – is it up from this horse's usual rate (**typically 35–45** beats per minute) by **10 beats per minute or more**?
- **temperature** – is it up from this horse's usual diurnal levels (**typically 37.8–38.3°C (100–101°F)**) by **1° or more**?

There are slight temperature variations between horses. Most have a diurnal temperature rhythm, with a slightly higher level in the evening; in some horses this will be up to 1°C (2°F). **If there is a rise of more than 0.5°C (1°F) from the horse's resting normal diurnal levels, take the horse out of work and carefully monitor for changes in other signs.**

Some infections stimulate a feverish rise on the day before reasonably perceivable (clinical) signs of infectious illness develop. In the case of high performance horses, the horsemaster will be well advised to pick up the warning signs of temperature changes by monitoring the temperature on the day before, the day of, and the day after exposing the horse to the stress of a race or a fast workout, and act accordingly.

Fever

In fever, the body core temperature control mechanism is working satisfactorily but the thermostat has been reflexly set at a higher level in response to infection. Many diseases lead to a fever. The responsible agents of the disease are presumed to produce a **pyrogen** in the blood which alters the regulatory centres to initiate conservation of body heat to raise the body temperature to a new level.

To assist this conservation the sub-cutaneous blood vessels are reflexly constricted to decrease surface body heat loss. The limbs and ears feel cold: shivering, even rigors, will occur.

Average fevers of 1–2°C (2–4°F) are said to be beneficial in the fight against the disease. Any attempt to reduce this too soon may be detrimental. Provided the animal is kept warm, a diagnosis sought and the appropriate treatment and/or nursing begun the fever will 'look after itself'.

Rises greater than 2°C (4°F) or more should be treated *per se* under veterinary management especially if appetite and thirst is lost, if lethargy is marked, and if signs of shock develop. Most equine diseases which induce fevers are associated with infectious diseases. Not all are specifically diagnosed but the syndrome of dis-ease – fever and illness – is easily recognised as a rule, so much so that vets use the initials 'F of UO' (fever of unknown origin) and 'NYD' (not yet diagnosed) in the early stages.

Most horses will naturally and successfully fight the infection. The use of antibiotics will only help if bacteria are involved. (In humans, antipyretic drugs, aspirin and its relations, will reduce fever and give a feeling of being better, but time must be allowed for the fever safely to run its course of usually three to four days.) There is a rationale for doing so in horses but this is a matter for veterinary decision. With horses the carer must be certain how to monitor febrile disease. In first experiences it is obviously sensible to seek professional advice, and especially if general illness is present or if signs of secondary complications arise. A simple example is when the appearance of a muco-purulent nasal discharge becomes complicated by breathing difficulties and marked coughing.

Infectious illness can affect various systems of the body but produces a central body core fever, more so if secondary toxaemia develops. Septic infections of wounds which are not brought quickly under control by treatment can release toxins which will produce additional fever. Pain, too, will produce a rise in temperature, simulating a fever; as the result of an increased metabolic rate as well as the effect of the basic pyrogens escaping from the damaged tissue cells – the primary source of the pain.

In all illnesses and injuries greater than minor, good nursing demands twice-daily temperature recording during the active phase and the early convalescence.

If clues point to a disease of the respiratory system
- lead the horse out
    - does it perk up a little, but
    - does it cough?
- try grazing in hand
    - does it eat?
    - does it cough more?
    - is there a nasal discharge collecting on the outside of the nostrils, or
    - does an opaque, slightly thick greyish white discharge appear at his nostrils, after his head has been down grazing or merely hanging dejectedly?

If all are affirmative, your suspicion of a respiratory disease is much stronger, but further help will be required to determine *why* and *what*. Clearly, *something is wrong, so no work today* – because these signs warn not only that the horse will be unwilling, unready or unable to work as efficiently as it had done but also, and *most importantly*, to try *to make it do so carries the risk that serious and perhaps irreparable damage will follow.* It may also be contagious to other horses. *The recognition of clues is, together with an efficient application of first nursing principles, of considerably greater value than working on until more specific diagnostic signs develop.*

In veterinary communication and case reporting it is usual to use the word which indicates the **organ, system** or **tissue**, and the **type** of dis-ease, for example

- toxic hepatitis (inflammation of the liver from toxin)
- bacterial lymphangitis (bacterial inflammation of a lymphatic vessel)
- metabolic myopathy (morbid change in muscles following a biochemical upset)

For the horsemaster, it is safer, easier and more explicit to talk about '*A suspected dis-ease of …, showing the following signs…*'

For example, *of the alimentary tract, showing*

- off food
- no faeces passed within last six hours
- dull
- some colicky pain

Or *of the respiratory system, showing*

- nasal discharge
- cough, even at rest
- laboured breathing
- fever of X°C

Or *of the locomotor system, showing*

- lame on left fore at walk on hard surface
- swollen distal cannon area, especially posteriorly
- no stone, or picked up nail, found in hoof
- was jumping yesterday, but
- not through a thorn hedge

The first two examples are clearly illnesses. The third is most likely a traumatic dis-ease, but it **could** be an infection – a hidden puncture wound. *All require further skilled attention.*

The veterinary surgeon perceives the clues as coming from particular pathological changes in specific organs. He is also dependent on good information from the handler, whereby his clinical assessment of *what*, *why* and *how* is added to the history of *which*, *when* and *where* (remember Kipling's '*Six Honest Servingmen*'!)

To the horsemaster, normal and abnormal signs should be obvious during routine daily stable management, and these chores should be seen as opportunities to practise such skills of perception, when mucking out, grooming, feeding, exercising or using.

With practice, the handler will graduate from being aware only of the obvious to having a quicker sense of less specific signs, for example: the horse becoming slower in eating up, or becoming more uncomfortable in accepting the bit, both of which signs could be indicative of a mild and not immediately serious mouth pain – which should nevertheless be investigated, rather than ignored until the horse begins to 'quid' its food, or evade the bit, thus showing a more advanced and so a more painful disorder – perhaps more difficult to treat successfully.

With further experience, the handler will for example automatically monitor loss of weight despite good appetite, or failure to respond to a training schedule, and will act expeditiously.

A basic objective of horsemastership is not only to recognise the fact of disease being present, but to minimise the risk of it worsening and/or spreading. Many 'dis-eases' are the result of man's 'omissions and commissions' in management.

It is *essential* for the horsemaster to learn the correct principles of, and quickly recognise and correct faults that might arise in, grazing, stabling, feeding, exercise and fittening, competing and transporting. Also, through regular discussion with the veterinary surgeon, to be up-to-date with preventative measures relating to **vaccination**, **worming, dental care** and **farriery**.

TYPES OF DIS-EASE

In practice, type classifications are not always clear-cut; inflammatory reactions are frequently superimposed on the primary structural changes of dis-eases of a non-inflammatory nature or type. The inter-relationship is discussed in the chapters following.

The major division between inflammatory and 'others' is related to and explained by **evolution** (over millions of years) and **domestication** (over two thousand years).

Present-day species of native animals, plants, micro-organisms and parasites owe their existence to

- ancestral changes which met evolutionary demands
- symbiotic co-existence and, in the case of animals
- survival despite the hazards of injury, infection, parasitism, malnutrition, predation

It is said that no parasite, adult macroscopic and larval microscopic organisms which can live only on or in an animal host, wish to kill the host. The host will fulfil its ecological functions by giving the parasites a 'home' provided it can control their numbers to a non-lethal level.

In situations where injury occurs or infection gets out of hand, the animal's survival and purpose in life (to reproduce the species) depends upon

- a defensive reaction – inflammation
- a native foraging 'cunning' – to cope with seasonal malnutrition, to avoid native toxic plants through recognition of 'warning off' taste and smell, and to recognise dangerous terrain

The basic hazards remain; fortunately, so too does the inherited natural response to them.

Inflammation is not *per se* a disease. It is a dis-eased state with a positive aim – to counter the natural injury or infection, whereby

- structural injury is limited
- bleeding is controlled
- infection is 'fought' and overcome
- immunity, to some infections, is stimulated
- parasitism is 'lived with' through a form of immunity and resistance
- repair is initiated

Nature is not always successful. For example, injuries can be fatal or disabling, making the animal exposed to malnutrition or predators; infections can overwhelm; and parasitism can be enhanced through unseasonal co-incidental malnutrition. But, unless a catastrophe occurs, sufficient numbers in the group or herd survive to reproduce, generation after generation.

Under domesticated conditions, 'other' factors are introduced and they are significant because in the relatively short span of exposure there was not sufficient threat to a species to stimulate evolutionary change. More significantly, there was not the time span for such changes.

Consequently the horse did not develop innate powers of resistance, a defence to them – and is not likely to develop them. If man can carefully breed for proven 'resistant' types and/or can carefully breed to avoid particularly 'susceptible' types, then the influence of these other diseases on the species' usefulness will diminish, though they will never disappear.

The Other Factors

Man has introduced, for his own ends, controlled grazing and conserved feedstuffs, stabling, controlled breeding, and work output, on top of '**maintenance**' energy costs.

These have disturbed the natural instincts of the horse, and so his behaviour; a grazing (and browsing) herbivorous diet has been

- time controlled, with
- altered constituents, albeit still 'vegetation'
- a nomadic existence seriously curtailed, with no opportunity to 'find' fresh pasture
- the gregarious nature interfered with – the 'lonely' horse
- the 'fright, fight, flight' response has been subjugated to alertness, obedience and performance, and these have been up-graded to athletic performance standards – greater work or '**production**' output

In addition, there have been introduced new environments, new contacts, rapid transport and no longer an established 'home' – therefore new infections and new stress factors.

It is worth remembering that had domestication, dominion over and commercialisation of the horse not been part of man's equine psyche the horse might now be an endangered species, even extinct. Man's conscience therefore must see the need for welfare considerations. Horsemastership is the first step.

Intelligent domestication has ameliorated the effects of the basic hazards and/or their effects. Understanding is better, diagnosis is quicker and more accurate, treatment is more specific and more supportive, surgery can be performed and rehabilitation can be achieved. Prevention is a management tool.

With experience, man has learned to understand these 'other', 'domestication' diseases and has constantly improved on his diagnosis and management, even if no preventative treatment or immunisation *per se* is possible in some instances. These disorders remain as evidence of his omissions and commissions – fundamentally a continuing, if diminishing, ignorance of how to balance management input and performance output. As in all productive (work output) domesticated species they are

- **developmental** diseases
- **allergies** – albeit some, such as urticaria, almost certainly existed before domestication
- **metabolic** – growth/performance related dis-eases
- **degenerative** dis-eases – especially wear and tear in the locomotor system, and often associated with developmental disorders

against which the horse has no innate powers of defence or repair.

Fortunately, few of them are fatal, but they frequently make the horse unusable, certainly in the domesticated practices necessary for optimal performance. Thus, as examples

- in **developmental** diseases the sufferer in the wild state would have died or become an easy prey. In domestication, there remains man's hesitation to cull, and his difficulty in accepting the need to change the breeding stock
- the horse affected by chronic obstructive pulmonary disease can be turned out and worked from grass, or fed and bedded differently, and/or kept on medication; nevertheless, it remains susceptible to further **allergic** attacks when unavoidably re-exposed to the allergen, for instance at shows, and is always liable to secondary (bacterial) complication. Once sensitised, it remains so; once affected, its respiration remains defective to some extent
- azoturia (equine rhabdomyolosis) cases can be relegated to slower, less exacting work, but 'no recurrence' can ever be guaranteed. The causal factors are not fully understood but there is recent evidence of genetic influences in certain types. Other **metabolic** conditions are more clearly related to malnutrition
- for the horse suffering from **degenerative** joint disease, medication, possibly surgery, and altered workload, can all reduce the 'progress for the worse'. Sometimes 'regeneration for the better' occurs, apparently in association with medication and overall better management. Other degenerative diseases, such as in nerve degeneration e.g. recurrent laryngeal neuropathy, are amenable to surgery to negate the effect, but for the 'wobbler' surgery is questionably cost-effective

On-going research often leads to classification confusion
- azoturia involves muscle dysfunction – a **myopathy**, to

which the name **myositis** is often given, indicating an inflammatory response. This is theoretically accurate, in as much as repair does involve an inflammatory intervention, but ER is primarily a metabolic disease; the inflammatory response is secondary to the structural change

- degenerative joint disease (DJD) can lead to osteo-arthritis – inflammation of the joint – which can also follow traumatic injury to the joint. Moreover, the start of degenerative joint disease almost certainly requires some trauma – persistent overstress with or without acute overstress (an actual sprain) – to be precipitated into clinical signs or to 'weaknesses' inbuilt with DJD, the seeds at least of which are often congenital and possibly hereditable
- laminitis literally implies an inflammatory disease of the sensitive laminae within the hoof capsule. Admittedly this is the clinical, invariably acute, marked, even dramatic, evidence of severe pain within the hooves. However, it is the end point of a management mistake, whereby the digestive system, especially of native breed ponies, is subjected to overloading and assault by unnaturally high levels of carbohydrate. The result is a two-stage toxaemia, finalising in dysfunction in the arteries and veins, which is most significant in the sophisticated blood supply to the pedal structures inside the unyielding hoof capsule. This is one scenario.

DEVELOPMENTAL DISEASE

It is more explicit to describe developmental diseases as abnormalities. They are not, strictly speaking, the result of injury, infection or parasitism on normal tissue. Nor are they primarily the outcome of the stresses of working, although they are usually worsened by these.

They begin at any time from fertilisation up to maturity of the tissues, which is reached in the majority by two and a half years as far as the abaxial structures (the limbs) are concerned. Some develop to a lethal stage in the foetus, which is then aborted. Some are congenital but permit of variable but usually short-lived existence. Others do not become clinical until neo-natal life or even later. Infection and malnutrition of the pregnant dam can be influential, and feeding mistakes may be involved during early foal life.

Those abnormalities which are present at birth (that is 'congenital'), may also be inherited, but few are known to be clearly so. The reproductive system would appear to have the highest incidence of gene anomalies or even whole chromosome abnormalities – as one might surmise. They are often found only in certain breeds

- cross influences of male and female **sex hormones**: affected offspring are sterile. Incidence is small. Professional advice is necessary regarding further parental breeding
- **cryptorchidism** is hereditable, most commonly in the Welsh Mountain pony. The male is usually fertile, but should be completely gelded. Its dam should not be bred from again
- **haemolytic disease** is an immune problem in which the mare produces colostrum with antibodies to the foal's red blood cells: there is evidence of a genetic connection

Four specific disorders of the immune defences are recorded. All are believed to be genetic

- in Arab horses, a combined deficiency of **B** and **T lymphocytes** – they cannot produce antibodies; death from infection is likely within five weeks
- **agammaglobulinaemia** (total absence of all immunoglobulins (Ig's), very rare. In the absence of **B lymphocytes**, death occurs within one and a half years after many debilitating infectious attacks
- in Arab and Quarter horses, a deficiency of **specific immunoglobulin**, from either a deficiency in the mare's colostrum or more probably an inability of the foal to absorb the antibodies from the colostrum. A decision as to future breeding along that line is not easily reached
- a more recent condition in which there is a failure of Fell foals to develop an immunity, the result of a genetic fault in certain lines in the breed. The lethal outcome is worryingly high

The **eye** has many developmental defects. One, the absence of the **iris**, is genetic. The others are suspected but not proven to be so. All are very rare. They range from

- no eye(s) at birth
- blocked tear duct(s)
- **cataract** (some forms), variable in importance and relatively common; true congenitals rarely worsen
- corneal growths
- detached retina
- ingrowing eyelids – **entropion**, operable

- eversion of eyelids – **ectropion**, operable but more difficult
- **glaucoma**, possibly treatable
- **night blindness**
- optic nerve defect

Hereditable diseases of the nervous and muscular skeletal systems are

- in the Arab horse, a mal-development of the cerebellum shows at about 6 months old
- hereditary **ataxia** in the Oldenburg shows at about 3 years old
- the **wobbler** syndrome shows between 6 and 24 months – the spinal cord is affected. Clear signs may not develop until 3 or 4 years of age. Seen in Thoroughbreds and crosses, usually the male
- in Arab horses, a fatal fusion of the head with the atlas and axis – the foal may be born dead
- **wryneck** – inherited; if congenital may interfere with delivery (often associated with 'fixed' limb joints)

Congenital musculo-skeletal disorders of doubtful hereditable cause are:

- hyperflexed, crooked, **fixed** limb joints from abnormal, irreversible relationship between bone and muscle/tendon length (a form of angular limb deformities)
- **contracted flexor tendons** (so called) – congenital and acquired. If able to be manually straightened on examination the congenital form is often self-corrective. The acquired form, in six weeks to twelve-month-old animals, can respond to corrective hoof trimming but may require surgery. ('Contracted flexor tendons' is a misnomer: it is not the tendons which are contracted)
- **patellar lateral luxation** in the Shetland – from birth
- **upward fixation of the patellae** – appears from any age to 5 years in warmbloods especially; in some cases, it is related to a passing mal-development of the distal end of the femur, which could be a hereditable condition. In others, it is a temporary weakness of the muscles which control the patella, and as such is developmental *vis à vis* muscle/bone length ratios and/or temporary muscle immaturity with lameness The 'straight hind leg conformation' theory has not been confirmed
- **laxity of joints** in the neonate – walking on the back of

fetlocks; a weakness, usually temporary. May be later complicated with angular limb deformities

Post-natal **angular limb deformities** are sometimes congenital in weak foals, such as twins which are more prone, but any weakness will predispose. They may develop in the older foal which is

- **top heavy**
- **lame in one leg** and so extra weighted on the other
- **over-exercised**, especially on hard ground

Those developmental problems found in the **digestive system** are all are thought to be hereditable

- **parrot** mouth
- narrowed diameter of the small colon, with obstruction
- absence of anus
- **white foal syndrome** – blocked bowel, as well as lack of pigment in iris and coat; fatal within a few days

There remain certain **miscellaneous** conditions, the most common are

- umbilical and inguinal **hernias** – known to be heredit-able in Quarter horses and probably in other breeds

It should be understood that with the exception of angular limb deformities, congenital limb weaknesses, the upward fixating patellae, the hernias and some of the eye conditions, the others are rare but also often lethal. Most foals, by far, are born normal and continue so.

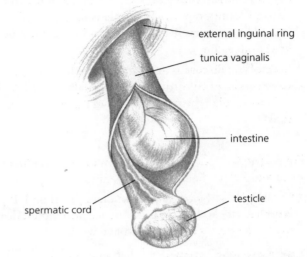

external inguinal ring
tunica vaginalis
intestine
testicle
spermatic cord

Inguinal hernia.

Umbilical hernia.

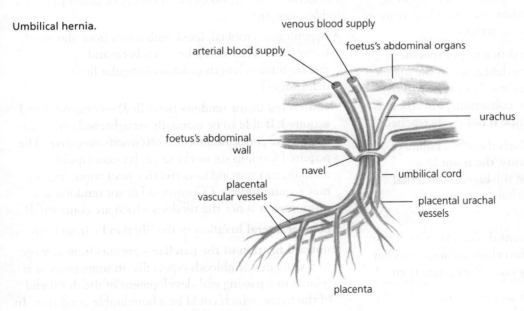

venous blood supply
foetus's abdominal organs
arterial blood supply
urachus
foetus's abdominal wall
navel
umbilical cord
placental vascular vessels
placental urachal vessels
placenta

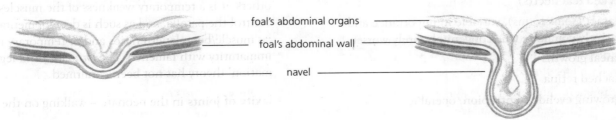

foal's abdominal organs
foal's abdominal wall
navel

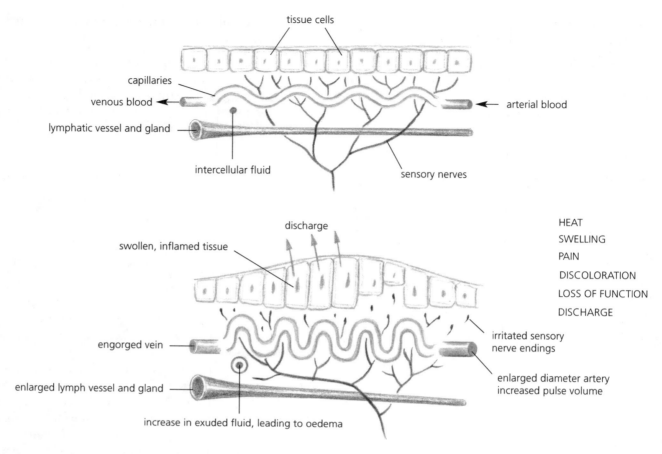

How the cell and its blood supply are affected by inflammation.

INFLAMMATORY DIS-EASE

Inflammation is a basic reaction to a not immediately fatal assault on tissues, irrespective of 'which' and 'by what'. It will not occur if the cells are lethally damaged, i.e. suffer necrosis or cell death; the ultimate is total cell necrosis – body death. Such 'fatal' damage to cells is said to have caused an irreversible disturbance of functioning whereby cellular metabolism ceases.

The main aim of inflammation is to initiate a primary series of events which will lead to a healing of the damaged tissues and a return to homeostasis. To this end there is, for example, in traumas

- an immediate but very short-lived constriction of the arteriolar blood supply to the area – presumably to minimise bleeding: colder when palpated

- a subsequent dilation of the capillaries to bring more blood to the area via undamaged neighbouring vessels:

warmer when palpated, with

- a concentration of white blood cells in the serum
- an escape of serum into the intercellular spaces
- the mobilisation of these cells there, and other anti-inflammatory substances around the damaged area
- the subsequent demobilisation of the blood cells via the lymphatic system

Much of this can be sub-clinical, unperceivable in part at least.

The mechanism is complicated but obviously efficient. The assaulted tissue cells release clinical messengers into the intercellular spaces

- **primary mediators**, which activate the two original vascular changes described above (the cold, then heat)
- other secondary chemicals which then
  - make the tissue cells adhere to the capillary walls

- cause capillary wall leakage, which allows into the affected area an outflow of plasma, and so serum, with white blood cells, proteins, anti-germ substances where relevant as in infections, and
- further chemicals which
  - 'call up' further white blood cells to mobilise at the site
  - initiate a chain of pain production

Inflammation is a necessary life-protecting reaction. Interference with it can be counter-productive, but is often necessary, if only, for example, on welfare grounds and in first aid. The unconsidered control of pain may lead to a false assessment of recovery and subsequent, injudicious, too early use.

The second response, as exemplified in a traumatised limb, is a rapid increase in the blood supply to the area via the nearby undamaged capillary system. *This hyperaemia is the basis of inflammation*. The related local pulse is 'bigger' and therefore, where palpable, feels 'stronger', but obviously it is no faster than the heart rate. The vein also dilates, often visibly and certainly palpably to accommodate the return of the increased blood supply.

Where pain is marked, for example in secondary infection, fracture or tendinitis, there will be a reflexly stimulated increased heart and pulse rate. Where secondary infection occurs, the degree will determine the degree of inflammation. In such cases the basal functions of sterile inflammation are necessarily aided by an inflammatory reaction capable of attacking, destroying and scavenging the germs involved.

The rationale for the increased inflammatory flow of blood is

- to make more blood plasma available where necessary for its clotting purposes and for its **fibrin** protective properties
- to make more serum available for exudation into the area to give a **lavaging** effect and to bring **humoral antibodies** where applicable
- to bring the various white blood cells, some of which are especially and reflexly mobilised, for **antibody** activity, **germ** capture and **debris** scavenging
- to prepare the self-cleansed area for repair, and special nourishment
- supply the required extra nutrients, including oxygen

Further enzyme activity stimulates the release of **modulators**

which direct the course of the inflammatory reaction to

- rapid resolution, or
- slow resolution
- suppuration in open infected situations, with eventual discharge through a skin wound or a body orifice, or the formation of an abscess
- tissue regrowth
  - sub-clinical minimal resolution deficit
  - a chronic state of partial healing with sub-optimal functioning, a fibrosing heal or 'in-filling'
    - in wounds, scar formation, repair with variable loss of functioning

Inflammation occurs irrespective of site and cause. Fundamentally, there is no difference between traumatic sterile, traumatic infected, and primary infected inflammation. However, the degree, the duration and the outcome will vary. Man can intervene to help (or to interfere) with natural recovery.

The clinical structural and functional signs, as distinct from the ongoing morbidity or pathology, can be perceived most readily in inflammation of the body surface, and understood most easily in limb cases – where temporary and permanent changes are visible and palpable. *In internal sub-types, the functional changes are seen as clues which suggest the underlying damage.*

Inflammatory changes are clinically perceivable by the five cardinal signs

- **rubor** – redness (first recorded in the 1st century AD)
- **tumor** – swelling, with
- **calor** – heat (first recorded in 1650 BC)
- **dolor** – pain (first recorded in the 1st century AD)
- **functio laesa** – disturbance of function (first recorded in the 19th century)

How perceivable they are varies. In pigmented skin with coat, the **rubor** will not 'shine' through, but it will do so in the bars of the mouth, the white of the eye, the bulbs of the heels, and the sole of the hoof if unpigmented.

The pain is 'recognisable' by how the horse behaves or, in the limbs for example, by how it reacts to digital pressure, and by its variably lame action.

Inflammation of organs, other than skin, is 'out of sight', but discharges will 'surface' at related orifices or via abscessed superficial lymph glands. Altered function will show in changes of '<u>A</u> <u>B</u> <u>C</u>'.

Trauma or Injury

Trauma is the result of the infliction of a force which is excessive for the natural and/or conditioned resilience of the tissues afflicted, as a consequence of which there is physical structural damage, and subsequent functional upset.

Where the force is **external** in origin – a blow – part of the horse (typically a limb) hits an unyielding object, or a moving object hits the horse. In both cases the skin takes the impact, but deeper tissues through to the bone are variably also affected. When the skin is not penetrated, such a trauma is described as 'closed', and by definition is a sterile injury; there is a variable degree of associated **bruising**. When penetrated it is an 'open' wound and therefore is usually infected.

Where the force is **internal** in origin, for example a strain of a tendon, a sprain of a joint ligament, or a tear of a muscle in part or all of a unit of locomotion, it is due to a functional over-stressing of the tissues under the skin. Here the resultant wound is sterile.

In both external and internal types there is to a greater or lesser degree a disruption of the connective tissues cells involved, as well as to the blood supply and nerve conductivity, usually with pain. Functional integrity will variably be lost: a ligament will fail to support a joint, a tendon will fail to transmit or to 'hold' muscle power, a muscle will fail to contract, a bone will fail to bear weight. The bleeding at all these levels will produce 'loose' blood, which will diffuse over and through the site and then clot – a **bruising**: the serum will separate from the clotting blood, and/or with other tissue fluids will concentrate in the area. There will consequently be swelling, loss of function, pain, and an immediate inflammatory response, which will result in more swelling, heat, and discoloration as seen through unpigmented, hairless areas of skin, more pain, and further greater loss of use.

Such changes can become perceivable at the body surfaces. Deep damage can be 'visualised' by knowing the cause, estimating the possible degree of the trauma, and from that appreciating the degree of pain, and assessing the loss of function.

In addition to the acute internal overstress traumas arising from 'accelerating forces in inelegant strides' (*see* Chapter 16, THE LOCOMOTOR SYSTEM), which whiplash the tissues, chronic repetitive concussion/compression/sub-acute strain will, eventually, produce inflammatory reactions in sensitive tissues such as the hoof laminae and corium, joints, muscles, tendons and ligaments, and all these can at any time translate into

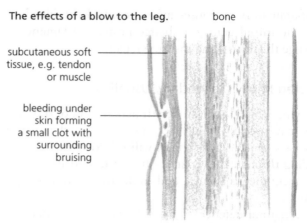

The effects of a blow to the leg.

bone

subcutaneous soft tissue, e.g. tendon or muscle

bleeding under skin forming a small clot with surrounding bruising

STERILE BRUISE – SKIN UNBROKEN

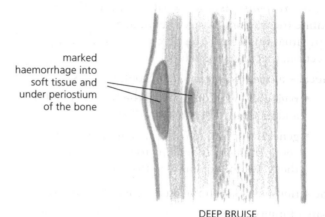

marked haemorrhage into soft tissue and under periostium of the bone

DEEP BRUISE

haemorrhage in soft tissue and around fractured ends of bone, and marked swelling of area

STERILE TRAUMA RESULTING IN FRACTURE OF BONE

clinical conditions or, in the case of compression and concussion, devolve into degenerative joint disease. In such limb traumas there is a variable exhibition of pain – lameness – with variable loss of use in the locomotor system.

Inflammatory responses aim to control the bleeding, limit the initial damage – hence protective lameness – scavenge the debris, and institute repair.

Infected Injury (Secondary, Usually Bacterial)

Following a blow associated with penetration of the skin, but not necessarily deep tissue trauma, the inflammatory signs associated with a 'bruise' will co-exist with signs of bleeding *through* the wound – from the skin itself, from the subcutaneous tissues, and from the relevant deeper tissues.

The natural defence of the skin against subcutaneous infection is breached, whereby bacteria and other germs can invade the sensitive tissues, and if they do *the inflammatory response is increased* to: **fight** the invaders, **confine** the area and **lavage** the wound.

In situations where the defence does not confine the infection, this may spread from

- **local** – along tissue tracts, to become
  - **regional** – with drainage to the lymph gland(s), and in some to become
  - **general** – spread to other systems, both by the germs themselves and any toxins produced by them and the traumatised tissue cells

The seriousness of such infected wounds depends on

- **site** of injury – worse if a joint capsule, tendon sheath or body cavities are entered
- **type** of infection – aerobic or anaerobic bacteria and related toxin, set against the
- **resilience** of the animal's tissues and local defences
- the **success** of their inflammatory counter-measures

As the inflammatory response does its work successfully, the clinical signs will diminish – the swelling subsides, pulse volume and vein swelling decrease (where they had initially been perceived, as in wounds of the extremities), discharge ceases, the wound visibly heals, and repair continues in deeper tissues.

Primary Infectious (Contagious) Dis-ease

An infectious dis-ease is one that develops in an animal following the

- invasion of a system's tract – for example, of the airway
- penetration of that system's surface defences

- overcoming that animal's blood-borne existing defences
- colonisation and multiplication on or in the system's cells
- stimulation of an inflammatory response
- interference with functioning of that system – producing a specific set of signs

by a micro-organism which thereafter may be excreted to pass directly or indirectly to other susceptible animals. The body may clear out the remainder or hold some in a dormant condition – i.e. the horse becomes a carrier.

Research continues into how pathogenic micro-organisms actually damage tissue cells. It is known that a pathogenic organism has a 'key' which enables it to attach to a susceptible tissue cell at a 'locking' point. The key and the lock are very specific. Not all tissue cells have the same lock design or 'receptor', and no germ species has the same pattern of key as others or even strains within. Some species of animals have no receptors for certain germs, and some germs have no key for any of the cells' locks in a species of animal. This is a simplified analogy. It must be added that a by-product of a key finding a locking point is the production of specific defences against that germ's key locking fully home in future similar infections. The primary locking will have instituted inflammatory reactions; a future locking will institute no or insignificant clinical inflammatory reactions, but will 'boost' or increase the initial immunity. In some situations the full locking may become reactivated with a return of the original sign of disease.

Few if any micro-organisms are 'new', but micro-organism may have altered over millions of years in order to survive. During these eons, environmental changes will have effected variations in the relationship between animal and micro-organism. Strains of a germ have 'got through' the defences of several generations of an evolving animal; some may have decimated a species before an immune status was built up, and in so doing have developed a greater pathogenicity – but a reverse capability, better immunity, can develop in survivors.

'New' germs, especially amongst viruses, have been isolated or 'discovered' in recent years – but this is more likely to be because research scientists have developed better means of isolation and identification of viruses which have been present and existed through the centuries, even if as strains in different species – for example, 'recent' strains of influenza virus are known to be 'drifted' strains of avian origin during the last hundred years. Even in more recent times, bacteria, readily isolated in laboratory samples, were given primary status when in fact they were secondary invaders to viruses which had not been looked for or could not be 'found' or isolated.

In historic terms, the primary invader may not have been clinically pathogenic, although present; the infected host remained sign-free, but its resistance could have been undermined. As a result, 'commensal' (secondary) invaders, originally harmless, now took the opportunity (**opportunist invaders**) and in doing so were perceived as primary agents.

For reasons which have stood the test of time, if not yet fully understood, appropriate 'key and lock' have *never* co-existed in some cases. For example

- species other than cloven-hoofed animals do not become clinically affected by the presence in their system's tracts of the several strains of the **foot and mouth** virus – a 'family-susceptible' disease
- close relatives of a particular virus will not cause a similar disease in two or more unrelated species of animal. Yet the viruses of, for example, canine distemper, human measles and seal 'distemper' are closely related but will not pass from one species to either of the other two – a species-specific resistance
- a particular bacterium *Streptococcus equi*, amongst several related streptococci strains, is the only one to produce the disease of **strangles** in horses, a disease not found in other animals – a genus-specific disease

In all susceptible mammals' systems there is a complex arrangement of defences to try to prevent even specific invading primary pathogens from gaining a foothold, i.e. colonising on the susceptible tissue cells which line their tracts

- physical barriers, as in the
  - respiratory system
    - the muco-ciliary escalator
    - the flow of expired air

which trap and expel germs before they can colonise on the mucous membrane

  - digestive system
    - the peristaltic pushing through of the ingesta and digesta
    - the varying electolytic and enzymatic digestive juice gut contents in different areas of the intestines
      - the associated varying pH of the ingesta and mucosal surfaces

- existing cellular antibodies
- coincidentally stimulated new cellular and humoral antibodies, to control the numbers in the invasion – the immune system activity

An infection reaches a clinical level when, for a variety of reasons, its pathogenicity (its ability to gain a foothold) is greater than the horse's natural defences. There remain many questions to be more fully answered – not least of which is 'where do "flies" go in winter?' Some answers are given later, where the more specific diseases of the systems are dealt with.

Viruses, and especially respiratory disease viruses, vary in this pathogenicity, as do the strains within a particular species of virus. This is further confounded by the individuality of the animal invaded, and particularly its age, temperament, work load, and management. Thus an infection by Herpes virus-1 is unlikely to inconvenience a 'school' hack but can be disastrous to the racing of a young Thoroughbred.

Specific infections usually found in organs/systems and are therefore called

- **systemic**
  - **primary** – as in viral respiratory disease
  - **secondary** – blood-borne from another structure or by direct spread along the mucosal surface in the same animal primarily affected. Such germs (usually bacteria) are said to be '**opportunists**'; they may be already on site, but inactive 'waiting' for primary (virus) damage
- **generalised**, affecting more than one system at a time as part of a
  - **septicaemia** – germ-spread, via blood
  - **toxaemia** – toxin-spread, via blood
  - **neoplastic** – metastises, via lymph or blood in the case of viral activated tumours

Grades of infection are reflections of
- the virulence of the germs
- their cellular destructive properties
- their associated toxin production
and are described as
- **hyperacute** – sudden marked signs
- **acute** – rapid development to marked signs
- **sub-acute** – slower development and/or less marked signs

- **chronic**
  - insidious development with less obvious or indistinct signs, or now in a
  - slow recovery state, with
    - temporary functional and structural changes

    These can be followed by
      - part recovery, with some permanent functional and structural changes, some related loss of use and scar tissue formation in the originally affected area
      - recovery

  In part or whole recoveries there usually is an immunity and a hypersensitivity in some
- **fatal infection** – no recovery

It would be an unusual horse which has no residual effects of a previous assault on its functioning and/or its structures which have been exposed to infections (and/or wear and tear) relative to age, type and work. The original reaction was to contain the damage of the assault, clean up the debris, institute some degree of repair and, in the case of systemic infection, give immunity against further attacks. An infected horse will remain variably susceptible to further similar infections and possibly be immune to their pathologic effects. In some cases this immunity takes the form of an allergic state.

The grades of infections can also be related to secondary bacterial infections associated with open traumas (wounds). The immune post-infection status does not seem to develop, perhaps a reflection of the bacteria usually involved, nor does allergic hypersensitivity, but there are exceptions. There is certainly no 'immunity' against repeat injury. (*See* skin infections, e.g. mud fever.)

Their athletic potential in all situations may have been reduced, but generally a clinical recovery from acute and sub-acute conditions, or a degree of regeneration, will allow them to adjust and/or to compensate. They will become, to all intents and purposes, once more '*at ease*'. Nature's purpose was to have them capable of living and reproducing; she was concerned only that the individual could keep up with the herd, graze, reproduce – not win a three-day event.

Whatever the disease, the inflammatory reaction is at cellular level as previously described. A condition such as pneumonia indicates a disease of the respiratory tract's lower airway. An inflammatory reaction therein is fundamentally no different from an inflammation of the intestines – an enteritis. Of course, the signs and effects will differ, but

- the cells which line the tract
- the capillary blood flow to and from it
- the nerve output and input and any intrinsic supply
- the supporting connective tissues

are *all basically similar*. The *consequences* are a disruption of their *specific cellular function*.

In the example of pneumonia there is an
- interference with gaseous exchange in the alveoli
- increase in breathing rate to compensate
- cough to help clear the inflamed passages
- possible fever, inappetence and dullness

In the example of enteritis there is
- interference with the secretion of digestive juices
- interference with the absorption of digesta
- an increase in peristalsis with
- a possible diarrhoea, which if severe leads to an alteration in body fluid volumes and electrolyte levels
- associated other systemic disorders

Non-Contagious Infections

Infections may be non-contagious, in the sense of the causal organism not being excreted as an integral part of the disease process, for example
- *Brucella abortus* (**brucellosis**) in horses – which can cause chronic lameness
- *Clostridium tetani* (**tetanus**) in all species – kills by its toxin's effect on CNS synapses, resulting in paralysis
- *Clostridium botulinum* (**botulism**) in all species – which invariably kills from the vascular spread of its toxin causing neuro-muscular paralysis

Brucellosis is primarily a contagious disease of cattle, and in pregnant cows it causes abortion. When that happens, and at subsequent normal births, the germ *Brucella abortus* is excreted with the after-calving, or abortion, fluids. It contaminates grazing and water and can be splashed into other cows' eyes (and into the stockman's and vet's) by a contaminated swishing tail. Thus it spreads and is contagious to other breeding cows, humans and some other herbivorous species – especially the horse.

In man and in the horse the germ affects connective

tissues around joints, but in getting to these tissues it may, in man, cause a bacteraemic undulating feverish illness. The horse invariably becomes intermittently lame. In closed situations such as joints and other connective tissues, the germ may remain for some considerable time, but as there is no route to any body orifice the germ cannot be contagious to other horses. The bursa at the poll and at the withers, one-time common sites for brucellosis germ multiplication – **poll evil** and **fistulous withers** respectively – could develop an 'abscess' which, when it burst or was lanced, released live germs to contaminate the vicinity. This situation was of limited contagiousness, as the quantity of excreta was minimal in comparison to that from an aborting cow's womb. Moreover, several cows in the herd could be contaminating the environment at one time. The bovine disease has been almost eradicated (certainly in the UK), and the risk to man and horse is now minimal.

Clostridial germs are characterised by their 'spore' existence in the soil. There they survive to multiply in an anaerobic and decaying organic material environment. When ingested as soil contaminents of vegetable material, they pass through the gut innocuously. They cannot multiply there in the absence of *dead* tissue.

Some clostridia gain entrance to the blood stream through an innocuous gut erosion and are soon wiped out in the spleen and other lymphoid areas, but should incidental inflammatory conditions develop in muscle and other connective tissues, as from tears or severe traumas, and the fortuitously 'infected' blood then haemorrhages into the injured areas, which by definition has dead cells, the germ will multiply and produce large quantities of specific toxin. Tissue gangrene occurs as well as systemic illness – a toxaemia.

Clostridium botulinum germ does not infect living tissue. Its toxin is secreted when this soil bacterium multiplies rapidly in anaerobic decaying vegetable and dead animal tissue. If this is fortuitously ingested, as when toxin contaminated food is eaten, there is a botulinum toxicity – botulism. It affects nerve-muscle complexes. An ideal situation for the toxin production is in damaged big bale silage which coincidentally may also contain dead birds and rodents picked up at harvesting.

The **tetanus** germ is introduced from soil or faeces (usually equine) into deep skin wounds. There it multiplies to secrete a toxin which exudes into juxta-positioned nerve tracts along which it spreads centrally. It is lethal to the neural synapses, including those of the brain's nuclei. There is no direct inflammatory or gangrenous reaction to the germ or to the toxin in the originally traumatised tissues, only this neural damage with resultant paralysis of various body systems; for example, when respiratory muscle is affected asphyxia will follow. Postural muscle involvement leads to recumbency, with pulmonary congestion, asphyxia and heart failure or, in the case of the muscles of mastication, death from starvation. It is the *consequences* which kill.

INFECTION

Some Definitions Regarding Micro-organisms

Invasion – the entry of potentially pathogenic micro-organisms into

- body system tracts, for example the upper airway
- subcutaneous tissues through a skin wound
- body cavities, for example tendon sheath, by a deep wound
- hair follicles with broken hairs – for example ringworm spores

Pathogenicity – the germ's capability of locking onto a tissue cell in a particular species.

Colonisation – this is the establishment on the living cells, having overcome the natural local defences.

Penetration – especially in the case of viruses, which require intra-cellular sites of propagation, when they penetrate the cells having avoided blood-borne defences as well as the local ones.

Multiplication – the increase in their numbers after invasion and subsequent penetration.

Incubation period – the time between invasion, often called 'being infected', and the development of signs of disease. This varies with the type of germ.

In day-to-day language, a horse is said to be **infected** – i.e. to have an infectious disease when it shows 'known' or recognisable clinical signs of an inflammatory response to the invasion and colonisation/penetration of one or more systems by a primary microbe that genetically is able to create such a reaction in a previously apparently healthy horse.

In the majority of infections the progeny of the rapidly multiplying invaders are discharged to the environment, whence they may be **contagious** to other susceptible animals.

All infections, by definition, may 'spread' from one

susceptible animal to another directly or indirectly. There must be some form of excreted contamination to make the link: droplets in the atmosphere, nose-to-nose contact, or through an intermediate inanimate contact contaminated by nasal or other discharges, drinking bowls, fencing etc. These last are known as **fomites**.

A disease qualified by the term infectious indicates that the cause is the active presence of a micro-organism in or on the tissue cells, the result of which is a **defensive inflammatory reaction**. The word 'disease' implies that signs of this reaction are perceivable, recognisable and, as such, 'point' to the system involved.

Diseases have two characteristics

- **infectiousness** is the ability to set up or to establish a disease; the infection may be of varying grades

- **contagiousness** is the ability to spread from one animal and gain entrance to another

These abilities are indicative of, amongst other things, the virulence of the germ. They relate to the number of the invaders, though such valuations are of little concern to the horsemaster. What is important to know is that a suspected infectious disease in one animal has the potential to spread to others. If it has succeeded in one animal it is almost certainly going to succeed in another susceptible and non-immune one. It is a reflection of its pathogenicity – its cell destruction potential set against the animal's

- physico-chemical **defences**

- its general **immunity** or **resistance**

- the previously stimulated **specific immunity**

- the **speed of stimulating** or boosting immunity

- the presence of any **debilitating factors**

The degree of the resultant illness will relate to

- the subsequent **spread** of the germ and/or its toxins
  - via the **lymphatics**, and
  - via the **blood circulation**

- their **final colonisation** on or in the tissue cells of the system evolutionarily predetermined

- the **secondary effects**, especially of toxins, on other systems

A successful germ strain usually 'leaves' (is excreted from) a patient

- in **increased numbers,** and often

- with **increased virulence** – the advantage to the germ of passage through successive animals

It is contagious via

- contaminated **air** – as an aerosol or a direct contact, colloquially an 'infection'

- inhalation of **dried discharge particles**, as in dust

- ingestion of **contaminated food and water**

- **contact** of the susceptible skin of one animal with the affected skin or contaminated objects previously in contact with infected skin – for example ringworm. Such a spread is colloquially described as a contagious one

In practice therefore any 'excreted' infectious microbe potentially able to infect (enter) and subsequently possibly affect another, must be *contagious*.

There are, however (see *Brucellosis* and *Botulism*), examples of infectious diseases whose causal microbes, although picked up from the environment, are no longer contagious since the horse is a 'blind' terminus for that disease.

The fact that **ringworm** can spread rapidly through a stable of horses would indicate that it is highly infectious (not 'highly' contagious; it is just 'contagious'). Nevertheless it does require a break in the hair and some skin abrasion to gain a foothold; most horses, through contact with each other and with tack and other inanimate objects, have a coat and skin micro-traumatised and so readily susceptible to this transmission.

Strangles is an infectious, contagious disease. It, too, can 'run' through a yard. It affects mainly the younger horses, but this is related to their having no innate or age-related immunity from prior exposure. As it passes from one to another it may develop an enhanced virulence, and so break through older horses' immunity.

A degree of contagiousness is difficult to evaluate. Usually the rate at which in-contact animals become infected is a reflection of

- the presence of primary trauma as with ringworm

- the overall lack of the various immunity factors

- its virulence *per se*

The initial invasion is insensible to horse and horsemaster; the horse cannot feel it and the observer cannot see it. Circumstantial evidence, for example one horse in a yard 'known to have an infectious illness', points to the strong possibility that other susceptible animals will 'catch it'. This evidence may be

- **presumptive** – the horse is showing signs typical of a disease which is invariably of an infectious type

- **definite** – the disease has been diagnosed

and, as more horses develop the same signs, the evidence is

- **confirmatory**

In adult horses, most infectious diseases are caused primarily by *virus* invasion and colonisation. Secondary invaders and/or **activated opportunist commensals** (simple 'commensalism' is an association of two species, in which one alone benefits but the other does not *normally* suffer) very often add to the inflammatory reaction. Recent work in in-training and in-work Thoroughbred racehorses has confirmed a long-held belief that inflammatory airway disease (IAD) is due to active infection of certain bacteria (see Chapter 24, DISEASES OF THE RESPIRATORY SYSTEM) and that viruses need not be implicated.

The easiest 'portal of entry' or route into the horse for a primary infection is via **inhaled air**. The gregarious nature of the horse and the volume of air inspired with each breath increases the chance of contagion by a virus in the air in droplet or aerial form.

In modern husbandry the first line defences are often undermined by management factors making the contagion more likely to be infectious, i.e. to **penetrate** onto the tissues of the respiratory system. The encapsulated virus particles, clumps of viruses in sloughed off damaged cells, are further concentrated in aerosoled droplets of expired air which can be spread downwind for many kilometres – distance dilutes numbers, of course, but the potential spread of the infection is important when *considering* isolation.

Other routes for entry of contagion are

- **ingestion**, with excretion in the faeces

- introduction via **other orifices**
  - **genital** – venereal disease
  - **ocular**

- insect **bites** (often called 'transmissible disease') – uncommon in the UK's temperate zone as far as specific disease is concerned

Some viral strains, especially of the **herpes** group, are further disseminated through secondary affected systems, and so 'leave' by the relevant route – for example, abortion discharges.

Reference has been made to what happens next, if and when the microbe penetrates the initial defences to colonise and multiply in the relevant tissue cells or on their surface and the subsequent stimulation of inflammatory reactions begins. This produces the clinical signs that the horse has been infected. In situations where it is important to be forewarned that there is an infection and that it is incubating (the incubation period), then twice-daily temperature recordings showing a rise would be the first clue. It need not be a marked rise, only 0.5–1°C (1–2°F), and it may subside within twenty-four hours (as in some respiratory viral infections) before the second wave of clues arrives – dullness, inappetence, reduced activity – they themselves can be missed; they may be too slight, the animal may not be under close supervision, and/or the horsemaster may be less than observant. The affected horse will very soon produce some more specific signs such as, in the case of respiratory disease, increased respiratory rate, coughing and a nasal discharge. Thereafter the disease will 'run its course' and some infected animals may develop complications

- secondary **bacterial infection**
- secondary **metabolic dysfunction**
- secondary **pathological changes** in unrelated tissues

Most infected animals will improve then recover; in specific circumstances they will become **immune** to that germ and some may develop a **hypersensitivity**. The germ is usually eliminated, but it can remain dormant to be periodically shed as a **pathogen** into the environment or be re-activated into clinical disease within the carrier.

In some situations the primary invader might originally be a commensal dormant germ (virus or bacterium); if the animal becomes debilitated, as by parasitism, malnutrition, overstress, or influenced by another low grade infection, the dormant germ may then become active i.e. pathogenic.

Stress, or, to be more correct, overstressful situations, will predispose not to the horse becoming invaded but to such a horse possibly succumbing to an invasion already there and so developing clinical signs.

The overstress can come from overwork, poor stable hygiene – for example, mould spore concentration – poor drainage and so collection of enteric pathogenic bacteria, chilling or intercurrent disease, as well as the other debilitating factors mentioned, which undermines an existing immunity or triggers the recirculation of dormant microbes.

A primary low-grade infection (usually 'common cold' viruses) will pave the way for more lethal ones. The damage they do is often short-lasting, but opportunist bacterial and fungal spores can move into pathogenic mode; with much more serious consequences in the original site, importantly so too can coincidental higher-grade viral infections.

Both grades of viral infections are potent stressors. Some can even be sub-clinical in effect. Failure to recognise this is excusable; failure to recognise and evaluate the secondaries is not.

Micro-organisms are programmed to survive through their generations, just as is the horse. They too must live to reproduce to do this predestined work – to invade and to traumatise tissue cells. They survive at the expense of the loss of vitality and functioning of the cells they attack; they live off them – they are parasitic. Their life span, especially in the active pathogenic state, is one of hours, but in that time they have replicated themselves a thousand-fold. During the horse's illness, and for a variable time afterwards, many of these progeny are dispersed into the environment – to infect other potential 'patients'. *Viral germs are said to be dedicated pathogens but not with lethal intent. Bacteria are often the reverse.*

When a host dies, the invader still within dies eventually, but may meanwhile continue to contaminate the surroundings for some time through secretions and carrion invaders of the unburied carcass.

It is rare for an infectious disease to wipe out a herd, let alone a whole species. There are historical exceptions but, even so, individuals survive and so does the germ, to continue to 'spread'. An infection may gain in virulence by spread or 'passage' through the earlier infected animals in an outbreak; conversely, even virulent epidemics 'burn themselves out' in time, allowing the later infected hosts to develop an effective immunity and so survive.

The germ's survival relates to its ability

- to live on the epithelial surfaces of systems' tracts, where they are accepted because they do no harm, but reproduce 'within reason', or because the host maintains a numbers limitation without inflammatory involvement. These are **commensals**, possibly opportunists in the nose, mouth, throat, gut or maybe the vagina. They can become active if the host's general resistance is lowered, if it becomes debilitated. It is possible that when their progeny are excreted these could be primary pathogens in a 'weaker' animal – the original host being a carrier

- to lie dormant in an animal's lymphoid tissues or in specific tissue cells, a latent state from which they are periodically excreted, directly or via the circulation, as potential pathogens – the 'carrier' or 'shedder' animal – and to perhaps re-colonise in the same animal: herpes is a significant example

- to survive host inflammatory and subsequent antigenic antagonism during an active infection in morbid cells, and be excreted therefrom as virulent pathogens – the contagious/infectious animal which is the potent source of further spread

- to exist outside the animal (the exception is a virus which requires live cells, certainly to reproduce)

The transmission keeps the germ 'in business'!

It is difficult to declare a once-infected animal as being free from contagion. In influenza where it is generally accepted that latent dis-ease is rare, the horse not only throws **off** the infection but throws **out** the germ; it 'disinfects itself'. Its naturally acquired immunity from the original infection does wane within a year or so. It does however retain a memory of it for rapid boosting at any subsequent re-infection. The influenza virus has an ability to mutate to produce new strains – this is called viral strain 'drift'. Although a recent example is now endemic in the UK, such new strains can set up epidemic outbreaks on their re-introduction or, indirectly but most importantly, if booster injections did not involve **updated vaccines**.

Within the category of primary pathogens, those colloquially and comprehensively called 'parasites' there is usually one stage in their development which is not microscopic. For this reason, and others such as their life cycle, these **ectoparasites** and **endoparasites** are described later. Here they are mentioned in passing because of all the pathogenic organisms they are the ones least anxious to kill their host, which harbours and nourishes them. If they did, several 'generations' or cycles of their species would die with it.

The viruses, which are ultra-microscopic, and the other microscopic types – bacteria, fungi, protozoans – are not so 'considerate'. Whilst many, especially the viruses, require the protection of the animal for their reproduction, others like some bacteria and some fungi can live away from animal tissue and to a varying degree survive and replicate themselves in the soil and in other organic materials – especially if safeguarded against the desiccation of wind, sun and high temperature.

It is the outwards signs of functional disturbances related

to inflammatory disease and the associated inner structural changes which enable the cause to be named or at least suspected. The signs are the disease. Several inflammatory germs produce similar signs in any one system; consider the clinical basic signs of pneumonia due either to a virus or to a bacterium. Conversely, the same germ can cause disease in different systems and so produce different signs. Diagnosis of the actual cause is not easy especially for the horsemaster. *Awareness that something is wrong is paramount*.

Domestication of the horse, and increasing knowledge in the horsemaster, have *minimised the effects of primary and secondary infections.* For example

- **vaccination** against influenza, herpes virus strains, equine viral arteritis and tetanus
- selective use of **antibiotics** in bacterial diseases
- improved feeding, housing, transporting, training and using
- improved sanitation and isolation
- improved import controls
- improved breeding selection

but it has *maximised the risk of infectious disease,* by

- housing
- increased national and international movements
- overstress generally

There is no practicable way of preventing germs from gaining entrance to the horses' body systems' epithelial tracts. If parasitic worm eggs are equated with germs, then, by preventing horses from grazing where eggs have been deposited, re-infection by the hatched larvae can be avoided. Only a few worm species eggs, those of the large white worm and a self limiting small roundworm of foals, can hatch in stabled environments. In no other disease in equines can it be claimed that germs do not exist somewhere. Where there are horses there are micro-organisms. Their clinical presence may not be apparent at any one time. Certain diseases exist only in certain climatic zones, for example the insect-borne viruses. Others may appear only occasionally, and in epidemic form, but they can, even must, be endemic elsewhere in the world.

The suspicion of the active presence of pathogens is based on clinical recognisable signs; confirmation requires

- **isolation** of the germ from the known predilection site – easier with germs other than viruses
- culture and **identification** of it in laboratory media

- **measurement** of antibody levels in paired blood serum samples (the titre)
- **comparable measurement** in two weeks – the convalescent sample – which should show a 'rise' in this titre
- rapid **reduction in the inflammatory signs**, following specific therapy in bacterial, protozoan, and fungal infections but not in viral disease: there is no commercially available anti-viral drug for internal use

In good stable management and horsemastership the basic skills are: knowing all is well, realising quickly when all is not well, and acting correctly. But it is equally important to know, in advance, what can go wrong, when it could happen, and how it can be prevented. In management, therefore, it is an essential background skill to know

- why do certain conditions arise?
- what actually causes them and, in the case of infections
    - where does the 'attacker' come from and how does it spread?
    - can it survive outside the horse?
    - where?
    - can it be 'disinfected'?
    - is there a cost-effective preventative?

but at all times not overlooking the skill of *recognising that something is wrong*.

Discussion with the veterinary surgeon is essential, and better still if it is done before disease develops, for example with regard to vaccination.

VIRUSES

Virus – from the Latin *virus*, a noxious slimy fluid.

The first viral disease to be **isolated**, that of the tobacco plant, in 1892, was described as 'a living infectious fluid', and the name 'virus' derives from the latin for 'a slimy, noxious fluid'. The plant sap contained billions of particles of what was eventually known as a 'virus'.

In the laboratory, virus particles are separated from larger micro-organic material by filtration of suspected fluid through ultra-filters – which the virus passes through with the filtrate, while bacteria or fungal spores are left behind.

Viruses are infectious; their pathogenicity or virulence varies.

Low-grade infections can so alter the structure and

Incidence of Microbes in Horses

	Foal	Adult 3–6yrs	Adult 6yrs and over
Viruses	+	+++++	++++
Bacteria and their toxins	++++	+++	++
Protozoa	+		+
Fungal	++		+++
Parasites			
Endo	+	++++	+
Ecto	+	++	+++

functioning of penetrated tissues that these become susceptible to other microbes.

Viruses are contagious, but they are very host-specific, i.e. they do not 'spread' to other species of animals; rabies is an important exception. Equine respiratory viruses are not infectious to other species.

Their contagiousness or transmissability varies with the species of virus but, generally speaking

- those in droplet aerosols are by definition more readily taken in by inhalation, where they are defended against by physico-chemical factors – the mucociliary escalator, the respiratory two-way flow and by on-site general immunity

- those which are readily passed on from animal to animal – for example venereal infections and diarrhoeic discharges on to food and water – but unless they are quick in transmission soon 'die' in the non-animal environment

- those which have contaminated inanimate objects, to 'await' being 'picked up' by licking, by skin contact, or by contaminated inhalation of dust, are least likely to remain infectious: they die

All are susceptible to various disinfectants, but the scientifically proven specific antiviral one must be used. In the stable, disinfection must be preceded by 'mucking out', cleaning up and high-pressure hosing, and/or warm water with 'washing soda' (NaCO₃), to dissolve organic material which might prolong the virus's extra-cellular existence.

Virus particles exist in an 'active state' rather than being 'alive'; chemicals and heat will destroy this activity. Viruses do not 'live' in the animal, in the sense that bacteria do, and consequently they are not susceptible to chemo-therapy or antibiotic therapy in the living animal; such anti-viral agents as are known are certainly of no practical and economic significance in the horse. The presumed rare cases of viral conjunctivitis will however respond to a specific anti-viral drug.

The pathogenic non-lethal types

- influenza strains
- herpes group
- viral arteritis ('pink eye')
- viral venereal and skin infections

are endemic in the UK. The more serious, often lethal types have not yet appeared in the UK with the exception of 'infectious anaemia'. A significant feature of this absence is that they are mainly insect transmitted and the British climate does not lend itself to these insects becoming established here.

Viral contagiousness is of importance, and **influenza** and some **herpes** strains do produce marked clinical illness; that is, they are of high pathogenicity.

The former can relatively rapidly develop new strains which are usually introduced from abroad. What is usually an endemic 'foreign' disease can then become epidemic with regard to the native horse population's immunity.

The latter virus also has the ability to 'drift' both pathogenically and immunologically, and it too can surface as an epidemic with particular regard to the non-respiratory strains. However, it is a truism that herpes germs are always present at some level of pathogenicity and of a persistently high infectiousness.

The virus which causes **infectious anaemia** in horses (EIA) has been occasionally diagnosed in the UK. Its re-entry and spread could become a serious epidemic. It is known colloquially as **swamp fever** and is transmitted not only by biting insects but also by inanimate objects contaminated with blood serum from minor surgical acts such as rasping of teeth.

Less pathogenic viruses do infect horses in the UK. Their importance is thought to be as either

- secondary commensals which can complicate primaries, or as

- primary mild pathogens in their own right which can trigger more serious infections

There are four; three of them are grouped as 'cold viruses' – **rhinovirus** strains 1, 2 and 3. As their collective name implies, they are found mainly in the upper respiratory tract. One strain is also enteric.

Rotavirus, the fourth, is associated with diarrhoea in foals up to the age of 5 months. It is a **collaborator** with the potentially pathogenic bacteria *Salmonella* and *E.coli*.

The majority of equine viruses not only infect via the respiratory system but they are also pathogenic to it. Moreover, they can 'escape' into the blood circulation to colonise in other tissues, to prolong the illness, and increase the range of organs which are attacked – heart muscle, skeletal muscle, kidneys, nervous tissue – and seriously affect their functioning. Most importantly is the need to monitor the secondarily *damaged tissues' recovery before athletic training is resumed.*

Such 'too early' metabolic demand becomes not only an important hazard to these structures, but also a stress factor predisposing to secondary invaders and to the recrudescence of herpes virus in convalescent lymphoid and vascular sites – an economically important feature in racehorse training.

The 'viruses' evolved to replicate themselves only in specific animal cells. To this end, they constantly strive to invade and to penetrate specific tissue. There are no grounds for believing that they evolved a pathogenicity sufficient to kill the hosts. Certainly they are often lethal to foals and to old animals. Their evolution paths were however not programmed to endure the other stresses of domestication. It is important that man is aware of this, and

- moderates his demands on the 'invaded' or convalescent horse

- seeks to immunise artificially where he can

- maintains a strict protocol against unnecessary or thoughtless spread, especially with venereal diseases and in sporadic herpes virus abortion 'storms'

Because of their ability to mutate and thereby produce new strains or sub-types with significantly different pathogenicity and immune bodies, satisfactory artificial immunity (vaccination) is not always efficient. Nor does this artificial immunity last; it requires boosting at regular intervals. The artificial immunity is humoral and so does not attack new invasions until the tissue cells have been invaded. The humoral immunity is, however, very useful against those viruses which 'aim' to become blood-borne. They are extremely **immunogenic**, especially under natural disease conditions.

Viruses will not 'grow' in ordinary media in the laboratory. They can be grown in live cell cultures or by being injected into live 'incubators' such as fertile hen's eggs. From these artificial multiplications a series of tests is available to identify them and their sub-types.

BACTERIA

Animals and germs have evolved together. The animal has developed defences against the germ, for example the epidermis. Germs must survive; bacteria do so on animal surfaces, 'internal' as well as 'external', where there is some multiplication, variable with the species but especially in disease situations, and in the soil. The common streptococcal bacteria of the horse are not good survivors 'off' the horse. They can live on epithelial tissues, especially mucosal, as commensals and as opportunists. Even strangles germs will survive in the guttural pouches long after clinical infection has subsided.

All bacteria are microscopic and require 1000x enlargement to be seen. They are much larger than viruses. They are everywhere – in the system tracts, on the hair and skin, and widespread in inanimate objects – and are teaming in the soil. Certain strains are essential, for example those in the large intestine of horses, for the breakdown of cellulose. Others are involved in the vitality of the soil and the decomposition of dead plants and animals therein.

Very few are directly or primarily pathogenic. Strangles is an example of a primary disease. The germs that can

Some Bacterial Diseases

Anthrax	Bacillus anthracis
Botulism	Clostridium botulinum toxin
Brucellosis	Brucella abortus
Leptospirosis	Leptospira species
Salmonellosis	Salmonella species
Summer pneumonia of foals	Rodococcus equi
Strangles	Streptococcus equi
Tetanus	Clostridium tetani toxin
Contagious equine metritis (CEM)	Taylorella equi genitalis
Other metritic diseases	Klebsiella pneumoniae Pseudomonas aerugonisa

Anthrax, from the Greek, *malignant pustule* (as in the human disease)
Botulism, from the Latin, a *sausage* (the original food product confirmed as the source of the toxin)
Brucellosis, after a Mr Bruce who 'discovered' the germ – *osis* means literally 'full of' the germ found in profusion at the morbid tissues
Strangles – describes the 'choking' signs of the related abscesses
Tetanus – describes the pathology, a 'tetany' or spasm of muscles

commensally exist on the epithelial lining of the systems' tracts may become active, being not only indirectly pathogenic to the original animal but also capable of being 'passed on' to their susceptible ones. Then their commensal character changes to infectious. It is believed that some strains of these commensals can actually become defensive against more virulent invaders. Bacterial survival depends upon the ability to reproduce without having to enter tissue cells of living animals, unlike viruses. Strangles once again is an exception: it requires living tissues, epithelial and glandular as a base. Strains eventually involved in disease do of course multiply rapidly in tissues but these, unlike viruses, can survive and remain infective for a year or longer in the environment after excretion. Such fomites become a hazard.

Disinfection of materials becomes essential in managing such diseases. It is of course impossible to disinfect soil, except under strict horticultural conditions. There are some soil germs, clostridia species, which exist there as spores in which they are 'weather proofed'. Naturally, these spores contaminate herbage and grown cereals (seeds), and consequently they are frequently ingested; some persist only in certain soil types, and so are of regional importance.

Ingested bacteria are usually passed through the gut. They do not multiply therein before being excreted onto and into the soil where, in the case of Clostridia, they re-sporulate. As a rule they do no harm in the gut.

Two situations can alter this

- **ulcers** in the mucous membrane – it is believed that if bacteria side track through these, into the blood stream, they are destroyed by the reticulo-endothelial system in a short span. If however the animal is traumatised, as by a muscle strain, or a kick, or even by a correctly made intra-muscular injection, any still surviving clostridial germs which *escape* with the blood into these tissues will become pathogenic there. They do so by rapid multiplication with the production of cell-destroying toxins – a local gangrene and an ultimate toxaemia develop

- **inflammatory** structural and functioning disturbances – in this scenario the primary inflammation, which need not be so serious as to be clinical, creates the ideal surface environment for **fortuitous Clostridia** to colonise and multiply, with the production of lethal toxins causing clinical toxaemia. A particular Clostridium, *Cl. perfringens*, is thought to lie dormant in the gut of foals particularly, and to become pathogenic under certain 'indigestive' conditions. An enteritis with secondary toxaemia develops and becomes clinical (*see also* Botulism and Tetanus).

Pathogenicity, the ability to cause an inflammatory reaction, develops when bacteria gain entrance to subcutaneous (and sub-epithelial) tissues from

Exogenous sources

- **penetration** of the surface of the skin or other tract linings by various species of germs common to them as commensals, for example, a penetrating wound. (When an animal bites, it inoculates the germs of its oral saliva into the bitten subject. Cat bites are rare in horses, but the feline does carry a 'nasty' which can cause 'cat bite fever' in humans.)

The subsequent morbidity is invariably followed by

- local **spread**
- a purulent **discharge**, with possible abscess formation if drainage is poor (e.g. in a foot abscess)

and possibly by

- **systemic spread** of germs and/or their toxin
  - via **blood**, leading to septicaemia and/or toxaemia
  - via **lymph**, leading to lymphangitis and to lymphadinitis with possible abscessation thereof
- the development of **immunity**
- the development of **hypersensitivity**

- **inhalation**, when they invade sensitive tissues by aerosol into the **upper respiratory tract**, especially in foals. Any associated nasal discharges are invariably purulent. In the healing stages this secretion is known as 'catarrh'. It may be an overspill from the pharynx and airways.

Those bacteria which are commensal opportunists of the respiratory tract include some eight or nine species. Their clinical signs serve to indicate an active secondary invader whose therapeutic elimination is possible, unlike a primary virus. To the horsemaster these signs, and especially the residual cough, are markers for a delay in return to work.

- **ingestion** onto the throat (the pharyngeal surface) with direct passage through that mucus membrane into the
  - regional **lymphatic system** and glands – and/or
  - the systemic **blood circulation** (as with the strangles germ)

- **direct** introduction onto mucosae, as in
  - **venereal disease**
  - **guttural pouch infection** – respiratory source

- **contamination** of the new-born umbilicus leading to
  - '**navel' ill** and possibly with spread to
  - '**joint' ill**

- **contamination of the eye** surface with local
  - **conjunctivitis** – this can also come from blood-borne spread as part of strangles and other respiratory tract infections

It is significant that most infectious diseases of the foal are bacterial. This is explained by the facts that

- a foal is born with no antibodies
- it obtains these from the dam's colostrum – *if* the dam herself has sufficient antibodies to the *local* environmental germs and *if* the foal sucks within 6 hours of birth
- a foal is programmed to sniff, lick, suck and eat whereby his gut is progressively populated with digestive bacteria: the dam's faeces are an extremely good source
- the outcome is a balance between the foal's congenital strength, its absorbed protection from colostrum, and the germs' virulence

Endogenous sources

An endogenous route is taken by bacteria within the horse's normal gut flora population to invade the gut wall and/or enter the circulation. This follows a direct change in the host's condition, not a change in the bacterial pathogenicity, as a result of

- overstress
- shock
- malnutrition

which all impair the natural general immunity, and 'magnify' the significance of gut wall minor traumas.

As with viruses, the family and species names of bacteria are of little help to the horsemaster – but see the chart for examples. There are however three categories relative to how and where they grow, which determine treatment, and so must be appreciated.

Those that require a good supply of oxygen to live and to multiply are **aerobic**. Those that do not appreciate 'fresh air' are **anaerobic**. And a particular bacterium, CEM, *Taylorella equi genitalis*, the cause of contagious equine metritis; is **micro-aerophilic** – i.e. it requires a particular 'half-way' stage environment.

These varied oxygen requirements apply to natural survival and pathogenicity especially in wounds, as well as to laboratory cultural requirements.

Generally speaking, the germs within each group are susceptible to different antibiotic (antigerm) treatment and to wound management.

There are three types of micro-organisms which are intermediate in size and lifestyle between bacteria and viruses. They are

- **Mycoplasma**
  - can be free living

  - can be a respiratory commensal
  - associated with **secondary broncho-pneumonia**
  - is aerosol spread

- **Chlamydia**
  - not free-living, found in several species of bird and animal
  - aerosol spread
  - not (yet) a proven equine pathogen

- **Rickettsia**
  - not free living
  - found only in association with lice, fleas, ticks and mites

Most bacteria are susceptible to **chemo-therapeutics** and to **antibiotics**, but

- the correct drug must be selected, as judged by laboratory sensitivity culture
- if chosen 'from experience' the response or otherwise must be monitored
- it must be given at the correct dose for the correct time
- oral drugs must be used with consideration for the essential gut flora (the veterinary surgeon will advise)
- none should ever be used on a 'fresh' case just because some doses were (wrongly) left over from an earlier one, unless under direct veterinary supervision (the vet will want to know why the original course was not completed)

All bacteria in the environment are susceptible to disinfectants but, as with viruses, some require special chemicals. Contaminated surfaces must be 'mucked out', cleaned up, and have organic material dissolved away and surfaces decontaminated first of all.

In-depth scientific knowledge may have limited practical value in everyday practice, but its implications should be appreciated. For example, when a wound is contaminated by bacteria there is a wide range of individual types involved, both aerobic and anaerobic, and there is little rhyme or reason as to which are introduced. Which survive to become predominant pathogens is a reflection of the type of wound. Sometimes, the type of inflammation points to the important ones, but most often not.

There are 5 aerobic and 7 anaerobic bacteria, all of which can be skin commensals, regularly found by laboratory tests to be wound contaminants, and another 2 aerobics and 1 anaerobic if an animal bite is involved or a thermal burn is the trauma. The veterinary surgeon decides from experience if therapy is justified, and which one. If there is doubt, or if results are sub-optimal, then samples for the lab will be required. Some bacteria are susceptible to simple antibiotics; others require more sophisticated broader spectrum drugs. A decision is a matter for the veterinary surgeon. *There is sound argument against the topical application of antibiotics to wounds.*

The first-aid management of wounds, and their subsequent nursing are dealt with in a later chapter, but it can be said here that when contamination of any wound is seen or suspected it is best to decontaminate by lavage. This also serves to aerate the wound, thus not only minimising infection but particularly minimising suitable conditions for anaerobic multiplication; anaerobic germs are often the more pathogenic.

As usual, it is very important to recognise that an inflammatory reaction is active, rather than to worry about what exactly is causing it, at least initially. It is important to know 'what can go wrong' or 'what has gone wrong' when

- the skin is penetrated – and, for example, the horse is lame
- a primary disease is complicated by secondary invaders, for example a 'cold' becomes a purulent nasal discharge, or a cough continues for more than 10 days
- a brood mare develops a post-mating discharge

It is essential to know *what you can do, what you should do,* and *what you must not attempt.*

Most bacterial diseases are self-limiting, due to the concurrent stimulation of *local* immunity. The presence of pus, as a discharge, is indicative of white blood cell aggressive action to contain and so expel the invader. An abscess retains it, but shuts it off; usually it eventually bursts or has to be lanced. (The pus is variously contagious.) Convalescence follows. Nursing aims to aid nature. *Antibiotic therapy, even when professionally administered, does no more than reduce the number of bacteria that 'nature' has to fight.*

Immunisation against the bacterial infection of strangles, *Streptococcus equi,* is not practised in the UK. The most useful anti-bacterial immunisations are those against their lethal toxins, usually of the Clostridia, when a 'toxoid' is injected, e.g. against tetanus. Some stables are recognised as being unusually susceptible to secondary Clostridial infections following wounds, even the trauma of intra-muscular injections or when blood escapes from an intravenous injection. Once this possibility is established, a specific anti-Clostridial toxoid immunisation programme has to be maintained. Research work is being done with regard to endometrial (womb mucous membrane) bacterial immunity.

In the UK, there are no equine bacterial diseases of a primary nature which are transmissable to man. Man and his horse can however be secondarily invaded by the same bacteria from various sources, which may or may not produce disease in one or the other or both. **Anthrax** can pass from abscess discharge, but is rarely seen in horses or in man. Clostridial soil spores and their eventual toxins are more likely to come from a common extra-animal source. Secondary **salmonellosis** can be transmitted, and therefore equine suspected cases should be handled with great care, as with all diarrhoeas especially in the foal.

PROTOZOA

Protozoa are the single-celled forerunners of mammalian tissue cells. An earlier-mentioned non-pathogenic example is *Amoeba proteus.*

Protozoan disease is not common in horses in the UK. A well-known lamb, piglet and poultry bowel disease is associated with large intestinal bowel wall-cell invasion by one species of parasite. It has been recorded in foals. It is usually a 'partner' in cellular pathogenicity. When present there is often a 'bloody' diarrhoea, as in **coccidiosis** which is spread via ingestion.

A disease not yet significant in horses, but present in sheep and man and 'carried' by cats, is **toxoplasmosis**.

The other strains are serious pathogens in the USA and in tropical and sub-tropical Africa. One type in America, equine myelo-encephalitis (EPM), has a predilection for the central nervous system. Protozoan disease, like several others, is insect-borne and transmitted. Worldwide, there are many, many species of free-living, non-pathogenic protozoa.

FUNGI

Like bacteria, fungi are part of our environment. Unlike them, their presence can become very evident in all nature, as distinct from the disease signs of morbid invasion of animal tissue.

The fungi are part and parcel of the recycling of organic

material, playing an important role in soil fertility and humus formation. The spores of some species and the mycelia of others spread into and over whatever the 'parent' yeasts and fungi contaminate. To multiply requires the correct combination of temperature and moisture. Thus, incorrectly harvested hay, or gathered and stored straw, helps multiply the naturally present fungi so that an obvious mould appears on them, and eventually breaks away in the form of dust and airborne particles. Moulds also appear on the walls of damp, ill-ventilated houses. The word 'mouldy' is used literally and metaphorically to describe an object as damaged and decaying.

The animal diseases associated with fungi are

- **ringworm** – a disease of the hair, the hair follicle and epidermis; a dermatitis spread by contact direct or indirect. Some species are communicable to man

- **aspergillosis** – an inhaled pathogen which colonises on airway mucous membranes and in the guttural pouches, causing a serious and often fatally ulcerative condition thereon

- **yeast infections** – most are ingested commensals of the gut, but may become super-active when normal gut bacterial flora are knocked out by injudicious use of antibiotics. Some species are involved in inflammatory reactions in the mouth, especially of foals and in the genital tract

- some species of fungi, mainly **micropolyspora**, contaminate hay and straw. When these bales dry out or are shaken the spores can become airborne and enter deep into the air tracts, to sensitise the alveolar mucosae and predispose it to **obstructive pulmonary disease** (OPD) when further challenged at a later date

- some fungi, when they multiply in badly stored cereals (over 14% moisture), produce toxins which contaminate feeds and remain even in the eventual absence of the mould. This is **aflatoxin**, which is fatally toxic on ingestion

- the **ergot of rye**, a mould which infects some pasture grasses. Equine toxicity from eating these grasses is not common, however consumption of badly infected rye grain can be serious. The rye grain when used as stock feed is *always* inspected for mould

- other vegetation can be affected
  - **lupins** are poisonous because of a mould

- very problematical, but is grass sickness a herbage (fungal) toxin, or a Clostridial bacterial toxin? Research continues.

PARASITISM

Ectoparasites
See Chapter 31, SKIN DISEASES

Endoparasites
See Chapter 26, DISEASES OF THE DIGESTIVE SYSTEM

ALLERGIC DIS-EASE

The word **allergy** derives from the German *Allergie*, 'a changed reaction', from the original Greek *Allos*, 'other and *Ergon*, 'energy' or 'normal activity'; hence 'altered activity' and so 'allergic reaction'. Colloquially, 'allergic' is used to imply 'having an aversion to' someone or something.

With reference to Chapter 21, IMMUNOLOGY, it is explained that animals have an innate ability, when their tissue cells/vascular systems are invaded, to

- recognise the presence of foreign, non-self substances mainly of a protein or polypeptide composition, and to

- react to their presence by producing anti-substances, which act as

- tissue/organ protectors

In the process of becoming immune (i.e. resistant to further similar invasions, by infection, vaccination or coincidentally) to potential pathological effects, the body systems become sensitised to the invader.

The desired benefits of this immunity, whether natural (subsequent to infection) or artificial (post-vaccination), are based on the formation of

- humoral immunoglobulins
- cellular (lymphocyte and other specific cells) mediated defences

Such an immunised animal is said to be capable of resisting colonisation and pathogenic effect of the antigenic substances. The degree and the duration of these resistance factors varies; most, but not all, will fade with time. However the primary sensitised state will permanently remain through 'memory' T lymphocytes.

In some cases a **hypersensitised** state will be present, with the risk of an altered, undesirable reaction to further antigenic challenge, by the specific protein, from

- inhalation
- ingestion
- skin contact
- (injection)

This reaction, or altered enhanced response, is an allergic one and the antigen is better known as an allergen. Such reactions' pathology varies with the

- animal species
  - anatomical/functioning parts involved
  - tissues/organs susceptible
- allergen
  - type
  - shock dose
  - type of antibody
  - degree of sensitivity induced

but non-protein substances, organic and inorganic, which have an affinity for the protein constituents within a tissue, can link with these – and the complex is antigenic – known as a **Hapten**. Once an 'immune' state is developed, the non-protein factor can thereafter remain as a sensitiser and be capable of stimulating an allergic reaction when it is reintroduced to the animal.

Allergic reactions vary with the route of the 'invasion' of the sensitising 'foreign body'. They can be

- localised, as in skin sites
- generalised
  - regional
  - systemic – often, in horses, with skin involvement

All reactions are of the *inflammatory* type of dis-ease, leading to

- tissue morbidity
- morbidity from other sub-types of allergic reactions

There is a similarity in hypersensitivity disorders and auto-immune diseases, which are functioning mistakes in innate self-preservation development. Hypersensitivity disorders are basically exaggerated immune responses of a clinical degree. True immunity represents a more refined, controlled response, usually with no, or at least only minor, clinical signs; there is still much to be learned, even in scientific circles.

The clinical reaction in allergic disease can be

- **immediate**, as in the **flush, flare and weal** type
  - obvious within seconds to minutes after the toxic

dose, known or unknown
- may last several hours
- is antibody-mediated along three possible effector pathways, which may overlap and, with the delayed type
- can occur in the absence of demonstrable confirmable protein antibodies – one example is anaphylaxis
- **delayed**
  - obvious, and usually progressively so in one to three days and time for effector cell recruitment
  - may last several days
- is a T lymphocyte cellular-mediated reaction
- is not always explicable in terms of primary sensitisation, but usually associated with infectious agents

The morbidity associated with allergic reactions is centred on the

- blood vascular system and, in particular, the capillary wall cells and blood vessel walls within this
- blood cells, especially the white and particularly the lymphocytes and platelets
- smooth muscle cells (the involuntary controlled system, especially the respiratory, in the horse)

By definition these cells have, at some time in the past, and usually not less than ten days previously, been invaded by an organic substance or by a Hapten, and so have become sensitised (or hypersensitised) by the antigenic (allergenic) properties thereof.

Anaphylaxis

This is a special type of immediate allergy, from the Greek word *ana*, 'against', and *phylassein*, 'to protect'. It is described as a perversion or an over-reactivity of a protective mechanism. It usually results when a 'shock' tissue is invaded by a sudden and relatively large eliciting dose which is 'received', as by injection of certain drugs, and the reaction is called a 'natural'.

In insect stings and snake venoms, the reaction is essentially to a toxic substance which is part of that attacker's natural aggressive/defence armoury.

The dis-ease is an **anaphylactic shock**. Death can follow quickly in some acute cases. Recovery may occur, and when it does there is a short duration de-sensitisation. The primary morbidity is in the capillary walls around the 'bite', or is diffuse when the eliciting dose enters the vascular system. There is fluid loss into tissues, with oedema, shock and haemorrhage, in the smooth muscle of the respiratory tract with respiratory distress, and in the pregnant uterus, with subsequent abortion.

The reaction follows the release of toxic substances such as **histamine** and **heparin** from mast cells and blood platelets.

The horse, as a species, is highly sensitive to histamine, and therefore reacts markedly to the release of this substance in anaphylactic and other acute allergic episodes; this reaction presents particularly with extensive oedema as the primary lesion.

The acute anaphylactic shock signs are

- whole body-surface oedematous plaques, 1–2.5cm (0.25–1in) in diameter, often running into one another
- cold, clammy skin and coat
- patchy sweating
- shivering, developing to rigors
- anxiety
- rapid and shallow respiration
- sub-normal temperature
- accelerated heart rate

A now unusual example is the reaction elicited when a warble larva was ruptured beneath the skin, from saddle pressure or from ignorant attempts to squeeze it out through a non-existent hole.

Purpura Haemorrhagica

This is a particular anaphylactic reaction to a primary or secondary infection which may itself have produced no clinical signs. Residual microbes or breakdown antigenic components still circulating can react with them (now allergens); there is an immediate obvious morbidity. The level of the original antibody is a reflection of the late stages or even the convalescent state; the purpura reaction can *only* occur then, sometimes up to two weeks post initial illness.

The common primary infections are by the streptococcal strains, especially of strangles, wound contaminants, and secondaries to virus infection. The clinical feature is described in a later chapter.

The 'Weal and Flare' Immediate Reaction

If man, previously sensitised by contact with or inhalation of the 'dander' from a horse's skin, as at grooming, has a subsequent contact, there is an immediate superficial skin reaction which shows as a

- central, hard, white swelling, the 'weal' – there has been an initial shutting down of local capillaries, a hypoxia, then
- a red flush, the 'flare' – from subsequent dilation of the capillaries, which also leak serum to produce
- local **oedema**, known as 'hives', which spreads
- **itching**, from the swelling pressure on special, as yet unidentified nerve endings, which lasts for several hours

Repeated inhalation of dander will produce characteristic signs of asthma. Such signs of hypersensitivity to contact and to inhaled allergens is an **atopy**, which is particularly hereditable. Most allergic conditions have some genetic component, thus explaining why not all horses in a similar environment respond to any allergens in the same manner.

In the horse, similar reactions occur from its own dander, with similar signs as in man *except* that skin pigment and hair hide the characteristic colours. It is now accepted that inhalation atopy does occur, and the reaction can surprisingly show as an **allergic dermatitis**. The **hives** are invariably well-marked, especially on the muzzle and face. **Hay fever** in the human, and **rhinitis** in the horse, are other examples.

Urticaria

Urticaria (from the Latin *urtica, nettle*) is characterised by the signs previously described as 'weal and flair'. It and other allergic skin conditions are arguably the most common equine hypersensitivities and, apart from ringworm, sarcoids and melanoma in greys, are *the most common type of skin dis-ease*.

The **pruritus** (itchiness) is sometimes accompanied by excessive loss of superficial epidermis and hair, producing a scurf and a flaking scab. The underlying morbidity is an oedema. The individual lesions are 1–1.5cm (0.25–0.5in) plaques. These can extend from the muzzle to the flanks, sometimes with extensive ventral oedema.

The various precipitating causes include

- high concentrate (possibly protein) feed in fit horses, as ingested allergens. This condition is colloquially called 'humour' (*see also* lymphangitis)
- other foods and grazings
- contact with saddle soap, detergents, chemical irritants, certain plants
- drugs – topical and systemic
- biting insects – gnats, flies, mosquitoes and mites (the

related disorder **sweet itch** is a well-known example)

• low grade chronic bacterial dermatitis

(in all of the above causes, urticaria is colloquially called 'nettle rash')

• nettle stings (a true rash)

• larval stages of endoparasites into or out of the skin

Common diseases of a specific nature are

• parotid salivary gland enlargement due to ingestion or inhalation, particularly of the oily pollen of buttercups which have contaminated the grazing, or of other ingested grass protein allergens

• mould spore 'allergy', as in OPD

• summer pollen 'asthmatic OPD'

• the various 'nettle rashes'

Delayed Type

There are several sub-types, but all are characterised by

• a demonstrable **reaction**, showing hours or even days after the eliciting dose, and lasting for many days

• originating in any **vascular** tissue, but usually that of the dermis

• basically due to an infiltration of **leucocytes**, following

  • the reaction between the allergens and a special type of antibody inside or attached to the tissue, called a **reagin**

  • there is no serum involvement, so it is *not transferable* via blood or serum infusion

The clinical exhibitions of allergic reactions, though given descriptive names as specific *diseases*, are more dis-ease *conditions*. As already mentioned, some are perverse immune states, and therefore associated with protective mechanisms. The human 'sufferer' is unlikely to see them as such, but rather as unpleasant and disconcerting handicaps – however much they are said to be related to his/her immune system. It is likely that in man and in animals some are genetically linked, and so 'run in the family'. Little research has been carried out in the horse in this context.

Some allergies when elicited can produce severe, even fatal consequences. In others, especially in infections which run a *chronic course* and so give time for hypersensitivity to develop *concurrently*, the reaction leads to tissue necrosis. In the human, **leprosy** is a classic example. In the OPD horse, the pulmonary tissue changes which develop, in a few mismanaged cases, to emphysema are reputedly due to ischaemia of the connective tissues from the pressure changes produced by persistent coughing. Perhaps there is a tissue necrosis factor as well?

Allergic syndromes in the horse are not the result of domestication *per se* except that, in OPD, the environment is worse in stables' ventilation (or lack of it), and because of modern hay-making techniques. Contact allergies are of course more likely in the horse which is working. The basic hypersensitivity potential is most probably as old as *Equus caballus*.

The Arthus reaction is a particular form of allergic reaction which presents as

• malaise

• fever

• urticaria

• arthralgia

• albumenuria

There is no histamine involvement and the pathology is confined to the synovia of joints and tendon sheaths, the kidney glomeruli and arterioles and venules.

METABOLIC DIS-EASE

Biochemical reactions occur within tissue cells – in cellular water. Collectively, they comprise the metabolic processes necessary for life. The term derives from the Greek *metabole*, 'change'; **metabolism** is the biological process which brings about change.

• **catabolism**, from the Greek 'throwing down', is the breakdown of tissue – of ingested food into smaller, absorbable and distributable elements which can be further absorbed into the animals' cells

• **anabolism**, from the Greek '*ascent*', is the rebuilding of these into 'larger', usable elements specifically required by the cells

Metabolism concerns nutrition of the cell; metabolic disease is basically a **malnutrition of the cell**

• the incorrect elements being digested and/or absorbed

• failure to deliver these at the right time, to the right cells

• failure of transfer from blood to the cells

• inability (e.g. enzyme failure) to make proper use of them

The elements are the usual nutritional ones, and particularly those minerals which become **electrolytes**. The clinical signs are fundamentally those of alterations in functioning, for example

- muscle relaxation failure in **azoturia**, leading to bilateral, usually hind leg, lameness
- nerve conduction failure, as in transit **tetany**

In some situations, the functional upset is subclinical and the effects, the structural changes, become clinical

- **Miller's disease**, in gross CaP imbalanced diets
- **Hyperlipaemia**, 'structural' change in the blood, following starvation of the fat pony

The liver is the major site of metabolism; it acts as a half-way stage in converting catabolised chemicals into more complex ones. Its property of detoxifying poisons is a life preserving feature, and of 'purifying' the blood of the waste products of cellular activity – for example, the conversion of ammonia into urea which is eliminated in the urine

- it modulates the potential toxicity of some drugs
- it manufactures the blood proteins from dietary amino-acids

Consequently, dis-ease of the liver can have far reaching effects whose recognitions (clinical signs) may not, at first, point to the basic morbidity.

Metabolic processes are also under the control of the endocrine system

- the metabolism of calcium (**parathyroids**)
- the metabolism of glucose (pancreatic **insulin**)
- the metabolism of urine (excess excretion from deficiency of output from the pituitary's **anti-diuretic hormone**)

From a practical point of view it is the horsemaster's skills in the application of good management to ensure

- adequate nutrients for the condition, age and work of the horse
- freedom from mal-nourishment (which does not necessarily imply starvation)
- absence of toxic factors
- seasonal and work output corrections in feeding
- early recognition of when mistakes occur

Horsemastership is the constant skill of balancing work output **by a particular animal**, against nutrient intake, and of avoiding overstress.

Horses evolved to survive in the total environment of their 'free' existence; they did not inherit any automatic defences or 'self cures' against the metabolic diseases imposed by domestication – wrong feeding (input) and wrong using (work output).

Basically, metabolic (domesticated) disease is neither traumatic nor infectious, so there is no innate healing inflammatory response, let alone a subsequent immunity. The diseased metabolism brings the animal to variable levels of unusability. The consequent drop in output can reduce the overstress and allow the metabolism to recover. Occasionally, tissues have been too badly 'burned' to recover, and death in part or in whole is the outcome.

There may be a genetic disposition, at least to some metabolic disease, or an individual or even a family tendency to be more susceptible to the effects of overstress factors. The disease may be more common in one gender than in the other; this would suggest a hormonal influence, e.g. azoturia.

Fortunately, man has learned to effect the necessary balances, and to act quickly when signs suggest that all is not balanced. Analysis of feedstuffs has played a big part in minimising the risks of malnutrition-based metabolic disease. Scientific and laboratory investigation has helped to explain the underlying causes, and management involvement has regulated overstress of growth and of work.

DEGENERATIVE DIS-EASE

From the Latin *degeneratio*, a morbid disintegration of tissue leading to a change in structure and functioning up to and including necrosis (death) of the cells involved.

This definition is a repeat of that given for inflammatory disease, to a lesser extent for metabolic disease, and is not dissimilar to the replacement of healthy tissue by neoplastic growths. *But in degenerative diseases the cause is significantly different*.

There are certain morbid conditions which, primarily or secondarily to other factors, cause 'disintegration' or loss of function. Such are *not* the result of direct infection or direct trauma, and are described as 'degenerative disease'; there is no inflammatory reaction, at least initially. This implies that there is no intrinsic ability to

- confine the morbidity, which is therefore progressive – to a variable degree or to directly

- instigate repair processes

But in some tissues, regeneration is possible provided not all the cells in an affected particular tissue or organ or unit of activity (for example, a joint cartilage) are destroyed.

Secondary and subsequent factors can and do occur; degenerative disease is often a complicated affliction as, for example, in the locomotor system. Structural changes are fundamental. In most cases the causative factors need not be *per se* destructive to the cells, but will induce a loss of vitality through malnutrition from

- nutritional imbalances at cellular level
- local interference with normal blood supply to influence cellular metabolism directly
- pathological changes in body fluids, for example those in synovial fluid associated with synovitis, leads to malnourishment of the avascular cartilage, causing deterioration in its structure

Subsequent functioning of such degenerated tissues will of course be altered in varying degrees.

It should be appreciated that degenerative disease can also be the culmination of

- inflammatory disease
  - traumatic – sterile or infected
  - infectious – primary or secondary
- allergic reaction
- metabolic disease, direct or indirect

superimposed on genetically weak and/or management weakened tissues.

To justify the descriptive title, the most important feature must be **structural degenerative change(s)**. In practice, these changes are often insidious and progressive. Acute forms do occur, but such are most accurately referable to the speed of onset of clinical signs, mainly functional, following subclinical structural morbidity from one or more causes.

Genetic influences are recognised, as in breed and family incidences, but whether entirely hereditable is disputed. It can be said:

- the **nature** of the horse *pre-disposes*
- the **nurture** of the horse *determines*, through
  - feeding
  - using – variable rates and degrees of wear and tear superimposed on growth rates and ratios, metabolic differences and acquired conformation defects

In the wild state, horses experienced the detrimental effects of wear and tear over the years. 'Survival of the fittest' would determine when, and natural span would reflect the end point whether or not by predators. Age would inevitably lower tissue resilience or vitality of structure and functioning. No doubt, developmental defects, congenital and acquired, played a part – but, again, these would be self-eliminating. Most animals would live to breed; in severe early degenerations they would not. Such tendencies would thereby be taken out of the genetic pool – the 'non-survival of the weakest'.

It is certain that the additional hazards of domestication – man's imposed extra stress factors, duress leading to distressed tissues and functionings – do play a significant role. Selective breeding policies to establish types for performance and quality characteristics do not always produce a physique and metabolism to withstand modern athletic forces and other management liabilities. In the wild and feral existences, improvement in functioning, let alone structural recovery, was unlikely in degenerative disease except in the herd as a unit through natural selection.

Occurrence in the domesticated, 'improved' horse is a different matter. Sensible, hard-hearted culling; more thoughtful, broader perspectives in breeding; artificial selection; and more careful using, are all essential to reduce the likelihood of non-age related degenerations, even at the cost of losing some youthful athletic success. The problem is not only an economic issue **but also a welfare matter**.

The majority of clinical cases do not show to the horsemaster as clear-cut, recognisable degenerative entities. They will in practice point more to the system involved than to the type of morbidity. Once again, it is the fact of 'something being wrong' which is important.

'What' and 'why' will originally be difficult to determine, and there is often the risk of a mistaken assumption or diagnosis.

For example

- a young 'light' horse develops a unilateral 'bog spavin'. There is a little lameness, but no history of injury. The possibilities for this distension of the joint capsule are
  - **idiopathic** – basically from no known outside influence
  - **traumatic** inflammatory
    - sterile, single, unseen sprain incident
    - infectious – direct or blood-borne
  - **insidious**, repetitive mild trauma – a chronic condition

- **degenerative**, associated with degenerative joint disease

'*What*' is obvious; '*why*' requires detailed investigation.

- a pony, grazing free-range on poorish land, becomes suddenly ill
  - it seems to lie down more than usual
  - when up, it walks stiffly
  - it has difficulty in getting its head low enough to graze – but is not off its food
  - heart and respiratory rate progressively increase
  - it cannot swallow offered feed
  - it has diarrhoea
  - it becomes recumbent

a wide range of diseases could be suspected in this syndrome, but the underlying condition is diagnosed as a degenerative condition of the musculature, **muscle dystrophy**, which is masked by the conflicting signs suggestive of colic, tetanus, azoturia, choke, grass sickness, pharyngeal paralysis, and even lead poisoning. The acute signs have been precipitated from an insidious degenerative condition possibly due to vitamin E and selenium deficiency, by sudden unaccustomed exercise – for example, being chased by, or chasing, newcomers.

- a two-year-old seven-eighths gelding is seen enjoying a free gallop. He skids into a quick turn and a sliding halt and fall, as his exuberance takes him too close to a fence. He rises with difficulty, and thereafter is ataxic, i.e. very weak behind. A severe back injury seems a reasonable assumption, but a condition called **Wobbler Syndrome** is diagnosed – a progressive nerve degeneration in the cervical vertebral cord of some duration from a developmental subclinical bone condition; it has been triggered into the acute clinical picture by the acceleration forces or whiplash of his fall. In this condition, a progressive undue pressure on the vertebral sensory (proprioception) neurones has induced a Wallerian degeneration of the structure of the nerve fibres, with a consequent altered functioning effect: the fall culmination precipitates an acute neural trauma

The most common, and in athletic animals arguably the most serious, of degenerative diseases is **degenerative joint disease (DJD)** – a complicated condition, in as much as there are four sub-types

- **acute**, as in the highly mobile, high-speed joints of knee and fetlock in young racehorses

- **insidious**, as in low mobility, low-speed joints of hock, pastern and hoof, the weight bearers in the more mature animal
- **age-related** articular cartilage erosion and disintegration – a true degeneration
- **secondary trauma** to the joint, precipitating latent **osteochondroses**

In all of these sub-types there is a primary traumatic inflammatory factor. Eventually, because of its influence on the functional integrity of the articular synovia, there is a secondary effect on the nutrition of the avascular cartilage – with subsequent degenerative changes, a chondrosis which is a usual precursor of DJD. The functioning of the joint is impaired, and other changes occur in the related bone, ligaments and synovial membrane.

Wear and tear, 'use', is the common traumatic feature of: biomechanical *compression*, *concussion* and '*sprain*'.

Compression and concussion are invariably repetitive traumas, eventually leading to DJD; but a sudden excessive (and usually inelegant) action may be an earlier precipitating factor. Tendon 'strain' is not directly related to DJD, but it is relevant to mention here that repetitive subclinical overstress of flexor tendons causes degenerative changes within which make an acute clinical strain more likely.

Degenerative diseases are seen in most systems, for example

- the locomotor – DJD
- the cardio-vascular – nutritional, parasitic, viral causes
- the neurologic
  - atrophy, secondary to bone pressure
  - idiopathic laryngeal haemiplegia

NEOPLASTIC DIS-EASE

From the Greek *neo*, new; and *plasia*, 'tissue growth'. By definition, a new or unusual 'swelling' is an abnormality and is described as a growth, a tumour, or, often erroneously, a 'cancer'.

In every-day work, such lesions are 'seen', as they are mainly on the surface of the horse's body – on the skin, in the depth of the skin, in the mouth, and within the orbit.

They also occur within the body cavities and in the mucosal or **serosal** surfaces of the systems' tracts therein. In such situations it is often their effect on functioning which is clinical.

The lesions are described as 'unusual' or 'disorderly', as distinct from orderly growth and regrowth of healthy tissue. A common example of disorderly regrowth of healing tissue is **proud flesh**, where the granulation of the sub-cutis, necessary to infill a skin wound before it can 'skin over', has 'got out of hand'. It is important not only because it hinders epithelialisation but also it is susceptible to further alteration into one form of **sarcoid** formation, a **tumour**.

Tumours are classified broadly as

- **benign** – not given to spread locally or to **metastasise**, for example **adenoma**, a 'simple' tumour of a gland

- **malignant** – given to spread
    - by local invasion and often thereafter by spread (**cancer**, Latin for crab or crawler)
        - by blood and lymph to other sites, there to metastasise and form secondary growths, for example **adenocarcinoma**, a malignant tumour of a gland with secondaries elsewhere

- **malignant tendencies** – given to
    - local invasion of the skin and epithelia generally
    - recurrence after surgical removal

    both are typical of a sarcoid

Surface, visible growths have certain characteristics of shape, growth rates and predilection sites to suggest a diagnostic name, but biopsies are generally required for histopathological determination of malignancy – or not. The various tumours are discussed in the relevant system disease chapters.

The actual cause is by no means understood, but

- a primary skin wound granulation may 'change' to become a sarcoid. A virus is thought to be implicated

- young horses have 'milk warts' around the muzzle. These are almost certainly viral in origin and a self-eradication immunity develops

- grey horses are prone to tumours of the skin – **melanomas** – where hair is sparse or absent these are usually benign, where there is coat they tend to be malignant and invasive, for example **melanosarcomas**

Endocrine glands are very susceptible to neoplastic growths: some mares, after puberty, become afflicted in one ovary with a granulosa cell tumour which markedly upsets their reproductive cycle; the geriatric horse with anterior pituitary adenoma.

Tumours of the nervous system do occur, but are invariably secondary.

By definition, neoplasms have no beneficial effect on or to the horse. They are not only parasitic but destructive as well. Fortunately, the most common are not life threatening, but those affecting the lymphatic system (and so having a fluid vehicle for spread) are quickly lethal.

The benign melanomata can also be internal, as in the guttural pouch and in the abdominal cavity; it is in the abdomen that a lesion on a long stalk can strangulate the small intestine or small colon. Those which 'mushroom' under the tail are liable to ulcerate and become susceptible to 'fly strike'.

Ever-present hazards of equine neoplasia are

- warts and sarcoids being rubbed by tack and harness; such trauma can stimulate further growth and open a way for infection and 'fly strike'

- eyelid tumours, subject to self-mutilation by rubbing or worsening by fly irritation

- hormonal imbalances, from interference with production, by under- or over-stimulation and subsequent target organ dysfunction

SHOCK

Shock is the systemic condition which develops, often very rapidly, when there is an inadequate flow of blood to meet the body's demands, and especially those of the vital organs, the heart, brain and kidneys. Adequate blood supply requires

- effective heart functioning

- unobstructed intact blood vessels, especially ultimately to the organs concerned

- sufficient blood volume to maintain flow **and pressure**, and so satisfactory oxygenation of the tissues

Thus, any condition which seriously and adversely affects these can lead to shock.

Causes

- **dehydration**, from
    - profuse diarrhoea (especially in foals)
    - excessive sweating, leading to heat stroke
    - haemorrhage

- **severe colic**
  - entrapment of water in gut lumen
  - endotoxaemia
  - pain
- **peritonitis**, especially if associated with a bowel rupture
- **septicaemia**, and direct germ damage to brain and heart
- acute **poisoning**
- sequelae to **travel overstress**
- major **trauma**, especially from road traffic accidents
- **electrocution** and lightning strike
- **anaphylaxis**

Effects

The lack of adequate blood flow for sufficient perfusion and oxygenation of the body tissues for efficient metabolism, will produce, clinically variable

- fast, irregular, weak pulse
  - pale gums
  - slow 'refill time'
- laboured breathing
- patchy sweating
- cold extremities
- rigors
- depression

Organ/system complications can be secondarily fatal

Treatment if attempted is a veterinary matter; for first aid, warmth is essential.

ANCILLARY AIDS IN DIAGNOSIS

Ancillary aids are employed by the veterinary surgeon to help elucidate and/or confirm morbidity of structure and functioning, and to make a diagnosis more accurately.

Most horsemasters will, however, wisely invest in a **thermometer** (or two). Recognition of a rise in temperature unassociated with exercise – a fever – is important.

Some may also use a **stethoscope**, particularly where heart rate and recovery times during fitness training are important to them. These owners may also listen to ('auscultate') the chest wall for respiratory sounds and the flank for intestinal motility rumbles. On his rounds, the veterinary surgeon will certainly use both of these valuable tools of his trade.

There is always a **hoof tester** and a **searching knife** to complement his shoe removing kit. Add an **ophthalmoscope** and **magnifying direct light** – and a lot of training, experience and common sense! These are his 'servants' for 'in the field' diagnoses. They are also the basic items used in pre-purchase examination.

There are several techniques or modes of further examinations which he can select to obtain further and better particulars of 'what is going on inside'. It must be remembered by the veterinary surgeon, and understood by the owner, that they are but aids; the information must be applied to the clinical diagnosis – and not the other way round. This is particularly relevant to what are called **laboratory aids**.

In practice, the veterinary surgeon can use

- **a stomach tube**, to (very carefully)
  - probe the oesophagus, for
    - difficulty in swallowing
    - foreign body obstruction
  - and into the stomach, to
    - drain gas and fluid, or to
    - introduce controlled amounts of glucose, for subsequent determination of gut and liver function from blood analysis
- **tapping** ('centesis') the two major body cavities
  - **thoracentesis,** to collect fluid (if any) samples from the chest cavity
  - **paracentesis,** to collect abdominal fluid

These are forms of biopsy and both will give *macroscopic* information:

- actual presence of fluid
- its colour and consistency (purulent, fatty etc)

and further *microscopy* will help to determine inflammatory, obstructive and neoplastic changes. In some cases **culture** will reveal bacterial presence.

- **fluid** can also be taken from abscesses (superficial), joint and other synovial cavities, the uterus, the bladder (by catheterisation or collection), the udder, the cerebro-spinal fluid – and, most commonly, blood from the jugular vein, for haematology and metabolic profiling.

- **flexible endoscopy** (direct visualisation of 'hidden' tracts) involves the insertion of a fibre optic flexible tube into:

- the upper respiratory tract
- the anterior end of the lower respiratory tract. The tube is introduced up one nostril and allows the vet to inspect the lining mucosae of nostrils, pharynx and recesses, including the ethmoid areas, guttural pouches, soft palate, glottis and epiglottis, laryngeal cords and ventricles, trachea and into the bifurcation of bronchi
  - into the oesophagus and the stomach
  - into the genital tract beyond the cervix

- **rigid endoscopy** is made into the thorax (rarely), the abdomen, and joint cavities (**arthroscopy**).

- **samples** can be collected via these instruments and 'damaged' tissue removed. These are known as
  - **biopsies** – samples of tissue, from the living horse's liver, uterus, lower bowel, upper respiratory tract, tumours, for laboratory histopathological examination to assess presence and type of cellular morbidity
  - or by indirect manual **recovery**, as with
    - **faecal examination** – for worm eggs, bacteria, other pathogens
    - **skin scrapings** – for fungi and ectoparasites.

- **analysis of grass**, fodder and forage – for nutritive content and ratios, as well as for
  - toxic elements
  - poisonous plants

- **analysis of stable air** – for dust, spores etc. Assessment of airflow rates and direction.

Many of the samples taken and tested will hopefully confirm 'nothing significant', but all findings will guide the practitioner regarding
- suitable **therapy**
  - drug sensitivity in bacterial diseases
  - nutritional amendments
- **prognosis**
  - is it serious?
  - how is treatment progressing?
  - should treatment be changed?
- **control of spread** to other horses

Many laboratory tests are now carried out in practice laboratories; this facility expedites results.

'Machine' modes of diagnostic technique

Radiography – X-rays

Röntgen rays are directed onto a sensitised plate placed on the farther side of the area to be examined. The rays are blocked to a varying degree, relative to the bone and other tissue density of the area. The contrast between densities, especially at the junction or interface of bone and soft tissue, shows as a line of demarcation, the outline of which is 'readable' on the subsequently developed plate. More subtle density differences within the bone can also be diagnostic for a variety of defects, not least of which is a fracture.

The technician who decides the settings, 'takes' the exposures and develops and 'fixes' the plates is called a Radiographer. The surgeon who interprets the plate is called a Radiologist.

Ultrasonography (Imaging Ultrasound)

Ultrasound scanning is the technique used to map, 'from the outside', tissues which are

- beneath the skin but not within the body cavity, for example tendons and ligaments
- inside the body cavities, for example abnormal fluid in the pleural cavities, the heart, and in the foal abdominal structures
- the ovaries and the uterus are visualised with the ultrasonic probe manoeuvred per rectum; these organs are not sufficiently radiographically opaque for well-defined interpretation by this mode, partly because of the distance between the 'camera' and the organ and the density of the tissues between
  - arteries and veins in the pelvic area
  - ligaments of the sacro-ilea

Very high frequency sound waves 5–15 MHz are pulsed onto the tissues under examination, and are bounced back onto a receiver, converted into electrical impulses, and displayed to the operator on a television monitor as shades varying from black (the waves met nothing of significance, such as the air round the outside of a limb), to almost white (the object met was solid, and most of the wave was reflected).

The 'picture' can be either a cross-section or a linear representation. A 'hole' can be seen in the core area of a tendon or along its length. The fluid in an ovarian follicle is almost black, as are the embryonic fluids in the uterus, whereas the foetus is greyer. Movement of the living foetus can be visualised from the altering position of the 'echoes'.

[NOTE: Scanning is not to be confused with ultrasound *therapy*, in which sound waves – travelling pressure waves at 1–3MHz frequencies – are directed at damaged soft tissues such as overstressed tendons or ligaments. The vibration induced at cellular level has a deep penetrating massaging and consequent heating effect. Such therapy can be dangerous to the horse if not used by trained personnel.]

Scintigraphy, or Nuclear Diagnostics

On the basis that inflamed tissue has a variably greater blood supply than normal, use can be made of the pharmacological fact that certain drugs, varying tissue to tissue, will concentrate in inflamed tissue; the drug is first made radioactive with isotopes selected for different tissues.

These isotopes are thus concentrated in the inflamed (traumatised) area, and the concentration can be read by a Geiger counter and comparison made of suspected and unsuspected tissue measurements. A high reading is a positive finding. In practice, bone is the most commonly scanned tissue.

Thermography

The infra-red rays given off by body heat can be recorded, and a picture (a thermograph) produced.

Inflamed areas are by definition warmer than normal, and will show up differently and diagnostically, in colour sequences, on the screen of the thermogram.

Scintigraphy and thermography are also of value in pinpointing areas which can then be focused on for more detailed radiography. They also pinpoint sites of trauma which cannot be diagnosed clinically or cannot be isolated by specific nerve blocks, and in particular can suggest the need for intra-articular anaesthesia.

It is now appreciated that chronic, fibrotic tissue which is functionally useful as in healing or healed tendons and ligaments have, by definition, a reduced blood supply. Scintigraphically, fewer isotopes will have concentrated there than in healthy tissue, let alone in acute 'hot' lesions. Thermographically, the temperature measured will be a reflection of the reduced blood supply, and thereby the compared other presumed normal leg will read as the relatively warmer one.

Ultrasonography, scintigraphy and thermography techniques of visualisation all require not only skilled application but also skilled interpretation. Printouts and clinical notes can be downloaded and, along with clinical notes, sent for consultative discussion.

[NOTE: The radioactivity in scintigraphic diagnosis requires very strict health and safety precautions and in the UK can be carried out only in designated premises.]

Doppler Ultrasound

A special ultrasonographic recording of blood-flow characteristics for measuring restriction to flow and elasticity of the arteries. It is mainly used as an aid in differentiating disease types in the equine distal limbs and in the heart.

Electrocardiography (ECG)

This is a printed record of the electrical activity associated with heart muscle contraction and relaxation. It measures rate, regularity and rhythm in the form of wave patterns.

Electroencephalography (EEG)

A recording of the electrical waves 'given out' by the brain's activity: patterns of healthy waves have been 'mapped' and those of dis-ease can be compared and an interpretation made.

Electromyography (EMG) measures the time taken for a motor nerve to act on a particular muscle and, indirectly, the degree of muscle response.

Auscultation, radiography, endoscopy, ultrasonography, and to a lesser extent scintigraphy, are the most commonly used physical aids to diagnosis.

It is generally accepted, although there is legal argument, that the X-ray plates, and the prints and copies from these and other diagnostic modes, are the property not of the horse's owner but of the veterinary practice or person prescribing the recordings and then interpreting them, the 'ologist'.

These are all, as has been emphasised, AIDS TO DIAGNOSIS – they are not diagnoses in themselves.

CHAPTER 21

IMMUNOLOGY

Immunity, from the Latin *immunis*, 'free from the burden of', is the study of how animals are, or can become, proof against dis-ease consequent on infection by potentially pathogenic micro-organisms which have been

- inhaled
- ingested
- 'introduced' into the (uro)genital system
- 'splashed' onto the eyeball
- carried through an open skin wound

and thereafter have aimed to colonise and to multiply on or in the cells of the related epithelial mucosal tracts or the sub-cutaneous tissues and organ systems.

Immunity depends upon the animal being

- inherently capable of inflammatory and subsequent antigenic response reaction to potentially pathogenic organisms, and
- subsequently capable of a rapid 'boosting' of, or 'topping up' (re-stimulation of 'memory' cells) of the original immunity when further challenged by the same infection. This acquired immunity is said to be **natural**.

(It should be noted that the horse is genetically non-susceptible to Foot and Mouth disease; this non-susceptibility is not a true 'immunity' state in the context of this chapter.)

The specific microbe has a protein component capable of active stimulation of the immune system. It is called an **antigen**, and the response to it is called a **sensitivity** leading to the formation of antigerm substances or **antibodies**. Any protein or protein-like substance which gains entry to the tissues directly or via the blood will stimulate antibodies to this protein which is not necessarily microbial in origin.

Some non-protein substances because of an innate ability can attach themselves to so-called 'carrier proteins' within the body. These inorganic substances, called **haptens**, have acquired the ability to stimulate the function of antibodies. There is rarely any definable reaction sign of this, which is also known as a **sensitisation**. Further exposure of the tissues to the hapten on its own will stimulate response of an allergic type.

The science of **immunology** includes the techniques of artificially supplying and stimulating an immunity to specific infections, commonly known as **vaccination**.

Before the significant research of Pasteur confirmed that some illnesses were due to infection by microbes, earlier medical observers were aware that

- recovery from a particular disease prevented a recurrence of the illness
- some people in a community did not succumb during an epidemic
- some people, affected by mild and local forms of a skin pox affliction, did not succumb to the lethal forms of systemic pox (smallpox). The dairymaid milker who contracted hand and arm lesions from the cow's teats did not get smallpox. (Dr Jenner used this observation; he scratched lymph from cows' teat pox onto the skin of children and, without knowing why, immunised them against smallpox. The Latin name for cowpox was *vaccinia* 'of a cow' – hence 'vaccination')

They concluded that some form of resistance was present or induced.

After Pasteur's discovery, and based on Jenner's work, research was directed to the explanation of these phenomena and to finding suitable, safe and effective means of replicating them by artificial active immunisation, or artificial passive (if temporary), protection.

It is now known that mammals survive despite the constant hazard of infection, because of certain innate factors

- a 'general' resistance to all, and especially to opportunist germs – in terms of overall health
- non-specific defences
  - physico-chemical barriers – the mucociliary escalator of the airway, gastric acid pH, peristaltic throughput of the ingesta and digesta, the cornified outer keratinised layers of the epidermis, and the pH of the sebum secreted onto the skin surface
  - blood and tissue first-line defenders – certain white blood cells and bio-chemicals
- specific defence mechanisms (**specific immunity**) generated by stimulation of the body's immune system by the microbe's antigenicity, via the
  - lymphoid cells of the reticulo-endothelial system, in the lymph nodes, the spleen, the bone marrow, the thymus gland (in the young animal), and the superficial lymphoid tissues of the the tonsils
  - the mucosal wall and related lymph cells of the respiratory and gastro-intestinal system's mucosae
  - the circulating lymph cells

The development of these is a complicated procedure, but when activated there results a mobilisation or presence of

- humoral immunity – circulating in the blood, **immunoglobulins**
- cell mediated immunity – local and circulating **special white blood cells** (lymphoid cells)
- secretory immunity – onto mucosal surfaces
- 'memory' cells, in these areas, capable of rapid re-stimulation of immunity

An ideal, perhaps idealistic, immunity complex is one which would *prevent* a microbe from

- penetrating the physico-chemical and other non-specific defences, to
  - colonise on mucosal surfaces, and to
  - multiply in or on these cells

An acceptable, or realistic, immunity is one that *minimises*

- damage by invasions of the mucosal cells
- penetration into the blood (and lymph) circulation, and so to subsequent other deeper cellular damage
- the need for an inflammatory reaction to subsequent re-stimulation of a primary disease immunity or of an established artificially induced immunity

Infection on top of immunity should

- boost the original immunity
- *not* produce clinical signs of this infection
- at the most, induce a sub-clinical response involving only a mild transient fever or a mild systemic functional disturbance which, if it did occur (as 'seen' by temperature recording), would be possibly significant only in the fit athletic horse

Active immunity can be the consequence of **natural infection** or of **artificial immunisation** – vaccination. The latter should at least aim to produce as good an immunity as an infection.

Passive immunity aims at minimising possible invasion, and/or penetration of the germ, both over a short period.

Some Definitions

Active immunity: the result of activation of an animal's immune system by antigens to generate antigerm substances. These are then available to the animal for a variable period (months to years). Can be boosted.

Active immunity is said to be **natural** when the antigen is part of an invading microbe, or is said to be **artificial** when the antigen has been produced in a commercial laboratory – a vaccine.

Passive immunity: the result of absorption of pre-formed antigerm substances produced in a donor animal's vascular system, into an animal's blood circulation. These are then available to that animal for a limited period (weeks).

Passive immunity is said to be **natural** when the antibodies have been produced in the recipient's dam and made available through the colostrum. It is said to be **artificial** when the donor animal has been artificially hyper-immunised by a vaccine, and its immune serum (rich in antigerm substances) is harvested from its blood for inoculation into another, the recipient – an **antiserum injection**. The horse is the usual source of antiseras for most animals. Tetanus antiserum is the most commonly used antiserum. There are risks attached to giving second or subsequent doses of antisera due to the formation of a hypersensitivity to the natural protein in the antiserum; the reaction is an **anaphylaxis**.

All immune levels tend to wane unless re-stimulated naturally by re-infection or artificially by vaccination.

Passive immunity should eventually be followed by active immunity either through exposure to endemic environmental infection, natural stimulation, or artificially by an appropriate vaccine.

Immunity can be undermined (*see* Chapter 20, DISEASE). Such a horse is colloquially described as having 'a lowered general resistance'. Some immune states are known as **tolerances**. An excessive immune response to a known or unknown antigen (allergen) will produce a **hypersensitivity**; if this is challenged, *usually* naturally, it will produce either anaphylaxis or atopy, both forms of allergic dis-ease.

Immunisation

A vaccine is manufactured in a laboratory. The antigen is produced from the cultivation of the germ

- viruses are 'grown' on live cell lines or in fertile eggs
- bacteria are 'grown' on artificial culture media
- toxins are extracted from bacterial cultures

There are three kinds of vaccines at present commercially in use which are administered intramuscularly

- **modified live** (MLV) – reduced potential virulence, slight risk of reversion to virulence, strongly antigenic
- **inactivated** (killed) – non-virulent but antigenic
- **'sub-unit'** – non-virulent but antigenic; with no risk of reversion. The sub-unit makes use only of antigenic particles of the cultivated, usually viral strain.

A further type of vaccine which has no risk of reversion is the **toxoid**. This is an attenuated form of bacterial toxin and is most commonly used for immunity against Clostridial toxins.

When inoculated into a specifically non-immune animal, a vaccine will

- if it is 'live'
  - sensitise and immunise the recipient to produce a cellular immunity, a humoral immunity, and possibly a secretory immunity
- if it is dead, or attenuated, or a toxoid
  - sensitise the recipient, which will require a second

dose before this sensitivity is converted to immunity (usually only humoral) and further doses to boost or to maintain this immunity

A subsequent natural infection will 'trigger' a memory faculty in all three immune states, which will immediately activate defences (boost them) so that the consequences of such infection are nil or minimal.

Present day dead or attenuated vaccines now aim to stimulate a cellular immunity as well as a humoral one. In herpes strains and possibly in EVA, where the virus of infection tends to be intra-cellularly dormant, this '2-in-1' re-stimulation is important.

Few present-day vaccines meet the ideal requirements for immunity, but in the dog, initial vaccination against distemper almost does; paradoxically, the antigen is that of the human measles strain. Where the morbidity is due to toxin from Clostridial spores, a very satisfactory immunity is obtained by injections of the relevant toxoid, as when used, for example, to protect against tetanus.

Research has recently developed an intra-nasal vaccine against influenza whereby the horse's immunological effort is concentrated at the points of invasion following inhalation of aerosoled virus particles – normally the nasopharyngeal and the rest of the URT. An inactivated vaccine is sprayed onto the nasopharyngeal mucosa to produce a virus neutralising effect.

The technique and the procedure for immunisation is usually the responsibility of the veterinary surgeon. Where proof of vaccination is required, the injection must be given by the veterinary surgeon and recorded on a passport or other document which can be identifiably related to that animal.

In practical terms vaccination relates to

- a sensitising dose – **first shot**, a mild response within 10 days
- a secondary activating dose – **second shot** (approximately 4 weeks after the first), a large response after 5 days
- a first booster – **third shot**, usually 6 months after the second shot, a large 'memory' rise at 5 days or less
- subsequent boosters, usually not more than 12 months later. With tetanus toxoid, the subsequent boosters are at 2 years' interval and/or whenever a 'suspicious' wound is present

Unvaccinated injured horses, or those of unknown immune status *vis á vis* tetanus, for example, should be given an immediate passively protective dose of tetanus anti-toxin. This should be followed in 12 weeks with the first shot of toxoid, to begin the active immunisation.

Why Artificial Immunity?

Most infectious contagious diseases of the horse are endemic, and are naturally protected against by the innate defence mechanisms supported by active immunity through exposure to the microbial antigens in the healthy horse.

These may or may not produce clinical disease. Where the virulence of the microbe is greater than the *general* immunity of the horse, then a clinical picture of dis-ease will occur; in most situations a subsequent convalescent specific immunity will develop.

In veterinary practice, most viral infections are sub-lethal. When they are lethal it is usually in the foal and the aged horse; usually due to secondary bacterial assault of the respiratory and the gastro-intestinal tracts. In the adult horse the infections are mainly viral. Whilst not serious in most cases, the effect of the illness on performance and on reproduction is financially important. Nevertheless, strategic active immunisation is cost-effective against

- Influenza viral strains

- Herpes viral strains, especially with the advent of the new herpes vaccine 1 and 4

- the virus of equine arteritis (EVA)

- Clostridial toxins, especially that of tetanus. It should be appreciated that, as far as is known, an animal does not naturally actively develop an immunity by exposure to these Clostridial germs *per se*. The toxins are produced by the parent bacteria only when these multiply rapidly. Such high levels of toxin are therefore the actual pathogens. The parent bacteria are not pathogenic in themselves. Artificial protection against tetanus, especially, is essential on an individual animal basis. It is rare for this toxicity to be non-fatal (normal treatment is usually ineffective), as natural active immunity to the bacterium is not a feature of such infections and it is unlikely that natural immunity to the toxin has time to develop before illness takes hold

Although diseases of the viral types, when endemic, can activate an immunity with or sometimes without clinical disease, artificial immunisation is essential for individual and population (herd) protection.

In any equine population, large or small, 70% of all the animals must be immunised to produce a statistically significant defence against being 'overwhelmed' by an outbreak of a specific contagious disease starting in a non-immune minority.

In artificial production of immunity the protection is either immediate and short-lasting, as from passive anti-sera, or slightly delayed but significantly long in effect, when actively induced against a specific disease – a vaccination.

It must be remembered that such immunity, particularly the active type, is without specific (and often uneconomic) tests and therefore is 'being taken for granted'. The 'proof of the pudding...' is in the absence of the clinical signs of infection and invasion.

There is always the risk that re-infection with sub-clinical effects on vital tissues may jeopardise a horse's fitness when coincidentally put to hard work. Attention has earlier been drawn to the value of temperature-taking in elite athletic horses; any rise is a significant indication that an infection has caused a reaction and it is the only warning that a trainer or horsemaster may have.

There is a constant but small 'voice' of complaint that vaccination against Influenza precipitates illness with 'flu. This has not been scientifically substantiated. It is recognised that in some recent vaccinates, within ten days a mild fever with moderate depression is noticeable, and a cough. This is more likely in horses in work

- they may be travelling (with attendant stress) and mixing

- they will in any event be stressed with work

In all vaccinated horses there is a post-booster drop in overall immunity. In some animals, commensal infections will 'take the opportunity' to become active, e.g. herpes 1 and 4, the cold viruses, and respiratory bacteria, to produce an indeterminate clinical picture.

In some cases (with veterinary input) it may be worth giving those horses antibiotic therapy for potential *bacterial* infection and resting all cases until the cough subsides. Ideally, horses should be vaccinated at rest when most pressures are off them, nor 'wormed' at the same time.

Cell Mediated Immunity (Cellular Immunity)

This is an important response against those microbes, most commonly viruses, which invade mucosal and vascular tissue cells. An initial invasion mobilises special blood cells which seek out infected tissue cells to 'kill' them, thereby exposing the microbes to other disintegrating action. All three cells – that of the host, the lymphocyte itself, and the virus particles – are killed: the loss of the few for the greater good! The quicker the natural control of the virus is activated, the less the illness and the quicker the convalescence. Early recognition to prevent misuse of the horse, and the subsequent nursing, are both important.

The defensive cells are lymphocytes which developed via the thymus glands and are known as **T lymphocytes**. They are not only 'killer' types; some control a humoral immune response, others become 'memory' cells involved in boosted immunity reaction, and still others modulate the cascade of biochemical activities involved in the complete response. Transplant rejections are brought about by a variation of these mechanisms.

Humoral Immunity

This depends upon the production of soluble antibodies produced by antigenic stimulation of plasma cells which are the progeny of the bone marrow's lymphocytes – the B lymphocytes.

They are called **immunoglobulins**, and are protein in structure. There are eight main types, each with several sub-types in the horse. Once formed, either specifically or as part of a general immunity development, they combine with or react to the microbial antigen. Specific antibodies use the 'key and lock' principle to combine and thus inactivate microbes, making them susceptible to other defensive activities. The immunoglobulins against bacteria are comprehensively efficient, whereas they require help from sensitised lymphocytes to mobilise and modulate a cascade of events to 'disintegrate' germs. The debris is engulfed by macrophages and transported to the lymphoid tissues for stimulation of memory cells and the production of more antibodies. Some immunoglobulins are involved in helminth 'tolerance' and 'self-cure' mechanisms, others with hyper-sensitivity reactions.

Secretory Immunity

This is a second line of defence to the physico-chemical first line. Some immunoglobulins, of which IgA is the foremost in the horse, are found on the mucosal surfaces of the small intestinal, mammary, and respiratory tracts. A precursor is deposited in special activated mucosal cells, and is there converted to active immunoglobulins which secrete or diffuse into the lumen. Immunoglobulins can be non-specific as well as specific.

The Mare and Foal

The level of the immune substances and their range of protection in **colostrum** is a reflection of the mare's immunity. It is advisable to have her 'exposed' to the germs endemic in the premises and/or fields in which her foal will be born, for at least 6 weeks before foaling is due, and also to have her actively **booster-immunised** against 'common' organisms such as

- Influenza
- Herpes viral strains
- Equine viral arteritis (on local veterinary advice)
- Tetanus toxin

no less than 10 days before foaling is due. These specific immune substances augment other important protein secretory substances in the milk's colostrum, which must be ingested within 6 hours of birth. Of course, it is essential that the foal sucks within that time; not only are there diminishing levels of antibodies with the passage of time, usually disappearing within 4 weeks or so, but over a shorter period the foal's intestinal powers of absorption are reduced, as the relevant absorption gland closes up and becomes impenetrable to the antibodies' relatively large molecules.

If the mare has been 'running milk' for several (over 3)

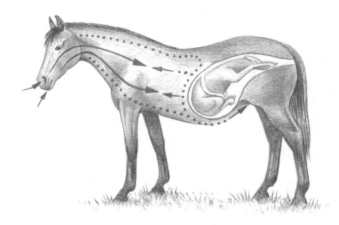

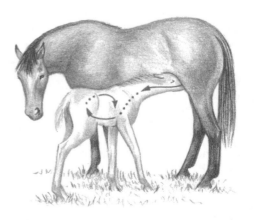

The mare's immunity passes to the foal in the colostrum.

days before foaling, veterinary advice should be sought on supplementary protection of the foal.

Later active vaccination of the foal is usually restricted to tetanus at 12 weeks of age and the three virus diseases already mentioned at later dates suggested by the veterinary surgeon.

Commensal bacteria and viruses, by definition, are those endemic to the stud in particular and, for that matter, to the equine world in general. Daily contact gives the opportunity for naturally controlled active immunisation as colostral immunity wanes, provided general health is maintained. The need for specific artificial immunity is related to the absence of natural exposures or to the particular virulence of the germ, especially herpes strains and EVA.

The presence of passive (colostrum) immunity in the foal's tissues can neutralise subsequent artificial vaccinations to a decreasing extent. Conversely, if vaccination is left too long after the foal's passive immunity has been used up, there is a risk of virulent infection in this 'immunity gap'. Although the immunity level can be monitored, it is more usual for the stud manager to work on the general principles suggested above.

A reverse approach to the study of immune responses is to see it as the study of the mechanisms which preserve the biological identity of animals – the recognition of 'self' and the awareness of something 'foreign' in the body fluids and tissues (compare transplant rejection in the absence of immuno-suppression, even for nearly identical genetic material, i.e. close matching between donor and recipient).

Certain processes – inoculation, inhalation, ingestion etc. of foreign non-acceptable substances, usually of a protein nature – will cause an antibody reaction to this stimulus and also create a 'memory' of it. (This is correctly known as **allergy**.) If the sensitivity response is protective in nature it is called an **immunity**, but if there is overreaction it is known as **hypersensitivity**. Further similar hypersensitive stimuli can create an **anaphylaxis**; the stimulus is then known as an **allergen** and the disorder as an **allergic reaction**.

The two states, immune and allergic, are related in as much as immunity is a health-preserving sensitivity, whereas allergic (and atopic) are potentially dis-ease-prone hypersensitivities.

CHAPTER

22 DISEASES OF THE CARDIO-VASCULAR SYSTEM

The cardio-vascular system's tissues are subject to the Types of Disease as listed in Chapter 20, DISEASE. Like that of the musculo-skeletal and the neural system, the cardio-vascular system has no normal access to the environment through body surface orifices, thus differing from the respiratory and digestive systems.

The cardiac functioning involves two inter-related double compartments, the *left* and the *right* 'heart', **systemic** and **pulmonic** respectively. Collectively they act as **intrinsic** muscular pumps with associated valves to maintain the circulation of the **extrinsic** arterial and venous blood, both systemic and pulmonary. Control is determined primarily by the vagus (cranial) nerve, by the autonomic nervous system, and by circulating biochemical factors. The rhythm is determined by an intrinsic 'pacemaker', and disseminated by the branching cardiac nervous system to the musculature. (*See* Chapter 6, THE CARDIO-VASCULAR SYSTEM.)

It is important to appreciate that this circulatory flow of blood passes along the endothelial surface of the heart chambers and over the valve surfaces. In doing so it is not immediately or directly concerned with cardiac tissue metabolism or oxygen supply to the heart itself.

The input of oxygen and nutrients for intrinsic cardiac use, and the reciprocal output, depend upon the heart's 'own' blood supply, the **coronary arterio-venous system**.

Disease agents, usually irrespective of the site of primary invasion, enter cardiac tissues via the intrinsic cardiac blood supply. They include potentially pathogenic

- micro-organism infections and their toxins, as a viraemia, septicaemia or toxaemia
- pathogenic antigens and allergens

- imbalanced serum levels of
  - electrolytes
  - minerals
  - hormones
- toxic substances
- (aberrant) parasites, usually the larval stages

Some germs may 'spread' across epithelial barriers, as from the pleura to the pericardium, and then to functional heart tissue.

Another significant route is by deposition of, for example, *Streptococci equi* (strangles germ) out of any turbulent extrinsic flow, as at the cardiac orifices, onto endothelial mucosae of the valves, where they colonise to produce local lesions.

THE DIS-EASES

Developmental

These are invariably congenital, but vary in the time of becoming clinically patent. This depends on their pathogenic effect on the dynamics of the circulation and the demands on the oxygen supply relative to neonatal and, occasionally, later exercise activity.

They are not (as yet) of proven hereditability. Basically they are unacceptable delays or frank failures in the programmed closures of necessary (if temporary) apertures originally present in cardio-vascular muscle and endothelia to permit foetal pulmonic by-passes. These can also be primary defects in structure; these acquired defects, although foetal in origin, never close, at least not as part of prenatal/neonatal requirements; they are essentially permanent.

Normally the temporary aperture closures are effected soon after neonatal respiration is triggered at birth with the placental separation and the consequent need for a pulmonic blood flow.

Developmental diseases include

- **persistent foramen ovale (PFO)** in the interauricular muscle wall. This foetal opening short-circuits the right ventricle (RV)

- **patent ductus arteriosus (PDA)**, linking venous to arterial blood flow outside the chambers, thus obviating full RV involvement in the absence of foetal pulmonic circulation. Rare in equines; it becomes significant, on average, from day four of life

- **ventricular septal defect (VSD)**. The most common interventricular septal defect; it is usually in the non-muscular part of the wall close to the aortic valve root, and less commonly the pulmonary valve. It is not always lethal; it is relatively rare. It is *not* a natural or necessary foetal feature, so technically it is an acquired defect. The mal-effect is often delayed until free exercise or even training has started; the prognosis, once clinical, is poor

- the very rare **atrial septal defects (ASD)** are faults in the foetal auricle structures and not a failure of closure as with PFO above

- the **tetralogy of fallot**, a complexity of failures of structure including VSD

There are others, usually acquired, including ruptured valve 'strings' or 'cords'. Overall, they are relatively uncommon. The incidence may vary with the breed, being greatest in Standardbreds and Arab horses. The ancillary diagnostic aid of echography has been particularly helpful, especially for differentiation between acquired defects and 'true' congenitals.

Clinical signs are

- respiratory distress

- early fatigue, as in postural requirements, e.g. at sucking and walking/trotting with the dam

- later, more complicated signs, especially of exercise intolerance

Compensation is possible, but decompensation is likely with time; congestive heart failure usually follows.

Murmurs are significantly present and can (at least) be pointers to the site and of the pathologic importance.

Traumatic

- direct, as from penetrating wounds
- indirect, from thoracic wall concussion with
- pericardial and myocardial bruising

as from road traffic accidents or kicks to foals especially. Echography may improve diagnosis and more accurate prognosis, otherwise they are suspected from history, auscultation and clinical circulatory and respiratory distress.

Inflammatory

Inflammatory disease can affect all structures

- direct via the intrinsic cardiac coronary blood supply
  - viral, bacterial (and their toxins)
  - endoparasitic thrombus-forming (aberrant) larvae
  - organic toxins
- indirect
  - onto endothelial structures. especially that of the valves from the extrinsic flow
  - via contact with pericardial penetration from the pleurae
- fungi and protozoa are not important cardiac pathogens in the UK. Some species' toxins act as organic poisons, e.g. aflatoxin
- fungi can colonise on guttural pouch mucosae and invade through resultant ulcers. There are two main consequences: erosion of the underlying carotid artery with possible fatal haemorrhage; necrosis of the sub-mural cranial nerves ix, x, xi and xii and the associated parasympathetic branches which control heart functioning, as well as varying degrees of paralysis of the throat area

Allergic

Allergic diseases are viral and bacterial hypersensitivities, which affect the muscular and valvular arterial walls' own capillaries, a vasculitis, to cause myo- and endo-cardial ischaemic changes, e.g. to

- viral arteritis and infectious anaemia
- strangles bacteria and toxin

A lethal complication is the generalised oedematous condition, associated with the myocardial vasculitis, of purpura haemorrhagica.

Metabolic

- effects of overstress, heat stress and shock on the electrolyte balance, and so on the
  - intrinsic myocardial activity
  - autonomic nervous system, with disturbance of the myoneural conductive system affecting contractility and so
    - rhythm
    - power, and so blood pressure
  - arterial wall with lumen diameter changes and so flow rate volume and pressure changes
- indirect effect of other metabolic pathologies, e.g.
  - acute rhabdomyolysis
  - secondary hyperparathyroidism

Degenerative

- thrombosis of minor branches of the coronary artery (see allergies above) and subsequent microscopic embolic formation with focal myocardial death
- toxicity, as in monensin poisoning

Neoplasia

These are usually only as metastatic lesions, and then rare

- secondary effects, as with myocardial lympho-sarcoma and alterations in calcitonin levels in the circulation
- intrinsic pressure effects of lipomata and haemangio-sarcomata

Any of these dis-ease conditions can adversely affect the cardio-vascular system to the detriment of its functioning capability. In most cases the pathological changes and effects are sub-clinical at least initially. The altered functioning can be suspected if heart rhythm and, more especially, rate are affected. Those are judged by the pulse or by auscultation and other aids by a veterinary surgeon.

The interpretation, as distinct from the fact, is not always possible. Suspicion is strengthened *if performance falls*. Even this loss is not emphatically, or always, attributable to heart disorder. Moreover the compensatory power of the heart muscle, 'the cardiac reserve' is usually quick to 'kick in'. Contraction power (systolic output) takes over from any failure of rate and rhythm, so performance usually continues up to a point. Compare fittening effects

(*see* Chapter 38, FITTENING) which can be equated due to the hypertrophic increase in the cardiac smooth muscle common to both dis-ease and to the increased effects of training and using.

Both situations cause an increase in the 'load' put upon the heart's pumping capability. Such stress can be reduced if

- in the case of suspected disease its sub-clinical nature is revealed by more detailed and specialist examination and treated where possible – there are few such types!
- the physical requirements' target is lowered to meet the 'new', perhaps less effective, compensatory power

This is similar to adjusting a training programme. An elite athletic horse has a high cardiac reserve, but whether induced or inherited is not (yet) clear.

The heart is said to have **compensated**. This is not always as simple or as successful as one would like. In compensation the ventricular muscle hypertrophy does not necessarily reduce ('recover') quickly, if at all, but the rate and rhythm are often eventually normalised and, with the hypertrophic enhanced power, maintain a life-saving level of output at least. The heart (muscle) becomes tolerant of the lowered demands with consequent reduction in any clinical abnormalities originally apparent.

Cardiac disorders are often secondary to dis-ease states in other systems; there is a knock-on effect. The heart disorder can worsen the primary condition or initiate changes in further systems; a vicious circle.

A significant feature of this primary, or more frequently secondary, other-system dis-ease is that it is usually clinical or becomes so before the heart shows signs of its pathology. It, or they, may resolve naturally or respond to treatment, as in respiratory conditions especially, even before the heart's involvement is suspected, let alone diagnosed on simple clinical grounds alone.

Conversely, rhythm defects, some potentially and quickly lethal, may, coincidentally or later, become active as, for example, in concurrent viraemia which itself, in many cases, is not even suspected. The seriousness of such viraemias is relative to the coincidental athletic demands put upon the horse. The associated arrhythmia itself could pass undetected or rapidly deteriorate into a fatal fibrillation. Veterinary help is often not called upon because of the suddenness of the disease, which is seen by the trainer as 'sudden heart failure'. He may seek an autopsy. Routine in-practice post mortem may not always reveal the full story.

CARDIAC TISSUE DEFECTS

Endocarditis – an 'inflammation' of the extrinsic blood flow surfaces with related valvular endothelial and underlying tissue pathology associated with

- immunologic reactions
- bacterial colonisation, as with Strangles
- verrucose (warty) growths on valves – cause unknown
- worm larval damage
- infarcts and other changes from microscopic thromboses
    - ossification in the right auricle
    - vasculitis, as with purpura haemorrhagia
    - equine infectious anaemia
    - paralytic myoglobinuria

Myocarditis

- inflammatory: post pyrexic conditions (respiratory)
- degenerative
- fibrosing lesions (also in the valves), all
    - associated with exercise intolerances
    - most often subclinical and self resolving unless coincidentally overstressed physiologically when the 'new' myocardial defect in the conduction system can be a complication, with
        - marked arrhythmia's
        - death from CHF (congestive heart failure)
    - an occasional stressless idiopathic decompensation with CHF

A particular chronic myocarditis of the right ventricle with marked hypertrophy is associated with COPD complicated by tricuspid valve incompetence with a loud murmur; CHF does not necessarily follow.

Pericarditis (rare – usually secondary to pleuro-pneumonic disease)
Acute inflammation of the outer covering of the heart and the surface of the myocardia; often with sero/purulent effusion and adhesions which can lead to right heart side compression with passive congestion.

There is a build up of pulmonic venous blood pressure with congestion of lung circulation and perfusion and so interference with airway gaseous exchange. May deteriorate to CHF (congestive heart failure). There is a characteristic friction noise on auscultation.

CONGESTIVE HEART FAILURE (CHF)

Many, possibly most horses which develop cardiac deficits are able to compensate by automatically invoking the innate cardiac reserve and coincidentally attempting to reverse the causative factors, direct or indirect, and so naturally reflexly reducing the work load of the heart.

It involves autonomic and reflex responses for

- peripheral vaso-constriction, which selectively redistributes blood flow to the vital organs at the expense of the locomotor muscular system
- an increase in ventricular distension to enhance pre-loading with relatively more blood
- ventricular hypertrophy to increase stroke volume
- an increase in heart rate to maintain output and so blood pressure
- sodium and water retention in the kidneys and so blood volume
- other homeostatic features

If these responses fail in collaboration and effect, the heart's pump action can deteriorate with reduction in stroke volume. There is a subsequent

- damming back of extrinsic blood into the veins
- a rise in capillary pressure
- a serum leak out into the extra-cellular fluid with
- oedema formation, which becomes a cardinal sign of the underlying CHF
    - this begins in the left side of the heart and so affects the pulmonary vein – giving rise to pulmonary oedema, with marked exercise intolerance, as well as altered respiratory sounds
    - there is a knock-on effect to the right side of the heart, with
    - systemic circulation back-pressure – giving rise to peripheral oedema, especially of the ventral trunk, brisket and limbs. This ventral oedema is usually the first clinical signs, especially to the layman. It is in fact a bi-ventricular pathology
    - there is a marked reduction in exercise tolerance

Therapeutic aids are few. However a complete cure is possible in certain situations, especially for some arrhythmias, particularly atrial fibrillation.

In any sub-clinical heart case incidentally exposed to

unaccustomed or unfit-for exercise, severe even if of short duration 'bursts' of strenuous activity, such as

- struggling in a frightening entrapment
- escaping from possible predation or malicious attack
- stud 'covering' work (the stallion)

with intercurrent disease, especially

- infectious, in which cardiac myopathy is likely, as in septicaemia or viraemia
- metabolic, as with exertional rhabdomyolysis

then the horsemaster will perceive the inevitable resultant progressive signs of

- fast(er) breathing
- coughing
- perhaps blood tinged nasal mucus

as respiratory distress, and seek veterinary help before

- inco-ordination (ataxia)
- and possible collapse

supervene.

Understandably, the horsemaster may not consider these specifically diagnostic of a (primary) cardiac dis-ease.

If disease such as primary viral or systemic bacterial strangles is diagnosed or suspected or is even just a possible contagion it is most important in athletic horses in full work that sufficient time is given to

- allow a possible incubating disease to develop – or not
- permit full recovery, with
- sufficient retraining and refittening after convalescence, during which there is
- veterinary monitoring of the heart (and respiratory) functioning put into action.

Cardio-vascular disease is mainly an interference with work ability, or at least one possible explanation of

- quicker fatigue with locomotor work, and
- respiratory embarrassment
  both progressive over several days

- a lowering of performance in speed, agility and endurance, i.e. 'a loss of performance', coincidental with other system dysfunctioning, possibly explicable by reduced cardiac-propelled perfusion of their tissues primarily of oxygen, and reduced removal of carbon dioxide and other waste products, and the clinical effects of such pathologies on them and on other systems *including the heart itself*

The heart can of course have varying degrees of sub-optimal functioning, yet does not necessarily do so overtly; as already described, such functioning failure remains sub-clinical at least to the layman and often to the vet undertaking an examination which is **not fully comprehensive** with respect to cardiac deficits.

'Heart failure' is an inexact term used to describe serious cardiac dysfunction. It is frequently equated with sudden death, presumably due to insufficient circulation of oxygen – particularly to its own muscles. This oxygen starvation, the deprivation of sufficient oxygen to the vital tissues of the kidneys, the brain and the heart musculature itself is, of course, an end point in all deaths. The syndrome begins first in the left side ventricular musculature with CHF and then in the right.

As already described, the heart, better than the brain and certainly the kidneys, has considerable power of compensation because, unlike the other two organs, it is significantly a muscular one. The fact that its muscle activity is autonomic is a 'saving' feature in both health (athletic work) and in disease. Neither man nor horse can directly control the rate and power. These are reflexes stimulated elsewhere as part of the vital body control system.

The grades of heart disease often relate clinically to its dysfunctional effects: its output is variably affected

- **direct** – intrinsic disorder
- **indirect** – extrinsic, other systems, disease

Grade I – sub-clinical, except perhaps for suspected reduced performance

Grade II – clinical, including
- reduced performance when measured subjectively or objectively
- signs of respiratory stress, a rate increase above the average normal for rest and varying exercise levels, and especially a delay in return to resting normal. If the cardiac dysfunction is direct, the respiratory increase is a physiological one in itself. If indirect and associated with a primary respiratory disorder, other signs including a variable fever would be present. So too with other system pathologies
- there may or may not be a coincidental heart rate or pulse rise. This is less likely if taken at rest: then there may even be a resting fall, a **bradycardia**

Special cardiology can of course discover cardiac pathologies which were sub-clinical at routine examination.

Grades III and **IV** are relatively uncommon in the equine, but clinical signs are then more obvious; other system involvement is more serious. However

- either the compensation feature acts so quickly that clinical signs are masked: the heart rate slows but gains power output to maintain blood pressure and circulation, and thus associated dysfunction may be prevented

- or the performance fall is so marked that the horse is taken out of work with consequent load reduction – as already described – and a convalescence follows which allows a compensation to develop with or without relegation to less exacting work levels

- Grade IV by definition is more likely to produce a failed compensation, a decompensation, with congestive heart failure and either sudden death or humane slaughter

The incidence of Grades III and IV varies with breed and occupation but generally is greater in the juvenile and the geriatric.

Acute heart failure – 'near' sudden death – is invariably a consequence of strenuous work, such as racing, on a (sub-clinical) compromised heart, and occurs most frequently at cooling off (warming down). It always involves a severe arrhythmia leading usually to atrial fibrillation and a lethal heart block. These may be missed if death follows quickly. The doomed horse may give a few minutes' warning before collapsing and dying; it starts blowing hard, becomes anxious and may whinny, there is a brief ataxia before going down. Resuscitation is hopeless. Should recovery follow it is either the nature of the heart pathology in this case, or it was not the 'heart' as such.

The quality of life considerations for man and dog, as distinct from the athletic requirements of the horse, permit greater acceptance of partial heart failure. The need to take a horse out of work at Grade II, even if only for economic reasons, paradoxically gives it a better chance of compensatory recovery. There are occasions, however, when slow recognition of Grade II or those warning suspicions of Grade I and, of course, the risks of not 'letting down' from a hard work programme when viral disease invasion is probable, can lead to an acute fatal failure. Hence the need for good horsemastership in all aspects of this skill.

THE HEARTBEAT

Heartbeat Sounds

On auscultation with an ordinary stethoscope several sounds can be heard in the area of the heart. These are **heartbeat** sounds, which are always present in health (and, in altered form, in most cardiac disease). They are called transient, and are associated with *tissue vibrations* produced during each cardiac cycle or beat; there are four such sounds, two are always heard, and possibly two more in the normal horse. The first two mark the beginning and the end of systole (contraction) and are described as '*LUB*' followed by a shorter '*DUP*', or '*LUB DUP*'. As a rule, the left and the right side mechanical events, which cause the sounds, coincide or overlap – synchronised rhythm conduction control. Heart rate increase intensifies their audibility. The 3rd and the 4th heart sounds can also overlap, especially at fast rates associated with increased stride rate. When this occurs it is called a 'gallop rhythm'. Recent terminology describes the 4th sound as the (atrial) sound as it is caused by the noise of the blood flow through the atria when they contract and other closely related electro-mechanical activities such as atrio-ventricular valve closure.

In general terms a heart rate of over 45 beats per minute at rest is considered unusual or even abnormal and possibly pathologic.

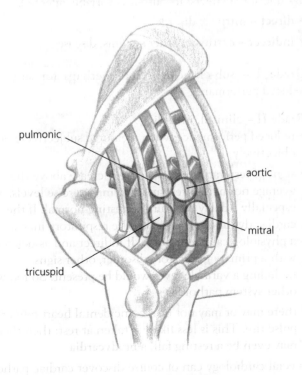

pulmonic

aortic

mitral

tricuspid

The valve areas – what the vet is listening to.

Heart sounds are a *composite* of

- electrical waves conducted through the cardiac musculature
- tension changes of contracting and relaxing cardiac muscle
- movement of heart valve leaves as they are opened and closed in response to heart chamber movement and the resultant changes in flow pressures
- movement of blood through the heart chambers and into and out of the 'great' vessels, and changes in flow rates as blood flows through from one chamber to another

Murmurs

Such sounds, distinct in character, origin and course from the transient heart beat sounds of cardiac muscle functioning, are produced by *turbulences in the blood*. There are resultant vibrations of the laminar flow through the several cardiac openings and of the related cardiac tissues.

In the normal heart, the flow rate is functionally altered by the marked changes between the valvular dimensions and that of the chambers as well as at the openings into the great blood vessels, the aorta and the pulmonary artery. The consequent changes in flow rate and volume of each stroke create the turbulent noise as the laminar flow is 'whirl-pooled' especially in the peripheral laminar currents (consider the 'babbling brook'!).

These normal changes also produce steady flow murmurs, which are functional and not pathologic and except in fit, slim, fine-coated horses and in foals, such noise does not always 'get through' to the body surface in sufficient intensity to be audible via a stethoscope.

When suspected of being associated with *some pathologic derangement* of the normal chambers, vessel surfaces and diameters, the murmurs are increased in pitch or intensity and altered in duration to become readily audible to the auscultating veterinary surgeon. Non-cardiac disorders can also cause laminar flow disturbance, e.g. the reduced viscosity of anaemic blood, which is more readily thrown into a turbulent flow.

All murmurs generally increase in intensity with increasing heart rate and the consequent raised stroke volume: physiologically, with increasing exercise demands for increased cardiac output, but significantly also due to pathologically induced ventricular hypertrophy as in cardiac compensation when power has fallen. Nevertheless, most pathologic murmurs can be detected by auscultation of the cardiac area sufficient to recognise

- their presence
- their identity as related to
- a 'diseased' valve *and* to the heartbeat sound
- other wall 'holes': faults in structure or neo-natal non-closures

The valvular deficits are usually insufficiencies of its seal's functioning

- incompetence of closure
- stenosis and narrowing of the aperture (rare)
- ventricular ring stretch (ventricular hypertrophy and/or atrial dilation)
- valvular cord (string) degeneration
- obstructive lesions on the valve endothelia

The most common sites are the
- mitral valve, then the
- tricuspid valve, then the
- semi-lunar valves of the
    - aortic artery
    - pulmonary artery

Apart from the congenital development defects, all types of pathologic murmur production are called **acquired valvular disease**. The majority of these are structural degenerations or physical defects, some inflammatory in origin. Some can be traced to myocardial defects, usually with interference in the contraction conductive system although this is more likely to cause arrhythmias.

Murmur production site and duration are closely related to the cardiac cycle of systole and diastole and their respective sounds, but are usually audible during the quiet periods between the heart sounds, before and after, but will continue to reverberate as the altered blood flow continues.

One example would be 'LUB brrrr DUP'. It is essential for the veterinary surgeon, with whatever aids he decides – stethoscope, ECG, phonogram, and especially the echogram – to determine a murmur's

- timing and
- duration relative to the heart sounds, with some five permutations of varying pathologic interpretation
- classification
    - innocent
    - pathologic

- quality
- pitch
- intensity (loudness)
  - variations therein
- anatomical point of maximum intensity (PMI)
- geometric radiation area from PMI

and so their significance.

Murmurs are graded **I** to **VI** according to intensity or loudness. For record purposes, innocent as well as pathologic murmurs are noted, because innocent murmurs can 'become' pathologic if disease subsequently develops in the related tissue sites. In general, murmurs by definition obstruct blood flow, and this reflexly stimulates a variable rise in heart rate.

Arrhythmias

Arrhythmia (lack of rhythm) and **dysrhythmia** (disorder of rhythm) are for all practical purposes roughly synonymous. Both are due to abnormal impulse conduction.

The cardiac pacemaker is in the right atrium at a sinus node, hence sinus rhythm, which automatically sets the normal pattern or rhythm of the heart beat, its atrial and ventricular cardiac muscle contractions. The beat is conducted by specialised 'nerve' fibres to ensure an 'all or nothing' contraction. Any variation from this species rhythm (to some extent individual horse rhythm) is said to be abnormal, an arrhythmia, which can be either

- regularly irregular, or
- irregularly irregular

in its

- rate of beats
- duration, and
- time intervals between beats

The atria and the ventricles beat synchronously in succession, atrias followed by ventricles. The duration of the contraction element of the beat (the **systole**) and of the filling element (the **diastole**), determines not only the flow rate but also the output volume. Together these develop a systolic and a diastolic blood pressure; the 'reading' between is the effective 'blood pressure' (BP).

As with all animals, in the horse there is a homeostatic low resting normal rate which, with the stroke volume, is sufficient to maintain a vital pressure and an adequate tissue perfusion. In the horse this rate is around 35–45 beats per minute.

First degree atrio-ventricular (AV) block causes a half-second delay in the sinus impulse going through the AV node to the ventricles. It is of little practical importance and is only detectable by an ECG.

Second degree atrio-ventricular block is a partial block, a missed or dropped ventricular contraction. In the resting horse, one in five beats miss – a regular irregular arrhythmia as part of homeostatic economy. The relatively capacious atria can remain functionally effective even when their rate is slowed under the influence of the high vagal tone and the associated parasympathetic autonomic nerve input.

When the sympathetic nerve 'alarm bell' rings, for *fright*, *fight and flight*, the heart rate automatically

- accelerates
- intensifies all elements of the beat, and so the
- stroke volume increases

until danger (excitement, aids to go forward etc.) ceases. Such an arrhythmia is rarely pathological unless the block is not eradicated by a physiological rate increase.

There are several types of functional arrhythmias, usually of short duration and easily 'lost' with work, but they should be noted when heard. In routine auscultation they are often missed – the very fact of this simple veterinary 'interference' is sufficient to speed up the heart rate and wipe out the block.

The pathologic, or potentially pathologic, can produce cardiac output deficits varying from lowered athletic performance (consequently not noticed in the average pleasure horse's activity assessment) to advanced CHF relative to the degree of exercise, especially if that is in excess of what was trained for.

The most common pathologic equine arrhythmias in the horse originate in the atria. They are

- **atrial premature complexes (APC)** which initiate 'early' systoles
  - occasionals – apparently of no significance
  - frequent
    - often fortuitously discovered
    - may be a sign of myocardial disease but also of electrolyte imbalance, toxaemia, septicaemia, reduced oxygen intake, or chronic valvular disease
    - associated with reduced athletic performance

- require ECG and other aids for confirmation
- when suspected or confirmed, a 4–8 week box rest is necessary
- an atrial tachycardia is present in persistent cases

- **atrial tachycardia (AT)**
  - not a 'true' arrhythmia
  - fast heart beat, 120–250 bpm
    - at any stage of exercise from rest upwards, i.e. not work related or necessarily associated with excitement
    - may be short lasting bursts – paroxysmal – or
    - sustained
      - regular rhythm or in association with a 2nd degree heart block
      - irregular rhythm
    - in association with chronic valvular disease – a weak pulse
  - four or more consecutive APCs constitute an AT
  - it can be confused with sinus tachycardia and ventricular tachycardia on auscultation, but these can be resolved on an ECG, especially if the paroxysm starts during the recording
  - may indicate an underlying atrial myocardial disease; this should be eliminated or treated where possible

- **atrial fibrillation** (fibrillation is defined as any local and uncontrollable twitching of some muscle fibres within a main muscle) – in the heart it is irregular twitchings of the muscular wall
  - the most commonly diagnosed equine dysrhythmia
  - it can be confused with 2nd degree atrial ventricular block
  - affects mainly athletically used horses
  - often an incidental finding
  - an irregular arrhythmia varying from slow, normal to accelerated, and is associated with
    - flurries of beats (paroxysmal) which are often fortuitously detected
    - cyclical in recurrence, therefore irregularly irregular
    - persistent when the horse is working
    - there is a loss of the fourth or (A) sound
    - reduced exercise tolerance, poor performance

- if work is continued there is
  - epistaxis
  - ataxia
  - tachypnoea
- intrinsic heart disease may be present
  - atrial dilation and associated
  - valvular disease
  - frequent APCs
- if there is no underlying cardiac dis-ease it will respond to treatment (quinine sulphate) and return to sinus rhythm

Prevalence of Arrhythmia
- heavy hunters in heavy going
- Draught horses in hard work, 10–15 years old
- Thoroughbreds in racing – sudden and unexpected deterioration in exercise tolerance (ET), 2–10 years old
- Thoroughbred crosses in fast work – vague earlier history of deterioration in ET, 8–15 years
- any horse with mitral regurgitation
- rare in ponies
- viraemia is a likely association

The cause of arrhythmias is occasionally inexplicable. Some are definitely associated with myocardial disease. Others are cardiac anomalies arising from

- electrolyte imbalances
- toxaemias

There is much still to be understood about arrhythmia. A significant number of any pathologic type are often sub-clinical, even in performance effect, until the horse is stressed.

Non-pathologic cardiac arrhythmias
- sinus arrhythmia
- wandering pacemaker
- sino-atrial lock
- incomplete AV block (2nd degree)
- first-degree heart block

Pathogenic cardiac arrhythmias
- atrial tachycardia leading to fibrillation
- ventricular extra systole
- paroxysmal ventricular tachycardia

- complete heart block with collapse and sudden death often associated with rupture of
  - valve leaf cords (chordia tendineae)
  - the aortic artery
  - the pulmonary artery

Non cardiac dis-ease with pathogenic effect including that on the heart, frequently causing arrhythmias

- metabolic
- hepatic
- renal
- endocrine

In many arrhythmic situations the significance can be determined only by ECG examination.

A (possibly pathogenic) increase in resting rate is called **tachycardia**. In itself it is not an arrhythmia, but it is usually indicative of cardiac pathology especially if it

- continues, or worsens, with exercise
- is accompanied by a jugular pulse

In general, most arrhythmias are associated with tachycardia of varying degrees, duration and irregularity. A secondary subsequent bradycardia is a possible sequel.

BLOOD VESSEL DIS-EASE

Thrombosis – macroscopic

- intra-thoracic aorta age-related wall thickening with associated necrosis and possible calcification with variable narrowing of the lumen. Possibly due to repeated strongyle larvae trauma. (The atheromatous cholesterol deposits of man are very rare in equines)
- intra-abdominal aortic obstruction leading to aneurysm formation and possibly to fatal rupture. Larval implications
- intra-abdominal distal aortic and its branches: the iliacs and femorals
  - bilateral, usually in young 'free' energetic horses in company, possibly associated with tearing of the related arterial internal lining resulting from pulsed rhythmic, hyper-dilation; may be associated with larval migration. There is a variable degree of ischaemia in the hind limbs and so in lameness
  - unilateral hind limb distal aortic branches partial

blockage, with repetitive ischaemia and consequent lameness during fast and/or prolonged work; the blood supply at rest is usually sufficient. The thrombotic obstruction becomes increasingly pathogenic with repeated and increasing exercise levels. May result in permanent muscle atrophy

- pain
- increased heart (and respiratory) rate
- variable pain-related fever
- marked sweating, but a cold affected leg
- severe cramping in the affected leg and marked lameness
  - recovery (diminishing over several episodes) with rest
  - the vein from that leg as seen on the inner thigh is significantly less distended than that of the unaffected (or less affected) hind limb
  - occasionally an asymmetric degree of lameness in the 'better' leg
- possibly associated with aberrant strongyle larvae. Infection and internal stretch trauma have been implicated, as has allergic induced blood platelet aggregation. In all cases there is frequently an associated embolism formation. A similar condition is seen in humans and felines. Surgery has been attempted; it is worthwhile to try for example Eqvalan (anthelmintic) therapy first of all

- jugular vein thrombosis – a traumatic phlebitis following intravenous therapy damage to the wall of the vein. The resultant thrombus is usually occlusive. There is no collateral circulation of immediate help; natural re-canalisation occasionally follows; bilateral occlusion is very serious. In some cases a persistent subcutaneous haemorrhage leak persists, with variable morbidity
- deep vein thrombosis in the proximal limbs, with emboli into the venous flow possibly affecting the bronchial circulation (uncommon, or at least rarely diagnosed)
- cranial mesenteric artery
  - a thrombo-embolic pathology of proven third stage larvae (Strongylus vulgaris) cause in their normal migratory pattern
  - embolic formation with varying levels of gut ischaemia to necrosis

- local sites, usually microscopic
  - intestinal wall vasculature: thrombosis associated with strongyle larvae migration into arterioles. A somewhat similar pathology is seen in Cyathostomiasis
  - laminar arterioles and capillaries, as in laminitis
  - podotrochlear arterioles, as in navicular disease and possibly in navicular syndrome dis-ease
- specific disease – lymphadenitis/lymphangitis
  - marked lameness
  - whole limb oedema with proximal cut-off line
  - engorgement of lymph vessel, painful to touch
  - high fever – pain related

possibly a bacterial allergic response originating in the proximal lymph gland.

Aneurysm

Intra-thoracic. Usually associated with major aortic and pulmonic vein damage close to the heart walls: thrombosis is usually a precursor. The human abdominal aortic aneurysm is not common in the horse.

REDUCED EXERCISE TOLERANCE

In the dis-ease situation, with appropriate care, management and, where feasible, treatment, the horse's innate cardiac reserve, its intrinsic ability to hypertrophy the smooth muscle, will come into play. Such a heart is said to have compensated.

Many physiological factors are involved. Not all are fully understood, but the basic function of this compensation is to maintain blood pressure, tissue perfusion and so 'living'.

It is essential when cardiac output deficit is suspected that a veterinary surgeon carries out a full examination of the cardiac and all other systems, to determine the basic cause of the reduced exercise tolerance. A secondary cardiac conduction problem will frequently develop into a more serious heart disease if the stress is allowed, or forced, to continue.

Some of these extrinsic pathologies may be sub-clinical in themselves, although possibly active for some time before the cardiac dysfunction signs appear. They may in fact have been self-cured but have left a legacy of myocardial disease and conduction defects or even valvular disease, showing as further reduced exercise tolerance,

which can be the forerunner of CHF with pathogenic murmurs and paroxysmal arrhythmias.

A feature of equine cardiac disease is the species' larger atria as compared to man and dog. The walls have more area to accommodate any conduction disturbances.

THE VETERINARY SURGEON'S APPROACH TO CARDIO-VASCULAR DIS-EASE IN PRACTICE

Unsuspected cardiac disorders may be discovered at
- pre-purchase examination
- insurance cover evaluation
- fitness assessment
  - in course of training programme
  - to satisfy official discipline requirements as, e.g. on Endurance competitions: 'Is it fit to continue?'
- investigating 'loss of performance' and/or suspected heart disorder specifically
- during a holistic examination for systemic dis-ease

It must be appreciated that there are other causes of 'poor performance' not directly connected with heart dis-ease. Some may produce coincidental cardiac disorders such as arrhythmias with loss of blood pressure and perfusion, or lower the animal's physical ability directly, e.g.

- respiratory dis-ease
- muscular-skeletal disorders
- neurologic deficits
- alimentary dysfunction
- nutritional deficits

In all such examinations, including other system appraisals, the veterinary surgeon will carry out a general clinical examination, which will include:
- the oral mucous membrane
  - colour
    - pale, as in anaemia
    - dark red, as in septicaemia and toxaemia
    - shades of grey or a bluish tinge as in endotox-aemia

    the last two with obvious more serious complications and verging on collapse

NOTE: cyanosis, severe oxygen depletion due to cardiac

dis-ease, is rare in the horse.

- capillary refill time (CRT) above the normal (less than 3 seconds) is basically a guide to peripheral circulation generally and so to possible tissue perfusion deficit.

- arterial pulse (usually the facial artery) as to

    - rate (beats per minute)

    - regularity (arrhythmic or not)

    - quality

    A weak pulse suggests congestive heart failure. Assessment is a 'practised' skill (and that applies too to veterinary surgeons!). When suspected as being deficit other parameters are required.

- jugular vein distension as an 'external' evidence of a cardiac disorder, e.g. a cardiac venous congestion and therefore a significant pointer to the presence of heart dis-ease. Usually right-sided but also to left-sided failure. NOTE: the head and neck should be freed to allow the horse to adopt a normal stance when assessing. There are other non cardiac obstructive causes

- jugular pulse – an apparent upwards pulsation (from the base of the neck, the thoracic inlet)

    - physiological if restricted to just the caudal end of the neck

    - suspiciously pathologic if continuing cranially often follows the CHF associated with tricuspid (right) atrio-ventricular insufficiency

- dependent (pitting) oedema in the

    - brisket

    - ventral abdomen

    - sheath (in males)

    - distal limbs from

    - right side heart congestive failure

    - other non cardiac causes

        - lympho-sarcoma

- palpation of the cardiac apex beat – similar to arterial pulse assessment but more accurate for ventricular power

- disorders of other systems in which

    - pain

        - acute lameness, acute digestive disorders

    - fever

are present, both of which will indirectly influence heart functioning

    - rate

    - rhythm

    - respiratory dis-eases

which reduce oxygen availability, will automatically (reflexly) increase cardiac output.

Both cardiac and respiratory disorders, clinical or sub-clinical, will lead to exercise intolerance, and they may be concurrent. It is certainly essential to investigate the possibility of cardiac disorders in both.

Ausculation is an essential, for the presence of

- normal heart sounds

    - heart rate: usually mirrored by the pulse

- abnormal sounds (usually murmurs)

- abnormal rhythm pattern (arrhythmias)

The ultimate veterinary requirement is to recognise the presence and the source of the murmur(s)

- which valve openings are involved

- qualify the

    - character – functional or pathologic

    - duration relative to systole (contraction) and diastole (relaxation, rest period)

    - relationship to rest and to exercise

- recognise arrythmias and, if possible whether

    - functional or pathologic

- relationship of both to cardiac functioning at rest and at exercise

In both murmurs and arrhythmias, the functional or physiological causes are very common in comparison to the pathologic. The effect *of* work is a very important consideration, the effect **on** work relative to depleted oxygen supply is a significant clue.

- heart rate (the initial estimation must always be gauged with the horse at a settled rest), as compared to

- resting normal for that horse (if known, otherwise the average for the breed)

- exercise induced normal for that horse's state of fitness in a known environment and 'going' (if known), as with

- time for return (towards) resting normal

With cardiac disorders these will change, usually to faster

rates, a **tachycardia** with or without a **tachypnoea**, and to a slower return to resting normal; the heart rate increase is to compensate for or to balance the deficits due to, for example, lowered output per beat with

- reduced forward flow
- less stroke volume per beat, and so quantity per minute from
  - ventricular weakness
  - obstruction to flow
    - valvular incompetence and regurgitation of flow
    - valvular stenosis (rare in horses)

As happens, the early, often sub-clinical pathologies produce changes in exercise tolerance. When a horse is exposed to an intensity of work that was 'normal' for that horse in the recent past before the disorders of the heart developed, it will now show as

- early tiring, especially in a usually willing horse
- loss of stamina, disinclination to jump, or just brushing through an obstacle, or falling after a jump as in racing
- dyspnoea
- epistaxis

In examination for loss of performance it is essential to have the horse ridden and reassessed after the canter and *again* after the believed level of fitness pace. In some cases a paroxysmal tachycardia, of which the average owner could not be aware, will fortuitously not show at veterinary examination with handling excitement alone, and can still be missing even at half-level intensity; hence the need for a full exertion to significantly produce the necessary fast heart rate and incidental arrhythmias.

Conversely, immediately after half-level intensity exercise under saddle, auscultation may reveal a sinus arrhythmia, which can be confusing. If of only physiological importance this transient sign will disappear as the heart rate decreases; confirmation can be obtained by working the horse to nearer full-level intensity, when such an irregularity will not appear after the exercise. The arrhythmia is said to be the heart conduction system 'hunting' for normality.

It may seem defeatist but it is important to appreciate that even with a comprehensive diagnosis of cardiac disorder or disease the subsequent veterinary input is limited to

- medical therapy, for
  - some auricular arrhythmias (ventricular fibrillation does not respond to electric shock as in humans)
  - some valvular endocarditic conditions (valvular replacement is not feasible)
  - limited to some contraction weaknesses, but digitalis-like drugs can be dangerous in the horse and Vitamin E benefits are anecdotal
  - other system disorders, e.g.
    - respiratory (especially)
    - hepato/renal
    - alimentary
  - muscular-skeletal systems as well as
  - electrolyte imbalances
  - nutritional deficits
  - obesity
- judicious re-training techniques

Cardiac disease is more rare than many owner/trainers believe. Most (apparent) sudden deaths are non-cardiac in primary cause.

Autopsy

In the horse, as distinct from other animal species, cardiac tissue changes associated with cardiac dis-ease, clinical or sub-clinical, which developed during life, are comparatively minor and relatively few. These are often missed unless post-mortem examination is carried out by a specialist in pathology.

Mild degenerative changes are common findings, but these are usually not significant as to the cause of death. Immediately after death the heart chambers are in diastole, i.e. relaxed. Systolic contraction is a rare finding, death from digitalis poisoning being an exception.

Later on there develops rigor mortis in the heart's two muscular groups, atrial and ventricular. This passes off. Rigor mortis in the RV passes off first and the chamber is usually filled with blood. The LV had the firmer contraction, which relaxes more slowly; its contents are usually coagulated serum, which may be blood-stained.

DISEASES OF THE LYMPHATIC SYSTEM

The lymphatic system's functioning is described as a 'fluid sewage system', which is

- **hidden** (except for some lymphoid tissues) as in the pharynx
    - there are no body surface orifices
    - in 'health', the superficial vessels cannot be felt, nor are they firm enough to 'stand out' under the skin
- **silent**
    - the flow is passive, being subject to other body 'forces'; there is no 'motor mechanism' or pump, and so no sources for the production of murmurs

Its passive purpose, within a broader homeostasis, is to

- **drain off** from all areas of the body
    - the physiological excess of interstitial fluid, plus
    - any 'escaped' protein molecules, and
- **return** these to the blood circulation
- **'pick-up'** foreign material, including microbes scavenged by white blood cells, for **filtering** out in the regional lymph nodes (glands) through which all lymph must pass

In this respect it serves as part of the body's defences, by

- **removal of microbes** via lymph-cell transport, for
    - further **destruction**
    - **immunity development**

The horse, as an unguligrade with 'elongated' limbs, has a proportion of its limbs distally devoid of muscle tissue – and therefore devoid of muscles' massaging effect on the passive lymph flow and also on the accompanying virtually passive venous return flow.

From the 'knee' and the 'hock' down, these return flows are therefore dependent on massage with secondary 'suction' occurring at the proximal areas of the limbs. This effect requires that such muscles are **actively engaged**, i.e. in locomotory work.

Venous and lymph fluid return flows are a reflection of the cursorial nature of the horse; athleticism requires

- relatively greater arterial blood flow
- relatively greater nutrient content in the blood

These, together with the anatomical factors, make the horse more subject to what is colloquially known as **filled legs** or 'humour' from **hydrodynamic dysfunction**, as in the heavier type which is well nourished but 'stood in' for most of the 24 hours (sub-optimal exercise). Minimal muscle-functional massage lessens the upward flows. A **back pressure** in both systems develops

- in the **venous capillaries**, so that more serum than usual transudates into the **interstitial fluid**
- in the **lymph vessels**, now with more lymph to transport but with decreased help

As a result, the excess interstitial fluid collects in, and distends, the interstitial spaces of the **sub-cutaneum** below the 'knee' and the 'hock' on the palmar/plantar aspect of the cannon (where there is more loose tissue than on the anterior) to produce a soft filling. The hind legs, further away from the heart, are affected more often than the forelegs.

In these hydrokinetic situations, the cause is **obstruction** based on failure to assist drainage

Basically this is **non-pathologic oedema**, as when

- **external** mechanical forces interfere with the flow
  - incorrectly fitted **bandages**, fastened too tightly just below the knee or the hock and/or with insufficient padding between the limb and the bandage
  - chronic (scarring) **inflammatory lesions** with tissue-thickening to give a 'too-tight-a-garter' effect (see also sporadic lymphangitis chronicity)
- **internal** mechanical forces
  - **neoplastic** adjacent external pressure
  - underlying 'new' bony prominences which induce clotting by partial obstruction in the compressed lymphatics
  - the heavily **pregnant mare** showing ventral oedema, udder oedema and filled hind legs
- **dietary** changes – a **biochemical effect**
  - **over-feeding** for work being done, especially of protein-rich nutrients. The protein leaks through capillary areas, with consequent vascular osmotic changes and, with any electrolyte imbalances, especially relating to sodium (Na) and potassium (K), will produce subsequent increase in interstitial fluid
  - the feeding of '**new hay too soon**', before the nitrogen is fully converted

A combination of the hydrodynamic and the biochemical types often occurs to add to the 'filled leg' syndrome.

Pathologically induced lymphatic flow dysfunction can be

- **obstructive** due to a diseased state within the system
  - lymph node enlargement and '**filter' blockage**
    - **inflammatory** – infection, via blood and/or lymph
    - **allergic**
    - **neoplastic**
- secondary **overloading** of the system (and so compromising its ability to 'drain' the area completely) from dis-ease within the **vascular** capillary system, by
  - **viral**
  - **toxic**
  - **allergic** dis-ease, causing
    - leakage of excess fluid, often itself diseased
    - leakage of excess protein through capillaries

Both of the above pathological types can occur anywhere in the body. The resultant excess fluid may collect within a body cavity, but frequently, because of the knock-on effect through the entire vascular/lymphatic system, it 'appears' in the dependent surfaces or the appendages of the body – the limbs first and especially (may affect one or all four); the head; the brisket; the ventral abdomen; and the prepuce/udder.

These observable signs are collectively called **oedema** – a sub-cutaneous swelling which distorts and stretches the overlying skin. It frequently percolates into the dermis. It is painless and slightly cold to the touch and it 'pits' on digital pressure. It should be distinguished from **inflammatory oedema** which is usually warm and non-pitting, and from **epidermal plaques** of allergic origin.

Oedema within the **abdominal** cavity is **ascites** or 'dropsy'. This is a transudate, an outflow from tissues into the peritoneal 'cavity' because of pathological changes within, e.g.

- **cirrhosis** of the liver – obstruction
- abdominal **neoplasia** – obstruction
- **peritonitis**, which adds its own serous/inflammatory exudate
- **malnutrition** – low blood-protein
- **wasting** diseases – low blood-protein
- **CHF** – obstruction to venous return

Advanced cases will produce a distended pendulous abdomen. The pressure itself interferes with diaphragm action in inspiration. It can produce hind-limb filling from the 'knock-on' effect.

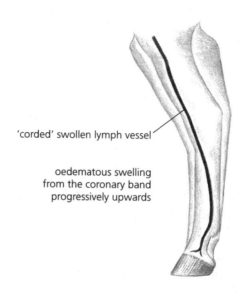

'corded' swollen lymph vessel

oedematous swelling from the coronary band progressively upwards

Ideopathic lymphangitis – hind leg, medial aspect.

The '**filled leg**' of non-pathological causes pits on digital pressure and refills; it also 'walks off' with exercise. The pathological types rarely do so, but certainly take much longer.

'Filled leg' is distinct from '**a leg**' – a term colloquially used when the posterior aspect of the cannon region is enlarged by sub-cutaneous local inflammatory exudate and associated oedema, due to sterile trauma to the flexor tendons and/or the suspensory ligament. It is painful to digital pressure and only variably pits. It is, in the early stages, hot to the touch.

The lymph vessels can themselves become inflamed, e.g. a **lymphangitis**, secondary to that in the tissues they drain; for example, a septic wound, or as part of a more general state as in some allergic reactions. In the limbs this is a '**big leg**'.

The lymph glands, an integral part of the system, are directly subject to those types of dis-ease of inflammation, allergy and malignant neoplasia; the inflammatory term is **lymphadenitis**.

Different clearly demarcated distensions are those of the **digital sheath**, or **non-articular windgall** and the **articular windgall** of the fetlock articular synovial sheath. They vary from soft to tense. They are not oedemas but protective over-production of synovial fluid. The overlying skin is generally at the temperature of the whole distal leg, except in acute trauma situations where there is a related acute 'picture' including increased heat. Infection markedly worsens this.

Inflammatory Dis-eases of the Lymphatic System

By definition, any infection of an epithelial surface

- skin
- mucous membrane

will be 'picked up' by the various lymphoid and scavenging cells, and transported to the regional lymph nodes and/or to other sites of lymphoid immune-stimulating tissues via the related lymphatic vessels.

Neoplastic malignant cells also travel this route. It follows therefore that a reaction will occur in the lymph gland tissue and, in some cases, in the lymph vessels themselves.

Some lymph nodes are visible in this otherwise hidden system

- tonsillar tissue in the throat protruding from the pharyngeal epithelial surface

Some are palpable

- submandibular
- retropharyngeal
- inguinal (by rectal palpation)
- mesenteric (by rectal palpation)

If there is little space between the primary invasion site and the regional gland, the fluid swelling, the oedema, will be limited – for example, in the submandibular gland, enlargement due to virus invasion of the nose and throat. In **Strangles-related lymphadenitis**, the duration of the enlargement and the degree are often sufficient to produce a distal swelling of the muzzle, more especially the lower-jaw chin area, a rostro-ventral area.

Examples of more focal types of lymphatic system clinical involvement with or without oedema are infected wounds where there is local bacterial activity, with regional diffusion into surrounding tissues.

If the microbe is invasive and 'spreading', the lymphatic vessel will become inflamed – **lymphangitis** (the red line up the human arm, from wound to armpit gland) – possibly visibly distended and painful to digital pressure. The regional lymph gland will also be involved, enlarged, obstructive and painful – **lymphadenitis**. If the wound infection is purulent in character, the gland will likely become abscessed and will eventually 'burst'.

If the first and perhaps the secondary lymph nodes contain the infection, all will become well; if they do not, the germ will go on to invade the main circulation – giving rise to **septicaemia** (blood poisoning) and widespread organ invasion.

As already stated, Clostridial **germs** do not *per se* create an inflammatory reaction, nor do they invade away from the original wound; their toxins, however, do so – for example, gas gangrene infections. Some toxins will be transported through regional lymph nodes, with varying degrees of lymphangitis and lymphadenitis, but they usually invade direct from site into the blood stream. Significantly, the tetanus toxin invades via nerve tissue, and so does not pass through the lymphatic system.

Any associated oedema, especially that around the *bacterially infected* wound which is also showing cellulitis with inflammatory exudate, is now called **inflammatory oedema**. It does *not* pit on digital pressure and is of course painful to the touch, and is warmer.

Viral infections will also produce a lymphadenitis, invariably **without** abscessation. The glands involved are those of the respiratory tracts, upper and lower. Pharyngeal lymphoid tissue, the horse's tonsils, are diffuse as well as local and will react, and in some cases remain, as a focus of a carrier-state or a latent-state infection – as in the herpes viral infection, in particular.

SPECIFIC DISEASE

Lymphadenitis

Enlarged tonsils and throat glands defending against a virus infection are examples of lymphadenitis without the clinical signs of lymphangitis. In a bacterial infection such as strangles, the affected lymph nodes, which lie between the jaws, are a second line of defence, usually resulting in abscess formation. Only in prolonged, severe cases before the glands' abscess 'bursts' is there a visible related oedema in the throat, but any lymphangitis as such is masked because of the particular layout of the structures involved. Secondary abscesses may develop in the throat lymph glands.

Lymphangitis

Sporadic (idiopathic)

In the equine limbs the regional lymph gland is proximal – as in the axilla ('arm pit') and in the groin.

If a lymph node is involved by infection carried to it by the lymphatic system, the inflammation causes a variable obstruction to the flow from the more distal areas and, consequently, a related swelling is usually seen in the dependent part of the related limb. There is usually a local sub-cutaneous inflammation associated and originating at the site of the original wound. Such secondary 'big' legs are part of true inflammation; the oedema does not pit and is painful on digital pressure.

Some horses with a sub-clinical but persistent low-grade obstruction in the lymph nodes in the groin from a previous infection, and which are, at any subsequent time, kept stabled from 24–36 hours (e.g. no work or exercise on a Sunday) and on a high plane of nutrition, can develop an oedema of the distal sub-cutaneous tissues, a primary 'big leg'. The lymph node dormant infection, having lost the flushing flow of exercise, 'flares up' to produce a more blocked gland, an acute lymphadenitis. The inflammation backtracks down the lymph vessel which, in turn, becomes

inflamed – lymphangitis. The original filled leg now becomes an inflammatory type, clinically a very 'big', painful leg. It is possible that the regional lymph gland reacted in an allergic manner to produce the acute blocking swelling, but rarely, if ever, forms an abscess.

It is very occasionally seen in both hind limbs and in either or both fore.

Signs

There will be a palpable, painful lymph vessel particularly in the thigh area – it stands out like a cord. The horse is very lame, fevered, up to 106°F and generally ill. It may stand 'holding' the foot off the ground; the pain may cause the horse to lift the leg violently because of the oedematous stiffness which interferes with flexion and induces abduction (beware handling!). Serum may ooze from the skin where tight over the bone as in cannon and inside low leg bone. Because it usually follows a period of rest, it is often called **Monday Morning Disease**, but technically it is known as **sporadic lymphangitis**. This is more frequently seen in the heavier type of horse than in the lighter breeds. The condition also occurs in the lactating mare, especially one on reduced exercise but on extra feeding for milk production **and** for condition (as in showing).

Diagnosis and Treatment

The pain and marked swelling are obvious and are usually much more extensive than caused by a primary or new infection of a skin wound (cellulitis) on the leg.

Antibiotic drugs are given in order to treat any possible infection, plus steroids in the early stage to reduce the inflammation, and the use of diuretic drugs helps to remove fluid from the legs. Pain-killing drugs are also given, and this should enable the horse to be given short periods of walking exercise at frequent intervals, to help disperse the swelling. Hot fomentation or hot poultices followed by massage and bandaging the leg from the hoof upwards, are also helpful.

Improvement occurs over two or three days and the horse's temperature and appetite will return to normal. Although the size of the leg will gradually reduce, some permanent, fibrosis thickening will usually remain. Unfortunately there is a tendency for the problem to recur in the same leg with ever-increasing thickening and eventual elephantiasis.

Bacterial

Glanders (Farcy) caused by *Pseudomonas mallei*
Up until the early to mid 19th century this was endemic in

the UK and western Europe but is now found only in the Middle East, Africa and India. It still remains on the British list of notifiable diseases. The infection rate is high and spreads by contagion to many species including man. It is often a fatal condition following systemic invasion with acute signs, as in asses and mules. The chronic form with lesions of ulcers and abscesses is common to the horse in which the skin lesions of ulcerating purulent lymphangitis usually in the hock and neck regions – areas of trauma and so a route of invasion – are typical. There is involvement of the regional lymph gland.

Confirmatory diagnosis is by the 'Mallein' intradermal test; isolation of the germ from the pus is highly suspicious.

Ulcerative Lymphangitis

Caused by *Corynebacterium para-tuberculosis*

A mildly infectious contagion – via injuries especially to the skin of the extremities, most frequently in the hind limbs. Once infected recurrences are common.

The onset is sudden with variable but often severe oedema spreading upwards as far as the stifle or the elbow. The leg is painful. A serum exudate soon follows with lymphatic cording. Discharging creamy green pus breaks from the skin in some cases. In the USA there are multiple small, draining sores.

In the chronic form the thickened lymphatics are scarred with granulating, scabbed lesions and entrapped oedema. Isolation of the causal germ determines treatment but eradication is frequently difficult because of the fibrosed pockets of infection.

Fungal

Epizootic Lymphangitis (Pseudo-Farcy) caused by *Histoplasma farciminosum* (mainly found in Africa, Asia and East Europe)

A rare, chronic, contagious notifiable disease, a suppurative lymphangitis of areas in contact with tack and other physically eroded areas. Thus the lesions are on the lips, neck, saddle area and girth, and hind legs.

There is a regional lymphadenitis with ulceration along the corded lymphatics. No systemic lesions as a rule but some lesions are found in the respiratory tract, eyes and joints.

It is more common in donkeys than in the horse. Treatment is not attempted: slaughter is usually compulsory. Spontaneous recovery with a solid immunity has been recorded.

Fungal granuloma/pythiosis (found in the Americas, Australia, tropical and sub-tropical areas)

An ulcerative granulomatous skin disease due to *Pythium insidiosum* infection which is contagious. Also known as 'bursatti', 'Florida horse leeches' and 'swamp cancer'.

Ulcerated lesions in traumatised, wet skin with marked pruritus and self mutilation. Systemic lesions are rare.

Single, usually unilateral lesions of masses of grey, necrotic tissue which later tend to spread extensively; when calcification develops it is called 'kunkers'. There is an intense eosinophilic infiltration of acute lesions.

Surgery is required with sodium iodide and amphotericin B supportive treatment. Bone lesion cases are usually fatal.

Lymphosarcoma

A **malignant neoplasia**, it comes in various clinical patterns. Relative to the lymphatic system there are

- space-occupying lesions within the abdominal cavity which, inter alia, affect the mesenteric lymph nodes
- space-occupying lesions of the mediastinum and/or the pleural cavities, which affect the systemic lymph nodes and the thymic area

  with effusion and oedema in both sites, for example ascites in the abdomen; excess pleuritic fluid in the chest

- generalised, including
  - bone marrow
  - spleen

There is a regional lymphadenitis in most situations; when the head and inguinal regions are affected there is an associated oedema.

From all of these, the 'seeds' of the tumour can spread to invade elsewhere, i.e. further metastasis with possible further lymphatic flow obstruction.

CHAPTER 24

DISEASES OF THE RESPIRATORY SYSTEM

Respiratory dis-ease is one of the most common reasons for a horse being 'off work'. It is certainly the most common of group or 'yard' disabilities when due to contagious infection.

Respiratory Sounds

A normal horse's breathing, as listened to from 'outside' it, i.e. not by stethoscopic auscultation, is

- at rest, quiet
- at exercise when fit, quiet on inspiration, a 'blowing' noise variably audible on expiration and more so with some 'high blowing' animals
- at exercise when unfit, and particularly when fat, an inspiratory noise is frequently heard which can mimic or confuse as being disease-produced

Abnormal sounds are said to be due to vibration of tissues of the airway tract, musical sounds produced in morbidly patent cavities (see **ideopathic laryngeal hemiplegia, ILH,** and **recurrent laryngeal neuropathy, RLN,** later in this chapter) and to sudden changes in airflow pressures.

Airflow is laminar, i.e. air layers glide over others, the layer closest to the wall is almost static, and the layer in the centre of a tract moves most quickly.

It should be noted that the curled turbinate bones of the nasal passages which form, bilaterally, three airway channels actually spin the air into non-laminar flow within the facial area. This normal 'turbulence' throws particulate material including inhaled micro-organisms onto the epithelial mucosa of the airway, especially the septum where, in most cases, they are trapped and carried to the throat and thence swallowed. This swirling of the air also brings it into greater contact with heating and moisturising surfaces.

Deformity in any part of the tract wall will cause an abnormal disturbance in the laminar flow and will result in abnormal turbulence. It is this which produces sound and interrupts rate of flow. Since there is a marked difference in flow rate at rest compared to at exercise, such turbulence becomes progressively more serious with the accelerated gaits, and so more detrimental to gaseous exchange. Exercise tolerance may even drop to the extent of a standstill in locomotion.

These abnormal sounds are

- an increase in loudness of normal sounds because of the effect of dis-ease influences
- a previously inaudible pathologic sound becoming audible, usually at inspiration
- a change in pitch from a vibrating organ obstruction, as with a displaced soft palate

Head carriage influences airway dynamics and so the possibility of turbulence. In 'testing' for abnormal noise the horse must be progressively exercised (exerted) until it is 'blowing hard' before being judged as negative

Inspiratory sound

- high pitch whistle, to low pitch roar
  - unfit
  - ILH
  - epiglottic entrapment
- irregular pattern, plus increased loudness
  - pharyngitis
- loud inspiratory/expiratory sound

- epiglottic entrapment
- nasal obstruction
- sinusitis
- sudden gurgling sound when under stress, e.g. near end of a race. Stops suddenly when pressure is ended, or if swallowing occurs
  - DDSP (dorsal displacement of the soft palate)
- stentorous loud noise on inspiration and expiration – a snoring sound
  - pharyngeal obstruction or cyst
  - guttural pouch empyema
  - tracheal collapse
  - tumours of the larynx and trachea

Coughing

It is assumed that horses in general

- do not have a communicative cough – *'Excuse me, but...'*
- do not need to 'nervously' clear their throat

that is, they have no voluntary control of coughing.

Throughout the respiratory tract there are areas which are particularly sensitive to 'unwanted' stimuli in the air flow. Special nerve receptors are activated by

- inspired
  - particulate material
  - marked changes in air temperature as at night and morning diurnal fluctuations or when meeting 'fresh', colder air on coming out of the stable
  - increased volume flow and rate associated with a rapid increase in inspiration as demanded by sudden exercise – colder air in consequence
- expired
  - muco (purulent) secretions
  - functional pressure changes in airflow, as in chronic obstructive pulmonary disease (COPD)

The exposure of sub-epithelial 'ordinary' sensory nerve endings when the protective mucous membrane is 'raw' from inflammatory and/or allergic morbidity is an additional source of irritation in itself and by the unwanted stimuli mentioned above.

The 'message' thus generated travels to the cough centre in the brain which reflexly motivates the special defensive mechanism of an increased expiratory flow rate and volume. When necessary these can be increased to become an explosive expiration which, on escaping through the mouth or the nostrils produces an audible cough or sneeze respectively. To the listener either sound indicates that the horse was reflexly 'aware' of the need to clear the airway forcefully, or attempt to do so.

The cough and the sneeze are clinical aspects of the airway defence system. The noise results when a volume of air travelling faster than normal along a relatively narrow diameter tube 'escapes' quickly into a much wider airway, for example

- trachea into throat
- throat into the mouth and the atmosphere
- throat into the nostrils and the atmosphere

The main respiratory reflex areas are situated in, and are relatively graded, thus

nasal passages	**
pharynx	**
larynx	*
trachea	*
carina bifurcation of the bronchi	***

Digital pressure down onto the space between the caudal larynx and the cranial trachea will stimulate a cough, especially if there is a sub-acute or chronic on-going respiratory dis-ease. Such a cough is often preceded by a reflex swallowing movement.

The cough followed by a sneeze is thought to indicate a naso-pharyngeal inflammation, primary virus or bacterial residual inflammation and, by definition, is a less worrying sign. It should be borne in mind that sneezing *per se* is a sign of rhinitis, **but** is also heard in herpes infections in which coughing is a less significant clue. (This cough-then-sneeze is not typical of OPD.) The combined sign is frequently seen at the start of exercise: a clearing of the tract. It is rare for them to be productive of a contagious aerosol.

A vicious circle obtains in chronic, unrelieved lung disease with persistent coughing; there is a build-up of intra-thoracic pressure which adversely affects the bronchiolar and alveolar blood supply; a subsequent cell wall hypoxia leads to an atrophy and eventual rupture – **emphysema**.

Where emphysema is present, expiratory flow volume rate emanating from ruptured alveoli is further reduced and coughing is even more required to assist in expiration.

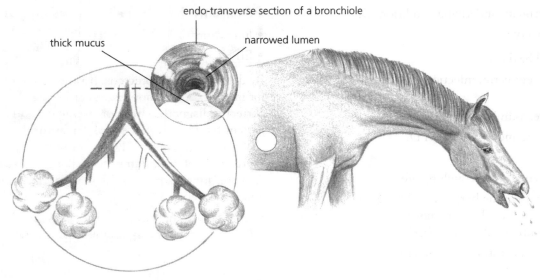

COPD – abnormal mucus in the lungs causes coughing.

To hear coughing should be enough to make the horse-master investigate **'who'**, begin to consider **'why'**, and decide **'what'** to do. It matters little in principle whether it is a lone horse privately owned or one in a training yard's new intake. If the cough is 'new' it is

- to the single owner, an indication that a forthcoming competition might be 'out' – for the horse's sake and for the welfare of the other horses it might contact
- to the racehorse trainer, a signal of a possible interrupted programme of training and racing – a financial worry

and that extra attention is now essential.

If a cough is 'new', it is described as an **acute onset cough**. It may persist in sub-acute forms of the underlying disease and if it continues for more than two months it is, not unnaturally, described as a **chronic cough**. Some coughs which are slow to 'build up' in degree and persistence are difficult to place as above. Their chronicity does require accurate diagnosis for effective treatment of the basis of the cough.

These facts should be noted

- coughs, as such, are not readily treatable. They are a reflex action following a primary condition
- this condition may be treatable (but not primary viral ones)
- certain drugs may ameliorate the cough
  - some reduce the inflammation – not to be

recommended, the cough is defensive

- some 'quieten' the cough reflex – again, not recommended – *the cough expels unwanted mucus, it is part of the defence mechanisms*

- a cough can be a sign of on-going infection. It implies a continuing aerosol spread of the germ and indicates that work is not yet advisable for that horse's sake

Acute onset cough can be age-related

- rhodococcal bacterial pneumonia of foals
- rotaviral infection of foals
- herpes viral infection of yearlings
- bacterial infection of the LRT in two-year-olds
- influenza viral infection at any age
- OPD, or spring grass associated obstructive pulmonary disease (SGAOPD) of older horses

It can be historically related

- recent contact with others away from home
- contact with recent imports; both point to infection, both with 'spread' within a group
- travel stress

And it can be environmentally associated

- OPD and winter housing/feeding
- SGAOPD, with pasture grazing
- lungworm disease with pasture and co-grazing donkeys

Cessation of coughing indicates

- response to primary underlying conditions therapy
- 'natural' recovery

A relapse could be due to

- a 'fresh', different germ, infection 'on the back of' the primary
- recrudescence, as in latent herpes infection
- failure of management, as in COPD

The causes of **acute onset coughing** are

- viral infections: equine herpes 1 and 4; equine influenza; adenovirus (less common); rhinovirus (less common); equine viral arteritis (EVA)
- bacterial infections: strangles; bacterial LRT infection
- oesophageal choke
- dysphagia (pharyngeal dysfunction), a difficulty in swallowing
- acute airway obstruction: OPD relapse or COPD flare up into a severe 'attack'; SGAOPD: sudden access to causative grazing; acute pharyngo-laryngitis
- lungworm infestation – early, larval migration stage
- exercise induced pulmonary haemorrhage (EIPH), possibly
- inhaled foreign bodies
- tracheal collapse/constriction trauma
- pulmonary oedema

The Causes of Chronic Coughing

- COPD
- post-viral airway disease: chronic exudative bronchitis
- lungworm infestation, the presence of the adult worm
- pneumonia – chronic with or without abscessation
- repeat episodes of EIPH – the free blood acting as an obstruction/ irritant
- tracheal cartilage ring nodule formation
- thoracic neoplasia

In all such cases, but to variable degrees, there will be obstruction, direct or indirect, to the airflow, with a consequent exercise intolerance and a greater susceptibility to new primary and secondary infections.

Some of the conditions and their management are dealt with elsewhere, and in particular

- the OPDs

- bronchitis
- lungworm
- EIPH

By definition, a chronic cough is one which has persisted for more than two months, either because it has not been correctly diagnosed, basically treated or managed, or the patient has become secondarily inflamed.

Nature of the Cough

A descriptive list of coughs can only be a guide to the underlying morbidity

- a **harsh, dry, hacking cough** is heard in dis-ease of the **URT** associated with virus infection or secondary bacterial infections
- a **throaty cough** of varying intensity is heard in minor viral infections and/or in restricted re-infection of a partially immune horse with influenza or herpes virus
- a **soft, deep and productive cough** is more often associated with **LRT** inflammations from virus infections and is usually followed by a **swallowing** action to dispose of the expiratory fluid collecting in the pharynx. In later stages, especially if secondary bacterial complications are present, the cough is accompanied by **phlegm** as expectoration or a nasal discharge
- a '**painful**', **hesitant, short cough** is associated with acute **inflammatory** reaction, as in acute **influenza** or **pleurisy**
- a **spluttering, wet cough** whilst eating, suggests secondary **bacterial infection of the pharynx and larynx**
- a cough associated with **inspiratory 'difficulty'** and '**noise**' or **expiratory 'difficulty'** and unusual 'noise' usually indicates some form of a non-infectious, non-allergic **obstruction**, a possible lodged foreign body
- a cough associated with marked *both inspiratory and expiratory difficulty and noise* indicates a severe **disturbance of both upper and lower tracts,** as in acute allergic reaction or severe pleuro-pneumonia as in **transit fever**

There are circumstances when the cough is required physically to clear the throat of inhaled irritants, but as a rule, *a cough should always be regarded as a primary clue of respiratory channel disease*.

Such disease is most commonly of the **inflammatory** type, particularly the **infectious** and **allergic sub-types**.

A particularly worrying aspect of hearing a cough is the knowledge that *most inflammatory infections are also*

Respiratory Diseases

	EHV	Influenza	Strangles	Bacterial LRT Infections	OPD	SGAOFD	Lungworm	Pneumonia
Age								
Less than ½ year	*	*	*	*			*	
Young adults	***	***	***	***	*	*	***	***
Mature	*	**	*	*	***	***	***	***
Contagious spread	**	***	***	*			(*)	
Environment								
Stable					**			
Pasture						***	***	
Donkey contact							***	
Stress		*	**					***
Season								
Spring/Autumn					**	***	***	
Autumn/Winter					***			
Cough								
Dry	***	***			***	***		
Productive	*	*	**	***	*	*	**	**
Painful	*	*	*					***
Inappetence	**	**	**	*				***
Weight loss	*	*	*					**
Nasal discharge								
Serous	***	***	*					
Muco purulent	**	**	***	**	*	*	**	***
Purulent			***					**
Foetid								
Food			*					**
Blood								*
Respiratory difficulty								
Inspiration			**					
Expiration			*	*	***	***	*	
Stridor			**					

contagious.

In the individual horse, such a cough may be and often is followed within twelve hours by some or all of a cascade of clues, such as

- altered **respiratory** rate and depth
- elevated **pulse**
- **nasal discharge** – sometimes with sneezing
- slight **ocular** discharge
- loss of **appetite**
- dullness and **lethargy**
- enlarged **throat lymph glands**

and possible signs of a similar infection in other in-contact, non-immune horses. These must be watched out for; *twice-daily temperature recording* is the one important parameter to be monitored in suspect in-contacts, *as a fever at the end of the incubation period invariably precedes the inflammatory response signs* and often drops within three to four days. Secondary bacterial etc. infections may cause an additional and/or secondary fever.

Coughing can also be a clue to respiratory dis-ease which is

- **non-contagious**, for example
  - **COPD**
    - other **allergic** and atopic reactions in which the morbidity obstructively interferes with expiration; the cough is induced as an extra aid to expel air
    - the cough of **OPD** is usually *quiet and restrained* in **acute** cases; the expiration cannot build up fair force and volume for high (explosive) pressure
    - in **chronic OPD** cases, the cough is *louder and 'hollow-sounding'*
  - **EIPH**
- **parasitic**, for example
  - **ascarid** larval migration in the foal
  - **lungworm** infestation in the adult
- **environmental**
  - excessive **dust** intake
  - **smoke**
  - **ammonia** (from ill-kept bedding and poor ventilation)

The rapid response reflex cough associated with stimulation of the pharynx and the glottis, signalling a potential respiratory choke and possible asphyxia is rare in the horse (compare with man).

The reflex sensors of the horse appear to be set at a high threshold, despite the apparent risk attached to high fibrous diets because

- properly masticated and saliva-lubricated boluses of food slide safely from pharynx to oesophagus over a closed glottis, therefore
- the risk of ingested 'irritation' of the pharynx, and even more so
- the risk of inhalation irritation, is low
- the flow rate and volume of expired air is a further efficient defence – they can be immediately reflexly increased to 'blow away' any particulate matter
- URT muco-ciliary escalator of the nasal region traps other inhaled particulate material and carries it to the throat for swallowing

However, there is an increased risk when

- a horse is allowed to eat hay when too closely tied, as in transport
- especially if before the post-exercise respiratory rate is back to normal
- if allowed to eat while bitted
- again, especially if tired or dehydrated
- if he snatches leaves from a bush whilst being ridden
- if startled while eating dry food
- if allowed to eat with restricting head bend

All these can lead to insufficient mastication and insufficient salivary mixing when, frightened or not, it swallows too quickly and the ingesta is not properly masticated. An 'anti-choke' cough will follow, which is

- often wet and spluttering
- followed by a compensatory forced inspiration and another expiration
- followed by a sneeze or a snort

The cough, which literally 'clears the throat', and the subsequent saliva swallow, helps the return of the throat tissues to their normal positions.

As often is the case, co-incidental dis-ease such as inflammation of the URT channel and appendages, even if sub-clinical, or neuro-muscular defects in the non-rigid structures of the throat can lower this threshold of defence.

Nasal Discharge

The horse, unlike in the bovine and canine species, does not normally show a constant fluid flow from the external nares or nostrils.

Nevertheless, there is a constant movement upwards along the entire respiratory tract of a thin sero-mucus fluid, over the 'sticky' mucus coating which forms the muco-ciliary escalator. The largest quantity of this emanates from the LRT, traverses the trachea and larynx into the pharynx, whence it is swallowed along with that arising in the rostral URT. This, the smallest quantity, comes from the naso-pharynx, from the guttural pouches, the paranasal sinuses and the nasal chambers themselves; it flows in the direction of the nasal escalator inwards to be swallowed. Some from both sources can go outwards to drain through the nostrils as physiological overspill.

The moist expiratory flow, and the airway warmth, minimise this exiting quantity to such an extent that it is not discernable as liquid but on the exhaled breath it is 'felt' as a dampness. This exhaled moisture will condense in the atmosphere and be recognised as such, particularly if the weather is cold.

Cold weather air temperature will mildly irritate the nasal mucosa on inspiration, so that excess sero-mucus will be produced – the 'drippy nose' of cold mornings, when the horse leaves a warm stable before body and airtract temperature rises with exercise.

At the start of exercise, with respirations at a slightly increased rate, more than resting, sero-mucus is brought up; not all is swallowed. That, along with an increased nasal flow, will cause the horse to snort, cough and sneeze.

After strenuous exercise during which the horse 'clears its tubes' the extra sero-mucus flow is aerated and often appears for a short spell as a fluid reminiscent of whisked white of egg.

The phrase 'give the horse a pipe opener' implies not only that it 'clears its tubes' but also recruits many more resting respiratory bronchioles and their alveoli from which a 'stagnant' sero-mucous fluid is expired. This thicker material is usually dispersed as above during the work.

In work there is possibly an increase in expiratory noise until the horse gets into a 'higher gear' and the mucus is cleared.

Wherever and whenever there is an inflammatory condition along the respiratory tract or its offshoots, the associated *increased* sero-mucoid flow has to escape. At rest, that produced in the larynx and trachea and in the LRT is swallowed. If marked or excessive, some may flow rostrally into the oro-pharynx and be coughed out; some will enter the nasal chambers and drain through the nares; because of its greater mucoid consistency it will, after two or three days of inflammation, not freely run but will stick to the external nares lining to form a 'dirty' or 'snotty' nose. The site of the muco-purulent production will determine whether the ultimate nasal discharge is unilateral or bilateral.

Unilateral discharge (consistent)

- nasal polyp in one passage

- nasal trauma to one passage

- para-nasal sinuses on one side (usually from tooth root infection)

Bilateral discharge (consistent)

- nasal polyps in both passages

- nasal trauma to both passages

- para-nasal inflammation (usually infectious) of both sides

- nasal inflammation of infectious origin

- lesions caudal to the nasal septum
  - bilateral guttural pouch disease

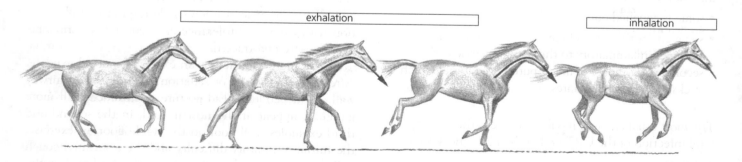

exhalation   inhalation

The rhythm of breathing in the symmetric gaits.

- unilateral guttural pouch disease discharge is mainly unilateral unless a severe often fatal haemorrhage occurs
- ethmoidal haematomata bleeding
- pharyngitis, laryngitis and tracheitis
- bronchial tree (lung) inflammation

The **appearance of the discharge**
- sero-mucoid
- mucoid, sticky
- muco-purulent, thickish
- purulent i.e. of increasing consistency
- colour – most often white through to yellow. Certain (secondary) bacteria produce a green tinge but not of diagnostic value
- blood tinged to 'all blood'
- foetid: nasty smell as in tooth root sinusitis, turbinate bone necrosis, guttural pouch mycosis, of some duration

It must be remembered that a persistent nasal discharge, whether unilateral or bilateral, is usually area 1 and 2 in origin; from the sinuses or from the guttural pouches. Lesions elsewhere have their discharges swallowed, unless

- a severe condition, in which there is overspill into the nose or mouth
- other pharyngeal conditions, in which swallowing is restricted
- conditions which directly or indirectly stimulate the cough reflex, resulting in expectoration of phlegm and expiration into the nasal chambers and subsequent discharge with sneezing sometimes

In oesophageal choke the reflux of saliva and post-choke ingesta is directed into the throat

- some is coughed out
- some enters the nasal chambers, and is sneezed out or becomes inflammatory to the nasal mucosae with secondary discharge of muco-purulent material which sticks to the external nares

The most usual cause of nasal discharge is the activity of a viral infection of the URT and of the LRT, and associated

- rhinitis
- rhino-pharyngitis

- laryngo-tracheitis
- bronchitis and broncho-pneumonia, especially if secondary bacterial infection has occurred when expectoration is more common

The most worrying conditions are bacterial or fungal in cause and are persistent, foetid, and usually unilateral discharges which do not completely respond to appropriate antimicrobial therapy. They will require extra veterinary attention for diagnosis and possible treatment.

In low-grade bilateral persistent discharge, the underlying cause is persistent post-viral pharyngitis or bacterial broncho-pneumonia, the healing/repairing phase of the inflammation, and this discharge is often spoken of as a **catarrh**.

In sub-acute or chronic conditions of the para-nasal sinuses, and guttural pouch empyema, the early production of the thick muco-purulent exudate is complicated by the anatomy of these diverticuli and especially of their relatively small orifices, which obstruct drainage.

Consequently, the pus builds up within, becomes inspissated, and may form hard lumps or chondroids which require surgical removal. The discharge may infrequently escape sufficiently to attract attention by its smell rather than its quantity. Secondary lesions develop in the cavities.

The free outward flow of serous or sero-mucoid exudate is helped by the natural action of the horse to 'eat off the ground'. The downward 'spout' of the trachea helps draw pulmonary fluid into the throat.

When he is tied up short and for long periods, during long travel, 'head down' is prevented, leading to sero-mucus stagnating at the base of the trachea and at the carina of the bronchi. There it acts as a medium for the propagation of commensal micro-organisms, usually bacterial, which under normal conditions would have been wafted or 'washed' away. The stress-related lowered resistance makes the horse particularly susceptible to these bacterial opportunists, **transit fever** may follow with pneumonia, or at least a low-grade respiratory inflammation with exercise intolerance and reduced performance, which is often protracted.

In chronic OPD there is an excess of mucoid exudate. After exercise, travel or sedation – relaxation of airway wall and dependent head posture, such mucus will more markedly appear at the nostrils and, in the second and third examples, will pool on the stable floor. In exercise, the initial respiratory difficulty and the associated cough will expectorate it, but at post-exercise feeding (on the floor) some will drain from the nostrils.

Strangles

Strangles is not a true respiratory disease; its essential characteristic signs include a **severe muco-purulent nasal discharge** and a **regional lymphadenitis**, which together with a naso-pharyngitis, interferes with swallowing and with breathing – hence the name indicative of choking or strangulation. Fever, inappetence and dullness are common. It is worthwhile describing here.

Cause

Infection by the contagious Streptococcus equi bacterium. This is a pus-producing germ with some toxin output which may circulate in both the vascular and lymphatic systems. It only affects the equidae.

Subjects

3 months to 3 years old, older depending on immunity factors, and especially immune depressant effect of some sub-clinical virus infections.

Source

Direct aerosol and direct nasal contact from carrier animals; also indirect inhalation and ingestion of fomites.

Site

The naso-pharynx, the regional lymph glands, especially the sub-mandibular.

Routes

Inhalation and/or ingestion of the germ onto the mucosa of the nose and throat and thence into the lymphatic routes.

Incubation Period

Two to three days during an outbreak. 'Second' case up to twenty days or even longer is a reflection of a 'chancy' picking up of the infection; a delayed contagion. Spread tends to speed up relative to immunity of the in-contacts.

Internal Spread

- rostrally onto nasal mucosa
- caudally into guttural pouches by airflow
- lymphatic flow with abscess formation in lymphatic glands
- vascular route, in just 2–3 days, throughout the body, both germ and toxin: subsequent regional development with secondary (usually) internal lymphadenitis is relatively slow

Diagnosis Based on Signs

The disease is a muco-purulent, fever-producing (up to 41°C/106°F) syndrome, with

- systemic involvement especially from the toxin (see later)

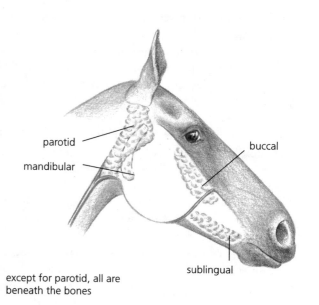

parotid
mandibular
buccal
sublingual

except for parotid, all are beneath the bones

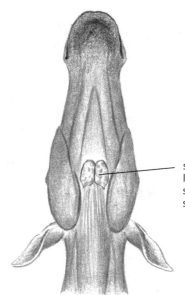

sub-mandibular lymph nodes, lying subcutaneously and so palpable

The position of salivary glands in the head.

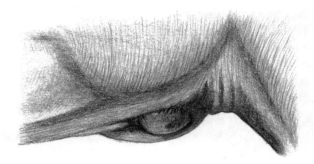

Strangles – the typical abscess under the jaw.

- inappetence; loss of smell, and so loss of 'safety' in eating which further induces inappetence
- soreness in mastication and swallowing
- obstruction and restriction to respiration
- some coughing
- depression
- **submandibular gland enlargement and abscessation**
- laboratory confirmation from germ isolation from high nasal swab and/or from pus from 'burst' gland abscess

In large studs with associated stock movements in and out, in competition yards dependent on competitors moving to communal venues, and in livery yards where movement can be at the owners' whim as well as their wish to participate outside the home territory, there is a need to identify convalescent and sub-clinical carriers. Nasopharyngeal swabbing is necessary for this. In the latter case with a percentage of clinically unaffected animals the swabbing is required to prove or disprove potential contagiousness before restrictions are lifted.

Duration
- variable usually until sub-mandibular gland suppurates and the abscess bursts or is lanced
- slow convalescence

Contagiousness
Whilst nasal and gland discharge is present. Thereafter the germ tends to 'hide' and survive; carriers arise in 50% of outbreaks, but the number of such animals in any one herd is unknown.

Most carriers harbour the germ not only in the lymphoid tissues but mainly in the guttural pouches. They are difficult to detect as the germ in the guttural pouches may **not** produce clinical signs of empyema, or will 'remain behind', after that has 'cleared up', in the chondroids.

Convalescent and later throat swabs are often annoyingly and surprisingly negative but hidden germs do escape at some time; the animal becomes a 'shedder'.

It is not yet known why some animals become carriers and whether they are persistent shedders of the germ or only under certain conditions.

In practice it is advisable, when an outbreak is suspected
- to consult a veterinary surgeon, especially re antibiotic treatment **or not**, and whether
- to isolate the yard
- to control staff movement
- to let the disease spread within the yard (arguable)
- not to contaminate grazing, where practicable
- to return to work carefully
- not to remove isolation for at least 4 weeks after last case's signs, the discharges, **have cleared**

Prognosis
- good in most cases if well nursed
- systemic spread of the germ via the blood (*most likely to follow incorrect antibiotic treatment*) will produce superficial and internal abscess formation; the latter potentially lethal
- beware purpura haemorrhagica in 3–8 weeks after start and convalescence of any case

Purpura Haemorrhagica
An anaphylactic reaction to the (toxins) of a Streptococcal infection. Fifty per cent of cases have a fatal outcome
- strangles
- secondary to a viral infection
- wound contamination with 'cellulitis'

In some cases there has been no perceivable morbidity.

Signs
Two weeks post recovery
- acute lesions
  - oedema of nostrils spreading to the whole head with
  - respiratory difficulty
  - dysphagia

- oedema of limbs – especially of hinds which 'fill' upwards with proximal demarcation, a 'bottle' leg
- oedematous plaques on body

all cool and painless, but some exude serum which crusts

- hyper-acute lesions
  - Petechial haemorrhages (echymotic in size) on
    - nasal, lip and tongue mucosae
    - conjunctivae, and with
    - blood-stained tears
  - anaemia
  - accelerated heart rate
  - temperature normal unless secondary germs become (re)active
  - dyspnoea from pulmonary oedema
  - serous nasal discharge
  - colic from gut oedema and subsequent wall necrosis

The other acute lesions will also be present.

Epistaxis

There are four types of bleeding from the various areas of the respiratory tract, the blood appearing at the nostrils as a nose-bleed

- trauma, in area 1
- ethmoidal haematomata, in area 2
- guttural pouch mycotic infection, also area 2
- exercise-induced pulmonary haemorrhage (EIPH), area 4

The first three are *not* associated with exercise *per se*.

Trauma

- usually at the rostral flexible cartilage end, the external nares
- occasionally from traumatised sinuses or turbinates
- polyps developing from inflammatory ulcers in the nasal passages or the sinuses, which have become eroded by sneezing
- other acute to chronic inflammatory reactions from primary and secondary infections which ulcerate the mucosa (and erode sub-mucosal blood vessels)

Ethmoidal haematomata

- idiopathic, progressive non-contagious, friable neoplastic thrombus in the ethmoidal region. The

bleeding is intermittent, rarely profuse and not associated with exercise; unilateral. Similar lesions are seen rostrally down the nasal passages. Rarely fatal but anaemia possible. Irritative to respiration. Surgery, where practicable, is 'curative'; relapses are possible

Guttural pouch mycotic infection

- guttural pouch mycosis with ulceration

Exercise-induced pulmonary haemorrhage (EIPH)

For over 200 years, horsemen have recognised epistaxis during or soon after performance work and in a (high) percentage of athletically exerted horses. This bleeding was usually

- bilateral during a race, and severe, with interruption of the fast gaits, to mild, with arguable effect on performance, or
- uni- or bilateral after a race, especially seen when the head and neck were lowered

With the advent of the **endoscope**, and especially the flexible fibre-optic models, used one hour or so after a race, it became appreciated that it is more conclusive to carry out this examination the following day if the first was negative

- blood could be seen in the trachea, suggesting that other blood had fluxed to the throat and been swallowed, or there was not sufficient to reach as 'high' as that so soon
- blood pigment could be seen in the trachea for several days after exertion, confirming that some bleeding had occurred

More recent research includes the use of radio-active red blood cells re-injected and their escape route from pulmonary blood vessels monitored by **scintigraphy**.

Three important conclusions were drawn from these findings

- many more horses bled sub-clinically than were seen as 'bleeders'
- in flat racing, most horses bled at least once in their career and many more than once
- the blood was coming from the lungs
- bleeding occurred only during fast work

The original research work suggested that this condition was exercise-associated pulmonary haemorrhage.

It is now accepted that it is indeed **exercise-induced pulmonary haemorrhage**, EIPH, and as such is related to speeds greater than 240m/min over a distances of more than 400m and their demands for oxygen (air), and so to near maximal respiratory and cardiac rates and flow volumes.

Type of Horse – Susceptibility

- Thoroughbred – racing, advanced eventing
- Standard bred – trotting/pacer racing
- Quarter horse – racing
- Thoroughbred-X-pony – advanced eventing
- Arab horses – racing

The 'trend' increases with age. It has not been reported in endurance horses.

There is **no** relationship with gender (geldings 'seem' to be affected more than mares and stallions), geography, climate, weather or 'going.'

Nor is there much substantiated evidence of coincidental acute or chronic diseases earlier established despite, as previously mentioned, the widespread herpes virus primary infection at some earlier time and subsequent 'flare ups'.

The bleeding is self-limiting, therefore non-lethal.

Associated morbidity, i.e. directly related to post bleeding tissue reactions: autopsy of confirmed bleeders (usually put down for other reasons) reveals

- bronchiolitis, but with variable inflammatory mucus: if this is absent rather rules out inflammation, or if present may suggest previous LRT primary viral, bacterial or fungal infection
- does not confirm any significant OPD findings
- the bleeding is from the pulmonary capillary system to the alveolar wall cells, and so into the airway
- it occurs invariably in the dorsal caudal area of the lung
- repeat bleeders do so from progressively more cranial (anterior), but always dorsal, areas. The capillaries in the originally affected (posterior) area become thrombosed and so cannot bleed again and the associated alveoli become atrophied and occluded with fibrosis

The condition is thought to be a dynamic stress, an internal trauma compression – a sports injury!

Epistaxis is better described as a 'dis-ease', and not as a 'disease'. In respiration, there is an ongoing rise and fall in

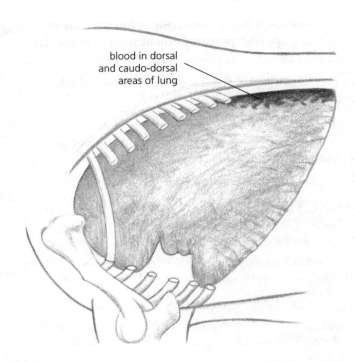

blood in dorsal and caudo-dorsal areas of lung

Exercise-induced pulmonary haemorrhage (EIPH).

intra-pleural, intra-airway and intra-capillary pressures. These increase in degree and in frequency with exerting exercise. The changes tend to produce greater across-the-lung pressure swings in the dorso-caudal regions of the lung. The greater the expansion of the respiratory bronchioles, the greater the risk of stress failure of the microscopic adjacent capillary walls already stressed by the associated high blood pressure of exercise.

The significance of the pressure changes being greatest in this anatomical area is perhaps explained by the caudal lung being between spine and antero-dorsal diaphragm, which in turn is pressurised by the return weight of the abdominal contents as the hindquarters swing downwards out of suspension in the asymmetric gait.

It is predisposed to by thoracic wall conformation, the dynamics of Thoroughbred galloping – on the forehand. Some recent work has extended the causal hypothesis of local compression discussed in the above paragraph to the coincidental effect of ground force reactions, especially from the forehand, on the chest through the scapular sling, and the cardiovascular and respiratory systems' need to meet the increased necessary gaseous exchange for the muscle metabolism at speed.

There is no satisfactory treatment. Prevention, if it can be called this, is management.

Some horses will not bleed again if raced within a week of the first episode without an intermediate gallop. They will, of course, be likely to do so in the future; perhaps it takes several build-ups of stress before rupture occurs.

There is no need for attempted first-aid treatment or subsequent special management of an actual epistaxis case. Other causes of epistaxis which are not exercise related or induced should be differentially diagnosed; treatment is essential for some of these.

FUNCTIONAL TYPES OF DIS-EASE

In domesticated circumstances the horse suffers from a wider variety of neuro-muscular functional dis-eases in the throat area than any other domesticated animal. Colloquially, the names used describe the signs rather than the underlying morbidity. As common currency they are gurgling, choking up, tongue swallowing, and whistling and roaring.

The first three are functional disorders which are not always distinct entities

- 'gurgling' is the descriptive short-lasting **noise** produced when the soft palate is displaced dorsally (DDSP)

- 'choking up' is the end result, a state, in which the horse is temporarily **deprived of air**

- 'tongue swallowing' is the associated displacement of the base of the tongue. (It is now thought that the physiological swallowing of saliva during work which naturally involves a lifting of the tongue does not induce DDSP.) This releases the cuff-like grip on the glottis whereby the distal, flexible soft palate 'flutters' or gurgles in the air flow which is markedly impeded. The soft palate and other musculature of the pharynx may be pathologically weakened from a direct viral megopathy or from related neuropathy induced in the guttural pouch or from focal fatigue. The resultant loss of tone allows the soft palate to dislocate. A horse affected with RLN (see below) may be so obstructed in airflow that the suction pressure adversely pulls on the pharyngeal walls and floor with consequent DDSP

These three are inter-related. They occur at or near the limits of exercise stress; they quickly resolve when exercise ceases. They do not regularly recur.

The excitement of racing and other fast and/or strongly contained or restrained work, and the variable influence of interference by the rider will induce them – in comparison to 'loose head', non-competitive speeds, which will not.

Gurgling, choking-up and tongue swallowing are so closely related functionally that they are often considered as mere variations in nomenclature to describe a composite state.

From drawings, the Greek pony, for example, was conformationally 'thick' throated and apparently over-bent. In modern horses such conformation, if rider induced and especially if congenitally present as well, can so alter the air flow that turbulence, with airway obstruction and noise at increased speeds, will occur. If there is an existing tendency to 'choke up' that is more likely to be exhibited. If there is an underlying laryngeal paresis the whistle/roar will be exaggerated.

- 'whistling and roaring' arise from a functional disorder of the glottis, due to a degenerative atrophy (structural change) of the left, recurrent laryngeal nerve which motivates the left arytenoid muscles to open and close one side of the glottis. The muscles progressively atrophy

Idiopathic Laryngeal Hemiplegia

The inspiratory abnormal noises of whistling and roaring are a sign of a disease called **idiopathic laryngeal hemiplegia (ILH)** or, as it is now more correctly called, **recurrent laryngeal neuropathy (RLN)**, a one-sided, invariably left, weakness of the activating muscles of the glottis due to the degenerating left recurrent laryngeal nerve, a branch of the vagus, cranial nerve X. This nerve, because it travels down the neck, round the aorta and back up the neck to the larynx, is a long nerve. It is relatively longer in horses over 16.2 hh, with conformationally elongated necks.

The dis-ease, arising from an 'inner' degeneration and not from an 'outside' influence in the first instance, has been recognised or at least recorded for 200 years, in the United Kingdom certainly since the Arabian stallions' influence.

It is still unknown in ponies and small cross-breds. It is more common in Thoroughbred and pure-bred horses, being apparently more so in geldings. In Thoroughbreds and Clydesdales at least there is a familial incidence: it is hereditable.

The underlying morbidity is a selective motor nerve fibre degeneration progressing from the muscle back to the nerve's branching from the parent vagus nerve. The muscles affected are first the glottis adductors and then the

Recurrent laryngeal neuropathy (RLN).

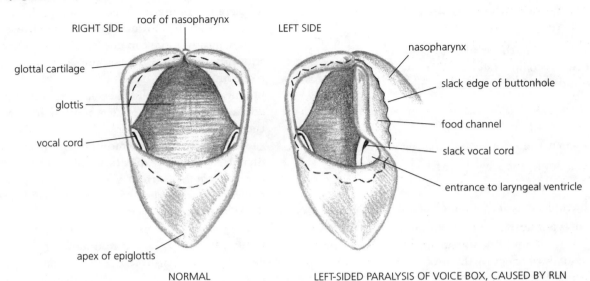

RIGHT SIDE   roof of nasopharynx   LEFT SIDE

glottal cartilage

glottis

vocal cord

nasopharynx

slack edge of buttonhole

food channel

slack vocal cord

entrance to laryngeal ventricle

apex of epiglottis

NORMAL   LEFT-SIDED PARALYSIS OF VOICE BOX, CAUSED BY RLN

abductors. The cause is unknown. Some investigators have shown that **30% of all horses** show some degenerative changes. Only those which fail to produce a regeneration become clinically paretic and potentially **'gone in the wind'**.

The pathological state can be recognised in the ages from six months upwards and endoscopic evidence of a slight tremor of the left cartilage is just recognisable, but the clinical disease of 'noise' and exercise intolerance may not develop for some time after that finding and then only with the requirement of a fully open larynx for strenuous exercise.

If the condition has not become clinical by the time the horse is 6 years old it is unlikely to do so later in life. Once developed, it may be progressive – whistler to roarer. It is suggested that an inter-current viral infection may trigger a subclinical to become clinical or to worsen. Since most horses are virally infected at some time this association requires further explanation.

The dis-ease is a permanent dysfunction of certain intrinsic muscles of the larynx and is not responsive to medicinal therapy. Surgery aims to mechanically overcome the loss of patency of the glottis.

Signs

The signs are the consequence of a failure to move the glottis widely open, and to maintain this maximal laryngeal diameter, for and during the period of increased air intake during strenuous exercise. The degree of failure varies with the animal's fitness and the degree of paresis.

The clinical effect is adventitious inspiratory noise from associated turbulence, possible insufficient air intake and so difficulty in maintaining or even attaining exercise potential.

The larynx is graded thus

Grade 1 – negative

• no clinical noise or exercise intolerance

• no visual (endoscopic) abnormality

• glottis opens and closes symmetrically on stimulation by instrument touch and by inference when stimulated by exercise need to do so

Grade 2

• no clinical noise or exercise intolerance – sub-clinical

• a visual 'flutter' of the left arytenoid cartilage

• glottis opens and closes symmetrically

Grade 3

• possibly a noise on exercise – early clinical

• a visually imperfect or reduced left-side opening and closing, a paresis, but artificial closure of the nostrils will induce a transient full opening at the subsequent 'forced' inspiration

Grade 4

• noise – clinical

- possibly some reduced exercise tolerance
- visually left full abduction is impossible
- adduction, which is the first movement to show paresis, is also marked in this grade; closure – for swallowing defence – is compensated for by movement of the right arytenoid over mid-line in an attempt to co-apt with the left

Grade 5

- noise – may well be a distinct roaring – clinical
- exercise intolerance may be marked
- visually no abduction or adduction
- true hemiplegia (paralysis of left side)
- if horse is put into forced inspiration the left side is 'sucked' across mid-line to narrow the glottis further (as on manually obstructing the nostrils with an endoscope in place)

The owner and the veterinary clinician are, in the first instance, attracted to a horse which makes an inspiratory noise at exercise. It must be appreciated that not all whistlers or roarers are so affected in the larynx, although some 90% are. There are other lesions between the nostrils and the caudal trachea which will create a turbulence and produce a noise.

The dynamic changes related to the inspiratory noise of a horse 'gone in the wind' can only be seen in action when the larynx is viewed through an endoscope. The normal resting horse's laryngeal rostral opening varies between

- fully closed, which it effects if touched by the endoscope when it reflexly closes for 'suspected' swallowing
- partially open, which symmetrical position it maintains for most of the time for the two-way passage of air

The flow rate and volume is minimal, laminar and inspiratorily soundless as heard when standing near by. Behind the vocal cords there is a lateral hollow or ventricle. Air obviously tracts into these but the laminar flow, although slightly disturbed, does not become so turbulent as to invoke a clinical noise.

In the unaffected larynx when the horse is inspiring air at a rate and volume to meet exercise requirements the vocal folds are pulled outwards and backwards to maximise the glottal aperture to equal the fixed diameter of the larynx body. Coincidentally the ventricles are folded over and effectively flattened: there are no hollows and so no noise. *At speed the normal horse produces an expiratory noise.*

In an affected horse at rest there is usually no need for accelerated inspiration. Depending on the dis-ease grade, and so the ability or otherwise to abduct the left side of the glottis, a turbulence can ensue. Only in severe paresis will this turbulence be audible at rest.

During exercise demands, a marked turbulence can produce not only a clinical noise but one which indicates difficulty in obtaining sufficient air; a 'roar' which typifies the severe mal-function.

An affected horse moving at speed produces an *increased normal expiratory* noise. This alternates with the *abnormal inspiratory* sound which, particularly, if a roar, together produce the biphasic sound reminiscent of wood being sawn.

In less affected horses a less audible, differently pitched noise is made. This is a resonance in the inspired air's greater flow passing over, not now a non-existent hollow as in the normal horse but a continuously present ventricle since the vocal fold has not been abducted.

The whistle is likened to the noise produced by a human blowing across the top of an empty narrow-topped bottle. The amount of turbulence, and so the obstruction to airflow, is not thought to be great *per se*. The effect of incomplete abduction on airflow, however, varies with

- air (oxygen) demand – and so more air, more quickly, at fast work
- the degree of restriction consequent upon the paresis

Thus, a Grade 4 is more likely to produce a more audible whistle at a slower rate of work than a Grade 3, whereas a Grade 5, in which the aperture is less than half because of the 'suck' effect drawing the paralysed left side beyond mid-line, will cause a roar quickly and at slower gaits even at rest.

An unresolved, important supplementary question relates to prolonged sub-optimal air intake on the onset of aerobic fatigue.

It is important to remember that roaring, more so than whistling, can be the result of other pathologic changes in areas one and two of the URT when severe turbulence is produced.

In area 1, the noise is usually persistent, varying with air rate since the obstruction is permanent – such as a tumour.

In area 2, whilst such neoplastic lesions may also be found, most of the problem is functional – as in soft palate and pharyngeal paresis and therefore often intermittent

There are other tests for external aid to diagnosis

- 'grunting to the stick' – the horse tries to hold the

glottis closed against the threat of being hit but fails to hold it shut. Air escapes as a grunt

- the slap test –this depends upon a loss of reflex arc because of the left recurrent nerve degeneration. The slap stimulus behind the right withers fails to complete the spinal arc circuit to the left laryngeal muscles. The ability to close the glottis by sharp snap action, which is palpable, is lost

Endoscopy is the only accurate means of determining

- the presence of laryngeal hemiplegia
- if the horse has been operated on for this condition
- if there are other lesions in the URT

Research is underway to estimate more accurately the detriment to airway flow by such partial obstruction. Some is based on the premise that inspiratory obstruction will alter the pressures necessary to overcome this. There will be a greater diaphragmatic pressure on the abdominal contents and so there will be an increased abdominal pressure measurable through a gauge inserted in the rectum.

Laboratory measurements of airflow have produced a table for 'obstruction or not' levels, and these have been graphed along with the rectal measurements. In practice, it is hoped that the easily recorded rectal measurements can be simply extrapolated to show obstruction 'yes', 'no' or in between and perhaps if surgery is necessary.

There is a school of equine specialist thought that believes many 'whistlers' do not benefit from surgery. Apart from the embarrassment of having the whistle readily pointed out by friends, the noise *per se* is not thought to be detrimental to the horse and the underlying morbidity likely to be exercise-tolerance-reducing only in a significantly small percentage of cases.

Surgery does not make the glottis work; it aims to keep it permanently open, which has its own disadvantages.

THE SURGICAL CORRECTIVE TECHNIQUES

Ventriculectomy – the Hobday operation – was first performed in Germany in the 1850s. An American veterinary surgeon refined the technique and brought it to the United Kingdom in 1900 or thereabouts, when Professor Hobday further 'improved' the technique by reducing the size of the laryngeal incision.

Although thousands of whistler/roarers, and even potential cases, have been 'Hobdayed' with supposedly beneficial effect – the noise reduces or ceases – there is much argument as mentioned earlier as to the functional benefit. In simple terms

- the larynx is opened by an incision underneath
- a burr is introduced to the ventricle (the right side is 'done', as well as the affected left)
- the mucous membrane lining is caught up and stripped off this cavity
- consequent wound contraction and adhesions in the ventricle draws the vocal fold (cord) and the arytenoid cartilage away from the mid-line
- the ventricle is ablated
- the glottis is expected to stay abducted (open)

This is not permanent and relapses are possible after one to two years or more. (With some operators the vocal fold is cut out completely.)

Abductor prosthesis operation (prosthetic laryngoplasty) – 'tie back' (A prosthesis is an artificially implanted material to replace a damaged or inactive part of the body.)

As the non-scientific name for this operation implies, it is the pulling back of the arytenoid cartilage of the larynx and the attached vocal fold, which cannot be naturally effected because of the paresis or paralysis of the usual muscles.

The 'tie' is a slightly elasticated man-made fibre, or even metal wire. Unlike the normal autonomic muscular action, it cannot relax to allow the side of the glottis to resume its normal resting respiratory position, let alone adduct to perform its role in the reflex safety closure of the larynx. The extent of the artificial opening is approximated to about half way, and hopefully is maintained permanently.

The operation was devised in 1970 by an American veterinary surgeon, Dr Marks who, like many other surgeons in different countries, was dissatisfied with the results of the Hobday operation. Today it is used in association with a unilateral 'Hobday'. Ironically, the 'Hobday' on its own still left the larynx with what adduction power remained relative to the grade of the nerve degeneration. The price for improved airway especially by the 'tie back' method was the variable interference with swallowing protection, the potential result of which was the need for greater and more frequent use of the cough defence.

We are still left with the problems, of not only estimating whether the horse requires surgery, but also determining if the result of surgery has been worthwhile.

The 'proof of the pudding' should not just be noise amelioration but a practical and reasonably accurate way of assessing improved performance – not an easy exercise, but, for example

- time to complete a set distance, as compared with pre-op performance
- ability to 'go a distance', i.e. stamina
- ability in speed and duration, compared with other horses which were better than it pre-op

All these are potentially variable *vis à vis* fitness.

The above-mentioned rectal pressure parameters, once fully evaluated outside research environments, would go far in answering the two basic problems. One authority is of the opinion that the first problem is answerable by endoscopy.

- Grade 4 probably to be considered for surgery
- Grade 5, certainly so

In both, there should should be no doubt that the visual findings would equate with persistently poor athleticism and that successful surgery should improve this. In both groups the noise would be a serious whistle or a roar, in which obstruction to airflow was definitely present.

The athletic disciplines involved would, of course, be taken into the original reckoning. Fast work and slower distance work are the most likely to be affected. The explosive anaerobic work of the show jumper is less likely. A roarer in any discipline must be under some distress and aesthetically would be seen to be so by spectators.

Soft palate paresis (from the Greek *paresis*, 'slackening') is a state of slight and/or temporary paralysis of the mobile floor of the naso-pharynx, whereby the flaccid tissue cannot be held down in place but gets sucked up into the airflow and taken above the glottis. In this position it 'flutters in the breeze'. Such related obstruction can be exacerbated if the pharynx is likewise weak, when the roof of the throat is sucked down to further obstruct the airflow. The horse 'gurgles' or 'chokes up'. Such weakness and flaccidity may be due to

- post-viral temporary neuritis and myositis
- simple muscle fatigue – unfitness
- a **mycotic condition of the guttural pouch** can erode onto the underlying cranial autonomic motor nerves

and induce a neuropathic true paralysis of the throat muscles. The effect is mainly on swallowing ability

It is said that some horses repeatedly affected with this gurgle at hard work have a too-long soft palate – which wrinkles sufficiently to become, paradoxically, easily sucked over the epiglottis. It is difficult to decide if this is the case, even on endoscopy.

Surgical shortening of the soft palate has been done with variable success. Hot laser surgical 'tightening' of the soft palate is a recent innovation. A similar method is used to ablate the ventricle on the paretic side in cases of RLN.

There is a specific group of disorders

- the horse that is evading the bit will often pull its tongue back (voluntarily or involuntarily) to get it over and onto the bit, and will likewise dislocate the soft palate
- in extreme poll flexion, the root of the tongue tends to bunch up, pushing the palate into the naso-pharynx with audible obstruction
- open-mouthed galloping horses run the risk of pharyngeal obstruction if inspired air escapes back from the throat under the soft palate to billow that up into the naso-pharynx, with severe gurgling and airway embarrassment
- where RLN (recurrent laryngeal neuropathy) is present there is stress on the pharyngeal musculature to overcome the altered aerodynamics. This can lead to pharyngeal and palatal fatigue weakness and subsequent gurgling
- a galloping horse, pulling hard, can disturb the balance between the pull of the neck strap muscles and the hyoid bone's rostral attachments. The strap muscles 'win', and the larynx is pulled back out of the cuff – releasing the palate into the airflow. It too is said to have **swallowed its tongue**

All such palate-involved conditions are collectively known as **dorsal displacement of the soft palate (DDSP)**. Importantly, even quick use of an endoscope in a gurgler immediately after exercise will not 'visualise' these structural displacements; they will have returned to normal when the 'pressure is off'.

Laryngeal and other pharyngeal loss of functioning is now being visualised by installing an endoscope in a suspected case which is exercised on a treadmill thereby inducing the physical factors associated with exercise.

There is a possibility that dental abnormalities making

the feel of the bit uncomfortable, or from excess saliva production as the horse tries to work the tongue free of mechanical irritation and pain, will induce DDSP.

There are two further conditions which not only impede airflow but induce noise on inspiration and even increased noise on expiration

- epiglottic entrapment. A fold of the mucous membrane from under the epiglottis is 'engaged' by that organ
- palato-pharyngeal arch entrapment. A fold of its mucous membrane engages the dorsal rim of the glottis

In both cases the glottal opening is restricted.

In addition, abnormal noise and possible airway deficit may occur in

- the over-fat horse, adipose pressure on the airway
- pressure from adjacent enlarged lymph glands
- pharyngeal (surface) lymphoid hyperplasia (**PLH**), is suspected of being detrimental
- tumours of the larynx, and congenital cyst formation under the epiglottic mucous membrane

It is presumed that all these disturbances are at least related to domestication and its effect through

- breeding and associated conformation and functioning weaknesses
- incorrect fittening
- incorrect using
- intercurrent infections and/or their legacy
- dental abnormalities' effect on bit acceptance

It will be seen that the least anatomically protected area is that known as the **throat** and the **windpipe**. Colloquially, 'going for the throat' is an aggressor's target for a quick kill by asphyxiation.

Although a safe supply route for constant air is vital, other essential life functions must be accommodated in conjunction with respiration's primary demands.

The throat and windpipe could have been encircled by bone, as is the neural canal of the central nervous system. However, such a cage would have represented

- a massive increase in bone weight, and would have necessitated a
- system of articulations additional to those of the skull and the spinal column, to permit the

- postural changes for, especially
  - grazing and browsing
  - sensory input and communicative output
  - self grooming
- 'local' changes for
  - deglutition (swallowing)

A compromise, not uncommon in nature, was reached as already described: the throat and windpipe is 'roofed over' and 'walled', in part at least, by extrinsic muscle.

In any aerodynamic situation, and especially in the 'to and fro' type, 'escape' facilities for changing pressures are necessary. Such valves need not be physical openings but merely functional 'give and take' areas. The throat is such an ideal area; it is 'mobile and flexible' due to its autonomic muscular components and its elastic connective tissue membranes, e.g. the guttural pouches.

This muscle complex, including that which activates the variable dimensions of the glottis, is adversely susceptible to internally produced

- paresis, as already detailed, and from
  - fatigue
  - possible metabolic influences
  - viral inflammation
- mucosal inflammation from
  - fungal
  - acute and subacute bacterial infection

with consequential effect on tissue functioning.

Any morbid influences which diminish the 'tone' of these autonomic muscles, and so allows them to become

- flaccid, weak, and unable to
  - withstand negative air pressure, and so be sucked out of position, or
  - controllably 'give' to positive pressure, and so create an obstruction to airflow, or
- paralysed (partially or completely through nerve atrophy), and so be unable, as in unilateral laryngeal paresis, to
  - close the glottis or, more, importantly
  - open the glottis fully

will be detrimental to a clear airflow. In addition, the functional changes and the associated turbulence will tend to produce abnormal respiratory noise.

Apart from the occasional bite or kick, traumatic

damage is rare. The initial inflammatory reaction can be serious but will subside. A crushed larynx is even more rare but is invariably fatal. Physical damage to the windpipe usually leaves a permanent variably obstructive scar.

Direct **functional** defects in the throat are not uncommon. They occur most frequently in the horse which is athletically challenged and/or posturally challenged by congenital poor throat angulation or discipline-induced 'wrong' throat angulation. The signs of their presence are

- adventitious noise
- interference with athletic ability which will become more noticeable with
    - faster work
    - post exercise, 'recovery' respirations

Conversely, the respiratory embarrassment during fast work – and asymmetric gait synchronisation – may be such as to bring locomotion to a slower gait or even to a halt, at which time

- the airflow rate and volume becomes no longer turbulent – the stress is relieved
- the displaced tissues are able to be re-aligned by reflex swallowing, whereby their obstructive interference ceases

Within the overall disease types, the respiratory system can be described as being affected by **structural** abnormality, or **functional** abnormality, or a combination of these in the

- upper respiratory tract – the ear, nose and throat, **ENT**, and the tracheal areas
- lower respiratory tract – the lungs and the pleura, **chest**, areas

and, in both situations, further qualified as being due to **inflammatory** changes or **non-inflammatory** changes to produce either

- a primarily coughing horse, with variable other respiratory clues, or
- a primarily respiratorily embarrassed horse, with variable coughing

At any stage in the disease progress, there will be altered patterns to meet the required air intake and output, by breathing **more slowly but more deeply**, or breathing **faster but more shallowly**.

The horse will involuntarily make these changes and

likewise change his activity, even to the extent of 'standing still and fighting for air' in extreme cases of, for example, pleuro-pneumonia.

The overall effect of respiratory disease is that of obstruction to the flow in one or other or in both directions, because of structural changes in the channel's *shape*, *diameter*, *and tone*.

These changes will compromise

- flow volume and rate
- gaseous exchange
- muco-ciliary escalator and other primary defences

and will coincidentally produce

- respiratory embarrassment
- adventitious noises

It has been stated that morbidity of the airway primarily affects the system's

- shape – as from abnormal 'angulation' (the resultant air turbulence is itself obstructive)
- diameter – a narrowing of the lumen – an obstructing effect
- smooth muscle tone, either a flaccidity, especially in the throat area (2) and as such a mechanical obstruction, or a rigidity in the 'bronchial tree' tissues from inflammation leading to an increased compliance pressure

FACTORS INFLUENCING AIRWAY RESISTANCE (AR) AND FLOW RATE (FR)

- mucosal congestion and oedema – thickening
- plugging of channel lumen, especially bronchioles, by mucus and exudates
- constriction of bronchial smooth muscle
- collapse and kinking of bronchioles due to loss of normal 'pull' of alveolar elastic fibres on their wall or to a loss of structural supporting tissues of bronchial wall as in pneumonitis
- thickening of bronchiolar walls causing compression
- cohesion of mucosal surfaces from surface tension failure

All these are the result of inflammatory or allergic reactions.

Bronchial obstruction.

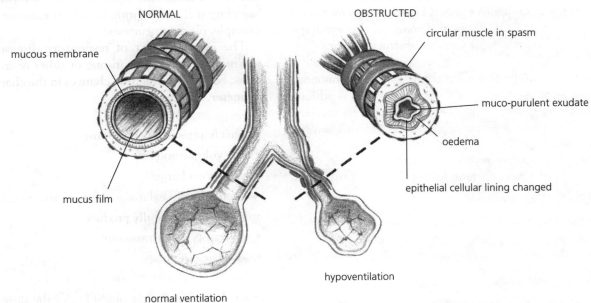

NORMAL

mucous membrane

mucus film

normal ventilation

OBSTRUCTED

circular muscle in spasm

muco-purulent exudate

oedema

epithelial cellular lining changed

hypoventilation

When compliance rigidity increases there is a consequent reduction in the air volume which can be respired.

The effort required to regain this compensatorily by deeper breathing is energy-expensive and self-limiting; it is more effective to compensate by increasing the flow rate – there is then shallow but fast respiration, as in the pneumonias.

With lumen obstruction, and therefore morbid interferences with flow rate, the autonomic response is for the horse to make use of the unaffected elasticity, that is deeper but slow respiration as in 'asthma' and COPD.

Difficulties increase dramatically when both compliance and obstruction are involved. There is also interference with thermo regulation, and to a lesser extent, sense of smell and phonation – communication.

In human medicine, dyspnoea is reserved for the emotional effect of 'difficulty of getting air', as in acute asthma; the patient compounds the effects of the morbidity by becoming nervous and 'uptight'. In equine medicine, the definition has been amended to suggest a physical disability displayed by the horse as

* exaggerated respirations not associated with exercise
* often accompanied by non-normal noise, and
* especially, if variably, interfering with exercise tolerance

Colloquially, non-contagious respiratory disease is often spoken of as

* 'broken wind' as in allergic OPD – some coughing, or
* 'gone in the wind' as in functionally obstructive conditions in the pharyngeal-laryngeal areas of the channel

Both are related usually to individual animals; an outbreak or spread is not likely but is not impossible in the former – several allergic horses being simultaneously exposed to inspiration of allergens.

When the signs of **contagious inflammatory** dis-ease start – a cough and/or other respiratory inflammatory clues – the day-to-day inferences are

* in a training yard of young horses – *'We've got the virus'* meaning that a herpes strain (1 or 4) of virus is active – and contagious

It is now believed that in some instances 'having the virus' is more accurately described as having a mycoplasma or other exotic types of bacterial infection primarily or more usually secondarily to a herpes infection.

* in a less elite situation, with older horses – *'We've got the cough'* meaning that one of the several types of virus has become active and that it too could 'spread' to non-immune animals

In the former situation, the trainer would know that

- not all horses are naturally actively immune
- those that were, could 'break down', and that
- both would be susceptible to a fresh intake of virus from new purchases – and *vice versa*

He is faced with the probability of
- laying off work
- turning out where feasible
- nursing sick animals
- using antibiotics for secondary bacterial infection particularly if identified, under veterinary control
- a slow, well-monitored return to work

He would be pleased to learn that there is a new vaccine against Herpes 1 and 4 which would at least help to prevent the breakdown of immunity, which is the main problem in this infection.

In the second situation, the owner/trainer would know
- that in most horses the cough would be the predominant sign, sometimes the only clinical one
- temperature-taking could forecast a new case or monitor an existing case which had become complicated by secondary bacterial infection, in which there would be other respiratory disease signs
- that there was no medicinal 'cure' for the viral infection
- that he must not return the horse to work until coughing had ceased (there are exceptions, for which veterinary advice is necessary)
- that, in general, a patient is no longer 'infectious' (i.e. contagious) after four days of coughing even though the coughing continues (herpes infection is a potential exception)

The signs which will direct the horsemaster to 'something wrong, and *possibly* respiratory' will vary with type of horse, age, use, fitness, immune status, as well as with the type of disease.
The basic signs of respiratory disease in general are
- **increased respiratory rate**, and/or
- **increased 'depth' of breathing**

as compared with the resting normal and with changes associated with excitement and work
- **coughing**
- **temperature** and **heart-rate** changes
- **nasal discharge**, possibly **sneezing**
- alteration in **sound**, as 'externally' heard

- **exercise intolerance**

These will vary with the acuteness of the infection, the severity of the infection, and the presence of systemic illness, especially when secondary bacterial complications follow.

DISEASE TYPES

Developmental

- 'wry face' – usually so marked at birth as to necessitate euthanasia
- cleft palate – really a digestive system disorder, but may lead to aspiration pneumonia, and will almost certainly be associated with secondary bacterial rhinitis and a nasal discharge
- cyst formation, especially in the nares, nasal passages, and in the mucosa of the soft palate adjacent to the epiglottis
- narrowing of naso-pharynx opening

By definition such animals exhibit these defects at an early age.

Inflammatory – Traumatic

Primarily Not Infected
By definition the following are the anatomical areas exposed to external trauma
- **nasal** region
  - laceration of external nares and underlying cartilage. The disfiguration and/or subsequent scarring may prevent dilation
  - external trauma, nosebleed (epistaxis)
- **facial** region
  - severe bruising
    - bleeding is usually confined to trauma to the soft areas, but the turbinates etc. are also fragile
    - some clotting may temporarily block one nasal passage
    - bone fractures are rare, but immediate disfigurement will interfere with breathing

- **throat** region
  - kicks
  - bites

    Both can even without deep penetration damage laryngeal cartilage, and subsequent bruising with oedema may interfere with breathing

    Penetrating wounds into the respiratory mucosa are prone to secondary infection with spread into the guttural pouches and into the LRT

- **tracheal** region
  - as for throat; if cartilaginous rings are disrupted, a semi-obstructive scarring with turbulent 'noise' and reduced airflow are possible sequels

- blow to the **chest wall** region
  - fracture of rib(s) and sternum – risk of lung penetration. Pain restricts breathing
  - open and penetrating wounds
    - risk as above
    - risk of pneumothorax
    - risk of lung collapse
    - risk of bilateral lung collapse – death
    - pleural abscesses if non-fatal

Secondarily Infected

- bacterial (and fungal) invasion from penetrating traumas – most will show as a nasal discharge, but there will be variable signs of airway obstruction
- commensal opportunists 'on the back' of primary viral infections

It is accepted that domestication has played a significant role in the prevalence of contagious respiratory disease

- housing
  - poor ventilation
  - high humidity associated with damp bedding
- nutrition
  - spores from mouldy hay fed from nets in underventilated boxes causing COPD and invasion of the LRT alveoli with allergic responses
- movement
  - young horses from studs to yards

- communal events: racing, hunting, and other competitions
- travel
  - stress
  - incorrect positioning of head to allow tracheal drainage

Primarily Infected

- bacterial and fungal – strangles; sinusitis; rhinitis; guttural pouch infection; other respiratory bacteria
- viral – influenza; herpes 1 & 4; EVA (equine viral arteritis); EIA (equine infectious anaemia – rare in the UK); the 'cold' viruses
- parasitic – lungworm; ascarid migrating larvae (in the foal); bot larvae migration through pharyngeal tissues

Allergies

- (C)OPD
- summer grass associated OPD
- hay cough

Metabolic

Of little practical importance; when there are homeostatic defects in the body fluids, gaseous exchange may be defective, but this is more likely at the site of systemic tissue gaseous exchange.

Fatigue may affect pharyngeal musculature and possibly the respiratory muscles.

Degenerative

- mainly related to nerve degeneration and, as such, causes an interference with pharyngeal tone and laryngeal opening
- associated with thoracic pressure induced hypoxia of the alveolar walls following EIPH and subsequent fibrosis
- post inflammatory cellular replacement by non-specific, non-functional tissue – amyloid degeneration

Neoplastic

- URT – cancers with lymphatic spread and bone distortion; nasal polyps (both of these are usually associated with a prior ulcerative inflammation); ethmoidal and other haematomas

- LRT – lympho-sarcomatous metastises; other rare types, such as pulmonary osteodystrophy (Maries disease). All will produce a chronic cough and 'make a noise' on respiration. Most will have signs from lesions elsewhere on the body

INFLAMMATORY CONDITIONS OF THE ANATOMICAL SITES

Upper Respiratory Tract

Areas 1–2

Rhinitis

Inflammation of the nasal passages (under the mucosa of the nasal passages there is a wealth of lymphoid tissue which is strongly defensive) from

- primary bacterial infections, e.g. strangles
- primary viral infections
  - the 'common cold' viruses
  - extension from the more virulent viral infections
  - secondary bacterial infections – 'snotty nose', and other purulent conditions, as from necrotic turbinate bone
- nasal mycosis
- usually associated with inflammation of related airway areas

Because of the functional need for constant *per nasi* respiration, the structure of the elongated nasal passages and the volume of air passing through mean that the nasal passages very rarely become blocked by inflammatory thickening of the mucosa or by excessive catarrhal secretions, as in humans.

Since the oral breathing which man finds a simple alternative to trying to breathe through his 'stuffed' nose does not occur, the equine 'nose' does not 'dry out'.

Diagnosis

- a discharge varying in amount, consistency, colour
- sneezing
- abnormal respiratory noise, especially on inspiration
- varying 'illness' and fever
- varying regional lymphadenitis

Prognosis

Usually good, but beware secondary sinusitis, guttural pouch involvement, U and LRT complications, and too soon a return to work.

Prevention Management

Vaccination for certain viral infections, and good and observant horsemastership.

Sinusitis

These are very much part of the airway – presumably as air heating and moisturising surfaces. Although large in highly vascular surface area, the bilateral entry is comparatively and significantly a small 'in and out' portal. They are seen as weight reducing areas within the skull which are possibly put to secondary respiratory use (natural economy). Certainly, their mucosal lining is continuous with that of the nasal passages. They are subject to inhaled irritants and pathogens and therefore potential areas of inflammatory reaction.

Furthermore, the roots of the upper 3–6 molar teeth project into the facial sinuses, both anterior and posterior maxillaries bilaterally (where they are covered by a thin, fragile layer of bone). Any infection of one or more of these roots will erode through the bony roof and inflame the mucosum. A necrotic, foetid secretion gathers; its pressure can distort the facial bones.

Signs

- foetid nasal discharge
- swelling of facial bone
- mastication difficulty
- possible fever

Diagnosis

- radiograph to display bone rarefaction over tooth root inflammation; pus fluid line
- tap sampling through bone into sinus

Prognosis

Guarded to good – dependent on early diagnosis, but possible recurrence, possibly in another molar tooth apical infection or new bacterial infection.

Prevention management

Better routine dental care; early recognition and treatment of naso-pharyngeal infection which can lead to a sinusitis. Unless a primary clinical URT inflammatory disease is present it is essential to rule out a primary dental complication. Fungal infection does occur with or without a primary rhinitis.

Pharyngitis

It is variably involved in infectious dis-ease of the respiratory system particularly perhaps primarily in those of the URT and secondarily in the LRT.

It is also involved in inflammation associated with secondarily activated commensals – bacteria, fungi.

Equine tonsils (superficial lymphoid drainage glands) are not 'concentrated' at the roof of the nose and at the back of the throat but are 'scattered' over the roof and sides of the whole pharyngeal and nasal mucosa (as shown below).

In the acute phase of any infection they show the characteristic signs of inflammation including a 'sore throat' and its effects. In sub-acute and the debatable so-called chronic phases they remain swollen but much less inflamed and eventually become only enlarged nodules (compare a child's 'enlarged tonsils'). They are then known as **naso-pharyngeal lymphoid hyperplasia (PLH)** – and are almost universal in young especially Thoroughbred horses, so much so that it is debated if they are a dis-ease state and not, in fact, an on-going defensive feature. They could be harbouring points for streptococcal and other bacteria and for herpes viral strains.

The ear may seem an unlikely component of the respiratory system but, as will be remembered, there are bilateral openings in the pharynx, leading to the **Eustachian tube**, a tract which opens into the middle ear, thus making a direct route from the atmosphere to what is otherwise a closed area, separated only by delicate tissue, from the inner ear.

In the equidae, the tubes have a diverticulum into a folded sac, an expanded area whose function, other than a pressure escape mechanism, is not fully understood. It is called the **guttural pouch**. These are incidental traps or depositories for

- bacteria from naso-pharyngeal inflammations which are air transported, or by direct mucosal spread and which colonise (usually unilaterally) on the pouch mucosa with the production of pus to cause an **empyema** – the strangles germ is a classic example
- fungi, Aspergilli species, by inhalation with subsequent growth of fungal plaques, a mycosis with subsequent mucosal erosion of the pouch wall to cause underlying nerve damage, leading to throat muscle wall paresis mainly affecting swallowing, and arterial damage, an often fatal haemorrhage, one type of epistaxis

Clinically

- **empyema** causes a visible enlargement of the sac, which becomes discomfiting and painful to digital pressure
- there is often a pre- or concurrent dis-ease of bacterial origin in the naso-pharynx
- the horse will invariably be ill
- **mycosis** does not usually distend the sac, but is suspected if
  - swallowing becomes difficult (pharyngeal paresis)
  - respiratory noise develops even at rest
  - epistaxis develops, often rapid and lethal but differential diagnosis in non-fatal cases is for traumatic bleeding; ethmoidal bleeding and EIPH

Prognosis

Guarded in all cases.

Management

Impracticable to a great extent.

In foals, a retained excess of air balloons the pouches, to produce an **emphysema** or **tympany** which is mechanically upsetting to swallowing and breathing

Functional disturbances of hearing are not well documented; a 'reverse' tinnitus has recently been reported in one horse, where a nerve-emanating whine was audible to the horsemaster when standing close to the

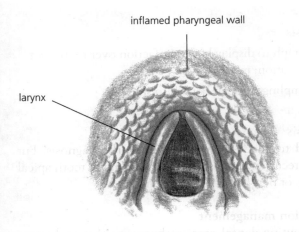

inflamed pharyngeal wall

larynx

Pharyngitis, also known as chronic pharyngeal lymphoid hyperplasia (CPLH) or lymphoid follicular hyperplasia.

horse's head. (Cause unknown; horse apparently unaffected.)

Soft Palate Inflammation

Secondary microbial inflammatory reactions of the dorsal mucosal lining; non-specific; may interfere with functioning temporarily, but related tissues similarly affected will confuse this. More important in functional disorders.

Laryngitis

Again, the lining is involved in infectious inflammatory reactions (the human altered or 'lost' voice); this is not so significant or clear-cut in the horse. Glottal pain may interfere with closure at swallowing and 'choke' cough may result.

There is variable obstruction to airflow from submucosal oedema and congestion; mucosal thickening; and excess mucus secretion.

The sore throat complex will interfere with exercise work – airway dysfunction; flexion of the poll, especially in dressage.

The neuro-muscular dis-ease RLN is much more important.

Tracheitis

- as for the larynx
- interference with muco-ciliary escalator
- purulent and inflammatory mucus produced in the LRT will be wafted up and into the trachea from which it will run (drain) only when the head is down, taking the neck below the horizontal, or where it is coughed up. When excessive it might 'narrow' the otherwise functionally almost rigid tracheal airway. At exercise, when blown up into the pharynx, it can require unusual rhythm upsetting swallowing which can interfere with the stride

Lower Respiratory Tract

Areas 3–4

This category mainly refers, in colloquial terms, to the lungs. Technically the LRT encompasses areas 3 and 4 of the airway both of which are within the chest cavity. Disease of these areas can affect the

- bronchi
- bronchioles
- alveolar ducts
- alveoli

and the related tissues

- interstitial; structural elastic connective tissue
- pleura
- vascular (bronchial; pulmonary, especially the alveolar capillaries)
- neural

Pathogenesis is related to

- inhaled material thus common to infection and allergy types
- blood-borne agents mainly of infections

Morbidity does differ between these two major types and further between infection and allergy.

Signs can be confusing but, especially to the layman and sometimes to the professional, in broad terms

- most infections present an acute picture
- allergies, usually present as a progressive, intermittently acute or marked expression of a basically chronic disease

Infectious inflammatory LRT dis-ease is often a sequel to a URT infection which

- 'spreads' down the airway by inspiration causing, en route, bronchitis, bronchiolitis, pneumonitis – some viruses have a tendency to this spread
  - influenza A (equine 1 types 2 and 3)
  - herpes types 1 and 4
- is disseminated via the blood – haematogenous invasion
  - herpes 1

Bacteria, especially when triggered into secondary invader activity, may also be inhaled from their URT sites into the thoracic areas. In the young horse especially the 2–3 year old Thoroughbred in training or in racing the most common and the most important (welfare and economics) respiratory condition is LR airway disease. This is confirmed by tracheal washings (airway lavage) revealing a compound bacterial infection with 50% of cases showing mycoplasma species as well as Streptococci, Bordetellae, and Actinobactus. It is these which are often erroneously referred to as 'the Virus dis-ease'. They will respond to antibiotics. There is a promise of possible-active artificial immunisation. There is often no systemic illness but poor performance is common.

Environmental factors commonly seen as stressors such as poor ventilation, cold and damp, fatigue, and transit may so weaken the horse's natural defences – existing specific and general immunity and airtract defensive mechanisms – that it becomes susceptible to its own commensal organisms (bacteria and fungi) and low-grade co-existent infections (viral).

The foal and the old horse, as well as a debilitated animal, are always more susceptible to primary infections and to subsequent secondaries with serious, often lethal, pneumonic complications.

Certain generalisations in horse management are

- pneumonia as a clinical entity *per se* is rare
- when it is suspected it is usually bacterial and then mainly secondary to stressor factors, e.g. transit fever
- as part of an overall respiratory disease it is usually viral and then susceptible to secondary bacterial inflammation

From a veterinary aspect the existence of a viral spread or a secondary complication is difficult to determine and to diagnose accurately. Its presence is signalled by

- respiratory embarrassment (dyspnoea) rather than by
- coughing as in URT dis-ease

especially in transit fever examples which is often complicated by

- pleurisy, a Streptococcal/Pasteurella commensal flare-up

Hyper-acute pneumonic complications follow the inhalation of gross foreign material such as food and drugs and smoke.

Pneumonia in the horse, therefore, unlike in the calf and the pig, is very much an individual animal disorder, an unlucky complication or an accidental assault on the airway. In URT respiratory dis-ease outbreaks or 'storms', pneumonia remains of low incidence and prevalence as a specific entity. It can often go unrecognised as a complicating pneumonitis in Influenza storms and, to a lesser extent in herpes, especially if the primary outbreak is in young horses. Nonetheless any evidence of an unnatural duration of an URT illness or of secondary flare-ups should be suspected as: pneumonic complications; secondary (bacterial) invasion; a superimposed different virus invasion.

Acute Infectious Inflammation of the LRT

Pneumonitis
An inflammation of the air tract's epithelium.

Causes
- a viral invasion, descending from the U to the LR areas
- influenza sub-types 2 and 3 and variants thereof
- herpes sub-type 1 and 4
- recrudescing herpes 1

The herpes direct, and the recrudescing, also spread via the circulation.

Pre-disposing Factors
- URT infections causing immuno-suppression
- inhaled particulate and gaseous irritants, for example, dust and ammonia

Pathogenesis
- usually a primary, direct invasion but possibly
- accelerated or made more invasive by a prior dis-ease of the area, or a coincidental or recent infection by Rhinovirus in the URT

Morbidity
- destruction in areas three and four of ciliated epithelium and mucociliary escalator
- alteration of the defensive ability of the white blood cells particularly in the gaseous exchange area 4
- subsequent secondary bacterial invasion with deeper damage to the interstitial tissues, muco-purulent exudates and abscess formation

Signs
- dyspnoea
- fever – if continuing for more than five days into the pneumonic situation it suggests secondary invasion
- cough
- nasal discharge
- (usually total lung involvement on auscultation)

- peripheral anoxia
- loss of appetite

Prognosis

In uncomplicated cases, good with correct nursing; a low-grade chronic stage can develop.

Pneumonia

An inflammation of the airway epithelium *and invariably of the deeper tissues*. Often associated with a bronchitis, but may also develop secondarily, a broncho-pneumonia.

Causes

Usually a bacterial infection flare-up by

Streptococci zooepidemicus

Pasteurella spp

Staphylococci

Bordetellae

Rhodococci (in foals)

Pseudomonas

Mycoplasma (recently thought to be the 'ring leader')

It will be remembered that these bacteria are present in the environment ubiquitously, in the ENT areas of the RT as opportunist commensals, and as latent infections. They are endemic to most large equine establishments with high throughput.

In addition to the bacteria the horse's respiratory tract can be invaded by the inhalation of

- fungi, to cause a direct mycotic bronchiolitic pneumonia (rare) or an allergic state (see COPD later)

and indirectly via the blood by

- migrating helminth larvae – ascarids in foals, lungworms in adults which develop into adult lungworm in the bronchial lumen

also by

- food aspiration secondary to pharyngeal deficits (DDSP, paresis, grass sickness, botulism)
- regurgitated aspiration as in oesophageal choke and gastric reflux complication of certain colics
- drenches 'going the wrong way'

These last three are obviously isolated hyper-acute cases.

It may be

- secondary to an existent viral LRT infection or
- predisposed to by stress, as in transit, malnutrition and debility, inclement weather and chilling, strenuous exercise whilst viraemic, as with Influenza, especially when 'thought' to be better

Signs in the acute cases

- a prodromal fever of 40–40.6°C (104–105°F) associated with
- an easily missed lethargy or conversely a 'high' from a fever stimulated increased metabolic rate
- in about 2 hours, marked tachypnoea with hypopnoea (fast and shallow) breathing and congestion of the visible mucous membranes (the hyper-acute)
- thereafter a drop in temperature
- 'lung' congestion (interstitial oedema and serum into the tract lumen) – dyspnoea and general distressed appearance and behaviour; moist cough, intermittent; nasal discharge, clear to mucoid or purulent; some cyanosis; inappetence
- increased heart rate
- depression – 'looks very ill'
- lethargy

To the veterinary surgeon changes in auscultated respiratory sounds not only indicate lung involvement (and pleurisy complications) but help in differentiating viral pneumonitis from bacterial pneumonia and these from allergic morbidity.

Diagnosis

By the horsemaster

- history
- clinical signs
- airway sounds not always audible even to the 'ear on chest'

By the veterinary surgeon

- as above
- auscultation
- ancillary aids – laboratory findings from tracheal swabs and 'washings'; white blood cell ratios; metabolic changes; possibly radiography; ultrasonography; thoraco-centesis samples to laboratory to confirm white blood cells of pleurisy, and to differentiate other causes

of 'fluid on the lungs' – oedema; air in the chest, pneumothorax; blood in the chest, haemothorax from severe rib cage trauma

Prognosis

Depends upon residual damage to the airway and complications – bronchitis persisting in a chronic form; emphysema, a permanent loss of air exchange space of variable extent; consolidation of the air space, a chronic fibrosing state with consequent reduced gaseous exchange; abscess formation. A persisting non-return to resting respiratory rate is a poor prognosis.

Bronchitis and Bronchiolitis

A more common complication than pneumonia and pneumonitis.

Acute stage

- as part of viral pneumonitis
- a primary bacterial descending invasion
- a secondary, to viral invasion, commensal bacterial inflammation

Signs

- as for pneumonia
- auscultation

Sub-acute and chronic stages

- the residual post-acute inflammatory changes until
  - the eroded epithelium regenerates
  - the muco-ciliary escalator reactivates
  - the sero-muco-purulent secretions decrease
- the lumen wall thickening may persist with consequent airway narrowing
- may be prolonged by the aggravation of inhaled stable dust and irritant vapours if these are not obviated

Signs

- muco-purulent nasal discharge especially after exercise
- persistent cough during the start of exercise with phlegm in some cases
- coughing at times of air temperature changes

- abdominal muscle effort on expiration
- (auscultation)
  - dry crackles over ventral chest
  - moist squeaks at distal trachea – noise of free, excessive sero-mucus
  - reduced exercise tolerance

Diagnosis

By the horseman

- persisting respiratory disease signs particularly 'keeps on coughing'

By the veterinary surgeon

- as above
- auscultation
- tracheal washings – white cell change including pus formation

Prognosis

As for pneumonia; poor if there is a history of LRT disease, infectious or allergic.

Pleurisy (Pleuritis)

An inflammation of the epithelial linings of the thoracic cavity and the outer surfaces of areas 3 and 4 of the RT. 'Pleurisy' is a colloquial term but it does suggest the often present increase in the nominal layer of fluid which bathes and lubricates the surface.

Cause

- a primary commensal bacterial invasion as in transit fever
- an extension of 'lung' inflammatory dis-ease
- (invasion through a perforating wound of the chest)

Predisposition

Stressors, especially transit, debilitation and chilling.

Signs

- mild fever (of the primary inflammation)
- higher in transit fever
- hypopnoea and tachypnoea
- inappetence
- stiff body carriage

- other coincidental 'lung' disease signs
- (characteristic pleuritic sounds on auscultation)

Acute pleurisy 'attacks' usually relate to overstress especially transit, when a purulent broncho-pneumonia may also develop – this can be fatal. Non-fatal cases may take many months to recover to athletic fitness. There is a risk of abscess formation in convalescence with secondary lethal effect.

Pulmonary Oedema
Often associated with

- aspiration pneumonia and its marked 'foreign body' irritation and the associated broad spectrum of invading bacteria
- smoke inhalation when the inflammatory fever develops in about one week after the exposure. The oedema may be progressive before that

Signs
Cough, dyspnoea and lethargy.

Chronic LRT Dis-ease
Apart from the chronic stages of RT infectious inflammatory disease there are certain conditions which are not infectious in origin. They may have acute phases but generally are persistent and in that respect, progressive, as in neoplasia or chronic, as in established lungworm in adults.

- lungworm
- neoplasia

The most prevalent and most serious is **chronic obstructive pulmonary disease**. This allergic state is chronic in that once a horse is sensitised it remains so to be restimulated into further attacks if exposed to the same inhaled allergen.

On rechallenge after a quiescent period the impression of an acute dis-ease does result. In many cases, even when re-exposure is prevented, a chronic morbidity may remain with compromised respirations.

It may have, in fact, already deteriorated into a permanent shutting off of areas of atrophied alveoli clusters and emphysema.

Inflammatory changes as they affect the respiratory system, especially the LRT

The acute and sub-acute stages of infectious inflammation result in epithelial damage, with

- loss of cilia
- loss of cells which produce the cilia
- increase in goblet cells with secretion of extra mucus of altered consistency
- hyperactivity in vascular/epithelial blood flow
- secretion of extra serum

These events weaken or destroy the muco-cilia escalator defensive capacity, causing excretion of white blood cells.

The combined effects are
- the production of a mucopurulent airway coating with
  - narrowing of the airway
  - plugging of bronchioles
  - loss of alveolar respiratory surface area
- erosion of the epithelial layer
  - exposure of sensory nerve endings
  - congestion of the tract's blood vessels
  - oedema of the airway wall with further narrowing of the airway
- loss of tone in the bronchi and bronchioles
- loss of elasticity in the airway and alveoli
- loss of surfactant
- increase in compliance with collapse of alveoli, anoxia of the tissues and further loss of respiratory area
- invasion of the supportive tissue (the parenchyma)
  - consolidation first from congestion, then oedema and finally the pneumonias and subsequent fibrosis

The accompanying signs are
- alteration in respiratory rate from the *normal resting rate of 10–15 breaths per minute*, and in breathing depth and rhythm
- increase in temperature and heart rate
- dyspnoea
- breathing pain
- depression
- cough
- nasal discharge

INFLAMMATORY CONTAGIOUS INFECTIONS

Viral Infections

Whilst intelligent assumptions as to which virus can be made, it is essential especially in racing and other group situations where health is an economic necessity as well as a welfare one that a differential diagnosis is made by laboratory assistance

- blood, for viral culture, from very early cases
- high nasal swabs essentially before secondaries develop
- paired serum samples at a 2-3 week interval for measuring a significant rise in antibody titres. The first is taken as soon as possible after initial signs appear. The second is called the convalescent sample on the assumption that a sero conversion or immunity has developed *specific* to the virus suspected

In the adult horse most respiratory dis-ease which proves to be a contagion – several horses serially affected – are caused by a viral infection. (But see also strangles bacterium.)

There is evidence that viral-induced disease was and is present in wild and feral animals including the Equidae. It is also acknowledged that pathogenic viruses are more contagious than virulent; they spread amongst susceptible species quite readily but their infectious virulence is not associated with serious lethal illness except: in the very young; in the very old, and in the debilitated individual, and when a new virus, or strain within, invades a population; producing an epidemic situation.

As already described the otherwise healthy mature animal has a range of non-specific defences which, whilst they may not stop an inflammatory response, will manage to contain it in most situations before serious illness arises.

There is reason to believe that in the non-domesticated scene secondary opportunist microbes did become active in virus infected animals. It is possible that it was these complicating infections which caused serious illness in some nomadic situations.

The domesticated situation is a different matter

- movement of young stock from a 'home' environment to the mixing environment exposing them to
    - new strains of primary and secondary microbes to which they are not immune
        - stress of transit
        - stress of mixing
        - stress of juvenile work
- national and international movement of competition horses
    - transit stress
    - poorer stabling and indoor working conditions
    - new infections
- stabling generally, home or away
    - stress of isolation
    - poor ventilation
    - respiratory irritants and 're-breathing' of infected air
- inefficient (unavailable or ineffective) immunisation

all combine to make

- primary viral infections more infectious and virulent and therefore often more contagious
- secondary microbial activity more active

Nevertheless, with only some exceptions, endemic viruses continue to be

- contagious problems and
- predisposing factors to
    - related functional disorders, especially in
        - brood animals
        - elite athletes

During tissue colonisation, i.e. virus replication, the infected animal can shed some of the viral particles to become contagious. Most viral infections are of short duration clinically and the germ is eliminated even before the illness subsides. Most develop a strong immunity response but of variable duration. Some are responsive to artificial immunisation.

The herpes group is a significant exception to the above in many respects. Its importance varies considerably with the type (and use) of the horses infected

Viral infections can have a profound effect in some situations

- morbid and debilitating and especially
- economic if in racing yards, competition yards and studs

At present it is recognised that in Great Britain the 'cold' viruses, influenza strains and herpes strains are all endemic.

Equine influenza virus has the ability to make strain 'drifts' or mutations in this country, but especially in others, which if they invade here act as epidemic contagion and as such are more infectious and potentially more virulent.

- equine viral arteritis (EVA) is factually endemic in status but because there is no endemic immunity and only limited artificial immunisation to this notifiable infection it is potentially an epidemic disease
- equine infectious anaemia (EIA) has been reported in this country but very rarely. It is therefore seen as a potential epidemic virus

Immunisation against these is discussed in the relative text.

It is vitally important in dealing with viral infections that the stable inmates' history is well documented:

- breed or type
- sex
- date of birth
- possible immune status, past infection and when, artificial immunisation and when
- how long on premises
- any known contact with viral infection, recent visiting horses, recent new horses
- recent movement off and back onto premises
- the signs of any illness – what, when, body temperature changes

As with all other living things viruses are classified into families, genus and species – and sub-species or types. Virology is a relatively new discipline: progress in recognition and identification has been rapid since the advent of

- the electron microscope – to see more detail
- laboratory cell-line cultures on which virus particles can be replicated
- a range of laboratory tests for identification, e.g. ELISA
- genetic (DNA) analyses of the germ

The importance of knowing not only that a virus is implicated in a dis-ease situation but also of identifying which one and being able to 'name it' scientifically varies with the 'interest' of the people involved, but the following are recognised in the UK:

Ortho-myxovirus	Influenza	A/equi 1
		A/equi 2
Herpes viridae	Beta (simplex) strain, as in man	
	Alpha strains, as in horses	
		sub type 1
		sub type 2
	(non-respiratory Coital Exanthema)	sub type 3
		sub type 4
Picornovirus	Rhinovirus	type 1
	The 'cold' viruses	type 2
Adenovirus Coronavirus	a 'diarrhoea' and respiratory virus	
Arterivirus	Equine arteritis virus	
	Several strains	
Lentivirinae	Equine infectious anaemia virus (vector spread)	
Reoviridae	Rotavirus (foals)	

Once a virus has been suspected and confirmed by laboratory aids the practitioner is more accurately able to advise on

- epidemiology – the pattern a particular disease will show in a stable or large group of susceptible animals
  - is it a typical one-animal species germ or
  - can it spread to other species including man, a zoonosis
- mode of transmission
  - animal to animal (direct, aerosol)
  - inanimate contaminant to animal (fomites)
  - insect vector
  - is the transmission vertical, one generation to the next, or horizontal within existing generation
- incubation period – often characteristic for a given virus and so useful information for an initial presumptive diagnosis
- duration of contagiousness – how long must a diseased animal be isolated as deemed dangerous to others
- virulence with particular regard to age, sex, breed of the patient and its environmental stressors as well as

directly the germ itself

- incidence – the number of new cases in a unit of time
- prevalence – the number of new cases at a specific time during an outbreak

All of the above helps in deciding on

- isolation or not
- potential for use of hyperimmune antiserum (foals especially)
- possibility of secondary invaders
- suitable medication for them
- nursing requirements
- 'turn out'
- possible duration of illness
- possible duration of convalescence
- future use planning
- future preventative measures

THE COMMON VIRAL INFECTIONS

Herpes

Herpes (from the Greek *herpo*, creep) so called because it 'creeps', slowly, relentlessly, often sub-clinically throughout most body systems even in the presence of proven developing active immunity. (It is said cynically that the herpes virus is like the poor – it will always be with us.)

Four sub-types are recognised in horses

EHV-1 associated with

- respiratory signs – sneezing, coughing, nasal discharges up to 'snotty nose' (secondary bacterial), bronchitis – possibly with secondary bacteria
- abortion
- neurologic signs

EHV-4

- respiratory as in EHV-1
- rarely abortion
- no neurologic involvement

Originally it was thought that 1 and 4 were synonymous; they were called the rhinopneumonitis virus (not to be confused with rhinovirus!).

EHV-2

- sub-clinical or non-pathogenic effects
- as a stressor factor precipitating 1 and 4

The above two are mainly spread by expiratory aerosol and by ingestion of aborted infection in contaminated food and water.

EHV-3

- coital exanthema ('spots') on the external genitalia of mares and stallions
- a venereal spread

The respiratory sub-types have a predilection for

- airway epithelia thence to regional lymph glands
- vascular endothelia to become
- latent within lymphoid tissue and cells from which they can again migrate via the blood to
- respiratory tissues and so to expired air
- reach the uterus in EHV-1 and/or
- invade the CNS tissue's blood vessels (a dead end?)

Consequently the infection may grumble on for years. During this time it is sub-clinical in all tissues or latent in all tissues but, subject to stress effect, able to recrudesce to produce further clinical illness and contagion, and non-clinical 'shedders'.

The cell-mediated immunity and antibody formation responses have a limited duration of no more than six months. Re-infection and 'new' clinical illness can, in addition to recrudescence, occur throughout a horse's life. The period of greatest morbidity and so the clinical effect in the respiratory system is from foalhood to 3 years and especially so in the training and working Thoroughbred.

The more extensive latency period and the recrudescences and the re-infections producing only mild, even sub-clinical, illness is thought to be the explanation of a group of 'below par' states:

- loss of performance
- catarrhal episodes and nosebleeds
- muscle stiffness

It is these factors which makes accurate diagnosis (and control) difficult.

The virus is very much endemic in the UK, consequently

most horses are infected when very young. The initial infections are the ones which causes the most clinical respiratory signs. Spread is easiest within collections of yearlings and two year olds, as in sale yards and training stables as well as at race courses. It is a disease of great monetary and of course welfare importance in the racing industry. Mares can be aerosolly re-infected like any other herpes-immunity-waning horse, or self re-infected by recrudescing virus, and theoretically can abort again. Most abortions are sporadic, individual occurrences. If a stud experiences more than three close together this is called a 'storm'. An arbitrary isolation of the stud farm of thirty days is recommended to minimise any potential aerosol contagion to cause new primary respiratory infection.

The high risk of recrudescing respiratory infection makes in-foal mares potentially aerosol contagious.

In studs

- **foals** in the acute phase of illness show
  - viraemia and fatal organ disease or to a lesser degree
  - acute eye lesions – a uveitis
  - variable fever
  - mild respiratory signs
  - colic
  - vague signs suggestive of prematurity maladjustment defects but can die from bacterial bronchopneumonia later on
- **mares in foal** are potential cases of abortion
- **mares with foal at foot** (a stressor) are liable to
  - other infectious respiratory disease and possibly inducement and/or exacerbation of OPD
  - neurologic dis-ease
- **stallions** during re-infection
  - rarely respiratorily affected
  - limb and scrotal oedema
  - ataxia, possibly progressive
  - loss of libido

Neonatal disease

This is seen in foals born to dams 'infected' late in pregnancy. All die within a few days from acute and severe respiratory disease and other systemic (usually liver) involvement. Those which survive invariably succumb to subsequent secondary bacterial infection. All aborted foals and dead suspected neo-nates should be examined at a laboratory.

Neurologic disease

This complication may affect horses of all ages not only brood animals. Elite athleticism or training may be the stressor. Nursing mares are particularly susceptable. These and other adults are more prone to recumbency which carries a very poor prognosis. The virus invades the endothelium of the arterioles to the brain and spinal cord causing neuronal atrophy.

Prevalence is usually single but 'storms', i.e. three or more cases have been seen in single yards.

As with abortion it is usually unheralded but serum titres invariably confirm an earlier (respiratory route) infection.

Signs

- altered gait
- weakness and
- hind-leg inco-ordination are the earlier signs over forty-eight hours. Some cases which show no worsening resolve over several weeks. These ataxias which have resolved may leave the horse with
  - a slack tail
  - toe dragging especially of the hind legs
  others progress to
- paralysis hind and/or fore and hind (quadriplegia)
- slow recovery over several months or
- death, usually by euthanasia

Nursing and veterinary support are essential. Isolation of the yard to prevent recrudescent nasal aerosol spread to other stables for thirty days after last recovery (or death) is recommended.

It is essential that when either (or both) of these conditions are suspected that laboratory help is sought. An accurate diagnosis, if possible, is essential to plan control methods to minimise the risk of endemic spread. This is so even if the prevalence of either does not always present as a worrying 'storm'.

It invades all breeds and types of horse. The intermittent even low-grade re-infections will interfere with use in all types but is variably so with the degree of exertion expected of the animal. It is of least importance in riding school horses – this does not preclude care and attention with especial reference to possible secondary invaders.

Sub-clinical animals are common and 'shedders' are potentially everywhere. Re-infected animals which are under stress are more likely to become clinical cases.

The actual viral particles are difficult to isolate in samples from nasal swabs or in 'fresh' blood except in very early infections. They can be isolated from

- aborted placentae
- neotal fatalities
- spinal cord nerve tissue on autopsy and an infection presumed from rising antibody levels in two serum samples two weeks apart, i.e. a serum conversion

The Respiratory, Primary Herpes Infection
Incubation period, 2–10 days

Signs
- serous nasal discharge
- fever: intermittent over several days 39–41°C (102–106°F), possibly biphasic
- sneezing
- coughing rarely on its own
- sub-mandibular (non-purulent) lymphadenitis
- mild inappetence
- mild depression

Duration
- variable, up to several weeks when secondarily complicated

Diagnosis
- suspicion, age and environment; needs laboratory confirmation. Ophthalmascopic retinal change

Complications
- secondary infections
  - bacterial
    - mucopurulent catarrhal nasal discharge from the URT secondary inflammation; the 'snotty nose'
  - may result in further spread to the LRT, with bronchitis and even bronchopneumonia with more marked coughing, respiratory embarrassment, fever and depression
  - association with other viral infections such as influenza

The herpes virus infection is immunosuppressant which makes these secondaries more likely.

Abortion

In-foal mares are always at a risk if infected, clinically or subclinically with EHV-1. Some incidents with EHV-4 have been recorded. The virus, when disseminated through the vascular system will invade the endothelial cells of small arterioles. Those of the pregnant uterus are no exception. Such morbidity

- may in itself so affect the womb wall that the placental attachment is lost and the foetus is aborted or
- may 'permit' the virus to cross the usually inviolate blood/placental barrier to invade the foetus which, depending upon the gestation age at the time of infection, will
  - abort dead foals, characteristically in 'fresh' afterbirths, suddenly from an apparently healthy dam which does *not* 'bag up'
  - be born very ill (neonatal herpes)

Most abortions occur in late pregnancy following a primary infection some two weeks to two months previously

- the mare has no serious or prolonged uterine discharge
- she does not become venereally contagious
- unless complications follow, her subsequent fertility is unimpaired

Pharyngeal Lymphoid Hyperplasia (PLH)

In the acute and sub-acute stages of herpes PLH is said to be present in 100% of all infected youngsters.

The morbidity causes
- disturbed laminar air flow
- adventitious respiratory noise
- discomfort (in swallowing as well as breathing)
- episodes of 'gurgling' (DDSP etc.) during training

The presence of *chronic* enlarged lymphoid nodules on the mucus membrane of the throat is dubiously important as a cause of sub-acute illness let alone 'poor performance'. It is usually a condition and subsides very slowly Abortion, neurological syndrome, and PLH are post viral, originally respiratory infections whether the initial inflammatory response is clinical or sub-clinical.

What has been emphasised is that their particular clinical expression is evidence of a herpes infection complication and the infected animal is almost certainly *contagious via the expiratory route* for a variable period (in addition to the shorter term per vaginal route following abortion). The isolation period of thirty days after the last case's resolution is arbitrary in abortion and neurologic examples, but is presumed to be a reasonable safeguard against spread especially to other stables, yards or other gatherings of horses. Isolation of PLH cases is a waste of effort.

As far as the particular complications are concerned

- the secondary contagion from abortion uterine fluids seems to cease with the post abortion end of discharge. The aborted foal and 'opened' afterbirth are potent sources of contagion and should be 'handled 'appropriately
- there is no evidence of a subsequent venereal spread
- in neurologically affected animals there is no outlet from central nervous system lesions. Some recent research suggests a retrograde spread via nerve tissue to the olfactory sensory nerve ending cells and hence to aerosol dissemination
- in throat lesions there is a direct exit route for aerosol spread but there is doubt if the virus is shed from these lymphoid locations as such

The throat lesions are now seen as a persisting defensive mechanism within the lymphoid tissues originally sensitised by cell mediated immune factors following the primary infection. How much a young horse, so affected, works below optimum is debatable but this lymphoid hyperplasia is not now looked upon as a serious morbidity but rather as protection.

More importantly is the latency/recrudescence aspect of herpes infection which can produce a clinical shedders of the virus.

The imponderables all serve to emphasise the difficulties in understanding and controlling the herpes infection and in particular in producing a vaccine which will

- extend the relatively short (six months) period of natural active immunity following infection
- hopefully prevent either
  - recrudescence or
  - stop such a viral awakening becoming
    - clinically active
    - sub-clinically active

- contagious to others

In conclusion

- herpes 1 and 4 infection is widespread. Clinically it is:
  - mainly a problem of young race horses, affecting them
    - acutely, and later
    - sub-acutely, chronically and with 'reduced performance syndrome' effect
  - a potentially recurrent infection
  - an occasional problem of older sports horses through nerve tissue damage
  - potential problem in pregnant mares
  - a low-grade often unrecognised problem in less athletic animals who are, nevertheless, a potentially dangerous source of infection to more susceptible (and economically more important) 'cousins'

In other words

- the germ is ubiquitous but
- its *serious* pathogenic effect is restricted to a small proportion of all horses but is especially significant in young racehorses as well as in neurological cases which are sporadic, particularly in competition yards, and abortion in brood mares

Equine Influenza (Strains)

These viruses are a cause of equine respiratory disease worldwide except in Australia, New Zealand and Iceland. They have been recognised, retrospectively, as being of avian origin in the 19th century.

Until recently the disease in Great Britain was epidemic in behaviour and particularly characterised by the emergence of new strains originating in different countries which resulted in these being designated by their origin.

The orthomyxo-viruses include influenza equine type A. There are two sub-types: 1 and 2 which are antigenically distinct but cause similar morbidity, although sub-type 2 is specifically more virulent and pathogenic and more likely to effect the LRT as well as the URT.

In addition the sub-type 2 has numerous strains which can 'drift' or mutate; these also have differing antigenicity. This determines the efficacy of vaccines. Sub-type 1 disease does not 'break through' correctly vaccinated horses, and, coincidentally or not, clinical disease due to it is rarely seen at present – but relevant immunisation must continue to protect against sub-clinical contagions. The strain drifts in sub-type 2 produce epidemics even in vaccinated horses injected with a vaccine deficient in a new strain.

It is now accepted that the strains can be grouped into American and European. Constant surveillance is maintained for emerging new sub-strains for vaccine updating.

Since 1956, when it was first confirmed that an A virus sub-type 1 was the cause of an equine respiratory disease (in Prague) and subsequently a sub-type 2 and its variants, influenza was seen as a 5–10 year cycling epidemic problem. Recently the comparatively few confirmed cases of sub-type 2 influenza have been in unvaccinated animals. One outbreak in a vaccinated group of horses did occur in 1994 (although all were up to date *vis à vis* Jockey Club Rules) in which the horses had been injected with various 'brands' of vaccine and the manufacturers' data sheet requirements had not always been followed. There were potential gaps of reduced immunity.

Most of these so called breakdowns were deceptively mild in clinical signs.

It is important that *suspected* cases, especially in vaccinates, should be investigated regarding an emerging new strain. High nasal swabs collected at the early stage of respiratory disease signs are a fruitful source of laboratory recognition of the virus.

Influenza is not only contagious but it is highly infectious. As expected it is primarily a disease of young (race)horses, but new strains can infect and affect susceptible animals of any age. It can, therefore be an economic problem in National Hunt racing, eventing, show jumping etc. – with their movement and congregation and their stresses and exposure factors.

Spread	aerosol, rapid, especially in close proximity and poor ventilation
Incubation period	1–3 days
Duration	7–10 days and variable period of coughing
Season	usually in cold, high humidity conditions but this is variable with seasonal sporting events' movement and mixing

Signs
- sudden onset

- fever – 38.9–41.7°C (102–107°F), lasts 1–5 days (so is easily missed) often biphasic, i.e. goes down then up again
- rapid spread in a group of susceptible horses
- harsh, dry cough, explosive, non-productive and frequent (see below)
- serous nasal discharge
- lethargy
- anorexia
- throat and glands 'sore' to touch (no marked lymphadenitic swelling)
- 'gags' when eating
- increased heart and respiratory rates
- eye weeping
- muscle soreness and stiffness
- secondary infections of both URT and LRT, possible pneumonic and pleura complications

Diagnosis
- suspicion
- rate of spread
- signs, but needs lab confirmation

Virus isolation is not easy. Positive sera conversions are the most helpful findings.

Beware if...
- fever continues for more than five days, and/or
- other systemic signs appear
- secondary infection is seen
- work is restarted too soon

Failure to obey these can possibly lead to
- relapse
- permanent damage to the heart muscle
- respiratory system complications
- prolonged exercise intolerance

Equine Viral Arteritis (EVA)

In the early 1900s a veterinary surgeon in Scotland recorded details of a respiratory illness with some abortions, which he considered was a separate contagion from those other respiratory syndromes which did not have the characteristic conjunctivitis, the pink eye, which

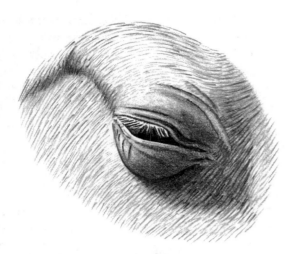

Swelling from associated conjunctivitis – equine viral arteritis (EVA).

gave this condition its then descriptive name. This appeared to 'die out' at least in his practice area. It is possible that for some time thereafter less observant practitioners did not recognise Pink Eye for what is was, or refused to accept it as such.

To confuse matters further, in the first few years after the Second World War some research workers were describing a respiratory disease, eventually shown to be equine influenza, as Pink Eye. Suspicion remains that the virus of equine arteritis may have been present in restricted areas or at low virulence levels elsewhere for some time.

A serious epidemic erupted in Kentucky in 1984 and this led to intensive laboratory as well as epidemiologic investigation. The disease is now recognised as having endemic status in the USA, and in Europe, a low-grade condition with epidemic 'flare-up' at five- to ten-year intervals. In the UK in 1993 an outbreak occurred which was shown to have been 'imported' via a European Warmblood stallion.

The outbreak in 1993 fortunately 'got away' to a slow start. When it was identified strict quarantine of all traced, affected and/or in-contacts kept it satisfactorily under control. In the year 1993 to November 1994, twenty-two sero-positive imported stallions were identified but only three of these were confirmed shedders.

In countries other than the UK and Ireland there is a high level of sero-positive mares and stallions. In the UK and Ireland equine populations have been shown to be almost wholly non-positive and therefore very susceptible. The overall UK sero-positive rate is less than 0.5%. Studs in this country are wide open to introduced (epidemic) infection from abroad.

Exposure to the virus may result in
• clinical respiratory disease
• sub-clinical respiratory disease
dependent on the
• strain of virus
• size of the 'dose'
• age and physical well-being of the infected horse
• environmental conditions
and it has been shown that
• infection, as judged by sero-conversion to higher antibody levels, can be high in mares exposed to 'shedding' stallions, i.e. venereal contact, but
• clinical respiratory cases can be low, almost sporadic

Transmission – Sources of Contagion

This is by droplet (aerosol) contagion via the URT. There are large quantities of the virus in coughed aerosol, sneezed or snorted aerosol, and nasal secretions

During this time there is a viraemia with excretion subsequently in urine, faeces, semen and aborted foetus and fluids.

After the respiratory signs subside the virus is found
• *only* in semen
• but *not in all stallions*, although such may be sero positive

Such 'shed' (via natural *and* artificial matings) has
• high concentrations during clinical disease
• thereafter still 'dangerous' for
• several weeks to many years
• can occur in originally respiratory sub-clinically affected stallions

A high proportion (*circa* 60%) are shedders for life. *Fertility is unaffected* (the virus does not locate in the testes). Infected mares translocate the venereally acquired virus to the respiratory system which then becomes aerosol contagious.

Respiratory Signs

These are variable, clinical to sub-clinical, but when clinical
• fever

- lethargy
- depression
- distal limb oedema
- conjunctivitis, hence 'pink eye'
- periorbital and upper eyelid oedema
- nasal discharge
- urticarial rashes and plaques
- oedema of the scrotum and udder
- abortion
- fatal cases in the young, old and debilitated have been recorded

It is important that any source of contagion must be contained if a devastating disease outbreak (in UK and Ireland) in the stud industry is to be prevented.

In the UK it is a notifiable disease: the EVA Order 010895.

Immunisation

This is possible but strict controls concerning sera-negative states being first confirmed.

Control

See (in the UK) HRBLB Code of Practice for Studs.

Acute Equine Respiratory Syndrome

In 1994 in Australia an outbreak of acute respiratory disease occurred in a training yard. The trainer and eleven of the fourteen horses died. Five other yards were affected with three out of ten horses dying. The dead trainer's vet and his head lad became quite ill from the same infection.

The fatalities occurred within three days in eleven out of the fourteen following signs of pyrexia, depression, shallow respiration and a frothy nasal discharge.

An autopsy revealed cyanosis of the mucous membranes (oxygen starvation) and severe lung oedema (obstruction to gaseous exchange etc.). The incubation period was eight to sixteen days and spread appeared to depend upon close contact (a fomites discharge contagion rather than an aerosol spread).

A 'new' virus was isolated; it is genetically similar to those already classified in the Morobillivirus family in which human measles, dog distemper, seal illness and rinderpest (cattle) viral agents are grouped. It will be remembered that in the first three there was no evidence of cross-species infection. Strict isolation and movement control seemed to contain this Australian infection whose source or origin remained a mystery until October 1995 when a case in another horse and a human, again in Queensland, occurred but on this occasion, there was no evidence of man and horse contact; they were five hundred miles apart. It is still not known where the virus came from or how it is transmitted; perhaps by an insect vector?

Non-Infectious 'Lung' Dis-ease

Allergic

The most common, by far, is **obstructive pulmonary disease (OPD)**, which rapidly becomes chronic **(COPD)**. It can affect horses and ponies of all types if they have been stabled, which is usually in winter time but not only then, fed on dry hay and (less importantly) bedded on straw. On the basis of opportunity of exposure to the sensitising agent it is more common in horses over 4 years, but is also recognised in younger (usually competitive or racing horses, which of necessity have been housed).

- a primary allergy
- not the same morbidity type as human asthma or 'Farmer's Lung'
- is invariably associated with the inhalation of
  - Micropolyspora and Aspergillus 'vegetable' hyphae and spores, which
  - sensitise the distal respiratory airway defensive cells in the alveoli, to
  - subsequent inhalations which produce clinical signs within 4–8 hours
- is possibly compounded by further allergic reaction by inhalation of
  - stable dust and horse dander
  - 'hay' dust (usually desiccated clover leaf)

  both of which are protein allergens, and
- is susceptible to secondary bronchial bacterial infection

Removal of the source of the allergens, as by turning out, will effect a clinical 'cure' in 4–28 days, but the *sensitivity remains* for further challenge.

A similar symptomatically presented condition is summer grass associated OPD **(SGAOPD)** due to the inhalation, perhaps even the consumption, of certain unidentified grass pollens. It is by definition a spring/summer disease. It is quite quick in onset, but again the horse has to be sensitised to the pollen – which can occur at an unknown time

	Degrees of OPD				
	0	1	2	3	4
Cough frequency	–	Occasional	Intermittent	Frequent	–
Duration of disease	–	0–3 months	3–6 months	6–12 months	12 months +
Dyspnoea	–	Slight	Moderate	Pronounced	Very pronounced
Respiratory rate at rest	8–15	10–14	14–18	18–22	22+
Auscultation	N	Just audible	Audible	Pronounced	Wheezing etc.
Work ouput	N	Slightly affected	Moderately affected	Greatly affected	Severely affected

after being at grass, and is obviously related to the presence of particular pollens.

Another spring/summer asthmatic-like disease can develop from tree pollens. Hay pollen induces an allergic pharyngitis, without pulmonary involvement, from the inhalation of dried grass pollens and possibly clover dust. Coughing is the only clinical sign, hence 'hay cough'.

Not all horses are predisposed to any of these allergies. No doubt there is at least a familial tendency, if not a true hereditable factor, in those that are.

COPD is also known as **'broken wind'** and **'heaves'**. (In fact, recent international discussions on respiratory disease have favoured the term 'heaves', largely on the grounds that COPD in horses is different from that in humans.) These two names 'recognise' the appearance of the double expiratory action in advanced cases with

- chronic bronchitis, and bronchiolitis
- recurrent airway obstruction: and the associated cough

If neglected, the horse may progress to severe respiratory distress associated with

- emphysema: as based on autopsy findings

Signs

- acute
  - dyspnoea (respiratory distress) with flared nostrils
  - coughing – soft, restrained
  - marked changes in respiration pattern, with abdominal muscular expiratory effort
  - possible elevated temperature in secondary infection involvement
  - wheezing or crackling noise when listening at nostrils
  - poor exercise tolerance, but
  - no emotional distress as in humans
- sub-acute
  - coughing – soft, restrained
  - altered breathing pattern is less noticeable
  - exercise intolerance, but the 'fresh air' environment necessary for exercise often ameliorates the active condition

- chronic
  - coughing – loud, explosive, paroxysmal
  - 'heave' line often well established
  - exercise intolerance is persistent

The morbid changes
- constriction of the bronchiolar airways from muscular spastic contraction
- plugging of the airways with abnormal mucus
- reduced ventilation area, and so reduced gaseous exchange

Differential Diagnosis
(as compared with infectious/inflammatory respiratory dis-ease)
- no fever unless secondarily infected
- no inappetence
- slow onset (slower owner appreciation!) but note the
  - dis-ease in brood mare syndrome
  - the neurogenic psychologic case
- seasonal and environmental connections are more remarkable
- usually in the mature and stabled and in the immature horse when stabling is part of the husbandry, as in Thoroughbred racing
- no loss of condition in the first few months at least
- in contrast the obese horse often 'shows' more clinically

Diagnosis
By the horsemaster
- coughing
- wheezing
- no 'illness'
- history re hay and straw use

By the veterinary surgeon
- clinical examination and history
- auscultation
- endoscopy
- tracheal samples
- ELISA tests to identify allergen

Brood mare acute OPD in late pregnancy and early

lactation, develops when 'brought in' at night
- a form of asthma of unknown cause but
- may be hormonal and
- neurogenic, triggered by
- idiopathic allergens in the stable

Signs
- as for acute OPD
  - more obvious distress possibly exacerbated by 'nursing' behaviour activity

Prevention
- do not use hay or straw
- if imperative, make sure they have been well harvested and **obviously** free of mould infestation. Visual freedom, however, does not rule out presently inactive spore contamination
- shake out hay down wind of the stables before filling nets
- better still, feed loose spread on the floor or
- soak the hay thoroughly for one hour before feeding but change from straw to paper bedding and
- do not fill nets or shake out onto the floor or make up the bed if hay/straw must be used, with the horse in the box at the time or
- do not use hay or straw but replace with haylage or the equivalents, use paper bedding and
- keep the horse 'at grass' for as long as possible in every twenty-four hours – upwind of hay/straw barn
- take care that the sensitised horse does not stand immediately downwind of other hay/straw users
- beware previous clinical signs of sensitisation from
  - tree pollen in the spring
  - other pollen sources in the summer
    - SGAOPD from grass pollens
  - hay may harbour the grass pollens which can induce an allergic pharyngitis without pulmonary involvement. Whether from inhalation or ingestion is unclear
    - a cough (hay cough) develops very quickly
- remember, some horses are allergic to their own dander. Clipping should be done in the open or in a separate box. Some animals need to be groomed in the fresh air and brushes knocked clean downwind from them

Another associated condition may be met – **Psycho-neurogenic OPD** is seen mainly in ponies and pony crosses which have been produced for active athletic work. Some are, no doubt, already sensitised subjects but this is not proven nor is the allergen known. By definition they are housed and dry fed. The act of plaiting the mane and other attention associated with hunting and other high activity, especially if done the night before, will induce a broncho-spasm. Significantly, the animal remains alert and bright with a good appetite despite the acute, often apparently severe respiratory wheezing. The horse suddenly develops

- accelerated respirations
- dilated nostrils
- sometimes a diphasic expiration
- wheezing
- coughing
- but is not respiratorily embarrassed

It will respond to symptomatic treatment and will resolve on arrival at the venue. Care must be taken that breathing has returned to normal before appropriate 'warming up' is begun.

CHAPTER 25

DENTAL PROBLEMS

Much of the 'Dawn' horse's original structure and functioning has been affected by evolution, not least the digestive system and the requirement to crop and to masticate the stemmy grasses of the 'new' grazing areas.

Organo-chemical features of these grasses determined the type of teeth necessary. The dental enamel had to be not only the prime material to act as a 'grindstone', but also to protect the other dental components. Its structure within the molar teeth was such as to make it

- prominent on the molar tables and in the vertical cusp tips
- more resilient to the masticatory wear and tear than the other constituents, dentine and cement

The basic feature of evolved herbivorous molar teeth is that they are

- so positioned that the four arcades each present as a contiguous platform with no interdental space
- so 'laid out' *vis à vis* top-to-bottom arcades as to form maximum grinding surfaces relative to the horizontal, semi-circular movement of the lower arcades against the stationary uppers and, from this 'work', they are
  - constantly being worn down
  - continuously exposing more residual crown to compensate for the wear, and continue to do so for many years after the true roots have ceased to grow (at about 6 to 8 years of age)

It says much for the functioning durability of the structures involved in mastication that the main requests for 'dentistry' are

- to maintain a minimally soft-tissue damaging molar table, or occlusal surface, by reducing the points and edges which are 'left' from the wear, and which varies with the type of nutrition
- to maintain a good grinding surface, with some cutting edge, by sensible (skilled) manual reduction – rasping **(molar teeth were never meant to have a smooth, rounded table)**
- to recognise abnormal developmental and eruption conditions and other morbidities which could
  - interfere with prehension (incisor teeth)
  - interfere with mastication (molar teeth)
  - predispose to trapping of food residues, so leading to fermentative damage to the enamel, dentine and the gums

Reappraisal of early twentieth-century veterinary dental knowledge indicates that there is much more to 'points' and hooks than had been appreciated. Moreover, some at least of the more serious dental disorders and subsequent dis-eases arise from the initial cause and later complications of these elementary deficits in molar occlusion. They require correct and detailed examinations. Failure to appreciate their presence and significance, and incorrect treatment, can cause economic and welfare deficits.

An owner's attention to the possibility of an oral problem arises when he sees signs of the horse

- evading the aids of the bit
- having difficulty in chewing
  - head cocked to one side, as though attempting to chew on one side
  - food uncharacteristically spilled from the mouth
- actually 'quidding' out part-chewed, saliva-soaked wads

of prehended food during mastication or soon afterwards

- losing condition

The time-scale of the last three can vary from immediate to progressive.

Loss of condition is not quickly recognised (recognition varies with management skill), and is often the consequence of incomplete mastication **without** a functional difficulty, such as quidding, being apparent

- 'bitting' evasions can be sudden, but more frequently are progressively apparent but usually before the eating difficulties
- regional lymph gland enlargements
- facial and jaw swellings – slowly progressive and, later, a
- discharge through a 'sinus' opening on the rim of the lower jaw
- foetid nasal discharge

None of these is **necessarily** preceded by clinical signs of mastication difficulty, although with hindsight there often will have been some indications. Seen in themselves, as a new 'something wrong', then the veterinary surgeon will at least consider dental disorders high in his list of differential diagnoses.

Dis-ease of oral structures, dental or soft tissue, even when inflammatory and so, by definition, painful, rarely overcomes the horse's survival instinct to eat. It is the **mastication which is compromised**.

In the common 'sharp teeth' situation, it is not pain in the teeth which affects chewing, but the **associated trauma of the tongue and the inside of the cheeks**, and the resultant discomfort or pain. As in all herbivores, horse dental nerve endings are within the pulp cavity, which is well protected by the surrounding enamel, dentine and cement. Penetration into this 'pulp' is, in comparison with man, rare but it does occur.

In the majority of oral inspections, a veterinary surgeon will use a gag to maintain an 'open mouth'. Without this, a full examination of all of the dental arcades cannot be made, nor can correct or even simple treatment of the lower jaw be carried out efficiently.

In many cases it is necessary to restrain the horse with a twitch, or to sedate it chemically – for the safety of the horse, the handler and the vet.

An owner should not attempt more than a superficial inspection of

- the incisors, by lifting the lips
- the tushes, by lifting the lips on that side
- the bars, by lifting the lips on that side, and by carefully palpating along the interdental space
- the first three pre-molars of the top arcades, by 'feeling' their edges through the facial skin

An ability to keep the mouth open, by a trained, skilled grip of the tongue, with thumb pressure on the hard palate will, in the well-held horse, permit

- a sight of the tongue and the rostral molars
- a feel of the inner borders of the first three lower premolars and the upper three molars outside edges

This skill is often learnt the 'hard' way; a crushed nail or lacerated finger is a not uncommon 'training fee'. Without a gag it is stupid to 'blindly' try to feel the back molars.

The veterinary surgeon working with a sedated and gagged horse must insist on the helpers being hard-hatted. Stout shoes are also advisable.

Several of the dis-ease types occur within and around the horse's mouth-parts, and variably require veterinary attention following the horsemaster's report that 'something is wrong' with the affected structures. Such less-than-common conditions account for about 10% of call outs for dentistry. These, plus the 90% for rasping and minor extractions do not, in practice, together exceed 10% of **all** veterinary input. Dental problems include

- **developmental disorders**
- **inflammatory conditions** – perhaps more common in the horse than suspected or even looked for, thus remaining as low grade but often slowly progressive discomforts, reducing
  - food conversion
  - balanced locomotion
  - exercise potential

  and becoming the cause of subsequent
- degenerative defects, and possible
- **neoplastic** disease

DEVELOPMENTAL DIS-EASE

Incisors

Inherited
Common, as in the Welsh breed, especially the pony

- **parrot mouth**, or forward shot **upper** jaw

Parrot mouth.

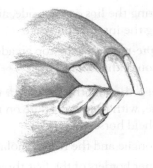

Sow mouth.

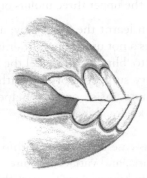

- **sow mouth**, or forward shot *lower* jaw (much less common)

There are anatomical variations to explain these

- an absolute developmental shortening of the receding jaw – the mandible in parrot mouth
- an absolute lengthening of the protruding jaw or a deficit in face/muzzle length

Little research has been done on the geometry of these abnormalities

- patently the articulations of the jaws are still functional
- there is little evidence of nasal defect in the upper jaw, or deficits in the maxillae. Cleft palate is not a concommitant, for instance
- there is a related mal-positioning of not only the incisor teeth but also of the opposing molar 'tables' or occlusal surfaces, making worse the natural effect of masticatory abrasion

The degree of imperfect incisor table occlusion varies from

- almost complete table contact, to
- incomplete, when
    - incision of short grass becomes difficult
    - overhang of one arcade in relation to the other as in parrot mouth, where
        - upper teeth traumatise lower inside lip

- lower teeth traumatise upper gums and hard palate

Congenital

Such rarities do not of course 'show' until eruption occurs: they are 'delayed'

Acquired

Abnormalities of eruption are due to trauma to the unerupted permanent incisor 'buds', from fractures, especially of the rostral mandible in foals and yearlings, leading to

- absence of one or more permanent incisor teeth
- displacement of growth direction, with
    - aberrant eruption
    - impaction

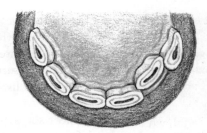

A common form of incisor mal-eruption.

- failure to 'displace' the related temporary tooth
- oblique mal-alignment of bottom jaw with top

These rarely interfere with sucking or eating, and are mainly aesthetic, but uncorrected overlapping of a retained temporary with the erupting permanent will form a food particle trap and subsequent gingivitis. A continuing gap between the top and bottom arcade may lead to overgrowth of the unopposed incisor. Both these situations require veterinary attention.

Canines or tushes

These are present usually in the male. They erupt between 4 and 6 years of age and are rarely 'misplaced'. Their normal position does not involve an upper and lower 'bite'. Smaller type tushes are sometimes seen in mares. Delayed but otherwise normal eruption in one or all four will cause 'teething pain' and, as this often coincides with initial 'schooling on the bit', an evasion is likely.

Eruption can be expedited by

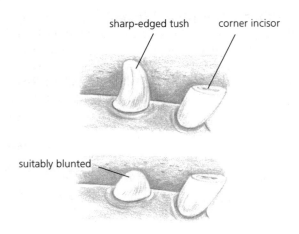

sharp-edged tush   corner incisor

suitably blunted

- gum massage
- veterinary 'lancing'

and followed by a period for gum healing before re-bitting.

In adult horses from 8 years upwards they become
- chisel-edged, when they may ulcerate the tongue, and the contact area of the lips, and must be suitably 'blunted'
- encased in tartar, which ulcerates the gum, causing a gingivitis which is occasionally painful to the point of causing bit evasion; the scale is relatively easily removed and this is effected usually when rasping is done

Wolf Teeth – The 'First' True Premolars

As a rule, these are situated close up against the next 'proper' premolar. When present (not all horses have them), they are most often seen in the top jaw, occasionally in both and, very rarely, only in the bottom. They are not always bilaterally similar in length of 'crown' and of root.

In a minority of cases they are situated well rostral to the premolar, and occasionally erupt somewhat laterally. In these forward positions they are more likely to be in contact with the bit, and so can be disruptive. 'Blind' wolf teeth are not uncommon and such un-erupted teeth are invariably forward. The teething pain is bit-evasive in effect. Veterinary removal is advisable when

- the consensus is that, although they do not normally interfere with prehension and mastication, arguably
- they might interfere with bitting. This is more likely to be the case when

- they are small and rooted superficially, so that they irritate gum nerve endings when a bit makes contact and 'vibrates' them
- double bitting (a double bridle) is used
- extreme collection is required, with associated head carriage as in dressage riding

Removal is usually easy, but it is essential to take the whole tooth out and not leave a root behind. Other than with small 'wolves', which can be 'knocked out' by a skilled person, such removal requires 'loosening' and elevation after gum incision. It is invariably done under a local anaesthetic of the gum and may require sedation of the horse, when local anaesthesia can be dispensed with. Several days or even weeks must be allowed for wound healing before re-bitting – otherwise further evasion may set in.

The Molars

The time schedule of molar teeth eruption is described in Chapter 8, TEETH.

In the maxillae, the roots of the permanent 5, 6 and 7 project upwards into the maxillary para-nasal sinuses, where they are covered and, in health, separated from the sinus cavities by a thin layer of fragile bone. A sinusitis can develop when the apices are inflamed.

In the mandibles, the erupting permanent premolars (2, 3 and 4) are doing so ventrally 'against' jaw bone which is narrow and shallow and is in fact almost totally occupied by teeth root and reserve crown. A sterile painless bone hyperplasia results and, in some cases, is seen as an irregular basal outline.

The reaction is most prominent under premolar 4. Recent research indicates that there is more to this than just downward pressure. The clinical signs 'smooth out' with time in most cases.

In horses with a 'short' head, really foreshortened nose and face, most frequently in crossbred animals a **ramp** formation between the last premolar and the first molar may develop with sharp edges as well as points on three sides of each.

Eruption Problems

The residual six temporary premolars over the erupting permanents are called 'caps' which are pushed out and disposed of orally on to grazing. It is doubtful if they are swallowed, and certainly not without being crushed into small pieces. Occasionally, a 'cap' is found in a manger.

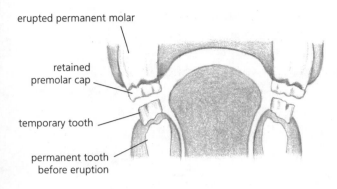

erupted permanent molar

retained
premolar cap

temporary tooth

permanent tooth
before eruption

Retained premolar caps may cling to the erupting
permanent molars.

Retained Premolar Caps

This occurs most commonly to 3 and 4 upper temporary molars, and occasionally also in the lower jaw

- the residual roots occasionally 'cling' to the erupting permanent molar
- with mastication they can be rotated horizontally and further jammed down
- the rotation leaves the sharp roots overhanging, or
- one or more may be driven into the cement of the 'new' table

Before they are dislodged naturally or by manual interference, they will

- irritate tongue and cheek
- cause interference with mastication and bitting
- predispose the 'new' tooth to
  - gingivitis
  - peridontitis and, less commonly
  - caries

Root growth, as distinct from on-going eruption, ceases around 6 years of age. By biodynamic means not yet fully understood, the root and residual crown are slowly and regularly 'lifted' or pushed towards the gum line to equate with the wearing away of the true crown by mastication. Thereby, until the late teens, effective overt crown lengths are maintained. From 20 years on, the residual crown is 'used up' and the inert true roots are all that is gripped by the alveolar bone. Eventually that is not enough, and molar tooth loss occurs. The mature horse's crown length varies, molar to molar and horse to horse. It is usually greatest in molars 3 and 4 but 'falling out' has no regular pattern.

Overcrowding of Erupting Molars

Especially in cross-bred animals there may be insufficient jawbone for the full complement of the total molar arcades, particularly when the permanent molars are erupting not only against the temporaries, but also the 4th against the same arcade's 5th. The 2nd and 3rd can also be involved between 3 and 4 years of age, all resulting in

- displacement laterally, to cause gum aberrant ulceration
- impaction, with subsequent damage to the roots, apical root/alveolar bone disease, leading to
  - sinusitis in the upper jaw
  - periostitis, jaw swelling, and sinus formation in the lower jaw

Surgical treatment is usually required, although antibiotic therapy may subdue a secondary infection until the jaw's growth accommodates the tooth.

Only in exceptional circumstances (old age) can molar teeth be simply orally extracted. In earlier years their root and residual crown length require surgical exposure through the bone to permit loosening of the alveolar 'hold', and then back-punching; or, if the bone is laterally elevated to expose the root, the tooth can be 'lifted out' sideways. Either way, a gap in the arcade is left, which prevents natural wear of the opposing tooth. Its resultant uncontrolled 'eruption' must be rasped away at frequent intervals.

More recently it has become the practice in cases of mandibular root inflammation, with possible infection, for the root to be exposed from the outside and the apex cut and drilled to remove the infection, and to allow the related bony swelling to subside (it is then 'plugged'). It is this swelling which is often the first indication of 'something wrong'.

Severe trauma to any molar tooth

- to the jaw externally, or
- on to the tooth, as by biting on a stone

can fracture (split) the molar down to its root, or indirectly split the roots, resulting in

- exposure of the pulp cavity, with descending infection and
- apical root disease subsequently

Impacted molar 7 (human wisdom teeth retention) is not a common abnormality in the horse.

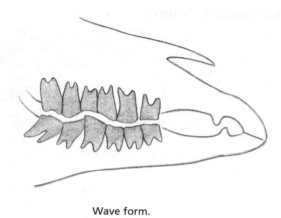

Wave form.

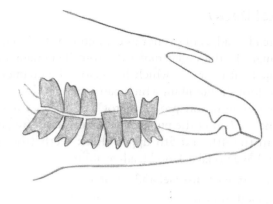

Wave form with a 'step'.

Abnormalities of Molar Wear

Irregular crown lengths can be seen along the whole arcade in some horses; the resultant profile is called **wave form**, which interferes with occlusion or apposition of top and bottom molars and, more importantly, with mastication.

It is said that in cross-bred horses there is a variation in eruption time and crown length between premolar and molar teeth which often results in a marked 'step' between premolars 4 and molars 5 and occasionally an interdental space. This defect exacerbates any 'waviness' coincidentally present.

As has been described, the normal chewing pattern causes incomplete wear of the tables, whereby

- the *outer* edge of the *upper* molars is left long
- the *inner* edge of the *lower* molars is left long, and
- the rostral occlusal surface of the upper 2nd premolar may be left as a **hook**
- the caudal occlusal surface of lower molar 7 may also be left as a hook (usually but not always in association with an upper 2nd premolar hook)
- in some cases, there is a reversal of the hook formation to lower premolar 2 and upper molar 7

Where there is a parrot mouth (or sow mouth) tendency there is often a mal-relationship between upper and lower arcades; wear becomes more abnormal and particularly exacerbates the formation of hooks and points. It is these projections of enamel which must be reduced and blunted. Failure to keep them as near normal as possible will increase the risk of low grade mouth discomfort but, more importantly, an altered pattern of chewing – which leads to

- torque and lever forces between adjacent molars with widening of the interdental spaces, leading to
- retention of food particles, and subsequent
- gingivitis, and eventual
- peridontitis
- overstress of the tempero-mandibular joint

INFLAMMATORY DIS-EASE

Gingivitis – Inflammation of the Gums

- usually in the interspace of two molars
- abrasive effect of putrefying trapped foodstuffs
- further erosion can lead to an interdental trough from lingual to labial borders, with further food entrapment

Once gum recession becomes established, a cure is not possible. Dental hygiene is then difficult to effect but must be continued regularly with saline lavage.

Peridontitis – Inflammation of the Related Gum and Bone

An extension of the above into the tooth socket, the alveolus, with involvement of reserve crown as well as the surrounding bone. This leads to apical root disease and so to

- **fistulous mandible**, from resultant purulent abscess formation
- **paranasal sinusitis**, and resultant empyema

Dental Decay

As already said, caries is not as common in the horse as it is in man. In the molar tables the so-called enamel lakes are filled with cement which lies below the enamel rims and so forms infundibuli which can retain food. Its subsequent fermentation products 'rot' the enamel and the dentine, and enter the pulp cavity. This is most frequently seen in the 4th and 5th upper cheek teeth (the lower molars have no lakes), and leads again to

- **maxillary root disease**, and possible
- paranasal sinusitis

It is recognised that such inflammatory and/or caried teeth are most likely to be associated with

- retention of caps
- development and eruption changes in the 3–5 year-old
- disorders of wear in the older (15-plus) horse

All are associated with a foetid smell, or halitosis (bad breath). These are all matters for veterinary attendance.

Most mandibular clinical swellings are not neoplastic but periapical abscessation associated with permanent molar eruption defects, caries and peridontal diseases, as well as from

- external trauma – reactive ostitis following a blow
- bit trauma to the mandibular bar – 'broken' or ulcerated – with secondary infection and periostitis. This only very rarely progresses sufficiently to distort the cheeks. Since it occurs rostral to the molars in the lower jaw there is no apical root disease. Bit evasion and altered head carriage are the presenting signs

Occasionally a sliver of surface bone will be discharged or have to be removed before the gum will heal. This is the result of traumatic thrombosis of the sub-mucosal arterioles which nourish the thin cortical bone; the related length necroses, and becomes a foreign body. The condition is sometimes referred to as 'broken jaw'.

In both situations the primary trauma is the result of excessive and/or prolonged bit pressure. It is more often seen as a unilateral condition, but some bruising at least can be detected in the other bar as well. Good healing requires

- saline lavage
- time
- awareness of the possibility of a bone sliver in the 'slow to heal' ulcer
- attention to future bitting and riding

Degenerative Defects

Dental tissue does not degenerate, in the sense of bone, cartilage and ligament changes in the arthroses. As described above under caries, dental tissue can be eroded by the bi-products of fermentation, and further destroyed by infectious inflammation. Long before a tooth degenerates, its supporting tissues, both soft and bony, will lose their grip and an obviously caried tooth will fall out either as a whole or as pressure-fractured halves (split between the roots).

Neoplastic

There are two main groups, but all types are relatively uncommon, especially the first group, even in humans

- **group 1** – basically developmental neoplasia, which can disfigure the surrounding supportive tissue, whereby it looks like the primary tumour. They are collectively known as odontogenic tumours and are usually intra-mandibular
- **group 2** – osteogenic tumours
  - mainly benign mandibular and maxillary growths of bony origin and, less commonly
  - secondary malignant mandibular cancers from the oral pharyngeal epithelium

Practical Observations

In the wild, a horse with poor dentition was likely to
- fare worse nutritionally
  - lose condition
  - become weak and subject to intercurrent dis-ease
    - be liable to predation

Hereditable perpetuation of this deficit was less likely because of loss of fertility and early death

In domestication, simple deficits such as excessive 'points' were reasonably assumed and readily confirmed and treated by rasping. Breeding from such animals was not contra-indicated.

The production of points is an inevitable consequence of normal equine mastication. Attention to feeding practice and routine dental hygiene care is capable of preventing most of the associated more serious disorder. Culling is therefore, theoretically at least, unnecessary except for severe conditions known to be hereditable.

The degree differs one side of the jaws to the other and is usually more marked in the lower (mandibular) left arcade. It is these 'normal' or naturally developing points which require routine assessment with regard to rasping, both for immediate reduction of irritation and for longer term benefits such as the prevention of non-natural, abnormal development of more serious morphological changes such as hooks, and better food conversion results, economics and better welfare.

On most normal teeth the sweep of grinding decreases towards the edges of the molars whereby the enamel cusps, buccal in the maxilla, and lingual in the mandible, are left with a narrow but extra sharp point. These are potential causes and often are, of irritation of the cheek and/or the gum mucosae.

In corn-fed horses the occlusal pressures continue but the range lessens (the feed is more easily and quickly ground). As a result the points are left more exposed, not only vertically but also further centrally. This results in

- sharper, wider, long points
- the formation of a continuous line to form a serrated 'edge'

Domestication has had its effects indirectly through
- younger horses in work
- more 8–15 year-olds kept in competition work
- older mares kept for breeding – 15 to 24 year-olds
- geriatrics over 20 years old kept as pets or as nursemaids

all increasing the duration of other more direct domestic influences on dental structure and functioning.

Dental disorders are exacerbated and more common in stall-fed animals. and of greater incidence in some cross-breds from, e.g.

- unbalanced skull morphology
  - incisor occlusion deficits
  - deficits in molar arcade configurations and occlusions
- mixed maturity ages
  - jaw size variations
  - eruption time differences

Most importantly, the management changes in domesticated nutrition and digestion, especially in working and performance horses, are associated with alterations to dental functioning and structures, e.g.

- interruption to natural 'continuous' grazing and mastication reduced salivation flow time and quantity.

Despite the close packed arcade, equine saliva must also have had a mechanical lavaging effect

- replacement of grass by conserved grass as hay, etc
- the energy demands requiring supplementary cereal feeds (chaff, chop and small particle-size grain pieces were more likely to get 'between the teeth') when trapped orally were more readily fermented with morbid effect
- the marked change in how the horse was fed was most significant
  - out of a net
  - out of a manger
  well off the ground and so not allowing it to feed naturally (when prehension, ingestion, mastication and deglutition took place with neck and head down and with the muzzle on the ground)

There is evidence that when a horse's head comes down its mandible moves rostrally relative to the maxillae, so bringing the lower incisor table partially in front of the upper.

This forward shift must bring the mandibular molars equally forward of the upper, which is said to be necessary for correct mastication and molar table wear.

There is evidence that when rostral mandibular maxillary apposition change is prevented by head-high feeding there is a deficit in the wear of the upper premolar 2 and the lower molar 7. Consequently, the overhangs develop as a hook. It is these hooks and other more minor irregularities which start off further molar table occlusal deficits and subsequent dis-ease as well as deficit mastication.

Differences in attrition wear is not due to dry feeding as distinct from grass; silica is present in all feeds and in grazing and relative to soil contamination as well as that within the grass. *It is the head position that matters.*

When not masticating, the more caudal position is assumed to be the most comfortable – and so too in equitation. Overbent head carriage is not just a respiratory problem but also a factor of jaw joint articulation.

Observation shows that with free access, hay on a stable floor is usually eaten in 10–12 sessions of varying duration once the horse has settled in, which reasonably simulates grazing.

Complete compound rations, offered at intervals, are much more quickly consumed per feeding and overall – leaving more time for boredom.

It has been found in research that over a period of time on an all-hay diet there is no adverse effect on molar table occlusion and attrition provided the horse is floor fed.

Compound rations do have an adverse effect, whether high or low fed, but again the effect is worse when fed high.

The incisor teeth, no longer needed for cutting, just 'grasping' hay, are noticeably less worn by attrition. Eventually their elongation has an effect on molar table occlusion – the molars cannot fully make contact; changes in wear pattern follow.

The oblique rotary grinding action and range of the molars in a healthy, normally conformed mouth whose tables paralleled at a horizontal angle of 10–15% is considerably reduced when concentrates are fed, especially alone or when the long fibres of hay are but a minimal proportion of the total feed intake or were chopped. There is a consequent reduction in the need for full-range mastication (and for the time spent, in doing so, *vis à vis* saliva production). The rotary cross-wear attrition of the tables falls shorter than normal of the buccal edge of the maxillary molars and the lingual edge of the mandibular. A molar 'vaulting' develops. It is the easier mastication of cereals which produces thicker points which give stall feeding the blame – not the feed itself.

Nevertheless the degree of attrition in **all** circumstances is due to the silica in grass **and** in herbage harvested and/or conserved.

Dental problems can predispose to other equine disorders
- directly related to deficits in mastication
  - indigestion and poorer food conversion
  - **impactions**
  - diarrhoea
  - **choke**
  - other colics and with
  - possible increase the risk of DDSP
- indirectly, evasions from bit aids
  - these often show more quickly than 'indigestion' and are related to the causes of, as distinct from actual deficits in, mastication
    - from mouth pain
    - uni- or bilaterally and subsequent
    - deficits in equitation control
      - indirect from evading head and from neck imbalances both possibly leading to
      - lameness (often subtle)

It is frequently necessary to manually structure a 'bit seat'

on the lower two 2nd premolars, and occasionally the uppers to prevent the bit riding up onto the table. 'Getting the tongue over the bit' then becomes more likely.

Management

Dental and oral health requires
- a careful, comprehensive examination of
  - all the teeth
    - the bony structures
    - the related tissues
- awareness that domesticated feedstuffs and feeding present the horse with
  - feed times which meet man's ideas, and so an irregular salivary flow with interruption to the otherwise almost continuous dental hygiene in grazing
  - concentrates, which more readily ferment in the mouth when trapped
  - chaff, chop and some concentrates all of small particle size, more likely to 'get between the teeth'

Veterinary inspection will in addition look for
- lip abnormalities, especially the commissures
- tongue injuries
- cheek abrasions, especially just inside and caudal to the commissure opposite the upper molars
- gum disorders
  - bit evasion
    - broken jaw
  - lower molar 7 hook interference with angle of the jaws
  - interdental inflammation
  - lower rami undulations
  - thickening on face over maxillary roots
  - sinusitis
    - by percussion
    - nasal discharge
  - throat dysfunctions
  - respiratory dysfunctions
- condition loss
- evasions
  - head carriage

In the United Kingdom the requirements of the Veterinary Surgeons' Act do not apply where routine work does *not* involve penetration of vascular tissue. Thus, subject only to the Protection of Animals' Welfare Acts, i.e. the prevention of cruelty, lay people may rasp the teeth of horses which are not their own or their employer's, and may do so for reward. They may also remove loose caps. This subject is covered in greater detail in Part 1, Chapter 8, THE TEETH.

CHAPTER 26

DISEASES OF THE DIGESTIVE SYSTEM

In man, a disorder of the digestive system is primarily associated with 'indigestion'; what has been eaten has not been properly digested. As a consequence, there are subjective signs (symptoms, the patient can describe them) not perceived when all is well. These vary from a 'touch of indigestion', flatulence, and some discomfort to severe stomach ache, with vomiting, diarrhoea or constipation, a disturbed appetite and thirst, and general malaise. The pain from the morbidity may originate in the

- distal oesophagus and the stomach
- small intestine
- large intestine and caecum

when it is called **alimentary pain**, or in one or other of the other organs and tissues within the abdominal cavity

- liver and gall bladder (but the horse has no gall bladder)
- kidneys and urinary bladder, and their ducts
- womb

when it is called **abdominal pain**

But disorders of the alimentary system as a whole refer as well to those related tissues '*outside*' the abdominal cavity. Such morbidity has an indirect effect on digestion, but does not, *per se*, cause indigestion.

EXTRA-ABDOMINAL SYSTEMS

Problems in the extra-abdominal system cause difficulties in obtaining nourishment – an inability to eat and/or to swallow

- **prehension**, involving lips and incisor teeth

- **mastication**, involving molar teeth and tongue
- **deglutition**, involving tongue, throat and gullet (or cervical and thoracic oesophagus)

The relevant tissues are in the head, neck and chest areas, all part of the single tubular digestive tract which runs from the mouth to the stomach. They are subject to most of the usual 'Types of dis-ease', both structurally and in functioning, just as the abdominal organs are, each in its own way.

An inability, despite a desire, to prehend, masticate and swallow food can be catastrophic. Where there is a less than total inability in one or all three, the effect can be 'under-nourishment'.

In the domesticated animal, the substitution of alternative 'suckable' ingredients such as liquid gruel and very wet mashes can maintain life if and until recovery from the disabling condition is effected if possible. Stomach tubing (nasopharyngeal intubation) is a passive method of ingestion where inability (and/or lack of desire) exists. Intravenous 'feeding' is a final resort.

Developmental

Inherited and/or congenital dis-eases are relatively uncommon. When they do appear, their severity very much determines survival of the foal both directly and on economic grounds.

The most common such dis-ease, 'parrot mouth', is the least disastrous, hence its constant recurrence in certain breeds – it is not 'lethal'.

Some inherited, latent congenital, or delayed, are recognised

- flaccidity of the oesophagus

- stricture (narrowing) in the oesophagus
- other acquired strictures may also develop in the gullet. These will progressively present as deglutition defects ('choke'), a temporary but in some cases recurrent condition, and ulceration from swallowed foreign bodies, and are often lethal from resulting permanent constriction

Inflammatory

Trauma

- severe lacerations of lips and tongue
- displaced fractures of incisor and molar lower arcade
- compressed fractures of molar upper arcades
- penetrating injuries (e.g. bites) of the throat and of the neck in the left jugular groove

Viral

- acute URT (upper respiratory tract) infection

Bacterial

- strangles as a specific primary disease
- paranasal sinusitis
- pharyngeal abscesses
- regional lymphadenitis
  these last three are also usually from secondary bacterial infection
- tetanus and
- botulism as specific toxin damage to the related motor nerves, the former a tetany, the latter a flaccid paralysis
- pharyngeal foreign bodies
- guttural pouch ulceration from
  - mycosis, with ulceration and
  - secondary nerve damage and subsequent throat paresis

Metabolic

- vitamin E deficiency myopathy preventing sucking and drinking in the foal

Neoplastic

- e.g. melanomata and external pressures onto the throat and intro-abdominally) as with
- lymphosarcomata

Functional

- oesophageal choke
- grass sickness
- motor neurone disease

Choke (Oesophageal)

The signs are usually dramatically diagnostic. The immediate history is often significant.

Treatment

- remove all hay, feed and water and replace straw bedding with paper, shavings and/or peat
- if behaviour is violent (subjects rarely lie down or go down as with colic) it may make handling in a loose box somewhat dangerous; remove any injurious objects and leave alone
- when quieter but still intermittently 'choking' lead out and walk around for 15–20 minutes. Most chokes are self-curing, and exercise helps soothe the anxiety and this in turn relaxes the gullet
- **do not** drench
- **do not** attempt to stomach tube
- **do not** attempt to massage any suspected obstruction down the neck

The veterinary surgeon will intravenously inject a smooth muscle relaxant. He may also decide that antibiotic cover is necessary against any coincidental inhalation of saliva and foodstuff.

He will later, when the horse is over the choke and relaxed, check its teeth, as imperfect mastication can be a contributory factor to choke.

Keep the horse off feed of any sort for 2 hours; thereafter off during next 6 hours, with small quantities of grass at 30-minute intervals. Grazing may be permitted the next day and a slow return to normal diet over 3–4 days, and work at a progressive level at the same time.

Make certain any management factor which is thought by the veterinary surgeon to be related is not repeated. Have the teeth seen to.

INTRA-ABDOMINAL SYSTEMS

There is an understandable tendency to see digestive diseases as being entirely related to this area. By definition, once ingesta has entered the stomach and beyond, any interference with its

- digestion
- undigested residue evacuation
- absorption of the digesta into the venous and lymphatic drainage to the liver (and onwards)

is considered to be a digestive disorder.

As such, there will be

- morbid changes in the relevant tissues
- disruption in digestion and absorption
- disturbances, direct and indirect, in vascular and neural systems
- changes in faecal consistency and quantity
    - more rapid evacuation – diarrhoea
    - slower and reduced evacuation regressing to **ileus** (obstruction resulting from lack of movement) and impaction
    - retention of gas with tympanitic distension
    - absorption of toxins from
        - altered digestion
        - enteric pathogenic bacteria
        - moulds

It will be appreciated that all animals 'eat to live'. Only man can afford the luxury of also 'living to eat', when pleasure comes before necessity. Like man, animals do go 'off their food'. In the horse, though relatively rare, it may be sudden and complete, but in less hyperacute situations it is more likely to be *progressive* and *selective* – first going off the hard food, then the hay, finally the grazing and succulents, before becoming complete.

Pica (depraved appetite) may develop at any stage, a taste for extra-sweet or extra-bitter feedstuffs, eating soil and faeces.

Equine instinct to graze and to browse, including tree 'barking', is a survival instinct. It takes much to put a horse 'off its feed'. Some feedstuffs will be refused because of abhorrent taste or smell, but increasing hunger, if grazing is scarce, can overcome these defences.

Progressive unwillingness to eat is also associated with dis-eases of other body systems, especially when their morbidity produces

- loss of the senses of taste and of smell
- severe fatigue
- heat stress
- septicaemia, toxaemia and poisoning

- hyperacute respiratory distress (too busy getting air!)
- shock, including that associated with
    - haemorrhage
    - severe trauma
    - central (cranial) nerve dis-ease
    - anaphylaxis

Such horses are clinically ill or 'sick' – right off their food – they are **inappetent**; the lack of nourishment can hasten the lethal outcome.

Inflammatory
- alimentary tract

Bacterial
These are an on-going possibility when one considers

- sources of food
- inquisitive licking
- self and companion grooming
- fomites onto food and into water

all of which can carry many pathogens potentially virulent to equines.

Several factors, genetically programmed, mitigate against the effects of such invasions

- ingesta is a constant and continuing one-way through-put; therefore time for bacteria to colonise is minimal
- gut environments of variable pH from the exocrene secretions are 'anti-sepsis'
- the mucous membrane is well equipped physically, physiologically and immunologically with defensive barriers
- the functionally necessary micro-organisms, plentiful in the tract, and especially in the large intestines, are themselves 'anti' potential invaders. Their own short life, disintegration and liberation of antigerm endotoxins cope under normal conditions. The risk is greater in the foal with its immature defences. (See also Laminitis and its relationship to sudden gut overloading with excess soluble sugars, and subsequent entero-toxaemia)

As will be emphasised under Diarrhoea, some virulent strains of bacteria can colonise with a severe invasive and toxic effect.

It is postulated that an undermining of the natural

defences is a prerequisite of such disease, e.g.

- malnutrition or mistakes in feeding and feedingstuffs
- prolonged stress being particularly important
- over-exertion
- intercurrent systemic disease
- current digestive disease, not necessarily infectious

Active infections lead to pathological disturbance of structure and functioning of the abdominal digestive tract, with

- altered rate of peristalsis, including atony and ileus, or conversely hyper-peristalsis with diarrhoea
- disturbed enzymatic and electrolytic content
- abnormal pH of the gut content, which can lead to upset of normal gut micro-organism flora
- ulcerative and erosive trauma within the mucosae, e.g. Salmonellae in helminth-induced ulcers
- Streptococcal abcessation of regional lymph glands and peritoneum
- Clostridial spores, gut-active in association with lush grass ingestion, and their subsequent endotoxin release
- food-borne toxin, e.g. botulism
- exotic potential pathogens such as listeria, campylobacter and toxoplasma
- fungal infections
- aflatoxins from mouldy feeds

with absorption to the liver – hepatoxicity is always a subsequent possibility, as is septicaemia in some types.

At one time it was argued that over-use of oral antibiotics, in dose rate and duration, could lead to opportunistic or coincidental pathogenic organisms replacing the essential micro-organisms. There is now a belief that a disease which specifically required such oral medication was itself a bowel stressor.

Endoparasitic infestations are perhaps the single greatest cause of gut morbidity, with variable consequences.

Allergic

Bowel-active conditions are not a direct problem, despite the oral being a simple route for ingestion of allergens

- diarrhoea can be an additional sign in purpura haemorrhagica
- extra-abdominal exhibition of secondary lesions in the
  - respiratory system
  - skin

from primary alimentary dis-ease.

Metabolic

By definition, this occurs following biochemical disorders associated with absorbed nutrients within other systems' cellular structures. The consequences may be spread vascularly to other parts, including the digestive system as a whole. Gut peristalsis can be speeded up or, more usually, slowed down, to full stop – an ileus.

The myopathy associated with low selenium and vitamin E intake, as in ponies on very poor pastures, or in old ponies with hyperlipaemia, can be clinically evinced in the muscles of prehension. Inappetence, as well as inability to prehend, is present. An ongoing thirst cannot be satisfied, as the sucking up of water cannot be effected. The pony just splashes its muzzle in the water but does not imbibe.

Degenerative

Aged teeth are a recognised problem of direct digestive disorder.

Neoplasia

Neoplastic changes, usually of **lymphosarcoma**, affect

- regional lymph glands, which can cause pressure obstruction on the wall of the digestive system from the throat to the small colon
- space-occupying lesions of the peritoneum where, in addition to lymph gland invasion, they grow on the mesentery and omentum

where they can become 'entangled' with the intestines and cause colic, or actually in the gut wall to be one cause of

- small intestine malabsorption syndrome, and
- large intestine diarrhoea from failure to reabsorb water

Melanomas – as the most common 'tumour', especially in grey horses

- perineal where, despite remarkable growth, there is little interference with defecation
- subcutaneous lateral to pharyngeal area, where pressure has effect on deglutition, usually minimal
- intra-abdominal; rarely life threatening *per se* but may loop around gut/mesentery and cause vascular strangulation and colic

ABDOMINAL PAIN

The *extensive surface area* of the gut, and consequent extensive vascular and nervous ramifications, expose it to

- over-dilation and stretch
- constriction and compression
- extremes of peristaltic movement which interfere with blood flow and hyper stimulate the sensory nerve endings

The resultant severe sensation of pain is the main cause of a horse's marked clinical reaction to 'gut' disorders. It is not an individual low pain threshold but is due, in particular, to the

- relatively small stomach, which is structurally incapable of regurgitating

  - excess gas
  - retained or refluxed fluid
  - 'irritating' ingesta

Even onward movement of these is often interrupted. The horse cannot 'belch' (eructate) or be sick, unless when the stomach has ruptured – with fatal effect from a septic peritonitis

- the relatively long small intestine, loosely suspended along most of its length – the coils of the jejunum and ileum

  - can be convulsed into a twist – or rotated around another part
  - pulled or pushed by peristaltic motion through openings in the mesentery, normal or acquired
  - telescoped one part into another – intussusception

- the voluminous caecum is easily impacted or gaseously distended

- the folded (four times) large colon is of varying diameters, with transverse and longitudinal motility and, on its left aspect, mesentery freedom, whereby

  - when distended and/or atonic in a length, can be twisted on itself – a **volvulus**
  - and become **impacted** at its flexures

- the on-going relatively slow fermentative large bowel digestion (up to 56 hours) of a basic 'ballast' of cellulose-rich roughage

  - the extensive serous (outer) coat, the visceral peritoneum, is rich in sensory nerve endings, and so very sensitive to over stretch

- the single access from the abdominal aorta to the greater part of the visceral blood supply, whose entire arterial component is subject to trauma from migrating strongyle larvae – seriously so, at the aortic junction – within the mesentery and within the gut wall

- the extensive 'end' artery system is subject to helminth (larval) damage, especially by thrombi

- the intrinsic and extrinsic neural control of

  - peristalsis
  - digestive enzyme secretion

  are particularly sensitive to

    - physical pressure, e.g. helminth larvae in the mucosae
    - inflammatory damage to the bowel mucosal wall with disturbed autonomic nervous system input
    - endocrine secretions from other organs and from electrolyte levels

When, for whatever reason, these structures and functionings are

- dis-ordered
- distended
- compressed
- obstructed
- inflamed
- metabolically and/or vascularly compromised

and directly or indirectly affected with

- hyperactivity, or
- hypoactivity

the sensory input to the CNS (central nervous system) is markedly altered, and registers pain. When this passes the arbitrary point of 'mild discomfort' it is called **colic**.

There is also neuro-hormonal positive feedback which further alters functioning.

Colic

The consequent reflexly induced response is mainly that of an *altered behaviour pattern*, primarily with

- voluntary locomotor activity
- involuntary 'other system' activity, or inactivity especially in other areas of the digestive system itself – a

secondary effect with

- hold-up of digesta – impaction and wall stretch and muscle spasm, with likely
    - subsequent further gas entrapment – dilation – further pain, or
- hyperpropulsion of ingesta with excess water output – **diarrhoea**

The veterinary surgeon, as clinician, as surgeon, or finally as pathologist, will sooner or later be able to describe the particular digestive organ affected and specifically what the morbidity is, or was.

It is not surprising that the horsemaster has considerable difficulty in even hazarding a guess. He has no need to try. *Recognition of the presence of colicky pain is itself sufficient*; observation could divide it into 'mild' or 'severe signs' as judged by the horse's behaviour, but even this is arbitrary, and is *not always of accurate prognostic value*.

However, statistically, the majority of colics, about 80%, are **simple** or **benign**, meaning self-limiting or medically remedial, unlikely to be life threatening and, by definition, not requiring surgery. They may develop

- acutely, suddenly and be noticeably painful
- sub-acutely, gradually, within an hour or so of first suspicions, with variable degrees and duration of pain
- chronically, developing over several days, when the pain is often low grade and variably intermittent

Vital signs as judged during these stages are

- increased heart rate up to 50bpm but dropping between bouts
- increased respiration rate, but often irregular, with dilated nostrils
- temperature usually normal – beware interpreting any temperature change; it is not too important and is often misleading. However, peritonitis and acute colitis will induce a fever
- patchy 'cold' sweating

The protracted condition is reasonably easily controlled, mainly by veterinary administered antispasmodics and analgesics, but may also require stomach-tubed medication.

The signs of pain relate to an irregular, in speed and intensity, peristalsis, caused by

- segmental over-contractions developing into bowel wall spasms with on-and-off pain

- gas entrapment, cranial to any obstruction or spasm, with serous coat overstretch
- possible cranial intussusception with physico-functional obstruction
- obstruction as with impactions which distend the related bowel wall

The obstructions can cause secondary ischaemia with cramp of areas of the bowel, whereby pain is much increased, possible further interference with vascular and nerve supply and so to more severe signs of colic and regression to complex conditions.

Hence the need to see all cases of colic as potentially serious. They must be veterinarily managed if persistent for more than one hour or are possibly mild but repetitive over 24 hours.

The use of analgesics is to reduce the pain-causing tensions

- permit the return of more normal functioning
- minimise the risk of self injury

A minority (some 10–15%) are **complex** or **non-benign**, often only surgically remedial, more likely to be seriously life-threatening unless recognised and dealt with surgically *within 8 hours from the onset*. More urgent surgical intervention is often required if such cases are only found when the onset was not witnessed, just the ongoing fact.

These are variably acute in onset, usually, severe

- may rapidly develop from a simple type to a violent state
- easily recognised, certainly as a colic, if not immediately as a surgical case
- not self-limiting, usually progressive. Analgesics etc. may give only temporary relief; approximately 50% will respond to intensive medical intervention

In both simple and complex states, despite a good initial response, there is always the risk of relapse to an acute situation or regression to a chronic state – beware!

The remainder are surgical cases with *a 75% success rate if undertaken before the onset of gut wall morbidity*, hypoxia and/or necrosis, hence the 8-hour protocol.

Some surgical cases are confirmed to be in-operable at the initial laparotomy, i.e. opening into the abdomen

- too much gut damaged – especially length-wise
- insufficient digestive system would be left for efficiency

- unrealistic and unfair (welfare grounds)
- 'shock' of surgery makes it not a viable proposition
- affected site out of operator's reach
- a·collapsed, toxic, shocked case is hopeless

If a 'no hope' case becomes obvious during surgery, euthanasia on the advice of the surgeon in charge **must** be agreed to. There is no question of a further referral.

The equine abdominal cavity permits two surgeons to work 'hands in', but also has several inaccessible areas.

Signs

Colicky pain, but this may be misleading

- a **benign** colic such as spasmodic can produce violent behaviour, disproportionate to the morbidity – the horse perceives it differently!
- a potential or early **non-benign** case, e.g. bowel displacement with, as yet, little vascular interference, may start with mild intermittent pain, even just a discomfort which goes unseen unless routine 'stables' skills are exercised, when changes in appetite, thirst, defecation and demeanour should be noticed at routine 'stables' or at work

Take no chances. See them as colic even in the absence of more specific signs.

In simple cases, recovery cannot be presumed until the horse is keen to eat with no subsequent (within 10 to 30 minutes) bout of pain, and/or is passing faeces normal in consistency if not in quantity.

In simple impacted cases, presumed recovery must await passing of faeces, successive excreta becoming more normally formed, softer and not mucus-coated.

In complex colic, but also in some acute benign cases, the horse will show other behavioural changes

- restlessness – pacing the box, dejected stance, ears back, stretching, going down, and getting up, anxiously looking round at flank
- abdomen – distension, tenseness
- as pain increases – pawing, adopting staling position, stales in early stages, variably repeated or prolonged after staling position, stretches into rocking horse position and looks round or kicks at abdomen
- patchy 'cold' sweating
- increasing restlessness and more severe pain – hesitant lying down, gets up quickly, goes down again; may lie flat, gets up, frantic stamping, crouching, kicking, circling, **profuse sweating**, more rapid but irregular respiration. The horse may collapse down with a grunt and a sigh where it lies on its sternum, head and neck extended, or lies on its side, swings head and neck off and onto floor, stretches them out flat, 'paddles' on its side with intermittent violent hind-leg movements, sweats more profusely – 'steams', rolls onto back, returns, goes the other way, may go right over, gets up, repeats going down, gets cast, prefers to lie on back propped up against a wall, or gets violent, hence head and leg injuries, very rapid irregular breathing, blowing and puffing, heart rate rapidly increases to 60bpm and then upwards, serious if above 80bpm especially if it does not fall to 50bpm or less between painful bouts. There may be intermissions of pain-free periods

In complex cases, surgical or otherwise, recovery occurs first with an end of pain, general appearance improvement, lessening of anxiety, increasing interest in environment, then defecation and interest in feed (preferably by very restricted hand grazing)

Beware the pain-free state associated with dullness, undue quietness and cold, clammy body extremities. These are bad signs of gut wall necrosis and massive toxin absorption, or rupture of gut with peritonitis – often accompanied by small quantities of diarrhoea, further toxaemia and terminal shock.

Management

If the horse is *down but 'active'* in intermittently getting up then down again, stay in the box with it and stay close, but do not bolt the door. Loosen out head rope, hold and be ready to try to pull head away from wall if and when it goes down again or to steady it when it gets up. Beware its sudden getting up. Do not be heroic!

If *down and quiet*, leave alone: don't get it up to 'see how it is'. Observe general demeanour; abdominal flatulence, defecation, urination if any, and breathing pattern. Catch to hold when and if it rises spontaneously. Let it 'gather its wits'. Walk it slowly round box. Offer from hand a little hay and hand-walk on a non-slip surface outside for 10 minutes at 10-minute intervals unless the pain returns to stimulate going down again.

Do not administer medicine, and certainly not by drench.

The food intake, despite keenness, must be restricted to small repeat offerings of hay or in-hand grazing.

With impaction, a straw bedding should be replaced with paper or peat but not shavings.

A benign case may have recovered within the unseen period. Evidence of an attack, and therefore the need for on-going observation and evaluation, may have been missed unless the presence of dishevelled clothing, superficial scuff marks on the head and limb extremities, bedding scratched up, excess bedding on hair or on rug, scuff marks on walls, less than normal droppings, are noted and assessed at the next 'stables'.

The at-grass horse so affected is more difficult to spot, but grass and patchy sweat stains or mud marks *unusually present*, and/or excessively rolled and pawed or scraped areas are seen. Remember, most horses at grass do roll and some dig a rolling pit for themselves, as normal activities.

Horsemasters require, in routine stable management, recognition of early signs of colic and immediate reaction to protect the horse against secondary injury and to evaluate progress. They need to decide about veterinary help – always better to 'play safe', consider differential diagnoses – no harm in trying, **but see colic as a 'first'**.

It is rarely possible for an owner/handler to determine exactly what type of colic is present. It is more useful for all concerned if, when the first three requirements above have been met, that he gives thought to

- is this horse subject to colic attacks?
- are there any recent changes in management or use to be suspected as relevant?
  - a recent acquisition to a sudden change of diet
  - possible access to new and/or excessive feedstuffs
  - changed grass growth rate
  - transit – prolonged, too fast
  - competitive use, over-strenuous
  - a recent (4–5 days before) worming
  - exposure to inclement conditions – wet and cold air *and* grass
  - recent hedging, ditching in field, or field applications and/or on land up-wind

The priority for the horsemaster faced with a horse 'behaving differently'

- in the field
- in the stable
- under the saddle, suggestive of sudden discomfort or pain

is to consider that the horse is **colicked**; see also rhabdomyolysis (ER), especially if during or soon after exercise.

At grass

- put on headcollar with shortened lead
- let go and leave in field
- carefully inspect others in the same field. Remove if thought necessary
- telephone for veterinary help
- stay on watch in field
- have someone to direct veterinary surgeon to field
- guide ill horse away from any ditch, if necessary
- if down in inclement weather, protect with sacks etc. but do not attempt to fasten rugs on, keep hold of head
- if New Zealand rug already fitted, make sure straps not too tight following rolling

If the horse is known to be difficult to handle at grass, slowly lead it if possible to a well-bedded box. Do this anyway during hours of darkness or in wet and/or cold weather. It is, however, safer for the horse to roll on grass, unless very hard and lumpy, than to risk walking over road or yard and have it going down there.

In loosebox

- put on headcollar, with rolled up lead
- remove all free-standing stable equipment
- if manger is fixed with space under, block that with bale
- quickly but safely 'muck out' obvious droppings (save for veterinary inspection as to consistency and amount)
- put down thick bed, heap up well round walls
- remove hay, corn and water
- beware violent activity
- secure door on exiting
- stay on watch
- send for veterinary surgeon as and when considered necessary

The ridden horse should be dismounted and the horse unsaddled and led to a stable or, if none nearby, off the tarmac into a field. When possible, exchange bridle for a headcollar. Beware rhabdomyolysis (ER) with misleading colic signs and the risk of further long walking.

There are other conditions which cause roughly similar

but confusing signs. Colic is always the most likely. All sudden-in-onset disorders are managed in the same way until a differential conclusion is reached by the veterinary surgeon.

Remember that 80% of colics are benign. A significant proportion of these, especially when the cause is circumstantially due to too much, too soon, cold, wet, or lush grass, will improve following a slow, short, 'walking around' between the bouts of spasmodic pain, whilst awaiting the veterinary surgeon. (Note: not the old-fashioned idea of walking for hours until the pain goes or the horse collapses exhausted!) Keep it near a straw or grass surface in case it wants to lie down to roll.

Do not allow eating or drinking until pain is well over, or until veterinary advice is given.

Types of Colic

Colics can be catalogued under which digestive organ is affected. Since there can be more than one directly and/or indirectly involved, and since identification is not for the inexperienced owner (and is often difficult for the veterinary surgeon) this is of little immediate practical importance.

The veterinary surgeon may list them as to what has gone wrong, e.g.

- 'the stomach with tympany'
- 'the small intestine with inflammation'
- 'the caecum with displacement'
- and so on

Mainly from information gained by a rectal examination and observation of 'vital and other signs' he can at least reduce the possibilities, if not immediately reach a conclusion. Repeat examinations are usually the rule. An essential investigation, certainly obligatory at a second examination, is the passing of a stomach tube to relieve reflux of gas and liquid excess, and determine the type of fluid, plus any retrievable contents which are guides to small intestine disorders.

An **acute abdominal crisis (AAC)**, is another name given for a colic of the **non-benign** type. As it is usually associated with severe blood-flow disturbance, the further description is **ischaemic bowel disease (IBD)**. As the title implies, it is

- sudden in onset
- invariably obviously abdominal in origin and must therefore show many of the signs of colic
- a crisis, therefore the signs will be inclusive of general

'unwellness', with markedly altered vital signs and usually severe behavioural changes from intense continuing colic pain and characterised by cardio-vascular disorder

As will be discussed under diarrhoea, the hyperactive stage of colitis X and its sub-types are also classic examples of AAC.

In terms of colicky alimentary disorders, AAC points to severe obstruction to blood flow and so to IBD with

- arterial obstruction, as from thrombo-embolism, strangulation of a length of gut or severe compression of a length of gut
- diffuse interference with gaseous exchange – arteriolar, capillary and venule 'shut down' – as from the effects of larval migration in the gut wall mucosa and resultant micro thrombo-embolism

Whilst *some* cases can be relieved by non-surgical release of the obstructions it is absolutely essential in most non-benign situations that veterinary diagnosis, even just suspicion, expedites referral for surgery and does not delay with vain medicinal therapy so that surgery passes the important 8-hour factor.

The following list itemises the morbid changes and functional disorders of the several parts of the abdominal digestive tract as the source of alimentary 'true' colic pain.

The Acute Simple Abdomen

The pain is not necessarily low grade in some types. Differential diagnosis with non-benign colic cannot be made on the severity in itself. Analgesic relief is still a vital therapy and is also of diagnostic value. Other significant features are

- variable intermissions from pain, and associated behaviour aberrations
- variable periods of return to appetite
  - especially with spasmodic
  - less so with flatulent types
- pulse does not rise above or, at least, does not stay above 60bpm, especially during quieter periods

Tympanitic or Flatulent Colic

Usually easily recognised on rectal examination by the veterinary surgeon.

Stomach – fermenting feed intake

- rapid in onset
- pain is severe
    - immediate, if temporary, relief via stomach tube

Small intestine – extension of tympany from the still fermenting feed intake

- rapid in onset, leading to
    - atony and possible serious worsening

Caecum – atony, especially of caeco-colonic 'opening'

- pain progressively greater, non-diagnosable except for right flank distension or from rectal inspection

Large colon(s)

- hyper-fermentation with excess gas production
- atony – thrombosis of capillaries with neural interference, as from
    - cyathostomiasis
    - neoplasia

and retention of 'normal' gas to excess degree

Not so quickly serious, as in non-benign cases, but if not dealt with quickly, can lead to serious complications.

Signs

A persistent colic with a variably tense abdomen. Less severe with atony, is short of ileus. Gut sounds, **borborygmi**, are by definition usually much reduced, and especially in the affected organ; what does pass to the small colon is passed out *per* rectum as flatus or wind.

Ingestive Factors

Such as sudden excess access to or unusual consumption of cold frosty or wet grass, especially if that includes lucerne, clover, lush grazing, or lawn cuttings, particularly if heaped and over-heated, are the most common, obstructions as suggested above can also cause this.

Spasmodic Colic (The 'Gripes')

Arguably the most common colic – about 75% of all cases. It is seen in

- tired horses, especially when fed hard feed too soon or allowed more than 4 litres/1 gallon of water
- irregularly fed horses
- unaccustomed feed intake
- those given to 'bolting' their food

- highly strung animals (psychosomatic colic) especially on arrival at new places or at imminent competitions
- tapeworm infestation
- larval stage 4 cyathostomiasis

The last two can also be involved in non-benign colics

Signs

- medium to severe pain, sudden attacks, intermittent, with the usual previously described behavioural changes
- extra audible intermittent gut sounds, but not necessarily with increased flatus
- frequently of short overall duration
- can be 'carefully' walked off

Chronic Simple Colic

- impaction

Cause

Mainly management 'sins of omission or of commission'

- sudden exposure to straw bedding following sudden removal of a production ration and/or grazing. This is the most common cause – eating the straw bedding
- poorly masticated coarse fibrous foodstuff, possibly associated with
- saliva deficits
- insufficient water
- intercurrent disease
- general malnutrition
- cyathostomiasis
- teeth problems

Signs

In general

- slow in onset
- diminishing appetite
- low grade to mildly severe pain
- diagnosis is difficult in early stages

Small Intestine

- associated with tapeworm infestation
- sand ingestion

The left colon – sites of impaction.

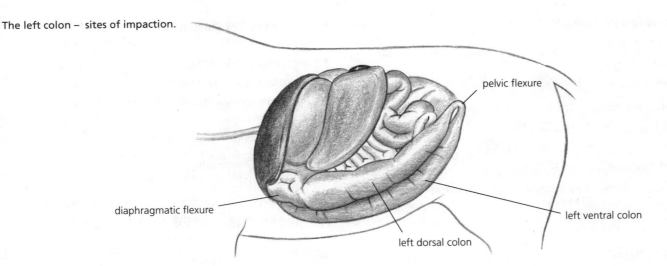

diaphragmatic flexure

pelvic flexure

left ventral colon

left dorsal colon

Colonic flexure impactions *other* than that of the pelvic flexure are

- more painful with some hind-leg striking at abdomen and tail swishing
- less easy to reach manually for diagnosis *per rectum*
- usually complicated by bloat in the anterior or cranial area

Pelvic Flexure of Left Colon, Impaction

A very common colic of the stabled horse.

Causes

- lack of water
- poor mastication – low grade but serious dental disorders
- sudden change to high dry material feed, e.g. grass to hay
- sudden free choice access to straw bedding
- presumed underlying atony – complication of parasitic larval morbidity or other causes of ischaemia usually localised so still generally viable
- adhesions are possible causes, but usually such a cause is non-benign in origin

Signs

- slowly decreasing appetite and thirst (possibly intermittent) and faecal output over several days
- slowly hardening (drying) of faecal balls
- eventually neither faeces nor flatus passed

- bubble blowing when horse puts muzzle in water
- eventual clinical onset of intermittent, low-grade pain – slowly worsens, horse crouches, looks at abdomen, paddles behind, postures into urinary position, no flow, occasional straining, carries tail high in anticipation of defecation or urination, yawning, 'smiling' grimace, no early signs of an acute abdomen: pulse 50bpm or less. Easily diagnosed on rectal examination, necrosis of wall can develop after 7 to 10 days, even longer, with toxaemia, peritonitis and shock – a truly non-benign state

This is a typical dis-ease which in the absence of good horsemastership, failing to see these progressive early signs, can be missed in its early, easily treatable days. *There is something different, therefore there must be something wrong, so get help...*

In this flexure fault, the faeces do not even enter the next area of colon in the complete impaction, let alone the rectum.

During and after this colic, veterinary advice about watering, feeding and bedding, exercising and teeth must be followed.

Repeat attacks despite preventative measures as advised by the veterinary surgeon justify further veterinary examination before the gut is fully impacted once more, when better information may be obtained by further rectal examinations.

Caecum, Impaction

Cause

- excess intake of lignous material. It may also but less commonly be due to peritoneal adhesions which interfere with peristalsis

The ileum to the large intestine, bypassing the caecum, may still be operative.

Signs

- mild, intermittent, low grade, occasional severe pain
- progressive over up to several weeks
- later stages, horse lies on back, legs propped against wall, head and neck curved into further balancing support. (Presumably this reduces the gravitational pull of the heavy caecum on its mesentery, and so lessens the pain)
- slowly diminishing appetite and faecal output, but
- slowly increasing softness to cow-pat consistency (the colons fail to reclaim much of the intestinal waters)
- diagnosis *per rectum*

It may become a complex non-benign abdomen because

- tissue changes have already or do occur, making surgery an economic and welfare no-go proposition in some cases
- loss of neural and/or vascular input – could be due to heavy tapeworm infestation effect

If left, or not considered by the layman, the usual necrosis and toxaemia follow.

It is the responsibility of the veterinary surgeon to attempt to identify what particularly is wrong, and to assess the severity and stage, as judged by

- pulse rate and feel, and whether deteriorating
- **rectal findings**
- membrane colour and refill time
- siphoning of stomach contents – fluid or gas
- peritoneal tap sample and to
- send for surgery if prognosis is not good, **earlier rather than later**. Better to find it doesn't require surgery in the hospital, rather than have it collapse in the stable

Chronic simple abdomen colics are, by definition, usually slow to show clinical signs and are prolonged in effect.

Another cause of chronic abdomen simple colic is hypertrophy (thickening) of the wall of the ilium, which

- can be associated with worm larval initial penetration and subsequent micro-vascular interference, or
- a chronic bacterial infection

- suspected by low grade pain and absence of other clinical signs
- possibly palpable *per rectum* by veterinary surgeon
- potentially an acute complex because of the risk of subsequent gas retention cranially, torsion and peritonitis
- potentially non-benign as not all cases are medically curable. Surgery is a high risk option
- confirmed on laparotomy or endoscopy

The Acute, Complex or Non-Benign Abdomen

Surgical in potential – a 'crisis'. The usual severe pain is a reflection of

- marked distension of a viscus by gas
    - a primary tympany of a severe nature, excessive fermentation
    - secondary tympany, usually cranial to volvulus, incarceration, strangulation, all with associated
- subsequent severe disturbance to the blood flow with ischaemia and congestion from thrombosis following macro-narrowing of the arterial flow and embolism (which is usually parasitic in origin) as with Strongylus vulgaris infestation and micro as with cyathostomiasis or from other causes most of which are confirmable at surgery
- the condition is usually in the large intestine but is also found in
- small intestinal reflex gut atony with tympany
- small intestine enteritis
- SI granulomatous inflammation, both extensive
- strangulation and volvulus of the small intestine

All these, except the first, usually lead to reflux of fluid into the stomach, attempted vomiting with liability of gastric rupture.

Intussusception

- a telescoping of one part of a viscus into another, as with
- small intestine, into a more caudal area
- small intestine, into the caecum
- caecum, into itself ('the outside-in sock toe')
- caecum, into large right ventral colon

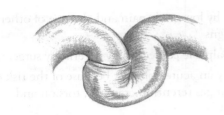

An intussusception.

predisposing to tympany, disturbance of neural control, and so to atony, interruption of vascular flows, necrosis with secondary endotoxaemia.

The variably acute signs require

- rectal examination
- exploratory laparotomy for diagnosis

Displacements

Hernias

- diaphragmatic, traumatic, or through the oesophageal hiatus
- scrotal (inguinal), especially in stallions, leading to strangulation. Externally palpable. Should always be suspected when an entire is colicked
- nephrosplenic entrapment of left colons over the ligament between the spleen and the left kidney

These three require rectal inspection and sometimes exploratory laparatomy for confirmation. The third can in

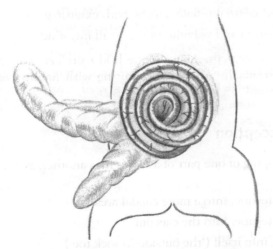

A volvulus of the small intestine.

some cases be reduced by casting and rolling.

- epiploic foramen entrapment of small intestine

All have potential for obstruction with subsequent tympany and/or strangulation leading to ischaemia then necrosis with toxaemia.

Torsions

A twist of a portion of part of the digestive tract around its own axis, as found in the small intestine, or at a flexure point of the large intestine – a **volvulus** – is a very serious condition rapidly leading to an abdominal vascular crisis from coincidental tympany, often severe blood flow strangulation, rapid and lethal because of the

- ischaemia
- enterotoxaemia, with
    - profound shock, eventual
- rupture, and subsequent
- peritonitis, quickly leading to death
- the pain until necrosis sets in is profound and violent

In the small intestine the effect is basically similar, but not so quickly profound and lethal. An atony of the rest of the small intestine with tympany is accompanied by reflux into the stomach. The small colon and the small intestine is liable to 'whiplash' into a 'half hitch' loop around themselves, or by strangulation by the stalk of a fatty tumour or melanomatous neoplasm.

The blood flow is again compromised, but more slowly, less severely, at least in the early stages. Many causes require rectal examination.

The causes of all these torsions, though difficult to determine accurately at the time, include increased peristalsis of a cranial length against a normal length caudal to it or to an atonic length because of

- enteritis
- obstruction
    - intra-lumenal (in the cavity)
    - intra-mural (in the wall) from focal chronic lesions
        - inflammatory
        - neoplastic
        - helminth larval damage to blood supply and nerve supply
- macro thrombo and embolism, especially in larval infiltration cases

Significant associated signs are

- the changes in respiration associated with abdominal pain
  - rapid, jerky sighing as in toxaemia and shock
  - intermittent rate changes, with sobbing, shallow and guarded as in peritonitis
  - fast, heaving and laboured with diaphragmatic hernia (rare)
- the changes in heart rate – the most important factor in assessing
  - seriousness of the case
  - prognosis
  - monitoring progress, or otherwise
  - under 50bpm (if not originally accelerated, and now down because of collapse) – is unlikely to be serious – should fall to normal when pain ceases
  - under 60bpm at time of maximum pain is not suggestive of acute non-benign abdomen
  - up to 80bpm is worrying, especially if it stays up under analgesic cover. If weakening and/or rising above 80+bpm – very grave
- rectal examination suggests to the veterinary surgeon 'where have the intestines gone?'
- rolling in health or during colic is **not** a prime cause of volvulus

The main reason for attempting to keep a horse from rolling is to minimise self-inflicted external trauma.

Assessment
Mucous membranes

- conjunctival
  - no worry if they **stay** normal
  - if blood vessels become engorged, and especially if scleral membrane becomes
    - brick red
    - dirty
    - plus a jaundiced colour

then they are progressive signs of gut circulatory damage when taken in conjunction with the pulse changes and other behavioural signs.

Gum membrane refill time

- in benign acute colics
  - on removal of thumb pressure, reddens quickly

- as circulatory damage develops (necrosis and toxaemia), as in complex cases, it takes progressively longer until the stage of cyanosis, associated with circulatory collapse, prevents pressure effect altogether. Cyanosis is not common in the horse

Musculature

- generalised muscular tremors, **fasciculations**, are very worrying

Faeces

- colour, smell, consistency vary with the diet
- all horses in the same regime should be more or less similar
- any change in one horse should be investigated: it may indicate an interference with digestion
- cow pat appearance is seen in caecal impaction and in parasitic conditions and in low grade bacterial infection
- gritty appearance or feel – excess silica (sand) intake (filter water-added faeces to confirm presence of insoluble sand)
- mucus coated balls in colonic obstruction
- blood stained and/or black mucus mixed points to ischaemic bowel disease (IBD).

When assessing the probability of colic or not, the horsemaster must take into account the immediate past and present situations of the horse in total. A horse at grass rarely gets colic, except

- within 4 days after worming, when a hypersensitivity reaction to dead helminths, especially larvae, and subsequent onward development of non-susceptible stages, may so irritate the bowel wall that peristaltic movement is altered with associated pain
- if turned out onto lush grass

A sudden rise in environmental temperature, and an increase in rainfall following a cold dry spell in Spring, and less so in Autumn, may, and usually does, produce a flush of grass, with the possibility of

- spasmodic colic
- tympanic colic in horses already 'happy' on such grazing

A sudden fall in temperature with persistent rain can have a similar effect.

Differential Diagnosis

- laminitis, the pain and posturing of which may simulate colic or, because of the enteric disturbance, it may be a coincidental colic

- access to poisonous plants, excess acorns, metallic poisons, can induce gastro-enteric disturbances often with diarrhoea (enteritis). Hypersalivation in addition could point to rhododendron and to organo-phosphate poisoning, as with access to sheep dip. Lead poisoning and its 'blind' staggers are also a possibility

- grass sickness, especially of the subacute and chronic types

- allergies which precipitate *acute* respiratory distress

- OPD of summer grass

- tree pollen OPD, and

- acute rhabdomyolysis in summer-pastured horses as well as at work

all with the associated distress, sweating, posturing and reluctance to move, present (or at least simulate) abdominal pain.

The horse which, ridden or loose, falls into nettles, will evince striking reactive signs suggestive of pain and 'trying to get away from it', so that colic is often suspected until the characteristic weals develop to point to the cause. A colicky horse may roll onto nettles!

At grass or stabled, the heavily pregnant mare can develop abdominal and alimentary colic, but she is more likely to be suffering low-grade pressure pain from foetal movement

- beginning (stage one) labour

- foaling (stage two) labour pains

- after foaling – showing non-alimentary pain from the stage three labour uterine contractions as she ejects the afterbirth

- experiencing distress and severe pain from haemorrhage with distension into the uterine broad ligaments

In the later stages of lactation when a mare is becoming milk-drained of calcium in her blood she can, especially if stressed by transport, coralling with others, fast-driven off hill and moorland (where grazing is often calcium deficient anyway), go into a hypocalcaemic convulsion reminiscent of acute colic.

Any horse, especially if of a hypersensitive nature, may develop transit fever with tetany. In the early stages, as well as in the later respiratory complications, colic signs can be imagined.

Heat stress patients progress through a cascade of syndromes

- off feed

- off drink

- increased respirations, pulse and temperature

- colic – atony of the bowel and electrolyte imbalance

- rhabdomyolysis: 'setting fast' stage

- rigors (tremors)

all of which are typical of true colic to one extent or another.

Gall stones and kidney stones although rare, with

- pain

- straining and posturing (kidneys)

- distress

are difficult to distinguish quickly from various types of colic, as can be polymyositis, polyneuritis (neuritis cauda equina, which simulates pelvic flexure impaction), tetanus, seizures and convulsions, botulism, uraemia, hepato-encephalopathy, chronic ragwort poisoning.

The most common cause of colic is parasitism, particularly (but not only) in the young horse, with lymphosarcoma a strong possibility in the old horse, in the absence of, or even as well as

- teeth defects

- low-grade liver disease

- malnutrition in its widest sense

The larval stages of some intestinal helminths, in particular that of Strongylus vulgaris, use the arterial system of the gut for migration from the penetration of the small intestine to the junction with the aorta and thence back to re-enter the large intestinal lumen as adult worms.

During this migratory stage there is damage to the intestinal blood flow, with

- reduction of supply of oxygen and nutrients to the gut tissues and especially to the digestive secretory glands, so that digestion and absorption is reduced

- ischaemia of varying lengths of the tract, which if not 'naturally' relieved of the end-artery thrombosis by the development of an alternative route's new supply quickly enough causes, in some cases, necrosis of the wall and ulceration of the lining leading to peritonitis and enterotoxaemia

- fibrotic healing with permanent loss of digestive surfaces – with reduced nutrient absorption, protein-losing enteropathy, and loss of condition

The widespread use of Ivermectin anthelmintics, e.g. Eqvalan, has so reduced the prevalence of this large red worm that its larval damage syndrome is now rarely encountered, certainly in well-managed horses. Its 'place' has been taken by the small redworms, the Cyathostomes.

They cause problems by

- extensive adult worm mucosal damage, but mainly by
- migration and encystment of larvae within the mucosum – cyathostomiasis, normal or 'inhibited'
  - surface damage
  - deeper damage, including to the capillaries and the glands especially by the over-wintering larvae
  - emergence trauma

DIARRHOEA

From the Greek *dia* – 'through', and *rhoia* – 'flow'. In mono-gastric, simple digestion mammals the inclusive term 'gastro-enteritis' means inflammation of the stomach and of the intestines, small and large. It denotes a syndrome with vomiting, inappetence, possible systemic unwellness and **diarrhoea**; it does not suggest a cause.

In the herbivorous horse, the complex alimentary condition is separated into

- gastro/small enteritis, usually just enteritis

Inflammation of the caecum and the large and small colon is 'large' enteritis.

In practice, both the anterior digestive tract and the posterior can be jointly involved. (The gastro-enteritis on its own is mainly but not always a foal disorder). Infection or a nutrient intake problem is involved.

The colitis syndrome, basically on its own, is the more important dis-ease, as the site of both acute and chronic diarrhoea syndrome in the adult horse.

The specific functioning of the horse's digestive system whereby the large gut is the fermentation vat with the caecum, and both the site of fluid reclamation, means that

- anterior inflammation's excess of inflammatory fluid is reclaimed (absorbed) in a normal large intestine so no diarrhoeic fluid escapes
- posterior inflammation not only produces excess fluid but is unable to reabsorb that and the normal fluids coming through it. The faeces becomes variably lower in dry matter consistency, it becomes watery or diarrhoeic

(Gastro) enteritis cannot induce vomiting in the horse to relieve the stomach of inflammatory fluid from itself or by reflux from the small intestine if and when ileus or atony develops with colic signs, as distinct from hyperperistalis and fluid throughput. This build up of liquid will in some cases overcome the natural obstruction of the one-way valve between gullet and stomach and so permit regurgitation of contents out through the nose (with the risk of inhalation pneumonia) or rupture the stomach causing fatal peritonitis.

In less lethal situations there will be reduced digestion and malabsorption of the 'soluble' digesta such as sugars, lipids, amino acids, minerals, vitamins, with disruption of electrolyte transport through the gut wall and subsequent alteration of gut content pH.

These have an effect on the functioning of the large intestine and the caecum. Although these organs can reclaim fluid they are not programmed to reclaim some electrolytes which will be lost via the faeces

- secondary systemic illness may result with loss of condition
- disruption of microbial fermentation
- low-grade inflammation
- changes in myenteric control
  - colic

Diarrhoea as such, therefore, is the sign of derangement of the functioning of the caecum and the colons due to inflammation from a variety of causes. It is essentially a loss of body fluids leading to

- dehydration – minimal in the adult horse unless the disorder is acute and prolonged
- loss of electrolytes and vitamins and other nutrients, especially protein
- alteration to cellulose fermentation with
  - reduced volatile fatty acid production
    - loss of condition
- variable and intermittent colic of a low grade nature

The most common cause is helminthiasis and in particular cyathostomiasis from which the diarrhoea may be chronically persistent; subacute to acute cases are also seen.

Chronic Diarrhoea

Defined as such if the diarrhoea persists for more than 28 days. It is usually a disorder of the caecum and/or the colons but abnormalities of the stomach and/or the small intestines may be contributory factors. It can be related to other organ dis-eases, such as cirrhosis of the liver or chronic bile duct inflammation from chronic small enteritis.

Other inflammatory factors are
- **infections**
  - bacterial
    - Rhodococcus equi (in the foal)
    - chronic Salmonellosis
      - incomplete recovery from the acute infection
      - intermittent recrudescence of infection from regional lymphoid tissue
- **infestations**
  - Ascarids in foals
  - the rare Strongylus edentatus larvae and adults
  - the once common Str. vulgaris larvae and adult, as well as the small red worms mentioned above
  - liver fluke
- **neoplasia**
  - lymphosarcoma
  - granulomatous lesions
- **ingestion 'mistakes'**
  - sand irritation of the colons
  - other rank, coarse, persistently wet herbage, e.g. Mare's Tail
- **non-inflammatory**
  - possible abnormal fermentation of cellulose
  - gut flora disturbance causing excess accumulation of gas, acetate and proprionate volatile fatty acids and sodium, all interfering with physiological re-absorption of water
- (suspected) idiopathic colitis
  - allergy
  - auto-immune disturbance
- 'growing-up disorder' in weanlings and yearlings: a persistent mild intermittent soft faeces with no apparent detrimental defect on growth, health generally or appetite. Gradually over several months becomes normal: the horse 'outgrows' the problem now seen as idiopathic; more worrying to the owner than to the horse

- gastric ulceration

Untreated dental disorders of mastication and coincidental consequent deficit in salivation can detrimentally influence the listed causes of chronic diarrhoea.

Other signs
- peripheral oedema in later stages (protein deficits)
- occasional variable fever
- secondary systemic effect is rare so there is no discoloured membranes, toxaemia shock

Chronic diarrhoea is difficult to explain and therefore difficult to treat and to manage.

Since it usually begins as it means to continue, that is as a chronic syndrome, the initial supportive signs of
- not ill
- not off food
- just loose in its droppings

do not encourage early veterinary help. It is the persistence beyond one to two weeks and certainly if beyond four weeks that really worries the owner.

Whenever the veterinary surgeon is called, the distinction between acute and chronic sub-types will be considered. It is easier to distinguish these than to explain the cause. In chronic cases the need for heroic supportive treatment is not nearly so great or so urgent as it is with the acute or the more serious hyperacute types in the adult horse at least.

There is time to investigate in some depth but even then the diagnosis is often vague or at the best presumptive
- appraisal of animal: clinical findings
- appraisal of its in-contacts
- history of environment and of the other horses
- laboratory aids
  - blood samples – protein loss and other variations *re* type of inflammation, haemoconcentration, enzyme levels
  - faecal sample – bacteria, helminth eggs, **malabsorption** findings by test feeding and blood glucose estimations at intervals following stomach tube administration of glucose

More often than not the negative findings are no more than that, e.g.

- faeces
  - no worm eggs (diagnostic level) would be expected if worm larval damage is otherwise suspected
  - Salmonellae, even in acute cases are but intermittently excreted with the faeces
  - sand in the sediment is certainly a pointer but is significant relative to grazing, soil structure and available grass length
- rectal biopsies
  - a negative for neoplasia only indicates that the rectal wall is not involved; lymphosarcomatous lesions are often in the rectum as elsewhere

Enteropathies will often reveal as

- malabsorption defects but not why
- haemoconcentration will confirm dehydration but not why

and so on, but helminth larval involvement can 'show up' in the blood, as will

- gut enzyme changes
- white blood cell level changes
- protein electrophoresis

However, these must be used with clinico-therapeutic value consideration for the cost, the results' value and that a significant number of the underlying causes may be incurable anyway due to the

- the primary nature, e.g. neoplasia
- the secondary damage, e.g. helminth micro ulceration, fibrosis of the gut wall (and the blood supply damage)

The veterinary surgeon will advise an empirical approach to the case in this order

- examine teeth and treat if necessary
- inspect pasture; if suspicious of
  - sand content or
  - indigestible nature
  - noxious weeds

and will rearrange feed intake, and if considered necessary administer bulk laxatives for sand ingestion

- give 5-day course of Panacur (or other small redworm larvicide) if the patient is a
  - recent incomer and/or it is October to March and not previously specifically treated

otherwise a simple dose of an adult worm anthelmintic

- administer anti-diarrhoeal drugs, this last after a reasonable, 2 to 3 day interval for the other treatments to show a response or not

During this time grazing will be variably restricted and balanced by a *gradually introduced* hay and oat straw diet with supplementary micro-nutrients as required.

The **acute** enteritis, typhlitis and colitis are much more serious. Whatever the cause, there are usually, in both small and large gut conditions

- changes to the micro-vasculature of the gut wall, causing
  - ischaemia
  - reduced absorption
- alterations to the mucosal cellular secretions
  - excess waters
  - reduced enzyme output
    - interrupted digestion

  associated with the influence of
- inflammatory reactions
- endocrine deficits on the
  - autonomic and myenteric nerve controls

The 'end' result is an accelerated gut peristalsis with the evacuation of variable percentages of water to faecal dry matter.

Causes of the diarrhoea/large bowel syndrome are often never determined, especially in life, but can be
- infections
  - viral: rarely implicated in the adult
  - bacterial
    - primary in effect, but with toxin production
    - Salmonellae sp. variably common
    - secondary from toxin release as from Clostridia sp or Escheiria coli species infections
- fungal – rare
- endoparasitic: most common 'infectious' cause except in the hyper acute conditions
- irritants
- dietary – too lush, too sudden, grasses and clovers
- toxic – vegetable alkaloids, chemicals, e.g. the organo-phosphates

All these can be associated with the gastro-small intestine as well; the lush feeds causing primary gastric tympany

- idiopathic
  - unknown factors
  - psychogenic

The various lethal effects especially those of infections are precipitated and/or exacerbated by various **stressor factors** which seem to be essential trigger factors.

Signs

- the faeces' water content

The consistency will vary with the diet, being wetter with 'all grass' than 'all hay and cereal' (there is no such thing as water-free faeces). The more water a horse 'eats' the more the extra intake, liberated during digestion, will pass through surplus to absorption requirements. Generally speaking, all horses on the same diet will pass the same consistency in the absence of bowel dis-ease.

In diarrhoea the looseness varies from cow pat to no visible solid, dry matter content. This is described as

- hose pipe, a steady stream or
- explosive, under considerable pressure as in hyper-acute cases
- persistent, not just a one-off, soft evacuation, often accompanied, in the acute syndromes, by
- changes in the vital signs – heart rate, respiration rate and temperature (taking this has difficulties and so may be falsely low)
- mucosal colour
- refill time after gum-pressure test
- variable changes in appetite, systemic disorder
- incidence – dependent on underlying cause it may occur in one animal, or two or more, or all but least likely in a stable or field

Travel and/or competition 'nerves' can cause diarrhoea which is non-persistent, usually limited in duration, but often repeated under similar circumstances; the horse, quite often obviously excited, passes normal consistency faeces (though less than usual), quickly followed by a very liquid, mildly explosive evacuation.

This is presumed to be a neurogenic functionally increased rate of peristalsis through the large bowels whereby the water content did not have the time to be reabsorbed. It is sometimes seen as a fear reaction within the fright, fight and flight complex.

Diagnosis

- the clinical signs in conjunction with speed of onset but
  - any alimentary or other systemic disorder signs
    - degree and duration
    - frequency
- laboratory aids
  - faecal sample tests
    - dry matter measurement
    - presence of abnormal digesta including sediments e.g. sand, worm eggs (**eggs per gram, EPG**), micro-organisms, toxins
- blood sample tests
  - haemoconcentration
  - white cell changes
  - serum – albumen/globulin changes, enzymes released from the gut wall, antibodies

Management

- isolate the individual case
- immediate removal of or from possible dietary and other causal factors
- ***seek veterinary advice***
  - appropriate antibiotic/anthelmintic therapy
  - rehydration and electrolyte replacement orally or intravenously
  - gut sedatives
  - absorbents
  - steroids

especially in

- young patients and in cases of
- diarrhoea with or following systemic illness and/or primary colics

It should be understood that diarrhoea may be secondary to systemic illness and/or disorders of the liver and peritoneum.

Colic may be an important sign within a diarrhoea episode.

Hyperacute Diarrhoea (Super Purgation)

Colitis X; as the colloquial name implies, the actual cause of this hyperacute diarrhoea is not immediately diagnosable, if at all. Invariably it is a fatal dis-ease. Not all the pathology is understood.

Suspected Cause

- neurologic-related stress, leading to shock as from
    - prolonged fatigue, engendered by travel or work
    - environmental change
- myenteric nerve 'stress' associated with helminthiasis
- dietary changes, especially on to lush grasses, e.g. rye grass
- secondary to bacterial inflammation
    - Salmonellae, with or without Clostridial toxins or associated allergic responses
- misuse of broad spectrum antibiotics

Signs

- a hyper (super) purgation of an explosive nature
- may contain blood, mucus
- a preceding acute systemic illness of 24 hours' duration usually with colic
- an early fever which rapidly declines to become sub-normal before death
- death **before** diarrhoea can occur, and autopsy reveals a liquid-laden bowel and other signs of 'shock'. This pooled fluid is just as much out of the circulation as is the lost diarrhoea water. Both cause a fall in blood pressure and a loss of electrolytes, both conducive to shock

In less quick, lethal outcomes

- muddy mucous membranes
- slow gum-refill time
- dermal pinch test variably positive
- heart rate up to 100-plus
- temperature rise, but only to 39°C (102.2°F) and falling fast thereafter
- respiration rate increased and laboured
- colic mild to severe, possible straining
- electrolyte and dehydration systemic signs
- progressive weakness often follows, leading to recumbency, collapse, death

Management

Very resistant, even to specific, if known, therapy

- steroids
- fluid replacement
- methylene blue intravenously for the often associated methaemoglobin as assessed from whole-blood sample especially in rye grass associated cases
- nursing

all under veterinary control. *This is hyper-urgent*.

The basic illness is an endotoxaemia with an enterotoxaemia associated with

- an infectious agent
- possible other toxic factors
- immune-related secondary morbidity
- micro-vascular thrombosis
    - ischaemia
    - venous obstruction
        - oedema
- exhaustion and shock

all presenting as an acute fatal illness. Salmonellosis is perhaps a possible exception.

Clostridial Enterotoxaemias

Some Clostridial (Cl) infections may present as a herd problem, but the prevalence is low in such cases as such an infection in many cases is or becomes chronic with intermittent relapses.

Causes

- Clostridia 'perfringens', 'difficile' and others
- multiplication of the Cl species in the presence of gut changes which are conducive to this
    - liberation of related toxins which
    - damage gut wall cells
    - an enteritis which liberates further toxins
- vascular absorption of both to produce
- systemic illness with endotoxaemic complications

Signs

- acute onset
- systemic involvement

- fever, rapidly falling as shock intervenes
- *no* respiratory embarrassment until shock intervenes
- heart rate falling as shock intervenes
- muddy membranes
- low-grade colic
- usually too quick to show dehydration effects
- profuse diarrhoea
  - watery
  - blood-stained, usually blackish ('digested' blood)
- shock
- collapse
- death

Very occasional cases die before diarrhoea develops.

Management

- oral antibiotics of doubtful value – the Clostridia germ itself is not dis-ease productive. Its toxins are; by definition, the illness once established is not responsive to antimicrobial treatment
- systemic (intravenous) antibiotics if used early enough might reduce numbers of germs still producing toxin
- specific antiserum subcutaneously. As this is 'made' in horses beware possibility of serum immune reaction
- steroids
- other antitoxaemia therapy
  - rehydration
    - non-steroid anti-inflammatory drugs (NSAIDs) such as phenylbutazone ('Bute')
    - dimethylsulphoxide (DMSO) – an antioxidant
- absorbents, by stomach tube – all under veterinary supervision. This must be urgently obtained

Anthrax

A *rare*, usually geographically restricted, septicaemic fatal disease

- lethal within 24 to 48 hours
- may show profuse blackish diarrhoea
- usually with throat abscess formation preceding the acute disease

It is contagious to man and is notifiable.

Salmonellosis

Basically an acute septic colitis. Some strains are pathogenic to man. It is advisable when managing suspected as well as confirmed cases that the handler wears protective clothing including gloves and gum boots, and carries out sensible hygienic precautions especially hand/food contact. Confirmed cases are notifiable.

Diagnosis is difficult in life as the germ is shed intermittently in the faeces. Conversely, confirmation that Salmonellae are not involved requires several 'clean' faecal samples over 7 to 10 days.

Causes

The germ is often opportunist, lying dormant in the digestive system. Colonisation occurs in damaged mucous membranes

- other bacterial activity
- ulcers caused by migrating helminths
- post-operative wounds
- weakened 'colic' tissues which
  - require surgery, or
  - are persistent effects of ischaemia

and are invariably the consequence of

- stresses and tissue fatigue as mentioned above, and/or
- prolonged exercise/heat stress
- concurrent respiratory illness
- other debilitating conditions

The germ may colonise in both the small and/or large bowels. Once active in the anterior gut it will wash through to the large with enhanced virulence. It is usually a primary colitis. From both areas it can invade the blood stream to cause septicaemia.

Signs

In association with immediate past history of the animal, has it been

- stressed
- recently undergone major surgery
- fatigued, and now is
  - systemically ill, has
  - an acute diarrhoea perhaps with blood and mucus
  - fever to 41°C (105.8°F), is
  - dull, depressed to become 'miserable'
  - heart rate increase

- respiratory rate up, becoming laboured and embarrassed
- colic
- dehydration – systemic (septicaemia) illness
- collapse
- death

There may be a pre-diarrhoeic phase of 2 to 3 hours, with
- colic, quickly lessening
- fever, quickly lessening
- rapid respirations and
- heart rate continuing increase, suggesting a poor prognosis

Management
Very resistant but
- steroids
- fluid and electrolyte replacements – oral and/or intravenously
- NSAID
- doubtful benefit from antibiotics
- nursing and supplementation with probiotics

A carrier state may follow in 'recovered' animals.

Excluding anthrax, these other three acute diarrhoeas (colitis, Clostridia, Salmonellae) present a confusing diagnostic picture. The treatment, even if usually hopeless, does require a similar approach to combat the
- septicaemia, in this case more a toxaemia
- dehydration
- electrolyte and acid-base deficit
- possible marked potassium deficit
- hypoproteinaemia, especially albumen
- excess mucous membrane secretion

Cost relative to prognosis is a very important consideration.

Purpura Haemorrhagica

As a sequel to its most characteristic signs of petechial mucosal haemorrhages and severe oedema, this anaphylaxis can develop bowel wall haemorrhages presenting with colic, blackish (blood pigment) diarrhoea. Internally there is subsequent bowel necrosis, all of which produce rapid toxaemia and death.

Peritonitis

That which follows colic surgery, but not only, will have developed from bowel erosion and show as the signs associated with the original abdominal crisis. It may originate from the other primary bacterial sources. There will be
- increasing pain, plus
- abdominal distension
- dark, sticky, not profuse diarrhoea
    - possible toxaemia
    - systemic illness and possibly leading to shock, collapse and death

Treatment is not satisfactory.

Poisoning

See also Chapter 28, POISONS AND POISONING

Organo-phosphate Poisoning

Signs
- salivation
- attempts at vomiting
- tremors
- colicky pains
- diarrhoea
- muscular weakness
- CNS damage – ataxia, bradycardia

Rhododendron Poisoning

Signs
Note similarity with the above; not unusual in many types of digestive poisoning
- salivation
- attempts at vomiting
- low-grade colicky pain
- diarrhoea
- CNS damage – ataxia

Constipation

Constipation is not an equine dis-ease as it is in man and dogs. Atony and subsequent ileus does occur with stasis of gut movement, e.g. in grass sickness. Impactions from a variety of causes do occur at various sites.

OTHER INTRA-ABDOMINAL ORGANS

The Liver

This is the largest internal organ – except for the advanced pregnancy uterus. It is one (the other is the pancreas) with immediate or direct connection with the digestive tract. Both secrete products *into* the small intestine.

The liver, via the venous and lymphatic outflow from the tract, receives digesta for metabolic processing. An important function is the detoxification of ingested potentially hazardous substances resulting from the horse's grazing and browsing habits. It is, therefore, subject to toxic damage itself. As a highly active organ, one with a considerable arterial input, it is also exposed to blood-borne

- infections
- toxins, as metabolites from other systems, causing morbidities within the liver
  - necrosis
  - excess fat deposits, lipidosis as in hyperlipaemia, and aflatoxicosis
  - cirrhosis
  - neoplasia, which

can all produce changes in activity and output. These can be measured in blood serum and plasma and in urine samples

- blood
  - liver function tests – Bromsulphalein (BSP) clearance test
  - bile acid concentration
  - enzymes specific to the liver
  - plasma level of ammonia
  - plasma level of glucose
- urine analysis
- by biopsy samples direct from the liver

Dis-ease of the gastro-intestinal tract, such as malabsorption, helminthiasis (some) and grass sickness can have a direct bearing on liver activity.

Signs of these liver deficits are: abdominal pain, sometimes diarrhoea, and weight loss, which are also some of the most common dis-ease signs of direct liver dis-ease particularly if of a chronic nature.

In this context the loss of weight (condition) should require consideration of diet-to-work-being-done, parasitic dis-ease in general, and dental abnormalities, before suspecting the less common possibilities such as liver disease.

In these less common cases the actual signs of the illness or dis-ease do not point immediately or directly to liver morbidity. There will be more specific signs of gastro-intestinal upset, metabolic deficits, and nervous signs such as ataxia when the brain is involved .

In many cases of liver damage the clinical signs do not present until damage affects more than 75% of the organ as the result of repeated intake of the toxin and the slow spread of an initial single 'dose' both producing chronic hepatitis, often called **cirrhosis**, during which time the specific liver disease signs might become clinical. But much more frequently a sudden illness develops, usually with severe CNS disorder, from ammonia toxicity, of secondary neurologic damage in the brain – the classic hepato-encephalopathy, e.g.

- ragwort poisoning, from continuing intake of dried plant in conserved hay, sometimes more acutely from ingesting the living plant
- other toxicities
- liver fluke infestation – rare and restricted to wet pasture land, usually causing
- bile duct inflammation and obstruction, as from ascending from the small intestine rather than hepatitis

Liver disease is usually suspected by signs of failure of its functions. Conversely, suspected blood samples may indicate liver pathology and deficiency before specific signs develop, e.g. photosensitisation.

Types of Liver Dis-ease

Inflammatory – non infectious

- acute – mild (stoppable!) or severe (irreversible – acute liver failure). Most are due to toxins at a level against which the liver's detoxifying powers are insufficient *per se* or, less usually, because of intercurrent morbidity from
  - pasture and hedgerow plants, including ragwort
  - others such as lead, arsenic, carbon tetrachloride, waste oils

Infectious

- viral
  - possibly hepatitis – as in hepatitis B
  - in the past via therapeutic viral antiserum of equine origin – a form of hypersensitivity with marked CNS disorder, once called **serum sickness**

Bacterial

- leptospiral infection

Fungal

- aflatoxins

Metabolic

- hyperlipaemia

- a post sub-clinical hepatitis, possibly of viral origin, in which the apparently recovered horse fails to respond to training after an acceptably reasonable convalescent period. With work it becomes lethargic and rapidly loses weight. If kept at work an irreversible cirrhosis develops

Laboratory tests which 'point to the liver' and **not** to another system will dictate a spring to autumn at grass, or an equivalent extended recuperation rest period.

Metabolic deficits in the

- anabolism of amino acids, fats and glycogen; specific proteins, albumen and some globulins; clotting factors; urea from ammonia; bile and its excretion
- catabolism of toxins; drugs

Liver fluke, neoplasia, and bile and pancreatic duct inflammation, are primarily obstructive disorders

- bile reduction and retention
- exocrine pancreatic juice reduction

Clinical Signs

- variable and often subtle
- usually non-specific but most common to all causes of morbidity and most marked
  - loss of appetite – capricious
  - depression
  - lethargy, especially with cirrhosis

- increased heart rate
- tendency to low-grade impaction
- intermittent abdominal colic pain
- weight loss
- yawning
- jaundice
- photosensitisation, especially following acute hepatitis when it is a grave sign, as also is
- ataxia, especially with cirrhosis
- behavioural changes (encephalopathy – wandering, circling, head pressing)
- ventral oedema (from hypoalbumenaemia)
- altered blood clotting (petechial haemorrhages), a poor prognostic sign
- occasionally diarrhoea

Most if not all these are non-diagnostic except for the suspicion raised by jaundice. They are seen in many pathological conditions.

Jaundice

Jaundice is due to

- obstruction to bile outflow with re-absorption into the blood from duodenal mucosal thickening of the common duct; chronic sternal flexure impaction; neoplastic pressure
- ragwort cirrhosis
- hyperlipaemia and the associated failure of the liver to excrete bilirubin
- acute destruction of red cells
- leptospirosis
- anorexia, associated haemaglobinuria and faint jaundice
- blood pigment absorption from a large haematoma
- acute rhabdomyolysis

As can be appreciated, jaundice is not liver-morbidity specific, but it is most noticeable where liver cells are destroyed, especially in acute necrosis, less so in the chronic types.

Management

Based on veterinary diagnosis and advice

- steroids
- anabolic steroids (as in post-hepatitis exercise intolerance but not in brood animals)

- probiotics if diarrhoea present
- control of metabolic acidosis
- vitamins, B group
- amino acids, and
- other trace elements
- specific antibiotics of correct duration and dosage rate (not potentiated sulphonamides)
- specific therapy for hyperlipaemia
- grazing, but beware sunlight and risk of photosensitisation
- rest

The Pancreas

This dual-role glandular organ lies alongside a bend in the duodenum encased in the mesentery which suspends the intestine and carries relevant blood, lymph and nerve supplies. Its secretory products are

- exocrene, secreted 'on demand' under hormonal and physico-chemical control, generated in the stomach and in the small intestine
- alkalising 'juices'
- digestive 'ferments', enzymatic, catalytic digestive juices, eight in all, which enter the duodenum through a short duct which exits in a mucosal projection of the gut wall in close apposition to the bile duct

At this point the ducts and their orifices are exposed to pressure and so to outflow obstruction by mucosal thickening, enteritis and neoplasia in the area.

Neither of these morbidities is frequent; nor are they easily clinically diagnosable. When obstruction does occur it can be significant in small intestinal digestion and effects, and indistinct signs parallel those of liver cirrhosis.

Endocrene is also secreted 'on demand' of changes in blood level of nutrients, in particular glucose, which is controlled by the hormonal product **insulin**. Its source is the pancreatic Islets of Langerhams, which are susceptible to morbidity necrosis from viral infection (blood-borne) and auto immune disease, possibly of genetic influence.

In simple digestive system mammals, such as man and dog, a disturbance in insulin production which results in an abnormal, high level of blood glucose, a hyperglycaemia, is known as diabetes mellitus Type I. Such a condition is very rare in equines. One such case of pancreatic necrosis was thought to be caused by Strongyle worm invasion.

A Type II diabetes is also seen in man and dog. This is called non-insulin dependent, i.e. it occurs in the presence of normal insulin production and does not respond to additional therapeutic insulin. The pathological hyperglycaemia of this Type II is said to be due to a failure of insulin receptors in the body's tissue and organ cells, or response by the cells' enzymes. There is an insulin resistance. This type is also seen as an auto-immune condition.

In recent years there has been growing evidence of somewhat similar morbidity in the horse, in which carbohydrate, fat and possibly protein deficits in metabolism are thought to be involved, e.g. exertional rhabdomyolysis, obesity, Cushings-like disease (pituitary tumour in origin), laminitis.

It is now recognised that equine Type II diabetes can occur as an insulin resistance *following and/or associated with increased blood levels of hormones antagonistic to insulin* such as growth hormones, cortisol, adrenalin, progesterone and glucagon.

Such homeostatic endocrine secretions are, to a varying degree, related to stressor states, especially of pregnancy and lactation, obesity and subsequent 'dieting', natural or forced, which leads to hyperlipaemia as well as to sudden dietary changes as seen in laminitis which, in itself, is 'stressful'.

With or without such background influences the hormonal cascade can be directly generated by neoplasia of the pituitary gland.

The important finding is the very significant difference in susceptibility to these in the pony as compared to in the horse. *The pony has a low glucose tolerance.* The neoplastic 'trigger' is, of course, especially prevalent in the geriatric pony; which is thought to have even greater cell insulin receptor deficits.

Insulin's role is not confined to carbohydrate metabolism; it is also involved in the control of lipids, again especially in ponies in which dieting for as little as 4 days can induce a hyperlipaemia and subsequent hepatic disease whereas it would take 21 days in a horse.

Amongst the several parameters analysed for reaching a diagnosis of Cushings-like disease is an abnormally high level of blood insulin.

In general terms it would appear that a sub-type within diabetes mellitus is involved to a greater or lesser degree in that complex of pony metabolic/hormonal disorders which include hyperlipaemia, Cushings-like disease, obesity and laminitis, when other hormonal products are disordered, usually by overstimulation, in a knock-on route.

In what was described as direct diabetes in a Shetland pony the presenting signs were

- chronic weight loss
- depression
- polyphagia – increased appetite
- polydypsia – increased thirst
- polyuria – increased urination
- persistently raised blood glucose levels with ketonuria (metabolic by-products in the urine)

all of which are typical of the canine, insulin responsive disease – but then Shetlands are perhaps the least 'horsey' of all sub-species of Equus caballus.

In Cushings-like disease, where thirst and urinary output also are, *inter alia*, markedly raised, the associated hyperglycaemia does **not** respond to insulin therapy.

Hyperlipaemia

Although this is classed as a sporadic, one-off disorder, the more animals under the same management and environment the greater the number of possible cases. Early recognition of the first, and appropriate preventative care, will keep the numbers down.

It is basically a metabolic disorder and so is not contagious. The condition is usually found in ponies, particularly in Shetlands, occasionally Welsh. It can occur

- any age over 2 years
- 80% or more are mares
- 10% barren mares, geldings and stallions
- 75% are pregnant in the last 3 to 4 months or lactating, the spread is that of the breeding year
- 60% are in good to fat condition, even obese
- 50% or more are under stress, i.e.transport, change of management, inclement weather, malnutrition, deprivation or underfed *vis à vis* pregnancy and lactation demands, restricted feeding for more than 3 days, as with prolonged choke and laminitis cases incorrectly managed.
- 60% or less have inter-concurrent disorders
  - gastro-enteric – cyathostomiasis, colic, grass sickness
  - Cushing's disease
  - metritis endotoxaemia
    - with or without laminitis
  - intestinal lymphosarcomata

It is a disorder of lipid (fat) metabolism.

In response to nutritive deprivation the fat stores are mobilised. The triglycerides are converted by lipase into energy and free fatty acids to the liver, where they are oxidised to glucose and ketones. The excess are re-esterified and then controlled by insulin. In ponies, insulin is blocked. The resultant very low-density lipid proteins re-enter the liver to cause hepatic failure, and then into the kidneys causing their failure also.

Signs

- initially vague
  - non specific – inappetent, dull, lethargic
- rapidly progressive – inco-ordinate, weak, muscle tremors, intermittent colic, pyrexia, increased heart and respiratory rates, jaundice, halitosis, ventral oedema, liver disorder – encephalopathy, abortion
- fatal within 6 to 10 days

Diagnosis

- blood samples for fat levels
- signs
- history

Treatment

- management of intercurrent disease
- restore energy balance, acid/base balances, electrolyte levels, orally or intravenously
- maintain blood pressure and potassium levels

all under veterinary input.

Management
Continue treatment.

Prevention
See to those intercurrent possibilities, minimise stress, maintain energy input whilst carefully controlling obesity and supply extra micro-nutrients as required to supplement diet.

PARASITISM

This condition was known to the Greeks, but much mythology existed. Ectoparasites were identified in the 18th century, but it was not until the 19th century that records of endoparasites appeared. Where they came from and went was not originally understood; their epidemiology was not clear. Advances in relevant knowledge paralleled the laboratory use of the microscope which, along with Pasteur's work on microbes, enabled researchers to divide 'foreign invaders' of animal tissues into the two main subjects of **microbiology**, the 'germs' of 'floral' classification, and **parasitology**, the endo and the ecto colonisers of 'fauna' or animal classification.

Of all the disorders causing ill-health and decreased overall performance in the horse (and other herbivorous animals), those related to parasitism, especially those due to 'worms', are high in the veterinary case list, both as an economic factor and as a welfare problem.

Most horsemasters know, if only from the indirect education of commercial advertising of 'worm remedies', that *horses do have worms*. It is these endoparasites which concern this chapter. The available drugs are on direct sale from licensed (briefed) sources. Their use and misuse should be explained in broad general terms. *Their correct, economic, and effective use on any one establishment is a matter for veterinary advice*. It is not a simple horsemastership requirement, as will be explained.

Effective worm control requires an understanding of the many species of parasite (worm), their life cycles, and how these relate to

- seasons
    - climate
    - weather
- available control methods
    - environmental, especially pasture, hygiene
    - therapies, and their
        - specific uses
        - dosage rates
        - repetitions
- the horse
    - its age
    - its related husbandry, either
        - stabled
            - privately
            - at livery (with others)
            - DIY
            - managed
            - at training yards (with others)
        - at grass
            - turned away

- part-time
- resting
    - at stud
    - in work

Control has general principles, a basic strategy. There have to be several variable tactics. It is these which require veterinary input.

Definitions

Helminth worms are endoparasitic, invertebrate animals, microscopic or just macroscopic, potentially pathogenic, which, for part of their existence and ultimate reproduction, require the protection and on-site sustenance of a larger vertebrate's internal organ, usually the associated tracts, mainly the gastrointestinal tract.

Parasite – a living organism which exists in a larger 'host' organism at the latter's expense. It confers no advantage on the host and may cause dis-ease in it.

The host animal frequently passively allows this protection but may actively respond to the parasite's presence. The host invariably 'suffers', but, for obvious reasons, the parasite has no wish to kill the host which it has invaded; it is a sub-lethal 'suffering', and in well-managed situations has limited ill-effect. The usual disease signs which can develop are

- poor doing or ill-thrift with anaemia
- weight loss
- diarrhoea
- colic

Parasitism – the state of being infested and of infesting – a host/parasite relationship.

Helminthiasis – infestation by endoparasites, colloquially known as 'worms' or helminths.

Infestation – invasion and colonisation by parasites; it equates with infection by 'germs'. **Infection** is often used for both.

Anthelmintic – a drug, usually given orally to horses, which will kill adult worms or possibly only temporarily reduce their fecundity or egg-laying for periods which vary with the drug used and, in some examples, also the larvae and even the eggs before their expulsion with the faeces.

Generally speaking a foal is not born with worms. One species of worm may be ingested via milk.

Important Worms of Horses and Ponies

Common Name	Latin Name	Organ
Redworms – Strongyles		
Large Redworms – important internal organs damaged by migrating immature larvae	Strongylus species	Large Intestine
Small Redworms – cause severe disease, especially the encysted larvae	10–20 species	Large Intestine
Roundworms – Ascarids Large white worm, particularly in foal	Parascaris equorum	Small Intestine
Pinworms Cause rectal irritation	Oxyuris equi	Large Intestine
Lungworms Coughing; association with donkeys	Dictyocaulus arnfieldi	Lungs (Bronchi)
Threadworms May cause enteritis in young foals	Strongyloides westeri	Small Intestine
Skin sores and stiff neck	Onchocerca species	Neck
Tapeworms Enteritis in young horses Colic in others No larval migration from gut lumen	Anoplocephala perfoliata	Around the ileo-caecal valve mucous membranes
Bots 'Numbers' may cause stomach ulcers	Larvae of Gastrophylus fly	Stomach

Life Cycle

Endoparasites have a cyclic regeneration programme

- egg
- larva which hatch from it: L1 which 'feed' off herbage micro-nutrients to become
- L2 which continues as above to 'moult' to become 'ripe'
- L3 which remains cocooned, surviving off the stored energy material, usually sufficient for up to 6 days, during which period it is said to be 'ripe' and so infective if consumed by a specific host. It daily migrates up herbage leaf blade but descends each evening, with the dew. If not swallowed it dies

Eggs and larvae 1 and 2 if consumed even by the correct, specific host do not develop further. Their required hatching and moulting are dependent on a prescribed temperature and moisture content in the micro-climate. Survival rates can therefore variably alter season by season and within these.

Pasture clearance of faeces – from which the larvae naturally can 'migrate' or be physically dispersed – is an essential horsemastership practice to reduce field levels of potential re-infestation. Desiccation by wind and sunlight play a part in reducing larval numbers but deliberate clearance – pasture hygiene – is most important.

Harrowing breaks open faecal pats and exposes larvae but also disperses them, which can be counter-productive.

Mixed grazing has a cleansing effect in as much as non-susceptible animals eat a proportion of eggs and larvae but also a proportion of horse grass feed. If cattle, as distinct from sheep, are used they will reduce the rough grasses which have grown in areas where horses have defecated and made them unattractive – hence the common problem in horse pastures of 'roughs' and 'smooths' leading to 'horse sick' grazing areas.

Horse worms are host specific except for liver fluke, which affects all grazing animals.

The Parasitic Period

When L3 is swallowed it moults and colonises on the intestinal tract and penetrates into the mucous membranes. Thereafter its migration pattern varies with the species of worm. Some stay locally, others penetrate further, even away from the gut via, for example, arterial walls and via lymphatic vessels to the liver and over the peritoneum. But all, after a further moult, re-enter the gut wall as L4 and subsequently develop to L5 before entering the large bowel lumen as immature and then mature egg-laying adults.

Some have predilection sites elsewhere, for example ascarids re-enter in the small intestine, lungworm enter the airways, and liver fluke can be found in bile ducts.

The pathogenicity varies with the larval behaviour and numbers and with adult feeding habits and numbers,

Some worms have an extra intermediate stage in the cycle during which time L3 or its equivalent inhabits an 'intermediate stage' host, another invertebrate in the case of herbivore parasitism. This life cycle continues when the intermediate host

- disgorges a new generation of larvae onto herbage, as with liver fluke
- is swallowed by the grazing animal and, on digestion, liberates the larva, e.g. tapeworms

Environmnent Conditions

Eggs require moisture and warmth which, when optimal, allows hatching within 7 days, but can also be much longer. It continues usually only from, in the northern hemisphere, April through to October. Larval levels on grazing are variably cumulative and are highest in late summer and early autumn. Larvae can go from L1 to L3 in approximately 20 to 30 days, but this can be delayed if climatic conditions are not favourable.

The adult (female) worm is usually a prolific egg producer aiming to make certain the regeneration of the species, despite many eggs on the pasture dying or their 'ripe' larvae succumbing to

- inclement micro-climate
- failure to be ingested by the specific host
- ingested by the wrong, non-susceptible host
- not ingested within their 6-day safety margin

It is believed that most adults live for one month in the host, but for various reasons, i.e. host (in)tolerance with some worm species, this varies. Some become quiescent or less fecund, especially in the winter months (no use laying eggs to exit into inhospitable external conditions!).

Host (in)tolerance is a form of non-specific immunity acquired by the host, subject to its constitutional well-being, in response to infestation, colonisation and subsequent morbidity by the parasite.

This tolerance determines parasitic levels during the larval development (migration), the adult establishment and its fecundity (the egg production). It can be considered as a product of the parasitism which controls the levels to prevent killing the host – as a rule. It applies particularly to adult worm numbers which eventually parasitise within the lumen or elsewhere within the body systems' tracts

- airways (lungworm)
- bile ducts (liver fluke)
- small intestine (large roundworm and tapeworm)
- large intestine and caecum ('large' and 'small' redworm)

In large white roundworms in yearlings, and in lungworms of all ages, a more specific immunity eventually ejects adult worm stages. Yearlings never again develop morbid levels of large white roundworms (ascarids) and horses generally maintain a resistance to repeat lungworm infestation. The redworm can persistently re-infest horses subject to the restrictions mentioned above.

It is involved, but even less explicably, in the onward migration and the hypobiotic-inhibited stages of some larval species, e.g. the Cyathostome small redworm. It is less effective in the immature animal, the old and the intercurrently dis-eased, all of which may be coincidentally **mal-nourished**, which factor is important in an ill-kept horse of any age.

Recent research suggests that tolerance is related to the nutritional status of the host, particularly in regard to the **protein level** of its diet, and so **its tissue amino acid levels**. Thus, those animals such as the

- yearling to 3-year old
- barren mare
- mid-pregnant mare
- outwintered stock, such as polo ponies
- pensioned-off geriatrics

all likely to be on 'economic' rations without supplementary feed, are most at risk. This becomes more serious, a more pathogenic life cycle, as helminthiasis increases, since the morbidity in the bowel wall is associated with reduced digesta absorption, as well as a protein-losing enteropathy and a further diminution in amino acids and globulin levels in the blood. **Hypoalbumenaemia** – low blood albumen – is a classical laboratory finding. Most species of worm benefit from this reduced tolerance, to the detriment of the host. The larval stages of Cyathostomes are most important in this relationship.

The important feature of helminthiasis, which has been mentioned earlier, is that it is seen as being dependent upon the method or manner of dissemination of the infestation

- the egg (sometimes, as with lungworm, the larva) via

the faeces in all common types of worm dis-ease

- the fate of the egg and of the larva during the free stage, or in an intermediate host (liver fluke and tapeworm) and its fate
    - their survival as influenced by external, environmental factors
- the larva, eventually the infective L3 by ingestion by a susceptible host grazer (foals can be infested by licking the mare and the immediate environment, as with the large white roundworm)

The factors that influence infestation of the host by ingestion of L3 are

- accessibility to contaminated herbage
    - direct
    - indirect via intermediate host's voided larvae
- grazing habits
    - close cropping
    - dislike of tainted herbage
    - nomadism

The factors that influence the host/parasite relationship during the parasitic phase are

- larval migration
- adult colonisation
- host's constitution

Under domesticated circumstances the horsemaster must accept that horses will be parasitised by worms and that pastures (and other sites) will consequently be contaminated by eggs and subsequently by larvae.

Strategic administration of suitable anthelmintics will control the output of eggs, and so the level of pasture contamination. This will reduce the level of larval build up on the pasture and their availability for ingestion.

It is possible to do this reasonably effectively if done correctly but **not always**. Some larvae get through. In mature grazing-horses in good nutritional status, any subsequent parasitism is of limited importance.

It is impossible to chemically disinfect pastures but **pasture hygiene, the physical removal of faeces from the pasture at regular intervals, is the most efficient way of minimising larval levels already there. Without it, anthelmintics can fail.**

Frequency of dung clearance reflects speed of hatching

and moulting of the larvae. In summer, twice weekly is essential. It must be done completely.

In practice, with well-managed horses of all ages and types, there is really no excuse for 'seeing' wormy horses – that is, those showing characteristic clinical signs of any degree. Enough is known about control methods that prevention is all but fool-proof. The weak links in this are

- development of **drug-resistant worm species**, most common in
- breeding and rearing establishments, which are often the most heavily larvae infested
    - mixed age group grazing
    - incorrectly wormed stock
- loss of tolerance associated with
    - overstocking
    - restricted grazings
    - over-used exercise paddocks
- *failure to control pasture hygiene*
- introduction of unknown stock without isolation and suitable larval and adult worm medication
- access to unknown pastures when horses are away from home which, on return, are not correctly dosed, e.g. Pony Club camps, overnight shows, at stud
- understandable attempts to cut wormer costs by reducing numbers of treatment without the back-up of EPG counts and pasture hygiene (over 2,000 EPG warrants treatment; this level and above can be associated with at least sub-clinical disease)
- failure to appreciate that the innate dislike of horses to grazing tainted areas, a natural protection against infestation, can be offset by the effects of
    - galloping hooves
    - 'picking' birds, and
    - vermin passively transmitting larvae onto acceptable grazing
- placing too much reliance on
    - harrowing before faecal pat lifting. Good as this is for pasture management, the expected larval number control depends upon dry weather desiccation of them
- mixed grazing; cattle and sheep will of course safely consume equine third stage larvae leaving less for the horse *but* it implies a greater area of grazing to offset competitive nutritional intake

Interval or coincidental grazing by cattle (store beasts),

whereby they consume coarse grasses growing in tainted areas which horses avoid, will help prevent horse-sick pastures. So too will cutting.

Diagnosis

- clinical signs, including loss of condition relative to possible presence of diarrhoea, and appetite-state relative to
    - season of the year – as with inhibited Cyathostome larvae
    - age of horse and its nutrition
        - weanling – source of large white roundworm eggs
        - geriatric – greater level of egg output
- EPG count
- blood samples for
    - white cell counts
    - albumen level
    - globulin level and electrophoresis thereof

Pathogenicity

The resultant morbidity is mainly functionally related to tissue damage which, although often clinical with other signs, *is not always characterised by diarrhoea*. Adult worm over-population and exiting Cyathostome larvae, especially the former, are more likely to cause diarrhoea; so too if inhibited larval emergence is delayed until April instead of the usual February, causing

- a severe 'shock' effect, when exiting Cyathostome larvae in the early spring cause marked enteric wall trauma as well as the loss of bowel absorption function, which can be on-going
- irritant hypermotility of the bowel
- failure to reabsorb gut waters, due to
    - increased speed of peristalsis
    - reduced absorption area in the damaged gut mucosae

As with other forms of gut disorders, the motility of normal peristalsis of the large intestine and the caecum, and indirectly of the small intestine, can be slowed to the extent of ileus or bowel paralysis in some stages of endo-parasitism.

Both this *hypo*-motility and the more usual *hyper*-motility (diarrhoea) can disorganise electrolyte levels in the body fluids, with subsequent systemic illness.

The worms whose L3 larvae migrate out of the bowel

wall can cause tissue morbidity elsewhere, e.g.

- the larvae of one large redworm, Strongylus vulgaris, was notorious (in pre-Ivermectin days) for blocking the gut's blood supply
- another Strongyle (Str. edentatus) larva produces peritoneal adhesions
- the lungworm larvae of Dictyocaulus arnfieldi cause lung connective tissue damage, and the adult induces inflammation of the respiratory airways
- the larvae of the large white roundworm, Parascaris equorum, produces asymptomatic lesions in the liver and, *en passant*, respiratory tissue and tract irritation, during its migration
- actual liver tissue damage by the liver fluke larvae is, unlike in the cow, sheep and man, sub-clinical but its entry into the bile duct begins the inflammatory changes therein which are worsened by the developing adult fluke to produce pathologic clinical signs including anaemia and diarrhoea

Anthelmintics ('Wormers')

There are three main generic groups of chemicals currently in use worldwide. These and the sub-groups, and examples of the trade names, are shown below

Benzimidazoles

Fenbendazole	Panacur	Hoechst
Oxibendazole	Lincoln	Battle, Hayward & Bower
Mebendazole	Telmin	Janssen

Tetrahydropyrimidines

Pyrantel embonate	Strongid P	Pfizer
	Pyratape P	Hoechst

Macrocyclic lactones

Ivermectin	Eqvalan	Merial
	Furexel	Janssen
Moxidectin	Equest	Fort Dodge

All, at the right dose and given at the correct time, will kill all the adult forms of equine helminths except Fasciola hepatica (consult veterinary surgeon *re* drug for this uncommon parasite). Their efficacy against worm eggs and the larval stages varies with the species of parasite. The 'age' of larval development knocked out will determine egg-laying intervals, as will deviation of activity of the various drugs; the efficacy of pasture hygiene will, to a significant extent, determine the likelihood of ongoing reinfestation.

Helminths can, and do, develop a resistance to anthelmintics. This usually is in the adult stage and therefore this plays an important role in egg level control. It is recognised with

- Fenbendazole, probably with
- Pyrantel, possibly in time with
- Ivermectin, and no doubt eventually with
- Moxidectin

In British parasitic control only Benzimidazole resistance is significant – so far!

A worsening scene is most likely in worm burdens in those groups of horses which are not all dosed

- at the same time, or are
- under-dosed
- paradoxically, dosed unnecessarily frequently, especially if also under-dosed per bodyweight each time
- are kept on the one basic (summer) drug for more than one year, except, so far, with the macrocyclic lactones

At least at the beginning of the grazing season, and again around half way through, random faeces samples from the immature, mature and geriatric horse age-groups, depending on the mixture of ages in any one total group, should be examined for EPG. If this level is 500 or less, at least one treatment can be left out.

Specific blood sample tests for antibodies to tapeworm are available. Where such infestation is suspected their use is advisable.

It must not be forgotten that the various levels of sub-clinical and clinical **larval** helminthiasis, especially cyathostomiasis, must be kept in mind even with a negative egg count. Veterinary differential diagnosis of lowered horse performance, mild unthriftiness or clinically 'wormy' is essential whenever these develop, to rule out helminthiasis or not. Egg presence or lack of them is no guide.

It is recognised that, given at routine dosage levels, Fenbendazole (Panacur) kills eggs, non-penetrated L3, emerging L4 and L5, and adults, and large and small redworms. Pyrantels kill adults, large and small redworms. Eqvalan or Furexel (both Ivermectin) kill L4 and L5 large redworms, adults, large white roundworm larvae and adults, and lungworm adults; and Equest kills late stage L3, L4 and L5 small redworm adults, but not the early encysted stage L3.

It is essential that the horse's mass (body weight at the

Chart of Anthelmintic Efficiency

	Panacur	Lincoln or Telmin	Strongid P Pyratape P	Eqvalan	Equest
Large Roundworm					
Larvae 4 & 5	✓	✓	✓	✓	✓
Adult		✓	✓	✓	✓
Large Redworm					
Egg (in rectum)	✓	✓	–	–	–
Larvae 3 & 4	–	–	–	✓	✓
Larvae 5	✓	✓	–	✓	✓
Adult	✓	✓	✓	✓	✓
Small Redworm					
Egg (in rectum)	✓	✓	–	–	–
Larvae early 3	✓ single dose for 5 days	✓	–	–	–
Larvae late 3	✓ single dose for 5 days	✓	–	–	✓
Larvae 4 & 5	✓	✓	–	–	✓
Adult	✓	✓	✓	✓	✓
Tapeworms					
Adult	–	–	✓ one double dose	–	–
Bots		–	–	✓	✓

The manufacturer's data sheet will suggest dosage regimes.

stance) is known to within 20kg and that the correct dose per kg is accurately administered, preferably in syringed paste form into an empty mouth, and seen to be swallowed; or a liquid or a powder form is thoroughly mixed into a small amount of usual feed and is 'seen to be eaten'.

All horses in the one environment, even if in adjacent fields, must be dosed at the same time and according to the prescribed programme for adult worms and/or larvae as well. Veterinary advice should be taken.

Beware when changing the 'make' of wormer that a decision is based on the generic and not just on the trade name. This is particularly so with the Benzimidazoles; Panacur is the trade name of but one of this group, the Fenbendazoles. Although the least resistance-causing of its group at single dosage rate, it is acknowledged as the next wormer most likely to become ineffective.

Paradoxically, but fortunately, in the 5-day course against cyathostomiasis it is still effective against parasitic larval stages even if resistance in adults has been confirmed.

The larval arterial stage of Strongylus vulgaris, a large redworm, is susceptible only to Eqvalan and Equest at routine dosage. With the widespread use of Eqvalan in British horses, the incidence of thrombo-embolism of the mesenteric arteries, especially the main branch from the aorta, has dropped almost to zero: so too have the often lethal associated 'acute abdomen' cases of colic.

Eqvalan is not effective against larval Cyathostomes, but its 'relation' Moxidectin (which is the chemical name for the trade product Equest and is one of the family of the Milbemycin group) is, *except* for early L3 which enters the bowel mucosal wall in late summer. It does knock out late L3, L4 and L5 but this leaves an infested horse with a morbid burden of early L3 in its large gut and caecal wall over winter – a low grade, debilitating parasitism worsened by constitutional factors and possible enteric and metabolic illness. This is a potential for crisis in February/March at L3 emergence time if treatment is not given with either drug or the spring dose of Equest is 'late'.

The time from larvae ingestion until the adult becomes egg-laying varies with the worm species; it is called the **prepatency period (PP)**. An early summer cyathostomiasis can have a PP of as short as 5 weeks. A late summer, early autumn infestation with associated hypobiosis, or arrested encystment, can be up to 5 months. The migratory period of the large red worm Strongylus vulgaris takes at least 8 months.

Such differences determine not only strategic worming but a tactical programme, as well as consideration of the **egg reappearance time (ERT)**, and so further pasture contamination.

Success of therapies both for established clinical helminthiasis and of prophylactic dosage for presumed sub-clinical conditions are judged by

- clinical improvement
- laboratory analysis of blood samples for worm burden presence and albumen estimation
- laboratory analysis of faeces for the number of **eggs per gramme (EPG)**

Remember that larval morbidity need not have a significant associated EPG (colloquially known, erroneously, as a 'worm count') for prevention of subclinical dis-ease, e.g. lowered overall performance or clinical disease with loss of condition.

Species of Equine Helminths

Scientifically, the large number of potential parasitic species are all members of the animal kingdom. Only a few parasitise British domestic animals and fewer still the horse. A brief catalogue includes specimens from the taxonomic classes

- Trematodes, or flat worms, e.g. liver fluke
- Cestodes, or tapeworms
- Nematodes, or roundworms – which are members of several different orders and families

The latter category includes the

- large white roundworm, the Ascarid: Parascaris equorum
- large redworm: Strongylus species
- small redworm: Cyathostomes
- lungworm: Dictyocaulus
- pinworm: Oxyuris equi
- intermediate stage of the dog tapeworm: echinococcal liver cysts
- ectoparasitic larvae
  - bots
  - warbles (now extinct in the UK)

With the exception of liver fluke and lungworm, whose adults infest the bile ducts and the airways respectively, the adults of the others mature and egg lay on the mucosal wall or in the lumen of the intestines; the large white roundworm in the small intestine, the others in the large and in the blind gut (the caecum).

Routine worming has 'taken care' of the pinworm; it will not be further discussed.

Liver Fluke

A rare problem in horses generally. Where it is recognised as a hazard of sheep, in which it is particularly pathogenic, or in the cow, where it is less so, then the horse owners in such districts must seek veterinary advice. In man and in horse, both unusual hosts, aberrant Fascioliasis has been reported as affecting the lungs and the subcutaneun, as well as in the bile ducts.

The few 'typical' liver migration stage and bile duct colonisation cases have vague signs such as

- weight loss
- increased appetite
- lethargy (possibly anaemia)
- poor performance

Diagnosis depends upon finding the characteristic eggs in the faeces; even a few are significant for diagnosis, unlike in other cases of helminthiasis.

The intermediate specific host snail in its restricted environment lends itself to effective husbandry control and chemical eradication.

Echinococcus

The cysts of this dog tapeworm, which develop in the equine liver which is a 'dead end' intermediate host site, is invariably discovered coincidentally only on autopsy or at slaughter. *Ante mortem* clinical signs are not recorded as such. Infestation in humans, especially slaughtermen and knackers, and even consumers, is a possibility.

Cestodes or Tapeworms

Anoplocephala perfoliata is the species most commonly discovered in the horse. It is a cream-coloured, short (less than 10cm, 4in) tape-like worm with a segmented body. Its eggs develop progressively with the age of each successive segment; the ripe segments break off to be voided in the faeces; the eggs are liberated onto pasture and, where relevant, onto grass subsequently cut for hay. There they are ingested by Oribatid mites which themselves are ingested. On digestion, they liberate the now developed larvae which mature on the gut mucosae of the distal ileal wall and around the ilio-caecal valve with the caecum.

It is only comparatively recently that any real significance has been paid to this helminthiasis even though, on routine post-mortem inspections, 80%-plus of horses have been found to carry sometimes many tens, even hundreds of them. Their longevity is unknown but re-infestation from horse-grazed pastures and hay fields is quite likely.

The ripe, gravid (full of eggs ready to hatch) segments, if present and looked for, can be seen in the fresh faeces. At autopsy, associated ulcers where adult tapes had established themselves are characteristic of their sucker attachment for feeding. When suspected, earlier researchers described

- general unthriftiness
- vague digestive disturbances
- blood in the faeces
- anaemia
- lowered performance, if on its own, was seen as possible evidence of sub-clinical infestation

Recently, with the increasing opportunity to surgically enter the abdomen more safely for colic-case identification and operative interference, especially where the caecum was the possible site of the morbidity, the presence of tapeworms was understandably associated with the colic. The pathology was often inflammatory with coincidental effect on the neurological network of the bowel.

Whilst the feeding ulcers could explain some of these changes, the causative derangement of the ilio-caecal valve function and the ileal and caecal peristaltic disorders are the more likely source of the colic causing pain and malfunctioning, producing variable types of colic such as

- spasmodic
- ileal impaction
- caecal intussusception
  - within itself
  - into the colon, possibly with associated vascular deficits

Such morbidity was thought to be due to toxic factors emanating from the worm and/or from the traumatised mucosae. Management was directed in the knowledge of the life cycle and efficacy of 2x dosage of Pyrantel. Since grass **and** hay could be sources of the infested mites, the horse, if treated in the autumn and again in later winter, could be kept reasonably clear of cestode infestation.

A serum sample can be tested for specific tapeworm antibodies; the interpretation is very accurate.

Apart from the above helminths, the horsemaster should be particularly concerned with the two main groups of nematodes (roundworms). Both are descriptively termed 'red' because of their blood-sucking stages.

The 'Large' Redworm

There are three species

- Strongylus equinus is rare in Great Britain, the male is 35mm (1.5in), the female 47mm (1.9in)

- Strongylus edentatus is more common, the male 28mm (1.1in), female 44mm (1.7in)

- Strongylus vulgaris was formerly the most common of the three, male 16mm (0.6in), female 24mm (1in)

Strongylus vulgaris and edentatus are now not so common – widespread use of Ivermectin has been so effective against the L4 in the thrombus it forms and against the adult that the life cycle has been critically interrupted.

It is advisable however not to ignore the possibility of a Strongylidosis involving both edentatus and vulgaris. Fortunately the adults are readily controlled by all the drugs in current use except that resistance may already be present to Fenbendazole. The ERT is short at 4 weeks with Pyrantel; the Ivermectins can keep the gut clear of adult egg layers for up to 6 weeks, Moxidectin for 13 weeks.

The 'Small' Redworm

Cyathostomes are less than 25mm (1in) adult size, of 10 to 20 species, and the 'fashionable' serious form of parasitism. The larval stage is **cyathostomiasis**.

There is a combined pathogenicity – adults attach to mucosae, suck blood, and eat epithelium and nutrients in the digesta.

When this sets up sub-clinical or clinical dis-ease it does so in early to mid summer, especially if the weather is mild and wet, when significantly large numbers of L3 have been and are being ingested to penetrate the small intestinal wall en route to the mucosae of the large intestine and the caecum. There they are temporarily encysted for up to 35 days. The actual numbers are a reflection of the daily intake. The progress in order of uptake, and consequently exiting the gut wall to become adults, is a steady succession.

Their intrusion, and their physical space-occupying infestation, can affect absorption of volatile fatty acids and the interchange of bowel fluids with mucosal interstitial fluids and the associated electrolytes. Pressure on the myometrial nerve tissue can also affect peristalsis, leading to a variety of mild colics, but rarely to the acute abdomen syndrome as no vascular crises seem to be involved.

It is difficult, especially in the absence of effective pasture hygiene, to prevent this infestation which in general has little **clinical** effect (but, by the numbers present, has sub-clinical **morbid** effect). If, for any reason, the larval and subsequent adult worm levels overcome host tolerance, then a state of clinical parasitism may

show. If larval, then an EPG count may be deceptively low in this stage. Worming with Ivermectin (Eqvalan or Furexel) or Moxidectin (Equest) will control the L3–4 and L5 if a differential diagnosis leads to such a suspicion (and so too will 5 x Fenbendazole – Panacur). Routine dosing (tactical medication) if the EPG is well into four figures, using one or other of the current therapies, will control the adult worms and the eggs.

Larvae ingested in late summer not only encyst but also are subject to metabolic disturbance whereby their further development is inhibited. (Some may remain so for years, but this is of more academic interest.) The causes of inhibition are postulated as

- environmental trigger, as with adverse cold autumnal weather; this suggests a 'sixth sense' decision. Such larvae are known as hypobiotic 'awaiting' the more favourable external conditions of next spring

- immunological trigger, to produce arrested larvae possibly for the same reason

Since it is impossible to differentiate, the description 'inhibited' is best used. There are two reasons for the seriousness of this inhibition

- the late summer build-up is on-going for several weeks at least; the total, said to be 1 million in some young animals, has a continuing and increasing pathologic effect

- the eventual synchronous emergence of all at (virtually) the one time, an *en masse* effect, causes severe bowel trauma and shock

It occurs primarily in February, with

- sudden weight loss (with ventral oedema)

- pyrexia

- anorexia

- depression

- occasionally a loss of thirst

- inducible flank pain

- evacuation of some reddish larvae L4 and L5 in obvious heaps along or separate from the faeces

A second syndrome is sometimes seen extending further than February, as far as May

- sudden onset diarrhoea (perhaps associated with adults in the lumen wall as well)

- weight loss and ventral oedema

- no pyrexia or anorexia

More serious colic, as from intussusception, has been

reported in yearling Thoroughbreds, and recurrent diarrhoea in aged ponies. It may be associated with chronic weight loss in adult horses, presumably from chronic enteric scarring and loss of effective absorption surface area.

It has recently been shown that Cyathostome larvae can not only overwinter on pasture as L1 and L2, but will become reactive even in reseeded pastures. Infestive L3 have also been detected in winter pastures with consequent risk to outwintered stock.

Management
As previously described

- Moxidectin (Equest) is larvicidal *only* for *late (L)* L3, L4 and L5

whereas

- Fenbendazole (Panacur/Panacur Guard) over 5 days is larvicidal for *early (E)* L3 *as well*

The use of this Fenbendazole course in October will kill bowel located adults (and 'new laid' eggs) as well as larvae in gut mucosal cysts, and this minimises the autumn adult parasitism and subsequent pasture contamination. Give at end of the grazing season, but no later than October for outwintered stock or when horses 'come up' in the Autumn, even though daily grazing is still on offer.

It will also **markedly reduce the risk of February acute emergence dis-ease** from inhibited larvae as well as later adult infestation and larval cyathostomiasis.

Moxidectin in February will also deal with the inhibited larvae and any Fenbendazole-resistant adults, or at least shut down on egg laying for at least 10 weeks, but the timing can be wrong for the former – the traumatic emergence may have occurred.

Strongyloids, which infest foals up to six months of age, may be associated with diarrhoea which is not usually serious. Most frequent at around the dam's 'foal oestrus'. The Strongyloides westeri inhabits the small intestine. Its life cycle includes larval stages in the dam's milk with subsequent oral infestation. These can also invade through the skin. They are usually self-limiting.

Endoparasitism

Recent research into the effects of anthelmintics (wormers), apart from their efficacy in killing adult egg-laying worms, concerns overall ability to keep the host's bowel clear of egg layers. This is a reflection of how far

down the life cycle they act. Immature adults can quickly replace the egg layers which were killed off; 5th stage, then 4th stage larvae move up the hierarchy.

Some wormers, as is known, will knock out these and the incoming 3rd stage larvae as well. There will be a gap of freedom from eggs in the faeces (and onto the grazing) accordingly.

This widespread kill is not a simple matter; it varies with the worm species and with the drug and its persistence in the gut. The gap, the period until worm eggs reappear, the egg re-appearance time (ERT), in practice appears to be fairly accurate although anything which undermines the general health of the animal may alter this.

The ERT determines the maximum interval between dosings for the commonly used wormers

Pyrantel	4 weeks
Benzimidazoles	4–6 weeks (subject to no resistance of the worm to this drug)
Ivermectin	8–10 weeks (the Ivermectins – Eqvalan and Furexel – have shown isolated pockets of this loss of usefulness. Others may follow suit in time, even Moxidectin – Equest)
Moxidectin	13 weeks

Resistance is most likely to develop in horse units where there are high densities, especially of

- juveniles
- and mixed groups following youngster sales and training intakes

Benzimidazole resistance was blamed on over-usage

- year-after-year dosing
- unnecessary dosing in any one year

Fort Dodge recommend 2 years' use of Equest gel (but this may have to be amended from manufacturer's experience).

These possibilities emphasise the need for

- veterinary input
  - faecal egg counts and their interpretation
  - recognition of genera and sub-genera within a programme (ability to 'read the label' correctly)
  - consideration for eggs killed in the rectum by some wormers
  - the feasibility of isolation of dosed horses off a

grazing for 48 hours. The practicability and economics compared with the risk of pasture re-infestation contained by hygiene

The advantage of worming to an ERT is that the number of treatments can be kept to a minimum, a strategy which works well with the seasonal strategies .

The risk of larval ingestion is greatest in April to October, and increasingly so during May to August.

The tactic of worming only if the egg count indicates a significant worm level is not foolproof. Certainly a count of more than 1,000 EPG is evidence of active egg laying; a gut parasitism is therefore assumed but usually of mild pathogenicity.

Lower than 1,000 is suggestive of low adult infestation *previously*. The level of current infestation is unknown. Absence of treatment therefore leaves some adults to go on laying, so pasture hygiene becomes more imperative. The level and the pathogenicity of larval stages in migration in or through the gut wall is often indeterminate during the spring and summer – again a reason for veterinary discussion.

The cost of faecal tests, especially if all horses are included, may well exceed the drug costs saved, but the risk of drug resistance is kept down.

Tapeworm control requires double dosing with Pyrantel; as there is yet no evidence of resistance to round worm medication this generic drug can be so used in the autumn and in the spring as coincidental roundworm control.

At present, Moxidectin is licensed to kill only the late stage of 3rd stage larvae of Cyathostomes. If given in February this will reduce the risk of *en masse* emergence morbidity, but it will have missed the overwintering inhibited 3rd stage Cyathostome larvae pathogenicity. In young (and old) horses and brood mares this may be dangerous: hence the advisability of **1 dose per day for 5 days, with Fenbendazole (Panacur Guard) – this should be done in late autumn and again in late winter.** This could be usefully applied to all horses who have been through a grazing season.

Suggested recommendations for **summer** worm control are
- strategic
  - restrict dosing to April to September inclusive, using the previously detailed intervals relative to the drug selected
  - change this basic drug each year, subject to
  - known resistance – consult with veterinary surgeon to determine this in your situation

- consider Eqvalan and Equest to be basically similar
- selective
  - if EPG is higher than 1,000, dose as above
  - if less than 1,000, do not dose but carry out EPG tests at 6-week intervals during May to September
  - if using Equest, dose 4 times per year as advised by manufacturer. No need for EPG unless clinical signs warrant it
  - dose for Cyathostome larvae as previously advised and for tapeworms and liver fluke if considered necessary on veterinary surgeon's advice. Other worms likewise
- any of the common anthelmintics can be assumed to be effective within the manufacturer's data sheet assertions provided that
  - the correct dose is given to an accurately assessed weight of horse (better to slightly over-estimate weight)
  - into an empty mouth if a paste or gel is used (check that it is not 'spat out')
    - left in manger if in a mixed feed
  - to a clinically healthy horse
  - all horses in a grazing area are dosed together
- hygiene
  - once-weekly pasture faecal clearance November – March. Twice-weekly pasture faecal clearance April – October
  - in routine situations there is no need to keep dosed horses off the pasture
  - it is beneficial not only to minimise the risk of infestation but when also to avoid overgrazing of pasture, to change fields, strips and plots regularly, relative to available grass
  - recent work has involved the supplementation of feed with a fungus which is known to live off grazing micro-nutrients, **including** endoparasitic eggs, but which is harmless to 'dung' beetles which are important in the degrading of faeces and withdrawal of the remnants into the soil

It is essential for both welfare and economic reasons that a veterinary surgeon is consulted with regard to the correct prevention and treatment measures of worm control.

CHAPTER 27
DISEASES OF THE URINARY SYSTEM

In veterinary practice, illnesses associated with dis-ease of the urinary system do not rank high in case lists, certainly not as primary conditions, although recent research work to develop more accurate diagnostic parameters has pointed to a higher incidence than was previously thought.

To the horsemaster, a horse which starts to hyper-react to being mounted (is cold-backed, or hunches up, even bucks), to be difficult to ride in collection, to refuse at jumping, or to resent grooming along the back, is often seen as having 'something wrong with its kidneys'. (Anatomically the kidneys are more or less under the post-cantle area!)

In reality, such a horse is more likely to be affected with

- neuro-muscular problems in the vertebral column – cord, bone, joints, ligaments, tendons and/or muscles
- lesions elsewhere in the locomotor system
- mouth, saddle fit, or rider problems

Nevertheless, it is good horsemastership to be aware (albeit the horse at grass, or partly at grass, does present difficulties in this context) of *any changes in the normal* <u>A</u> <u>B</u> <u>C</u> of urine excretion, such as

- frequency
- approximate quantity, each time and over 24 hours
- times and places when and where done
- relationship to feeding, work and grooming
- posture

There are explanations for some of these changes which are not indications of abnormality. Thus, variations in daily routine can be associated with time away from the stable, at work, being in transit, having altered work loads, and work-related sweating, and this *vis à vis* weather conditions.

There is the undeniable fact that urination cannot always be witnessed and, unlike defecation, the result is not 'left behind' as a factual indicator. Despite this, the attentive horsemaster should be aware of

- wetter or drier bedding than is customary
- an absence of staling at a usual time for a particular horse – for instance, when a new bed is put down, or on coming in from exercise

Some signs can be misleading to the inexperienced

- the urinary posture being maintained for what seems to be longer than necessary after the stream has ended
- 'winking' of the clitoris (in the mare) during this post-urinary period
- grunting, more common with the gelding, being mistaken for vocal evidence of pain

These can be normal for the in-season mare, or as an individual peculiarity, but they can suggest a defect elsewhere, e.g. locomotor system pain exacerbated in the stance or posture, which hurts at the time, or causes stiffness and difficulty in relaxing from the posture.

As with all signs, the horsemaster's skill is in *recognising that something is 'newly' wrong*, i.e. *different*. Actual diagnosis then depends upon more experienced knowledge.

The indications that a problem in the uro(genital) system is more than a dubious suspicion are that urination seems to be

- incomplete, or much reduced
- an intermittently interrupted stream

- accompanied by obvious straining, sometimes unproductively
- more frequent, with less volume at any one time

and, in the male

- without 'dropping' the penis, so that the flow is 'through' the sheath orifice
- 'dropped', but followed by an unusual delay in retraction
- of greater volume of clearer urine and/or more frequently in any given time period
  - this is **polyuria** following **polydypsia**, i.e. more water out because of more water drunk
    - psychogenic or idiosyncratic
    - a failure to concentrate naturally, from a defect in ADH (antidiuretic hormone) production following anterior pituitary tumour, usually in the older animal (see Cushing's disease in the older horse)

or that urine shows changes from the normal in

- **colour** – usually pale yellow to amber, but there are individual variations, and nutritional-effected variations
- **consistency**
  - clear, to opaque (cloudiness relates to dietary calcium levels)
  - becomes turbid at end of stream
  - is slimy, which varies with the level of mucus necessary to prevent aggregation of calcium crystals and so facilitate passage of them (it is produced by special glands in the kidney pelvis)
- **smell** – is 'strong' relative to varying levels of ammonia

It is such *abnormal variations* in any horse, occurring within a matter of days, which may be noticed by the owner/groom.

Further changes, in pH and specific gravity, are measurable by tests on a sample.

How to Collect a Urine Sample

Samples are usually requested

- when any of the warning signs already mentioned are reported to the veterinary surgeon
- when a metabolic profile is to be effected which requires complementary blood and urine samples. The

veterinary surgeon will instruct concerning the time scale or interval between samples

- when the veterinary surgeon requires urine to augment his examination of other body systems

To collect the sample

- be ready for donor at its known time of urination
- have a wide-necked jar, non-glass, in hand, already thoroughly clean and heat dried, sterilised (scalded) if such a sample is requested, with folded 'loo' paper (or sterile cloth) in the bottom to deaden stream noise (an abnormal noise will startle the horse into stopping the flow)
- be apparently occupied as usual, make bed, 'gentle' horse
- keep collecting jar in hand, but out of sight
- let horse begin to urinate
- quietly and slowly place jar in position – the later the stage the better, especially if a sterile sample is required
- remove before horse finishes
- beware swish of tail (it may undo your good work!)
- cover jar with clean cloth
- store as advised

Morbidity of the urinary tract can result in the presence of 'whole' blood (the red cells give the dominant red colour), when it is known as **haematuria**

- evenly distributed throughout the whole sample, but more usually as
- streaks of partially clotted blood
- discrete clots – intermittently throughout the stream, towards the end, or after the flow, when it is 'pushed' out or 'drained' out

Such bleeding can occur anywhere along the urinary tract from the renal (kidney) pelvis to the end of the urethra. In the collected sample, or on centrifuging, the cells settle to the bottom to leave a normal coloured urine above.

Blood pigment, discolouring it red – **haemoglobinuria** – throughout the stream, with even colouring and *no clotting*, is indicative of kidney dis-ease *per se*.

If the sample stays mainly discoloured even on centrifuging

- brown tinged to dark walnut – **myoglobinuria**
  - throughout stream, with no clotting – is indicative

of muscle (myoglobin) pigment, usually from **equine rhabdomylysis** (ER/azoturia), excreted by the kidneys which may secondarily suffer renal tubular disease from obstruction by this breakdown protein if it is excessive. In indeterminate cases of ER the veterinary surgeon may require laboratory tests to distinguish between these pigments in a sample

- pus (sometimes with haematuria)
  - clots scattered throughout stream
  - clinging threads of pus on lower commissure of vulvar lips
  - clinging drying streaks on backs of thighs and points of hocks
  - purulent deposits on bedding or ground, left behind from drained away urine (compare with phlegm gobbets in manger, water bucket, wall and floor outside stable door in chronic respiratory tract dis-ease)

Such inflammatory exudates will originate from the urinary tract or, more frequently, from the genital tract, especially that of the brood mare after 'covering' or foaling; and the stallion, in which the discharge arises from lesions on the end of the penis or on the lining of the prepuce. An ascending infection of the urethra and into the bladder may follow

- abnormal leakage
  - incontinence following foaling trauma to the pelvic nerves or uro-genital tissues
  - retention with overspill – neuritis of cauda equina; sacral nerve damage, as in sacral bone fracture and displacement from falling over backwards onto a hard surface; EHV-1 neuropathy
  - there are postural and behavioural changes as well as the more obvious defects in urine and faecal excretory control

Secondary signs are wetness on thighs, hocks and sometimes tail which, in some dis-eases, loses its tone and so cannot be elevated clear; and dried urine streaks on these areas.

The kidneys, under hormonal, enzymatic, neurogenic and blood pressure influences, determine whether body water should be conserved or the excess voided, and what electrolytes and other, more compounded, substances should be retained or disposed of.

Defects elsewhere in the body's control systems can be more definitely suspected by the results of aberrant effect on kidney functioning. Conversely, altered function of the kidney's filtration and/or concentrating mechanism will permit unwanted excretion or retention, with feedback effect on other organs. In both these situations any underlying cause may be sub-clinical except for the animal's failure to grow, or maintain condition, or reproduce, or athletically perform up to expectation.

The urinary system is responsible for

- the maintenance of water and electrolyte homeostasis
- the excretion of metabolic waste products
- the kidney's endocrine functions, producing
  - the hormone erythropoietin, for red blood cell formation in the bone marrow
  - the enzyme renin which is used by the adrenal glands, and
  - the active metabolite of vitamin D3

Sometimes, morbidity within the system is discovered during veterinary investigation of suspected renal disease, following routine blood and urine test indicators, other dis-ease, or at autopsy – said to be the most common source of information.

In addition to the signs related to micturition (passing of urine) and the urine itself, other clues of a less directly related nature may be exhibited before the more obvious appear, if in fact they ever do in life

- loss of appetite
- dullness
- lethargy
- fever
- anaemia, from loss of erythropoietin formation
- loss of condition

and, later in the course

- oedema along the ventral abdomen and legs
- uraemic halitosis – blood urea level increase

When kidney excretory function begins to fail at any stage, but usually later, the resultant ammonia reflux to the blood and so to the brain leads to **encephalopathy**.

When signs are acute and associated with pain, especially due to

- inflammation (bacterial infection) and/or
- obstruction

the picture can be confused with

- acute colic, as in digestive system crises
- ER (azoturia)
- bilateral lamenesses
    - laminitis, acute
    - back, pelvic, or hind-leg trauma

DIS-EASE TYPES

Developmental

(No hereditary factors have been confirmed – as yet!)

- congenital, including
    - open urachus at umbilicus (leakage at navel)
    - ruptured bladder, from parturition trauma – can be surgically corrected

Trauma

- rare; the kidneys' position gives good protection
- vertebral column injury could fortuitously interfere with vascular and neural control, but little information is available
- vaginal (urethral) at foaling
- vulvar at foaling and from external sources
- penile and preputial

Inflammatory Infections

The terms used usually end in 'itis'. Thus there is

- **nephritis** – of the kidney and its different 'parts'
- **uretritis** – of the ureter from kidney to bladder, usually in association with a kidney infection and thus a 'descending' spread
- **cystitis** – of the bladder. May be descending, fulminating there, or ascending from external sources via vagina and urethra
- **urethritis** – of the urethra. May be a further descent, especially associated with 'stones', but most frequently an 'ascending' infection

Kidney inflammation can arise from

- blood-borne infection and larval infestation
- secondary to other causes of morbidity

The primary infectious agents which result in nephritis are

- viral
    - equine infectious anaemia (EIA) (rare in Great Britain)
    - possibly equid herpes virus (EHV), indirectly through arteriolitis
- bacterial
    - streptococcoi (St. equi) causing suppurative obstruction, especially pyelonephritis
    - actinobacilli, and
    - corynebacteria, in foals
    - leptospiral – suspected, but not proven; many horses are serum positive for leptospirae, clinical signs are rare
- fungal
    - mycotoxins

Parasitic

Aberrant strongylus vulgaris larvae have caused renal vein obstruction with massive swelling and degeneration of a kidney, with haematoma formation and considerable pain.

Allergic

No specific condition has been documented. The auto-immune and allergen antibody reactions, as seen in man and in carnivores are, however, being investigated at present.

Degenerative

- kidney tubular nephrosis, following
    - infectious nephritis and pyelonephritis
    - obstruction from myoglobin
    - chemical poisoning – rare in the horse, except for excessive acorn ingestion, possibly bracken consumption, and chronic lead toxicity

There are no specific clues, but the morbidity can be such as to cause, sooner or later

- acute renal failure, or at least impaired renal function and consequent

- uraemic poisoning, from the associated loss of functioning
- generalised electrolytic imbalance
- death or euthanasia

- chronic wasting disease of the old horse, associated with interstitial nephritis, leads to
  - chronic renal failure
    - generalised electrolytic imbalance
    - uraemia and secondary further loss of condition
    - possibly encephalopathy
    - death or euthanasia

Neoplastic

Neoplasia is rare and when it does occur is secondary. Benign melanomas, fibromas or lipomas situated alongside the urethra in the mare may stimulate irritation of this part of the tract to such an extent that intermittent, irregular attempts at urination may stimulate intra-tract inflammation and/or partial obstruction and vague 'in oestrus' signs, out of cycle.

Urolithiasis

The formation of urinary calculi (stones) 'begins' within the kidney system, resulting in excessive amounts of insoluble minerals in the urine. These aggregate or concrete in the kidney pelvis, and either

- enlarge there, usually without signs, unless so big as to block outflow, when either
  - intermittent colic pain develops. Usually one kidney is affected, consequently urine production and output is unaffected, but some haematuria may be exhibited. If the affected kidney's production is completely blocked from the entrance to the ureter, a back-pressure build-up will occur with morbid effect on the kidney's functioning including nephritis and eventual degeneration
- or are extruded into the ureter, with inflammatory reaction, and become obstructed, or more commonly are washed into the bladder, which is the most common site for calculi

Vesical (or bladder) calculi invariably causes cystitis, with secondary bacterial infection. Signs are

- frequent micturition, and so repeated small volumes
  - pain at micturition
- prolonged posturing with straining
- haematuria, possibly pus – white blood cells (WBC), bacteria and bladder cells
- sometimes fever
- inappetence
- stiff gait

A straightforward ascending bacterial infection will produce somewhat similar signs without calculi formation.

Urethral calculi are

- rare in the mare, with her short straight urethra, but produce
  - occasional mild pain
  - limited straining, but perhaps more frequent until they are passed
  - some haematuria if 'stone' is big (they are usually smooth)
  - rarely with fever or 'off food'
- more common in the horse and gelding, with his long and 'bent' penis as it turns round the ischial arch, and with its relatively small urethral orifice
  - signs are more pronounced

In general the signs associated with these dis-eases are either

- too vague to be readily perceived and evaluated when the tract is affected
- or are those of a non-specific nature such as
  - poor performance
  - inappetence
  - wasting

when the kidney itself is affected.

If either or both of these are suspected, as during a non-specific investigation, the veterinary surgeon will make use of back-up laboratory aids involving

- blood changes
- urinary changes

Very often the first finding is that of anaemia in chronic, sub-clinical 'poor performance' syndrome.

DISEASES OF THE REPRODUCTIVE SYSTEM

INTRODUCTION

The domesticated horse's environment is an opportunity for man to, *inter alia*, decide which horses to use for breeding, the reproduction of the species, and thereby to enhance or improve the quality of his stock. Sometimes he succeeds, other times he fails.

Such aims may be within a breed or they may depend upon crossing a recognised pure (and better?) or established thoroughbred line with a non-pure bred or 'type' of horse. It is seen as an up-grading. It is usually based on a wish to obtain an improvement on the non-thoroughbred in terms of

- conformation

- temperament

- performance

  - ability

  - durability in speed and endurance

Rarely is it directly concerned with improvement in fertility which, generally speaking, is not seen as an immediate worry. Paradoxically the well-attested fact of hybrid vigour and related fertility gained by outcrossing – usually from a narrow or inbred line – is often overlooked.

What is more relevant is the risk, even within a thoroughbred line, of selecting a mare and/or stallion for their genes for e.g., speed only, to find that those for conformation related locomotor soundness have been lost. Even more worrying would be incidental loss of fertility. Coincidental locomotor problems, for example, can be later overcome or avoided by farriery and training; but poor semen quality or ovarian dysfunction are not so readily, if at all, correctable.

Unfortunately, stallions are invariably and primarily selected on their performance records. Equine semen samples are not simple to analyse, and it can be one or even two years into stud work before a suspected sub-fertility can be confirmed by results. These genetic faults are by then bred into at least a small number of future athletes. Whilst mares have their part to play the potential damage is limited just to their offspring; this possible sub-fertility, a 'slowness to get into foal', can be taken out of the genetic pool on an individual basis.

It should be noted, however, that in the Thoroughbred world maiden mares out of training may have an average conception rate of 90+%, thus genetically determined sub-fertility is not a likely problem. Nurture influences and future foaling traumas can substantially alter this. It is found that this 90+% drops when judged by subsequent pregnancies of e.g. 100 animals, to reveal on average

- 25 barreners

- 10 dead foals – a form of sub-fertility in the mare's records

- 65 to go forward for training

It was on these figures that the stallion's fertility rating had to be based and so his retention. Obviously his earlier athletic performance rating was important but only to around 33%.

A brood mare is judged

- firstly on her pedigree, or 'line'

- next on her performance results

- eventually, and hopefully, over several years on her fecundity

Because of the inevitable wear and tear of pregnancies and the repetitive unavoidable, albeit usually transient, genital infections, her fertility tends to fall. Eventually there is the infertility, even sterility, of advancing age. Whilst an annual foal is an ideal the mare is not a commercial milk producer and so has no urgent need for this annual lactation requirement. The cost of one year's barrenness is relatively small. The 'cost' of sterility is another matter!

There is little evidence that sterility was a serious genetic problem at wild herd level. No doubt there was in the females a percentage of poor breeders as well as permanent barrenness, but there was no evidence that any natural recognition of these occurred. A few causes of such infertility must have been associated with systemic illness and the risk of death or debility, which led to predator disposal of them. Unresolvable **dystokias** (birth difficulties) and their septic sequelae would have been exceptions; the majority remained in the herd but of course made no real contribution to that group's or herd's overall survival. Whatever the cause of their failure to breed they self eliminated; their contribution to the genetic pool was stopped: nature was taking no chances.

Reproduction disease in domesticated situations is either

- primarily functional with no readily discernible, if any at all, predisposing structural abnormalities, or
- begins as a structural disorder, the effector factor, with associated secondary
  - deficits in reproductive functioning either in the
    - affected animal(s) or in the result of the mating, the conceptus – a future brood animal

In comparison with other system dis-eases on which structural changes are present as the primary foci, traumatic and/or infectious, those of the reproductive system are often dysfunctions and usually of hormonal origin. They are often related to or precipitated by environmental nurture influences. Moreover there is no room for compromise in the outcome: it must be a return to fertility or at least to sub-fertility (intermittent fertility, the 'difficult to get in foal mare' which is not synonymous with the chronically poor performance athletic horse).

In the sub-fertile animal there is of course the additional question of

- hereditary implications
- economics

Sterility is finality in breeding, although such an individual perhaps can return to its original athleticism even if the reason for sending her to stud in the first place was because of a lack of athletic success.

PREGNANCY

Pregnancy of 320—355 days from the date of the last 'service' is known as **full term**. Foaling can be expected from 320 days and forecast by external structural signs in the mare and biochemical changes in her foremilk. If greater than 355 days, a prolonged gestation or pregnancy, she is said to be **overdue**. That offspring is rarely oversized but does have a reduced expectation of survival.

If less than 320 days it is said to be **premature** and invariably is under-developed in size and defective in the vital organs. A full-term but weak and undersized foal is classed as **dysmature**; such is indicative of a damaged, compromised vascularity of its placenta.

The actual date of foaling is determined by hormonal change influences in the foal when, it is thought, intrinsic factors associated with foetal maturity and possibly reflecting much earlier biochemistry in the womb have come 'ripe' to trigger the correct foaling signals, which start with

- increasing tone of uterine smooth muscles
- placental changes, especially the produced and secreted progesterone
- ripening, slackening and lubrication of the birth canal and its valves
- changes in the tone and the tensions of the pelvic striated muscles and associated ligaments
- secretory changes in the udder; altering colostrum consistency and its levels of calcium, sodium and potassium. It is these levels which change within the last 48 hours and are useful pointers to imminent foaling

The mare herself tactically selects the beginning of the second stage of labour to coincide with, as a rule, darkness – an atavistic precaution against predators.

Embryonic death at less than 4 months pregnancy is followed by

- **resorption** of all the fluids of the conceptus into the mare's blood stream or
- degeneration of the residual placental and foetal tissues (no bony skeleton has been formed at this time) which remains in the womb where it delays the return of oestrus. When this does occur the unrecognisable vestiges are expelled, often unnoticed during the next heat period; this could be delayed until the next year. Routine, or on suspicion, ultrasonography would of course reveal the pathology

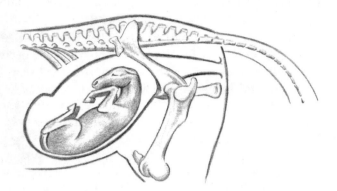

before the first stage of labour

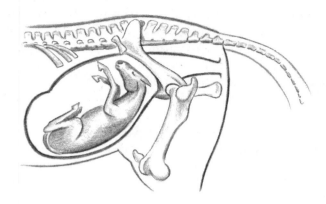

during the first stage

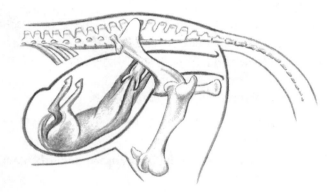

first stage, continued

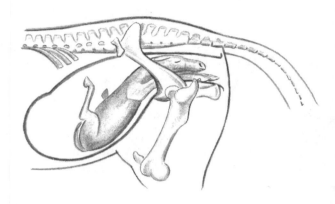

early in the second stage

- **mummification** may follow foetal death after 4 months when a calcified skeleton has formed. Some resorption and degeneration occurs to leave a 'mummy', a skeletal object, which reflexly stimulates persistence of the ovarian corpus luteum and ongoing dioestrus. On some occasions the cervix will relax to initiate mild straining leading to an investigation. In most cases it is the suspicious signs of the pregnancy not developing and or the failure to come into oestrus the next year which causes concern

- **abortion** (miscarriage) is the unwanted expulsion of a foetus before full term, usually before 300 days. Immaturity at the time invariably results in non-survival and often death before abortion. It is usually associated with placental circulatory deficits from a variety of causes, for example, in viraemias, i.e. blood borne to the foetus, which dies and is then expelled as a foreign body. Few abortions cause the mare much distress. Half of all abortions are spontaneous with no stage 1 signs. The rest show some mammary changes and she will 'run her milk' as after foaling. This is common when twins are aborted. Dystokias are sometimes a complication if presentation is wrong or with simultaneously delivered twins. There is more risk of post abortion problems such as metritis, laminitis and later sub-fertility. (Viral herpes 1 abortion is of serious contagion importance.)

- **still birth** – the expulsion of a dead foal after 320 days of gestation. There are various causes not least important a disruption in the birth process, often with failure of the foetus to begin extra-uterine breathing quickly enough

Fertility – Status (Male and Female)

At or below the average time (one or more successive ovulatory periods) required for conception in any one breeding environment, e.g.

- a private stud (closed to outside mares)
- a public stud (open to outside mares, usually with certain hygiene requirements or veterinary conditions)
  - in-hand service
    - teaser used
    - teaser not used
  - free running (open – a stallion with a group of mares on e.g. mountain or moorland or closed – restricted to enclosed fields)

and is relative to
- the breed (particularly the stallion)
- nurture
  - climate
  - grazing
    - supplementary feeding
    - handler skill and experience

Sub-fertility

Is above this average, but the eventual conceptus will go to full term to produce a live foal. (In some studs the stallion's fertility is ultimately based on the number of offspring, which get to training (or using) age irrespective of the number of ovulatory periods involved.) This status is perhaps better described as 'difficult to get into foal', or to be an inconsistent breeder e.g. less than four foals in five years, although there may be secondary reasons which are not of genetic importance.

Infertility – A Fertility Which Can Vary Year by Year

Is often used instead of 'sub-fertile', but does imply that she is more likely to return to services in any one breeding year. The cynic might say 'change the horse'; incompatibility is not an impossibility.

Female Influence

Physiological *vis à vis* the ovulatory cycle. Hormonal inputs and disruption thereof are relatively common but reasonably mild. The fertility consequences can be
- temporary during an ovulatory cycle
- temporary during a breeding season – sub-fertility
- permanent (sterility)

Such hormonal imbalances, as a primary cause, are not themselves diagnosable on the blood levels in the mare in a routine stud situation. Deficits or excesses can be assumed from related clinical assessment, as judged ultrasonographically and/or manually of ovarian structural changes such as follicle ripening, ovulation and corpus luteum formation as potential causes of infertility and sterility.

It is accepted that the influence of
- environmental factors such as daylight hours and temperature, and
- pathological factors such as infections isolated from the genital tracts are of greater importance as associated with
  - pneumovaginal pathological inspiration of air into the genital tract through faults in the perineal area
    - inherent
    - acquired
  - other traumas of coitus and foaling. These all contribute to infertility
- development abnormalities such as
- granulosa cell 'tumour' of the ovary
- hypoplastic ovaries with chromosomal defects

both result in sterility and are thought to be possibly hormonally related
- imperforate hymen is a minor developmental problem, easily treatable

- **twinning** – a non-identical pair from two ovulations at the same ovulatory time is a cause of at least temporary infertility. (Low incidence *per se* but a nuisance particularly in the Thoroughbred where the breeding season is tight.) It is understood that one of the pair may die 'naturally' so permitting the survivor to proceed to full term. More commonly, the death of one from placental starvation and its expulsion causes the other to abort. Unless early in the breeding season a fertile return to oestrus is not always possible that year.

If retention of both occurs, birth is usually early with high risk of immaturity. Survival is unusual. The advent of ultrasonography enables
- early recognition at 15 days gestation
- per rectum manual dislodgement of one foetus, up to day 21
  - success rate is 90% if each is in a separate horn
  - success rate is 50% if both are in the same horn

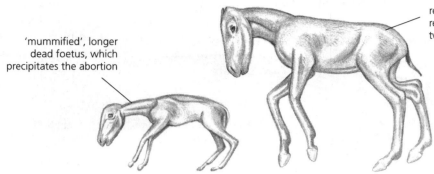

'mummified', longer dead foetus, which precipitates the abortion

recently dead but reasonably nourished twin

The difference in size and development of aborted twins.

even though there is always a separate placenta

Some stud owners prefer drug abortion of both foetuses to be effected if digital dislodgement proves impossible. Prostaglandin before day 35 (start of endometrial cup formation and secondary progesterone production) is the drug of choice. The primary cause is hormonal but why is unknown; there may be a genetic explanation. The incidence of twin ovulations, 30% at the height of the breeding season, is much greater than that of actual twin pregnancies.

DISEASE

Coitus provides an opportunity for micro-organisms commensally or opportunistically present in the

- male's urethral glans and the preputial fossae
- female's clitoral sinuses

to be cross-transferred and the mixed flora to be introduced onto the anterior vagina and into the cervix. Some are deposited into the body of the uterus, some are eventually withdrawn to reinfect the

- preputial sheath environment
- clitoral area environment

In both sites the smegma also becomes contaminated.

There is no doubt that these micro-organisms, even if of low virulence, can create an inflammation, especially on the mucosal surface of the uterus, the endometrium. The resultant endometritis is quickly brought under control by local

- cellular immunity which prevents deeper invasion

- oestral mucosal flow, and any resultant discharge is quickly washed out onto the vulvar lips

but there is no total destruction of the organisms. The visible signs usually clear in 24 hours post coitus. The stallion rarely exhibits clinical signs.

When more virulent (more pathogenic) organisms are involved or there is susceptibility in a particular mare's tract to the usual type of flora, the reaction is more intense and intrusive. Such inflammation is potentially

- spermicidal: a sterile service and capable of causing a
- metritis, which uterine inflammation can lead to a
  - more obvious post service, discharge and, if not resolved naturally, or more often therapeutically
  - chronic infertile state with the formation of
    - uterine cysts and/or fibrosing of the mucosae

The virulent organisms' source is usually in (and some will return to re-populate) the male prepuce and urethral glans or they may be dormant in the clitoris and return there in a more active state (having infected the male). Some may, for a time, remain as in infection on the female's perineal skin and in and around the male prepuce. A contagious, venereal situation has been potentially established. A similar situation can arise in the mare at foaling but because of the normal amount of lochia (post stage 3 uterine fluid) the resolution and end of discharge follow after about 6 days, and infection can be active for up to 10 days. (E coli and fungal, straw and dust-borne, organisms are common here.)

The pathogenic organisms of equine importance are

- certain virulent strains of Klebsiella (capsular types)
- certain virulent strains of Pseuodomonas
- Taylorella equigenitali (known as CEMO) of the

Vulvo-vaginitis.

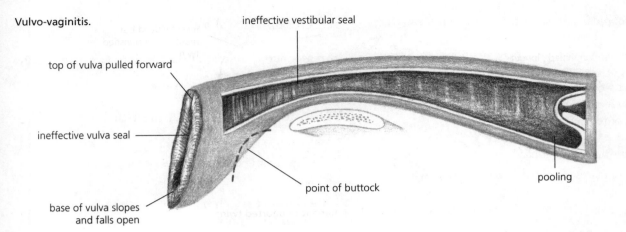

Haemophilus species which is a pure venereal organism

The stallion is usually asymptomatic, but becomes a carrier, as do handler's hands.

The degree of endometritis and duration, and the possibility of an extension to metritis, can be influenced by

- lowered local resistance

- trauma

- enhanced organism virulence. If conception is established despite the initial inflammation, there can follow

- an uterine 'environmental' risk to the conceptus, possible

- premature lysis of the corpus luteum, with loss of progesterone function or even in late pregnancy from a placental source

- placentitis (frequently associated with secondary fungal toxicity) and abortion possibly repeated in subsequent pregnancies

The associated organisms when present in a stud, usually initially in the stallion, generally are almost unavoidable invaders at coitus.

Ascending **vulvo-vaginitis** with pooling of associated infected vaginal mucus just caudal to the cervix is the common outcome of pneumo-vagina, usually the result of non-specific but occasionally of more serious specific pathogenic organisms. Until pooling is prevented and drainage effected the condition will remain to become chronic and possibly with a secondary ascended endometritis and/or a metritis. The original air, which was sucked in, remains and as a consequence the subsequent discharge is often frothy. A characteristic feature of the

associated loss of vulva seal is the whistling noise of aspirated air into the vagina when the mare moves. The acidic vaginal pool leads to infertility or even sterility and is also lethal to spermatozoa.

The Male

The associated problems of

- insufficient libido

- failure to maintain an erection or

- other coital disorders e.g. no pulsating contractions and no ejaculation – after two attempts

may be psychological in origin or from

- memory of previous painful traumas associated with service

- penis

- back

- abaxial tissues

as from slipping and/or female aggression

- sperm deficits
  - production, quantity and quality
  - maturation or ripening
  - vitality and
  - viability
    - on reaching the oviduct (fallopian tube)

These are possibly of genetic origin or determination: there is little evidence of them being hereditable (*cf.* ovaries of the mare). Certain stallion 'lines' have been identified as below average 'begetters of foals' and these have been linked to such sperm deficits. For example, semen quality and so fertilising capacity is variable and, often, microscopically looks sub-normal. This can vary from day to day or breeding season to season yet results are often up to average over time. There are, however, degrees of sub-fertility; overuse plays a part. It is usual in Thoroughbred work for a stallion to impregnate 40–50 mares in one breeding season, covering 2–3 mares on some days inclusive of repeat services.

Statistically this reflects *inter alia*

- the number of mares involved – more than 40 will lower results
- their age spread
- their number of previous pregnancies – mares with many lose some fertility
- their previous breeding history: how many e.g. 'difficult to get in foal' status
- the number of services required (including repeats) for total mares found in foal
- how his fertility is assessed
    - number of **positive pregnancy** (PD) diagnoses
        - when tested post-service, at less than 40 days
        - number of foals aborted
    - number of foals born dead
    - number of foals alive
    - number of foals which survived
        - until when
            - weaning
            - enter training (sold or kept)
            - start racing
                - number found unsound before and after then
                - number found 'useless'

In non-Thoroughbred yards such statistics are not always available or accurate. Nevertheless, statistics showing the

- number of pregnancies recorded
- number of coverings in total
- number of mares at stud and covered at least once irrespective of PD

do give significant breeding information about any one stallion. More than 65% would be acceptable, even praise-worthy!

SPECIFIC DISEASES

In reproductive tract and system disorders many of the catalogued dis-ease types are recorded

Hereditable and Developmental

- male
    - hypoplasia of the tract, especially testicular
- female
    - defective sex chromosomal content in the ova, causing sterility
    - structural faults
        - hypoplasia of the tract
- imperforate hymen (not a big problem) its hereditability is uncertain
- intrapelvic malalignment of the rectum/anus with the vagina and consequent tipping forward of the vulval lips with resultant
    - pneumo-vagina, is relatively common

The last is surgically correctable by the Caslick's operation (after the American veterinary surgeon who pioneered the technique). Under sedation and local anaesthesia a narrow, shallow strip of skin and mucous membrane on both sides of the vulval lips is removed. It is extended from the dorsal commissure down to below the level of the pubic brim (in some cases the opening left is quite small). The two raw surfaces are brought together by in-dwelling

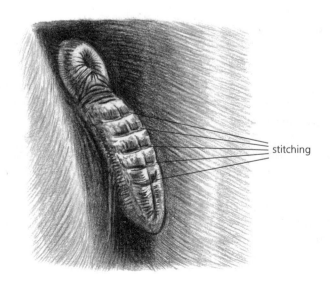

stitching

Caslick's operation – malalignment of anus and vulva, corrected by stitching.

sutures: the stitched lips remain 'sealed'. The aperture can be proportionately enlarged for mating and entirely for foaling. The suturing is always re-done

- after mating and, at the veterinary surgeon's discretion, 28 days later after a positive ultra-sound pregnancy diagnosis
- after foaling when birth swelling has resolved

Heritable occurrence of intrapelvic malalignment can occur in successive generations and is a serious nuisance factor. The pneumo-vagina is the only one to be suspected before sexual activity begins. Sooner or later all become perceivable at stud and are then accessible to diagnosis and possible treatment.

Inflammatory

Apart from the usual traumatic risks of equine life those associated with reproduction are specifically important but are not very common. Nature did not intend mating to be hazardous nor birth particularly traumatic, but there can be

- aggressive male physical behaviour, and female fierce resistance against mating at the 'wrong' time
- aggressive protection of her foal against acquisitive other horses, which sometimes results in injury
- the stallion's use of his forefeet and teeth, both in attack and in the limited foreplay on the neck and the tail-head of the mare, and his
- exuberance and weight to obtain submission into the mare's static posture for intromission

He may be thrown off and/or slip with contusion and/or strain damage, and before or after coitus be kicked or bitten. Damage here can be permanent as far as future service; the memory of the pain of the various sites of injury (particularly the testes and the penis) can even put him off altogether.

Soft tissue tears to his genitalia and bony pelvic damage at service can be the cause of a sterile service and/or subsequent interference with mating.

In comparison, the mare uses her

- hind legs in defensive action
- teeth, especially with foal at-foot

Apart from the possible paralysis from vertebral column and pelvic injury during coitus, the resultant internal exostoses and possible structural disorder can compromise foaling

- **foaling injuries** – all degrees of dystokia (difficult birth)
  - soft tissue tears and bruising
  - to the uterus, with possible opening into the peritoneum
    - haemorrhage into the broad ligament(s)
  - cervix
  - vagina and (vagina into and through rectal wall: recto-vaginal fistula)
  - vulva and (damage to the urethra) tears
  - vulval lips (leading to distortion) on healing and pneumo-vagina
    - haemorrhage – to the outside
  - fracture of the pelvis, especially if she slips down during a standing delivery
  - injury to the abaxial skeleton

Such traumas can occur in even the best-regulated studs. Many can be avoided or minimised by trained caring and careful attendants and good management.

Incidentally, it is believed that the mare 'decides' the ultimate size of the foal to complement her own pelvic dimensions.

Infections

The genital tracts, due to their respective functions and the almost certain environmental bacterial and fungal contamination from the stallion's abdomen and preputial skin and from the mare's perineum, clitoris and tail, are liable to intromissively transmit commensal organisms. Foaling also presents similar opportunities in the mare for commensal ascending infection, and temporary tract inflammation but possible chronic sequelae. Trauma has a complicating influence

- the cross-transfer of bacteria and fungi and possibly viruses some of which can be
  - primary pathogens, i.e. venereal, and most of which are
  - opportunist commensals

Bacteria

The majority are controlled by in-built defence mechanisms and the flow of genital fluids to the outside and to the recesses in the clitoris and in the prepuce as earlier described. Some may linger in and around the cervix. Both areas are thereby coincidentally reinfected.

In the presence of mild trauma and in the older animal, the commensals set up a low grade inflammation in the various sites mentioned – an endometritis/cervicitis in the mare and urethritis in the male. Their presence can be inimical to conception or to a subsequent pregnancy through a subsequent placentitis. The primaries are directly pathogenic

Fungi (in association with environmental dust)
Usually introduced at foaling with no, or rarely, clinical signs. A placental deficit abortion can follow in the middle third of pregnancy with a subsequent metritis which is difficult to clear – an infertility even sterile situation.

Viruses
Herpes (equid herpes 3, coital exanthema) – a one true venereal infection: the cause of blisters and subsequent ulcers on the

- external penis
- vulval lips

It is not a prime cause of infertility except that soreness can 'dissuade' a stallion! The lesions heal in 10 days and contagiousness ends in about 2 weeks. Sexual rest is necessary for 2 weeks to avoid further transmission and to allow complete healing so avoiding secondary inflammation. The mare may be a recrudescening carrier.

Other viruses
Equid Herpes 1 and 4. The respiratory and other diseases of herpes 1 and the lesser infection of herpes 4 can have a detrimental systemic effect on the conception, but the main concern is with herpes 1 (rhinopneumonitis) and its association with sudden, 'clean' abortion at 7–9 months. A late infection can see the birth of a sickly, infectious foal, which usually succumbs. An abortion eliminates any latency in the mare. It is highly contagious to foals and yearlings (usually in Thoroughbred studs). In studs, abortion storms can occur. There may or may not be premonitory signs of the primary disease of respiratory signs including a 'snotty nose' let alone more systemic invasion. It is not spread venereally.

Equine Viral Arteritis
- infection at coitus – venereal or
- via the respiratory route
  - abortion at any time – vaginal discharge for

3 weeks, unlike herpes 1 which is 'clear'
  - the stallion can remain as a 'shedder' in 34% of cases

These viruses, if active during a stud season, should warrant a temporary shutting down of breeding activity. Any in-foal mares should be revaccinated (or begin vaccination) where feasible especially for herpes 1.

- Endo and ectoparasites will have only an indirect effect on breeding. Their prevention and control are one aspect of good stud management for adult and foal health and condition

Metabolic disease
It is unlikely that the overstresses associated with athleticism will affect brood and in-foal mares, even if clinically recovered cases are eventually bred from

- e.g. exertional rhabdomyolysis; previously severe cases should be carefully monitored before and during the exertions of foaling
- nutritional secondary hyperparathyroidism is rare generally and should not be a problem in studs or in veterinary supervised private situations
- hypocalcaemia is a risk in the late stages of lactation in Mountain and Moorland pony mares especially if transport or other distance movement is required when grazing nutritional levels are falling especially calcium which is already being drained off in the milk
- vitamin E and selenium deficiency in pregnant or nursing pony mares 'at grass' on poor, coastal soils has been recorded
- preventative nutritional care should always be taken on veterinary advice re
  - late pregnancy feeding
  - laminitis risks
  - milk production sufficiency
    - mineral supplements for mare and foal

Degenerative
- not specific to fertility in the usual sense of the word, but
- malfunction of erection
  - paraphimosis – failure to retract the penis, a not uncommon cause is misuse of some tranquillisers; where persistent engorgement (tumescence) is

present the condition is called priapism

- senile mares become progressively less fertile
  - more subject to uterine, degenerative cysts

Neoplasia

- the stallion is subject to tumours of the penis which are often malignant. It is certainly a serious morbid disability to reproduction. Squamous cell carcinoma is the most common

- other lymphoid tumours and metastises in the abdominal cavity may cause genital serous coat involvement disabling the ovaries, the fallopian tubes and the wall of the uterus

- granulosa-theca cell tumour – this is not a true neoplastic disease but is a result of a hormonal dysfunction, which has a knock-on sterilising effect on the other ovary. The cause is unknown and so may be developmental or due to later altered feedback influences in the hormonal 'orchestra'. The dysfunction can take several forms of altered behaviour including aggression to other males and females dependent on which sex hormone becomes dominant – oestrogen, progesterone and even testosterone; some affected mares show oestrus but do not ovulate. Surgery is usually essential to remove the affected ovary. Three other ovarian tumour types (all rare) have been recorded, one being malignant.

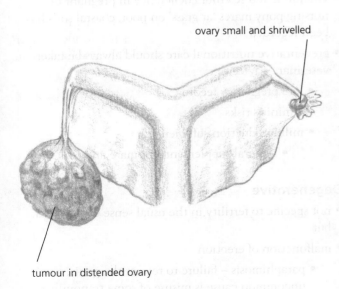

ovary small and shrivelled

tumour in distended ovary

An ovarian tumour.

Management

In the 'domesticated' reproduction environment the stud management aim is to keep the fertility rate as high as possible. This is a reflection of the stallion's fertility, as judged above. It should also reflect the number of services per mare, and take into consideration the ratio of stud females and the number of visiting mares.

These female statistics may vary year by year as the stallion's fertility gets better known – and advertised – as a consequence

- more mares up to the ideal 45, some of which may be compromised
  - when, as the average mare age increases so does the likelihood of some of these becoming 'difficult' breeders

- some of the added mares are recently out of high performance work and may have at least a temporary lower fertility

There is a risk in persevering with infertility treatment; a low or sub-fertility can then be bred into the offspring subsequently born; the gene pool for fertility is thereby hazarded. In commercial cross-breeding studs this is not so important: the gene pool is deep anyway. The mare owner's requirement is a foal – even if this will have required expensive therapy and have been a drain on the stallion!

An on-going rule was to develop and maintain a system of husbandry as near to the 'wild' as possible

- a gregarious 'out of doors' existence
  - with an accompanying stallion for herd groups of 10–15 mares

- freedom to roam and to trickle feed off
  - successive pastures for
    - more varied herbage
    - natural worm control

As the system became progressively more 'domesticated' stud management had increasing responsibility for its dominance over the stock. In terms of breeding this was to

- select a suitable stallion and a suitable larger harem of mares
  - monitor and maintain general health *vis à vis*
    - nutrition: grazing and fodder with appropriate supplement

- worm control, pasture management
- artificial immunisation against tetanus, influenza and possibly herpes virus strains
- freedom from toxic substances
- maintain specific health; an extension of the above but particularly with regard to
    - transmissable disease agents in
    - general as with herpes strains and equine viral arteritis
        - coital contact especially
            - commensal organisms
            - pathogenic germs by
                - variably controllable 'normal' introduction
                - associated with (and made more invasive) with coital and birth trauma
- recognise the sexual behaviour involved
    - readiness of the mare's sexual rhythm
    - activity of the stallion – and where practice determined know when and how to safely present him
    - pregnancy behaviour
    - foaling behaviour
- be aware of possibly abnormal genital structures and functionings in both the male and female

and be quickly pro-active with veterinary help when necessary

It is easy to pick out a stallion of poor fertility; this will show in the majority of his mares sometime in the season, usually sooner than later. The decision to geld him is made on the grounds of

- why is he sub-fertile?
    - what are the clinical findings?
        - are they treatable?
        - will they resolve?
            - economically?
            - permanently?
    - is there a possibility of a genetic cause?
        - are there any tests?
        - or is he sterile?

One must just speculate about a similar situation in the wild. Unless associated with illness he would have gone on covering and re-covering the harem throughout the breeding season. The physical exertion effect of this would make him a target for take-over by a young horse possibly attracted to the group by the unusually high number of in-heat mares towards the end of the season.

The veterinary surgeon today can explain several disorders of the ovulatory cycle. Some he can confirm by analysis of the mare's serum, others he can help correct by appropriate therapy. He and the stud manager can in fact enable (or try to enable) a mare to be bred when nature intended otherwise and thus possibly perpetuate a genetic weakness or to recognise when the fertility deficit is due to man's interference and so not inheritable.

Such disorders are likely the more management has deliberately

- hastened the onset of the cycle
    - artificially increasing daylight ahead of nature
        - warmth outdoors by rugging, indoors by heat source
    - specifically increasing conserved (out of season) feedstuffs, especially protein
    - 'therapeutically' introducing hormones
- failed to appreciate how far domestication has otherwise overstressed the mare (and the stallion)

Some disorders likely to be causing sub-fertility can be better identified and corrected if the mare, usually a barren but also a brood mare with a foaling dysfunction, is examined by a veterinary surgeon

- post partum and, if passed fit, with or without treatment eventually
- monitored as to the rhythm of the next cycle's
    - transitional oestrus
    - actual oestrus
        - before going to stud

these will save costs and the stallion's efforts!

CHAPTER 29

DISEASES OF THE NERVOUS SYSTEM

In day-to-day horsemastership the suspicion of a neurologic disease being the cause of 'something wrong' is basically just that; that there is 'something wrong' but no ordinary clear-cut clinical signs to explain it.

The worrying 'something wrong' may be of sudden onset or slow to develop

- the behaviour has changed, yet there has been no known change in management – feeding, housing, or use (bit/saddle/rider)

- the posture has changed, with no apparent explanation – at rest, a slight 'head tilt', e.g. on being made to 'move over' in the stable, a possible neck stiffness; in getting up, a possible hindquarter weakness

- altered action – dynamic changes are seen in the various gaits in limb flight and/or foot fall

yet there are no signs of related injury or pain; nor does it look like actual lamenesses; the signs are peculiar, they are *bizarre*!

It is then that the veterinary surgeon is usually called to decide if there is a primary other-system condition present. If not, an overall neurologic examination is begun but with the proviso that, in the horse, many very helpful tests possible in other species are neither feasible nor practicable.

For example in man, sensory input can be checked by

- stimulating the skin, a 'tickle', skin prick, or variable pressures on focal areas

- initiating various reflexes and replicating them – patellar and other tendon/muscle tapping, e.g. the 'knee jerk' reaction

- estimating muscle tone – flaccidity/spasticity

all with the co-operation of the patient. In addition, man can be requested to test his sight (blink and fixating reflexes), hearing, olfactory and gustatory senses, touch, and co-ordination – and to comment on the results.

In the dog and the cat the evaluation of the special senses is clinically useful information but only up to a point! Proprioception can be tested by involving 'placing' reflexes with the patient held off the ground or table. The horse is a different matter, but changes in its mental state, behaviour and posture can be discernible after close observation.

Such can be associated with morbidity of the sensory cranial nerves

I – sense of *smell*, the **olfactory** nerve

II – sense of *sight*, the **optic** nerve

V and IX – sense of *taste*, the **gustatory** nerves

VIII – sense of *hearing*, the **acoustic** nerve (**auditory** branch)

VIII – sense of *balance*, the **acoustic** nerve (**vestibular** branch)

The ability to smell, taste, see and hear, however, are not only difficult to confirm in the horse as distinct from man and dog but can also be masked or altered by

- dullness and fever associated with active systemic illness

- lack of interest, or more interested in some sensory input other than that being tested

and might also be due to morbidity at the source sensory organs from, say, nasal catarrh, recent overpowering taste as from a medicine, eyeball defect, or inflammation of the inner ear.

Balance, however, can be impaired to varying degrees in the dynamic gaits and can be associated with other signs such as head tilt, a postural change, from morbidity in the vestibular sensory organ; in other words, it shows as a deficit in the standing animal as well.

A dis-order of balance in a gait can be exaggerated (or confirmed) by masking the sensory input of sight, as by blindfolding.

To the horse these nerves which register smell, sight and hearing and give information as to spatial facts (balance) are extremely important as *urgent* as well as routine messengers.

Those which monitor the involuntary functionings, in association with the autonomic nervous system, of airway muscle patency, cardiac muscle power and rate, deglutition, digestion and excretion, are relatively slower, less urgent in many cases, but are nonetheless vital.

Visual defects of neurologic origin are usually associated with a dilated pupil, whereas when they are due to inflammatory impairments in the eyeball itself there is usually protective behaviour indicative of efficient protective reflexes

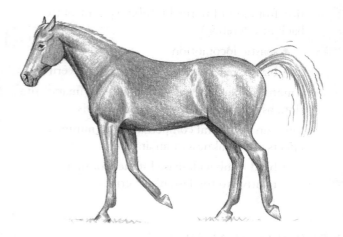

Shivering.

- blepharospasm

- photophobia

- constricted pupil – to protect the retina and the optic tract, and excessive tear formation or even a purulent discharge

Such a horse could still have its optic centre stimulated if ophthalmic instrument light rays could get through to the back of the eye and onto the retina.

It will, in either surface or in depth (neurologic) blindness

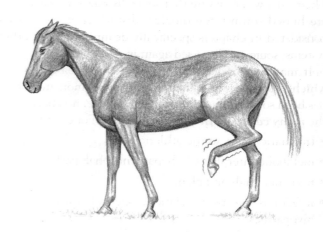

Stringhalt.

- turn its head to accommodate the restricted vision if that is unilateral

- increase ear movements, especially if a bilateral blindness exists

- have locomotor problems in negotiating terrain changes and obstacles

whereas with low-grade balance difficulties the horse's gait is more likely to be spastic, hypermetric (high stepping) – he cannot correctly judge spatial relationships.

The nervous system reacts to inflammation resulting from trauma and/or infection in four basic ways

- negatively, usually as a direct result of trauma, e.g. paralysis, motor nerve dysfunction

- positively

  - due to release of subordinate functioning innerva-

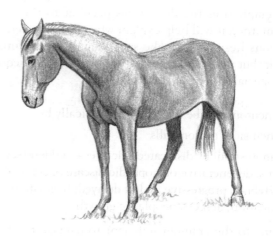

Hind limb wide-based stance – a functional postural compensation.

tion from loss of normal inhibitory control (feed-back interference)

- spastic locomotion
- bizarre reactions, e.g. stringhalt, 'shivering'

- a motor nerve's altered response to a primary irritation, as seen in epilepsy with meningitis
- functional postural compensation to minimise the effects of a weakness or an ataxia
  - hind -limb wide-based stance for support relative to the lesion's severity

NEUROLOGICAL DISEASE

The reader will be aware that some disorders whose defects are biased toward neurological disturbances have been considered in chapters specifically dealing with the other systems; some are discussed again in this chapter.

It may be wondered why neurologic disease as such, which is said to be comparatively uncommon in horses, has been so extensively written about here: it is because of the *many causes with a common effect*. For example

- traumatic injury in the athletic horse
- metabolic interplay, e.g. hepatoencephalopathy
- toxic materials and plants
- infectious dis-ease association, especially the neuro-myopathies
- specific CNS (central nervous system) disease, and
- much that is not yet fully understood

If it emphasises the difficulties peculiar to the nervous system, then it will help explain why practising veterinary surgeons hesitate to make spot diagnosis of neurologic deficits but rather carry out a strict work-up and frequently seek specialist help.

The neurons can be damaged traumatically by

- concussion, as from falls
- compression, by dislocated fractures – sudden (severe) signs; degenerative orthopaedic disease of cervical vertebrae, progressive and/or delayed; haematoma formation; abscess, neoplastic growth

Trauma to the cranium sufficient to damage the brain is relatively rare except in road traffic and similar accidents, and through shod kicks to the fallen horse or intentionally by an adult horse to a shorter, annoying or aggressive one.

Spinal cord disruptions are the most common cause of motor tract and LMN (lower motor neuron) damage. The signs will depend upon the site affected but generally

- behind the site, will lose motor activity
- in front of the site, will lose caudal sensory and especially proprioceptor communication
- simple spinal reflex arcs centred on the
  - cervico-thoracic and the
  - lumbar cord enlargements; the area of emergence of the respective fore and hind limb nerve plexuses will remain operative provided they are not the site of the trauma itself

Peripheral nerves can be traumatised as they pass

- over bony prominences which are anatomically exposed to blows
- through **spinal foraminae** which are affected with osteoarthritic exostoses, i.e. new bone outgrowths
- between muscle bundles with fibrotic adhesions which 'trap' the nerve

In addition to the traumatic effects, sudden or progressive, mentioned above, other inflammatory conditions do occur. Due to the nervous system's ramifications and its several sub-systems, such morbidities can be

- focal
- multifocal, and therefore diffuse in effect, as in the
  - central areas
    - brain
    - spinal cord
  - peripheral nerves when several are affected
  - autonomic nervous system and its subsidiaries

or combinations of these.

They can be

- primary, e.g. tetanus toxin paralysis
- part of a systemic illness, e.g. herpes virus allergic effect on the vascular capillaries in the CNS
- secondary to a primary illness elsewhere, e.g. guttural pouch infection

and can affect the

- neuron
- its vascular supply, and so cause ischaemia with oxygen

and nutrient (especially glucose) deprivation, and can affect
- the connective and supporting tissues

The signs may be
- easily recognised and
    - easily located as to the origins, e.g. the 'whistler'
    - not easily located, e.g. the ataxic horse
- difficult to relate to the nervous system *per se*, e.g. the 'head shaker'

The resultant malfunctioning becomes clinical in the
- efferent system, and so in the
    - locomotor system's activity
        - voluntary
        - reflex with
            - flaccidity – loss of resistance to passive movement
                - atrophy of related muscles
    - other systems' motor involuntary activity
        - respiratory
        - digestive
        - vascular
        - excretory, with or without loss of voluntary control
    all of which may be
    - altered
    - interrupted
- afferent system, and so in the
    - receptors of information from the above systems and the body surfaces. Their input may be
        - cut off
        - misinterpreted, and consequently
        - 'mismanaged' efferently with resultant
            - changes in activity and behaviour
                - loss of awareness and/or reflex withdrawals
                - presence of gait deficits

There is usually a two-way effect and especially so when peripheral nerve-carrying afferent **and** efferent fibres are affected, e.g. Polyneuritis equi.

Morbidity of the autonomic system's ganglia, especially the sympathetic sub-system, tends to 'spread' or have a common widespread distribution with consequent widespread effect.

Peripheral nerves can be biochemically compromised by intracellular and intercellular electrolyte imbalances associated with inflammatory oedema. Damage to the capillary walls, from whatever cause, allows the escape of protein-carrying serum with consequent formation of osmotic oedema.

This intercellular, traumatising pressure on nerve tissue is a serious cause of neural dis-order, especially in the confines of the skull and to a lesser extent in the vertebral column. The brain is also very sensitive to decreasing uptake of oxygen and of glucose.

The site and the extent of the damage will determine the
- distribution
- degree
- implication of the neurologic deficits

The nervous system is hazarded by
- traumatic damage through injury to the
    - skull, enclosing the brain
    - vertebral column, enclosing the spinal cord
    - limbs, along which the peripheral nerves 'run'

When non-traumatic dis-ease, infectious, allergic and metabolic, affects the nervous system the morbidity is usually
- microscopic, even
- ultramicroscopic

and consequently 'inconceivable', especially to the layman in the first instance.

In all nerve system dis-ease including trauma, it is its **body control function** which is altered or lost. It is this mal-functioning which produces the **clinical picture**.

In dealing with suspected neurologic dis-ease, perhaps more than in other system's dis-ease, there is a close relationship between
- perception of the signs and the need to know the
- underlying morbidity – what and where within the central and/or the peripheral systems

There is still, however, much to be learnt about

- neuro anatomy – especially the neuronal tracts within the CNS
- neuro pathology – how disease alters neuronal functioning *vis à vis* the integration of sensory input and motor output

From a veterinary point of view, pathological knowledge can and is being built up from

- extrapolation of other species' information (but this can be misleading!)
- electronic neuromuscular conduction measurements
- autopsy samples analysis (but not commonly of nerve tissue *per se* in life – biopsy), but
  - the amount of suitable specimens is limited since, fortunately, in Britain neurologic epidemic disease is relatively uncommon and so of limited economic importance
  - apart from the neurologic complication of herpes viral infection, the likelihood of viral neuropathy at stud/herd incidence level is rare
  - access to post-mortem nerve tissue is laborious and costly, especially of the brain and of the spinal cord
  - permission, and willingness to pay for a post mortem is often withheld
  - toxic neuropathy (in multiple animals) via grazing and conserved foodstuffs is not unknown but these are basically seen as poisoning

Research funding from commerce and the horse industry is therefore not seen as a pressing necessity. Grass sickness research is a notable and a praiseworthy exception.

There is one important characteristic of neurologic disease

- the relative constancy of certain clinical signs to a known morbidity, e.g.
  - grass sickness and its three or four levels of illness all show as an interference with swallowing and gut peristalsis; the morbidity is always seen in the autonomic ganglia at autopsy
  - spinal cord trauma always shows as locomotor weakness which may progress to paralysis. The basic picture is constant
  - some disease is only *intermittently* manifested but because of its nature, e.g. seizures, is more patently

of neurologic origin. The morbidity or deficit factors must have *always* been there or possibly for some time; a trigger factor is necessary to produce a clinical picture or 'attack' or fit

Signs of Nervous System Disease

These signs are

- loss of awareness – consciously, i.e. centrally and peripherally from negative reaction to skin stimuli and/or noxious (painful) input
- unusual behaviour perhaps *including* gait abnormalities when situated
  - at conscious level
- altered actions within otherwise *normal* behaviour
  - at lower brain stem levels
  - at spinal cord level
  - at peripheral nerve level

To the layman the horse is seen to be

- acting peculiarly, 'seems wrong'
  - in the head
  - in its balance, and/or it is
  - lame

Many illnesses which present with features suggestive of neurologic dis-ease are not primarily neurologic

- acute limb trauma with protective muscular spasm and tremor
- limb fracture with apparently complete loss of use
- ligament/tendon injury which mechanically interferes with action to such an extent that the horse panics into abnormal behaviour, e.g. Achilles tendon luxation off the point of hock
- fibrotic healing of stifle flexor muscles, 'ossifying myopathy', causing an apparently unco-ordinated movement of that leg in locomotion
- muscular, nutritional or metabolic dystrophies causing weakness but no disturbed sensory input so no reflex ataxia
- exercise-induced temporary muscle disturbance
  - aorta-iliac thrombosis – vascular related
  - acute rhabdomyolysis (ER) – metabolic related

All *simulate* loss of neuro-muscular control. Some other

metabolic/nutritional disturbances do produce neurologic deficits.

There is increasing evidence that *psychological aberrations* occur in the horse. When behaviour is affected yet there is *no organic disease found in any system* to account for it, then attention should be given to mistakes in training and the need for retraining to overcome persistent fear and evasive fight and flight. There is a need to restore confidence. Some saddling up difficulties and mounting are cases in point.

Contradictorily, however, there are some incidents of 'something wrong' when the owner initially perceives the signs as being those of neurologic dis-ease or damage

- acute trauma as in the fallen, temporarily recumbent cross-country horse which eventually rises but is then seen to be 'on three legs'
    - it is then seen as having
        - 'broken down'
        - 'sprung a joint' or
        - fractured a bone

Any nerve involvement is coincidental.

All these incidental to, or causative of, the fall will produce a 'loss of use' picture in which the horse cannot bear weight due to the pain and/or loss of structural integrity.

On the other hand, such malfunctioning in one leg could be due to

- short term nerve damage as from a direct blow with nociceptor sensory input – pain – as in polo stick or ball blows
- some can be potentially long-term nerve-damage with decreased
    - motor output – weakness to paralysis of a limb

Nevertheless, structural (axial) damage and specific nerve damage can be co-existent. The fallen horse which remains recumbent is more likely and more worryingly to have a 'broken back', with a potentially vital effect on the enclosed spinal cord. Due to the understandable hope of the owner or the misguided zeal of onlookers, such a horse is optimistically seen as 'just winded' which of course, until differentially diagnosed, it may well be.

An attempt to 'force' the patient to rise without professional assessment may eventually be successful but

- if the horse struggles before it has fully got over the

'shock' this may

- exacerbate a coincidental limb wound, or the horse may
- fall again and inflict further injury to itself and other people
- if in fact 'broken backed', it may suffer much unnecessary pain and fear by such a crude 'diagnostic' technique before rising is obviously an impossibility

A fractured vertebral column in the horse is

- in most cases associated with an immediate dislocation compression of the spinal cord; such necessitates euthanasia. In some incidents a delay is necessary before such a diagnosis can be made
- in some cases where the trauma is restricted to a non-displacing fracture of the body of the vertebra or the lateral facets when there is no cord or nerve root damage there must be time given to recover from the shock and acute pain. Such will get up, eventually. Thereafter if not given sufficient recuperative healing time then, with the lack of practicable immobilisation in the horse, there is a *serious* risk of fracture breakdown to
    - involve a joint and subsequently a nerve trunk or root
    - involve the cord itself

Apart from box rest there are few preventative measures. The owner must be made aware of the risk. At best there will be some locomotor deficit; at worst a hopeless paraplegia.

At the level of practical horsemastership the acute or sub-acute appearance of

- lameness at stance, walk and trot, quite understandably suggests a painful limb; common things are common!
- weakness in all gaits, but perhaps more so in the asymmetric ones, does not initially suggest possible neuropathy
- reluctance to perform could suggest
    - low-grade unlocated pain
    - intercurrent illness
    - nappiness
- inability to perform to expectations suggests
    - intercurrent illness

- infectious
- metabolic

but

- peculiar behaviour, uncommon and often indeterminate in its clues, is the one most likely to suggest a brain disorder (but see also true 'nettle rash')

The ambiguous 'back problems' are seen as painful, traumatic muscular conditions *per se* (which some may well be) rather than reflex protective spasm for pain coming from bone/joint lesions, often with compression of central or peripheral (neural) elements close to the vertebral column or to proprioceptor upset from lateral articulation torque mal-alignment.

It is when locomotor disease as such or intercurrent other system disease cannot be

- perceived or
- retrospectively associated with the voluntary locomotor system

and especially if the

- condition is marked at the onset and/or thereafter
- is deteriorating (with muscle wasting)
- showing no signs of recovery

that lay and veterinary attention is directed to the possibility of a neurologic disease. So too with involuntary motor deficits in other systems.

Conversely, it does happen that during a

- work-up to diagnose (or to eliminate) a systemic disease or at
- a pre-purchase veterinary examination

signs suggestive of neurologic deficits may be recognised, such as

- alteration in (normal, average equine) mental attitude
- behavioural changes
- loss of menace reaction, the blink reflex
- poor pupillary responses
- cranial muscle tone loss including tongue weakness and facial paralysis
- slap test deficit (see also Laryngeal disorders)
- focal (local) loss of skin sensitivity

- abnormal sweating patterns
- nasal discharge which **might** point to guttural pouch mycosis and suspected or potential pharyngeal nerve weakness
- head, neck, body and limb postural abnormality
- gait deficiencies (lamenesses) and bizarre gaits
- muscle group atrophy of trunk and limbs
- altered tail and anal sphincter tone

Then the next stage is for the veterinary surgeon to determine if the **neurologic deficit disease (NDD)** originated in

- a localised part of the nervous system
- a diffuse area of the CNS
- an inflammation of multiple cranial and spinal nerves – a polyneuritis
- the autonomic system directly, as in grass sickness

or if it is a

- quasi-neurologic condition, originating in another system, such as with hepato-encephalogy, which interferes with the smooth functioning of the central and peripheral neuro-system

It will be seen that all NDD involve motor (muscular) activity directly or indirectly; i.e. somewhere there is interference with UMN (upper motor neuron), LMN (lower motor neuron) or peripheral nerve **afferent** output.

The anatomical distribution of the nervous system is reasonably clear cut. The functional distribution is not. Hence the difficulties in diagnosing and localising the origin of the functional deficits.

The veterinary surgeon must, once he has

- identified the significant signs and
- the most likely locale to be dis-eased, then
- relate what diseases he knows may be associated with that anatomical site
- differentiate this short list by
  - clinical acumen (learning, experience – knowledge)
  - on-site tests
  - using ancillary aids when necessary and where practicable
    - blood samples
      - haematology

- metabolic profiles
- serology
- cerebro-spinal fluid analysis
- electric modes
  - radiography for
    - bone lesions
    - space occupying lesions
      - neoplasia
      - fluid retention
  - scintigraphy for inflammatory 'hot spots'
  - thermography for inflammatory 'hot spots' and chronic 'cold spots'
  - ultrasonography for soft tissue disruption
  - **electroencephalography (EEC)** neural activity
  - **electromyography (EMG)** neuro-muscular
  - muscle response to stimulation
    - faradic, where nerve supply is intact but there is muscle action response deficit
    - galvanic, where there is primary motor nerve deficit
  - nerve conduction times
- biopsy

It will be appreciated that this range is rarely fully employed and that much of it requires specialised skills – and expense.

Professional clinical diagnosis in itself is time-consuming and variably difficult in the horse

- equine size, weight, strength and temperament cause their own difficulties when applying manual stimuli
- the normal reactions of fright, fight and flight to unusual handling make the stimuli not only difficult to apply but the responses difficult to interpret

Consider passive lateral flexion of the neck. Is any stiffness due to

- 'stiff' musculature – spasm or strophy?
- 'stiff' joint(s) with or without spinal cord involvement?
- pain from nerve entrapment?
- 'cussedness', or merely 'natural resentment'?

even comparing left with right can be misleading; most horses are 'one-handed'.

The patient must be given time to relax and to accept the investigator's presence and activity.

Conversely, the horse's natural rebalancing reflexes do lend themselves to human diagnostic interference (stimuli)

- forced lateral displacement at a stance of
  - forequarters
  - hindquarters, to elicit support muscle ataxia or weakness
- extremes of vector locomotion in hand
  - up hill, down hill, cross hill
  - serpentines and varying radii on both reins
  - (manual) displacement upwards of head and neck to minimise visual aid
  - repetition of the above under blindfold to elicit ataxia and visual and balance deficits
- when testing total spinal (head to tail) joint ranges it may be necessary to overcome natural muscular guarding resistance by sedation/tranquillisation

Historical information is always necessary, just as in all system examinations, perhaps even more so in neurologic problems

- was the onset sudden or slow?
- what were the *first* signs?
- what other dis-ease is known in
  - the patient?
  - the in-contact animals?
- have there been recent environmental changes?
  - movements onto premises?
    - aggressive two-way reaction leading to
      - trauma?
      - stress?
  - on-site grazing
    - recent fertiliser applications?
    - ditching to bring some plant roots up?
    - weed control?
    - dumping of unknown vegetation and other material by a neighbour?
    - access to unknown grazing?

- effects of seasonal or unseasonal weather?
    - lush grass growth?
    - failure of growth?
        - access to toxic plants?
        - nut and fruit windfalls?
    - 'new' bought-in feedstuffs?
- have any of the signs, especially behavioural, been triggered by any particular sensory inputs? For example
    - sight, sound or smell of
        - other horses
        - humans
        - animals
        - machinery
        - places or 'fear' when close to electric fencing

Diagnosis, and especially prognosis, are both important *vis à vis*

- welfare
- economics

Many neurologic diseases can be

- prolonged
- often permanent
- frequently incurable

It may well be that there is worthwhile benefit in 'waiting to see' in some cases, where immediate welfare is not a concern or can satisfactorily be controlled, before unnecessary diagnostic expense is incurred.

When the signs are

- sudden in onset
- acute/severe as in suspected
    - EHV (equid herpes virus) neuropathy
    - tetanus, botulism and grass sickness
    - cranial and spinal trauma nerve damage

then appropriate therapeutic and supportive care becomes urgently required and the progress carefully monitored, if considered justifiable on welfare grounds

- tetanus is common (but shouldn't be!). Once seen, the signs are readily recalled
- botulism is not common, and in its *early* stages the signs can be indistinct; diagnosis is not always easy. The type of 'long' feed is often a pointer, i.e. big bale silage

- grass sickness and its geographical frequency is a constant fear to some horse owners, but an unknown fact to many others

A combination of **cranial nerve** and **autonomic ganglionic lesions** will give rise to

- swallowing difficulties
- phonation changes
- airway obstruction
- behavioural changes in cranial 'damage' in general
    - head pressing
    - compulsive wandering
    - circling
    - licking
    - aggression

all of which are so sufficiently persisting as to be readily perceived

- seizures (unless triggered by handling, e.g. tacking up) may be so irregularly intermittent as to be missed
- persistent yawning is less readily evaluated

The mental state of the horse, its level of awareness and consciousness varies in dis-ease states from

- lethargic
- somnolent
- depressed
- stupored
- semi-comatosed (or alternatively delirious) to
- comatosed

These states may also be part of another system's illness with secondary effect on the brain.

Concussion

Concussion, e.g. as a direct cause of a neurologic deficit, causes

- a transient loss of some cranial reflexes
- variable loss of consciousness in depth and duration
    - following a blow to the head which may have permanent effect on cerebral functioning in part, especially if
        - intra-cranial haemorrhage and/or

- ischaemia, following vessel damage and leakage with subsequent oedema
- head posture changes
  - tilt of poll to one side, muzzle and neck normal as in vestibular disease
  - head and neck turn to one side (with or without poll tilt) as in unilateral focal damage to cerebrum

Such deviations of the head and/or the neck are fixed more or less and are most obvious when viewed from in front of the horse. They must be differentiated from bit evasions in locomotion or mastication induced pain whereby the horse chews 'on one side' with muzzle deviation – a rostral distortion. The body appearance changes are

- focal muscle atrophy
- localised sweating
- changes in pain perception
- response to pain as it influences
  - behaviour
  - action

Gait and Posture Aberrations

These are suggestive of neurologic disease. The most common CNS morbidities are

- weakness – in general there is a motor tract deficit up to just short of paralysis
- paresis with
  - knuckling
  - stumbling
  - toe dragging
  - dipping back on first mounting (could be hyper-reaction to spinal stimulus) – 'cold-backed'
- dysmetria – any disturbance in the range of voluntary (limb) movement, the stride phase
  - hypometria – spastic-like limb movement with lack of flexion – a deficient step length
  - hypermetria – a high stepping and exaggerated joint movement – an over stepping length
  - spasticity – stiff flexion – rare in the horse
  - easily pushed sideways (laterally displaced) – ataxic lack of reflex centre balancing but otherwise not a weakness

Ataxia (bizarre gaits)

There are many degrees ranging from subtle to recumbency

- a proprioceptive (sensory) nerve tract and/or receptor end of dendrite deficit
- a motor tract deficit originating from
  - centres in the brain
  - possibly spinal motor tracts
    - the ventral roots
    - the peripheral nerves, all with variable signs such as
      - toe dragging
      - trunk sway
      - muscle tremor
      - exaggerated hind limb 'swing' phase abduction (on circling and turn on the forehand in hand)
      - turning difficulties, on a turn on the quarters, will not cross inside leg in front of the other
      - crossing fore or hind limbs at walk, and especially
      - insecure balancing reaction against manual pressures

A concurrent weakness is not uncommon, but whether
- constitutional
  - disease
  - malnutrition or
- neurogenic

is not always easily determined.

In practice the commonest neurological disorders most readily seen by the horsemaster are those which involve the motor innervation of the locomotor system, whereby the horse seems to have a lameness in as much as there is

- difficulty in moving a limb or doing so but in a peculiar fashion
- weakness in standing on a limb which assumes an unusual posture

In some cases there is a history
- of a fall

- having been cast

In some there may be signs of
- trauma, but the
- degree of associated wound pain is not in keeping with the defective action

Frequently the signs 'just appear overnight'.

Motor output can be compromised by
- sensory input – wrong information, especially via proprioception
- wrong interpretation in the higher brain
- interception of the transmission from the upper motor neurons
- interruption of the transmission from the lower motor neurons

and especially by damage to
- the nerve trunks somewhere out-with the cranium and the spinal column

Proprioception input can be altered at the site of the receptors, e.g.
- those of the lateral articulations of the vertebral column, whereby a reflex protective muscle spasm develops which imbalances the horse's action
    - the spinal tracts can be compromised by pressure whereby the input from the hind legs is altered, with consequent altered output instructions, as in Wobbler disease and the associated bizarre gait of ataxia
    - the occasional complication of EHV infection which produces an encephalomyelitis of vascular origin resulting in brain and more usually spinal tract disruption, will show as variable limb defects from subtle to recumbency

Subtle Gait Deficits

These, distinct from one-leg lameness, can be seen in horses which are not neurologically impaired, as when attempting to
- guard against locomotion pain
- compensate for locomotor disturbances

of which most are 'wear and tear' (chronic) inflammatory and/or degenerative changes, e.g.

- myositis of recurrent 'azoturia' (ER)
- lumbar muscle pain, direct or indirect
- spavin, especially if unequally bilateral
- navicular syndrome, especially if unequally bilateral
- in spinal arthrosis, especially, but not only, cervical,
    - lateral articular facet osteo-arthritis – cervical and lumbar
    - kissing dorsal processes – thoracic
    - spondylitis – lumbar ventral surfaces
    - lumbar transverse process arthrosis

They can also arise from
- bitting problems
    - sore mouth
    - 'bad' hands
- unlevel rider
- ill-fitting saddles

It is important that such peripheral problems and conditions as described under 'subtle gait deficits' are given prime consideration and ruled out before a true neurological dis-ease is assumed. They are much more common in everyday horsemastership situations.

Nevertheless, the compensatory rebalancing induced by these non-neurologic conditions can have a torque effect on the spine, with resultant proprioceptor deficits. This may require physiotherapeutic 'mobilisation' or 'adjustment'.

It is such 'vicious circle' situations which create questionable descriptions of 'the back being out'. The underlying condition must be recognised and identified where possible.

The morbidity inducing neurologic dis-eases of reasonably significant importance in the horse are found in the
- cerebrum
    - acquired at any age
        - unilateral
            - trauma
            - focal abscess (neonate foals)
            - aberrant strongyle larvae
            - neoplasia

- bilateral
  - trauma
  - hepatic encephalopathy
  - aberrant strongyle larvae
  - EHV-I neuropathy

If the cerebellum, the brain stem and/or the spinal cord are also affected, gait abnormalities and weaknesses will show. Cerebellar abscesses with variably diffuse secondaries and persistent fever are examples

- spinal cord
  - acquired at any age
    - trauma
      - vertebral fractures
      - luxations with
        - cord compression
        - vascular deficits

The level in the cord determines the limbs affected with the associated ataxia, weakness, spasticity and possible paralysis

With roundworm aberrant larval migration into the central nervous system (and if the spinal cord in particular is focally affected), then a single leg ataxia may follow, otherwise the results are invariably bilaterally asymmetric in degree and type.

Most mineral, chemical and 'vegetable' toxins give rise to generalised neurologic signs

- chemical
  - organo-phosphates – peripheral nerve morbidity
  - monensin
  - lead – **peripheral autonomic nerve morbidity** – recurrent laryngeal neuropathy (RLN) with inco-ordination and weakness
    - arsenic
    - strychnine
    - Ergot of Rye – peripheral nerve morbidity
- thiamin deficiency
  - following prolonged ingestion of bracken fern and/or horsetail grasses when on unusually poor diets. Responds to thiamine therapy. Signs are ataxia, depression, weight loss, sudden heart failure.

SPECIFIC DISEASES ASSOCIATED WITH LIMB WEAKNESS AND ATAXIA

Degenerative Neurological Disease

Grass sickness and motor neuron disease can also be classified under this heading.

Cervical Vertebral Stenotic Myelopathy

- distortion of spinal vertebrae alignment, causing a narrowing of the spinal canal and pressure kinking on the spinal cord with eventual neural degeneration from the periphery inwards of the white matter, the spinal tracts. Usually at C3 and C4 but can be at C6 to T1
  - a congenital condition of fast growing Thoroughbreds and Thoroughbred crosses, usually geldings. Progressive wallerian degeneration from 1 to 2 years but clinical gait deficits sometimes delayed until 3 to 4 years when triggered into an acute dis-ease following a fall – neck whiplash. There is then marked ataxia and inco-ordination – 'Wobbler'. The 'slap test' reaction is usually disrupted

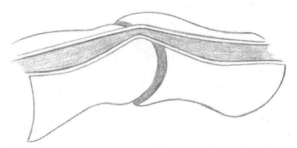

Distortion of spinal vertebrae alignment causes pressure kinking on the cord.

Degenerative Myeloencephalopathy (EDM)

Young light breed horses can be affected. Reported in zebras and Przewalski horses (also llamas, wildebeest and camels). Signs in horses usually begin before 6 months of age and up to 3 years. There is evidence of familial incidence.

Signs

Ataxia, weakness often sudden in onset; progressive until maximum at maturity; found in all four limbs. Apparently in good health otherwise.

Autopsy

Spinal tracts in mid-thoracic region are most affected by the degenerative changes.

Cause

Unknown but could be, in addition to familial tendencies

- toxic
- nutritional, especially vitamin E deficiency. Some cases respond to this therapy
- metabolic

All of which have been incriminated in other species

SPECIFIC INFECTIONS

Bacterial

Meningitis

Mainly seen in foals. Pyrexia with skin hypersensitivity, neck pain, depression, anorexia, seizure and blindness.

Tetanus

Causes paralysis of specific interneurons of inhibitory pathways in the CNS which would normally limit the degree of muscular contractions and thereby prevent spasm which myopathy is a cardinal sign of tetanus.

Botulism

Interferes with release of acetylcholine at nerve-end synapses with resultant muscular weakness both voluntary and involuntary.

Vertebral Osteomyelitis

Infectious inflammation of the spinal vertebrae, a sequel to blood or lymph spread of

- Mycobacterium (tuberculosis)
- Brucella abortus bacterium (contagious abortion infection of cattle)
- Corynebacterium (now rare in foals)

progressive with sudden clinical signs.

Viral

- EHV-1 myeloencephalopathy
- EIA (equine infectious anaemia), an ependymitis meningitis

Equine Protozoal Myeloencephalitis (EPM)

Suspected cases of this **protozoan** infection of the spinal cord and occasionally the brain have been reported in the UK

- it is particularly common in Eastern North America, but identical parasites have been recorded in other parts of the continent
- imports from the USA to the UK have exhibited clinical and autopsy findings
- young to adult light horses (Thoroughbreds and Standardbreds in particular)

History

Clinically, any part of the CNS can be affected with multifocal, necrotic, non-suppurative myeloencephalitis. This wide distribution of lesions, invariably asymmetric and of variable progression, produces a wide range of signs.

Signs

Basically a mild lameness. Sometimes there is an acute onset of

- ataxia
- head tilt, facial paralysis
- weakness – recumbency, and later
  - muscle atrophy
  - sweating
  - bowel and bladder defects

Overall a wide range of CNS lesion signs. A particular lesion of the caudal cervical cord produces a horse which

- moves with extended forelegs (flexor muscle weakness)
- low head and neck carriage

Diagnosis

There is no specific ante mortem test available

- elimination of other possible causes
- cerebro spinal fluid (CSF) examination may show an inflammatory/necrotic alteration of the white blood cells

Treatment
Is possible under a veterinary surgeon's control.

Allergic

To bacteria and/or primary to a virus such as adenovirus

- neuritis (Polyneuritis equi, 'Cauda equina neuritis')
  - neuritis of the cauda equina
    - atrophy of gluteal muscles with hind-leg weakness
    - paresis of facial and trigeminal cranial nerves

In addition to trauma, infection, allergy, neoplastic and degenerative conditions, some of which have already been described, two other dis-ease types have a marked influence on nerve system functioning in the CNS and particularly in the brain.

Metabolic

- electrolytic at cellular level
  - hypocalcaemia – deficiency of calcium in the blood
  - hyperkalaemia – excess potassium in the blood
  - hypokalaemia – deficiency of potassium in the blood
  - hypomagnasaemia – deficiency of magnesium in the blood
- metabolites
  - hypoglycaemia – deficiency of sugar in the blood
  - hyperglycaemia – excess sugar in the blood
  - uraemia – presence of urea in the blood
  - hyperammonaemia – excess of ammonia in the blood

Endocrine

- pituitary adenoma

Hypocalcaemia (Eclampsia)

An *absolute* deficiency of blood calcium, as distinct from that in 'milk fever' in the cow where it is a temporary deficit

- in the eclampsic mare, usually on non-supplemented diets
  - seen at end of lactation rather than the beginning

- especially if stressed as by unaccustomed transit

Signs
Fundamentally due to lack of calcium, affecting nerve and muscle functioning

- apprehensiveness
- restlessness
- sweating
- increased heart and respiratory rates
- unsteady stiff gait
- some unilateral contraction of lips, a **trismus**, with staring expression
  - difficulty in swallowing
  - reduced defecation
  - collapse
  - convulsions
  - coma

Some, if not all these, at different times during progression of the cascade of signs are also suggestive of

- abdominal (colic) crisis
- respiratory crisis
- acute laminitis
- tetanus – but history, blood sample and response to treatment, differentiates

Transit Tetany

A *temporary* unavailability of calcium and magnesium (they are 'locked up', possibly under hormonal influence)

- in **lactating** and/or **in oestrus** mares but, also in other horses
- following *prolonged transit* and undue, associated fatigue, hence the descriptive name

Signs
- tetanic spasms
- trismus
- stiff-legged gait
- heart and respiratory rate increased
  - profuse sweating
  - distressed
  - collapse

- convulsions

Differential diagnosis again relates to history, blood analysis and response to intra-venous therapy. Secondary complications of **bacterial pneumonia** are common (transit 'fever' and subsequent endotoxaemia).

Synchronous Diaphragmatic Flutter
(thumps or hiccoughs)

A synchronous contraction of the diaphragm with the heart beat

- as seen in the fatigued, sweating horse especially the endurance competitor with electrolyte imbalances

Signs

- diaphragm 'snaps' to produce audible as well as visible thump
- obvious sweating
- the fatigue signs (not invariably marked) can progress to other more serious signs of heat stress with increase in temperature to 18°C (110°F) with
  - staggering
  - frothing
  - collapse
  - convulsions

Hepatic Encephalopathy

Subsequent to acute and chronic liver disease, and *particularly due to ragwort poisoning* of the chronic type. The faulty liver function allows

- an excess of ammonia to leak into the circulation
- the hyperammonaemia leads to
  - encephalopathy with
    - ataxia
    - leaning on walls
    - head pressing
    - aimless wandering and yawning
    - hyper-excitability which becomes dangerous (delirious)
      - collapse
      - convulsions
      - death

Uraemia

Following acute renal failure (rare in horses) will act somewhat similarly when the associated ammonaemia increases and circulates to the brain.

Neoplasia

- brain tumours (rare) but
  - pituitary adenoma indirectly
  - lymphosarcoma

COMA AND ALTERED STATES OF CONSCIOUSNESS

An alert state, fully *compos mentis*, is maintained by

- multiple sensory inputs from all sources traversing the spinal and cranial nerves to the
  - cranial nervous system and in particular to the
    - brain stem
    - thalamus
    - cortex, the 'seat' of consciousness

When some or all of these three higher centres are deficient in reception and/or in transmission then awareness decreases from

- depression, to
- semi coma, to
- coma, during which cascade other signs such as
  - behavioural
  - visual deficits
  - seizures

dependent upon the related CNS defects are usually seen.

All diffuse brain diseases invariably lead to coma prior to death. Coma is a state of recumbency with unconsciousness and total unresponsiveness, and is primarily associated with deep changes in the

- mid brain
- fore brain, from
  - head trauma and haemorrhage. Recovery is possible within 24 hours – 'comes round'
  - meningo encephalitis

- parasitic invasion
- liver disease
- in any poisons

Collapse

Technically 'a sudden inability to stand up'.

Acute Collapse

Without immediate coma, this is seen in

- hyperthermia
- shock
- hypoglycaemia
- hypocalcaemia
- hypokalaemia
- endotoxaemia
- exotoxaemia (e.g. gas gangrene)
- anaphylaxis

many of which will rapidly progress, but not necessarily so, to

- comatose, then
- 'in a coma', before
- death

There is a compound hypoxia, malnutrition, especially of glucose, and toxic effect on the brain as the basic pathogenesis.

Other episodes of 'collapse' with immediate unconsciousness are seen in the **syncopes**

- cardio-vascular altered functioning, fainting
  - non-serious, recoverable arrhythmia
- cardio-vascular disease, more rare, with usually ultimate syncope – heart failure
  - atrial fibrillation
  - ruptured valve cords
  - aortic endocarditis

all leading to hypoxia of the brain and collapse.

In **fainting** there is no warning sign. Some struggling may occur during recovery. In the other types specific signs are often present if not before, then during recovery from the collapse as perceived at the post-attack veterinary examination.

To the layman, a collapsed horse is seen as a crisis even if it does quickly recover – with or without loss of consciousness

- will it recover?
- if it does
  - will it collapse again with me on it?
  - will it collapse again and fall on me?
  - why did it collapse in the first place?

By definition, a collapsing horse has no control over

- its going down: it is unconscious, and has reduced control on recovery, over
- its getting up: it is still dazed

so it can be dangerous to the handler. It rarely collapses 'under saddle' but gives some warning by slowing down, but this is not a strict rule.

Causes of Collapse

With or without loss of consciousness (i.e. in a coma or not) are

- acute airway obstruction – usually fatal
- acute severe (usually internal) haemorrhage – usually fatal
- cardiac arrest – usually fatal
- pain induced convulsive collapse – usually conscious, e.g. colic
- cranio-spinal trauma
  - cranial: goes down – often becomes unconscious
  - spinal: traumatised by falling over an obstacle 'goes down' – no loss of consciousness

There are associated deficits in

- sensory input especially proprioception
- motor output and so motor paralysis

Other causes of *apparent* motor paralysis include

- acute exercise induced ER
- Quarter horse **hyperkalaemic periodic paralysis (HKPP)**
- cataplexy/narcolepsy
- seizures loss of consciousness with
  - nystagmus
  - opisthotonus

- incontinence

In all collapsing episodes, the outcome is
- recumbency but gets up
  - fully recovered
  - with gait deficit
- possible repetitions and then as above
- fails to rise (euthanased)
  - or eventually dies
- sudden death

Narcolepsy

An episodic sleep 'attack' usually accompanied by cataplexy.

Cataplexy

A profound loss of muscle tone (power). These have been reported in
- Suffolk foals and horses (familial)
- Shetland and Welsh ponies (familial)
- Thoroughbreds
- Standardbreds and Quarter horses
- other light crossbreds

Signs
during an episode
- the 'sleep' rapidly passes from
  - very drowsy to
  - asleep on its feet to
  - knuckling in distal forelegs

This knuckling is the failure of the stay suspensory apparatus because of the motor paralysis (minimal as that muscle effort is, in the asleep, standing horse). This is an initial
- cataplexy, but there is still a proprioceptive awareness and the horse may now snap out of it, become awake and stand upright again

In some cases, full narcolepsy occurs and the horse collapses to be
- recumbent, mainly without response to reflex stimuli

except for
- some facial responses

without other signs of neurologic deficits or other diseases.

The sleep is of the deep, rapid eye movement type and comes on immediately, unlike ordinary sleep in which the shallow, slow eye movement sleep begins first. The recumbency is often called 'inappropriate'; there is no reason for it. Arousal is possible with variable difficulty. Rising is eventually done quietly and easily.

The basic causes are unknown, but a biochemical defect of the brainstem sleep–wake control centres is thought to be present. In some cases other trigger factors are involved
- in the foal, when the handler holds it tightly in his arms
- prolonged 'gentling' and petting of the head and neck in adults seems to induce a soporific state
- slow hosing-down of the horse tied to outside rails
- tied horses sunning themselves

It does not occur at exercise or in the presence of stable yard activity. Between attacks, unless these are frequent, there are no clinical signs. In between frequent attacks, especially in the foal, there may be drowsiness.

Diagnosis
Differential between this and epileptiform convulsions and cardio respiratory causes of collapse and **mild electric shocks** from an **underground source**.

Treatment
Episodic intervals can be increased by specific drugs. Usually necessary only in a very few cases of this uncommon condition.

Seizure

A fit, **ictus**, or convulsion, an abnormal behaviour. It is relatively uncommon in the horse. Those which do, usually have a recognised cause
- metabolic
- traumatic
- infectious
- developmental

an idiopathic (i.e. cause unknown), occurs in young horses, usually Arabians, called **idiopathic epilepsy**.

Seizure is the clinical expression of abnormal electrical discharges from neurons, a dysrhythmia, in the

- fore brain which 'descends' to the
  - somatic and
  - visceral motor end-plates, and there initiates
    - spontaneous
    - paroxysmal
    - involuntary movements

these tend to have a

- sudden onset
- a definitive duration
- sudden end, but are often preceded by a
- pre-fit 'aura' of variable depth and duration
- post-fit 'aura' of decreasing depth but longer duration

during which time the horse

- becomes distracted and less aware
- restless
- has muscle spasms before the fit proper when it
  - falls to the ground
  - rhythmically thrashes

The post-fit aura may have blindness of a temporary but, in the foal, several days' duration. Younger animals have a lower threshold to a trigger factor. The benign epilepsy of the foal is usually in animals with an intercurrent disease such as pneumonia. In the adult, seizure is usually associated with other brain lesions and accompanied by varying degrees of loss of consciousness. Quasi-seizures are seen in the violent reactions associated with

- acute colic
- pain of femoral fractures

THE NEUROMUSCULAR DISORDERS

Botulism

Usually in association with plastic-wrapped silage (an on-going risk. Each big bag, before being used, should be checked for

- appearance – tears will expose contents
- smell
- pH

Definitive lab diagnosis is difficult. Serum from severe early cases for toxin tests.

Cardinal Signs

- salivation
- tongue paresis
- dysphagia
- inco-ordination
- progressive cranial to caudal paralysis

Mild cases – still walking and swallowing, respond to supportive care. In mild or early cases **botulism anti-toxin (BAT)** is helpful but not available in the UK. More severe – seldom survive. The toxin damages the cholinergic neuro transmitter activity throughout the body.

Equine Motor Neuron Disease (EMND)

This is usually a sporadic disorder affecting horses of all ages and breeds as well as ponies. Epidemiologically it is seen

- mainly in adults
- more common in those horses kept
  - short of grazing and/or on alfalfa hay in parts of America
  - fed on pelleted concentrates
    - deficiency of vitamin E. These are the putative causes
- an eastern states of USA disease
- more recently recognised world-wide including the UK
- not thought to have been recognised pre 1979
  - marked increase since 1984
  - recorded in the UK first in 1993

It is a pure motor neuron acquired degenerative disorder confined to the LMNs (lower motor neuron systems) in the ventral horn of the spinal cord and those of the medulla's cranial nerves V, VII and XII. Its ultimate effect is a progressive degeneration of the related muscles usually those involved in posture and stance which have a high percentage of slow twitch Type 1 fibres which are highly oxygen dependent. The *autonomic system is not involved* (compare with grass sickness).

In the USA it could be confused with

- rabies

- equine protozoal myeloencephalitis

and anywhere that

- EHV myeloencephalopathy is found

In the last few years the degenerative morbid changes in the LMN in this disease have been likened to those of the autonomic sympathetic ganglia morbidity in grass sickness (EGS). A similar toxic pathogenesis has been suggested. In the USA both diseases have been suspected in the one animal.

Signs
An acute onset of

- trembling
- excessive voluntary recumbency
- almost constant shifting of weight in the rear legs when standing
- progressive muscular atrophy
- low head carriage
- high tail/head carriage in later stages
- leaning-over-the-forehand stance
  - walks better than it stands

all due to

- postural muscle/stay apparatus weakness
- good appetite which because of inability to get about is possibly augmented by dung-eating causing black dental tartar
- in stabilised cases
  - bizarre gait abnormalities, e.g. stringhalt-like action
  - some horses regain muscle mass
    - but few survive and none are satisfactory athletically
    - euthanasia is the usual outcome

Diagnosis
- history of management (see above under epidemiology)
- clinical signs
- tail/head muscle biopsy
- spinal accessory nerve (XII) branch biopsy

both these for degenerative changes

- autopsy

Differentially

- acute cases with
  - laminitis
  - colic (except appetite is good)
  - ER
  - botulism
  - EPM (equine protozoal myeloencephalitis)

Neuritis Cauda Equina

In the earlier days of investigating this condition, it was commonly seen as being confined to the nerve roots of the sacro-coccygeal spinal nerves in the cauda equina of the spine, and affected them external to their dura-mata covering. At the present day it is known better as **polyneuritis equi** since it is now recognised as a diffuse polyneuritis.

It is characterised as a chronic granulomatous inflammation of many peripheral nerves, spinal and cranial.

Cause
Still not fully determined but

- possibly a virus infection, e.g. an adenovirus or more likely
- immune mediated – an allergic neuritis – based on a prior viral infection

Subject
Usually in **mature** animals, horses and ponies of both sexes

Pathogenesis
Progressive, insidious involvement of peripheral nerves with

- initial hyperaesthesia
- then anaesthesia
- then paralysis of affected musculature

Signs
relate to

- damage to cauda equina nerve roots with
  - hyperaesthesia – tail rubbing and
  - hypersensitivity to touch over the perineal area, progressing to
  - decreased sensation to skin touch

- analgesia of perineal area

including the penis but not the sheath (different nerve trunks) followed by

- weakness or paralysis of the
  - tail
  - rectum, with retention and overspill to a limited extent
  - anus
  - bladder, with incontinence and overflow
  - urethral sphincter, with leakage dribble down the thighs (in the mare)
    - cystitis
    - skin scalding
- mild pelvic limb weakness
- ataxia when disease spreads to lumbar nerves
  - involvement of cranial nerves
    - V, VII, VIII with
      - weakness of masseter muscles
      - facial paralysis
      - vestibular disease
    - IX, X
      - difficulty in swallowing
      - XII tongue paralysis
  - involvement of autonomic nervous system

Diagnosis

There are no specific tests except for possible importance of increased serum titre levels to a nerve protein

- differential
  - sacral fracture
  - sacro-coccygeal dislocation from trauma and
  - history
  - EHV-I neuropathy (serum titre levels and history)
  - EPM (imported USA horses)
  - EMND (equine motor neuron disease) a general but progressive muscle weakness

Neoplasia

- Pituitary adenoma – reference has already been made to the endocrine secretions (hormones) released from the pituitary gland because of its

- anatomical position just beneath the brain
- functional relationship with the brain through the hypothalamus-pituitary-infundibulum neuro-stalk
- 'master gland' reputation

Any disease of this gland can have a widespread effect

- direct and pressure influence on the hypothalamus and adjacent brain tissue
- endocrine malfunctioning

and they both involve neuro disease one way or another.

Tumour formation mainly occurs in the central part of the anterior pituitary whose particular output is ACTH (adrenocorticotrophic hormone), which is essential for the functioning of the adrenal gland.

This formation causes an excess of this hormone and prevents any feedback control to regulate the outflow. The pressure damages CNS tissues such as the hypothalamus itself, so interrupting 'release' messages to the pituitary and to its thermo-regulatory function, to the optic nerves and the secretions of ADH (antidiuretic hormone). Consequently there is a wide range of signs. The condition is seen in old horses and in ponies, male and especially female.

Confirmed cases have been recorded as young as 13 years. A possible primary viral infection has been postulated as a trigger factor in these comparatively young animals.

Signs

- weight loss
- muscle wasting
- hirsutism – retained coat which becomes shaggy and curly – this is the common finding and as such is symptomatic of the tumour and its site
- sweating
- laminitis
- polyuria and polydypsia
- ataxia
- blindness, and apparently excess supra orbital fat
- hyperlipaemia which may be associated with
- hyperglycaemia and low glucose tolerance especially in ponies

those directly attributable to excess ACTH are collectively called **Cushings-like** or **Cushingoid disease**

Diagnosis
Lab tests on blood.

Prognosis
Poor. Welfare considerations are important.

Treatment
Possible but expensive.

Originally the hyperglycaemia was seen as Diabetes mellitus but the common human type of this condition is very rare in the horse, nor does Insulin have any beneficial effect in this condition. There is still much to be understood about fat and glucose metabolism in the horse.

Diabetes insipidus is due to a failure of the kidney to concentrate urine because of a lack of ADH or an insensitivity to it. The polyuria and polydypsia in pituitary adenoma is due to pressure interference with ADH production.

CRANIAL PERIPHERAL NERVE DAMAGE

A detailed discussion on causes, effect, signs and the inter-relationship of one nerve with some others and with the brain and with the autonomic system will not be attempted.

It is unlikely that the horsemaster will find it necessary to examine for deficits. He may, of course, come across the more patent effects of some nerve damage. As with the spinal nerve conditions, the interference with sensory input, the loss of skin sensation over the face, head and anterior neck, can originate along the sensory nerve trunks or within the integration areas of the brain. The nil muscle reaction or motor output, a necessary clue to the input failure, could also be a failure of that side of the circuit in its own right.

In cranial nerves, some are only sensory, some motor, and some dual. There is, moreover, a greater involvement of the autonomic system with associated involuntary muscle action.

The horsemaster may be alerted to an apparently sudden loss of unilateral, possibly bilateral visual activity. In the absence of superficial lesions with clinical signs of

- acute eye injury
- acute eye ball inflammatory lesions (usually unilateral)

the cause will be more central and will usually present with other signs of brain disorders.

More subtly, however, some disorders of

- pupil size and/or
- eyeball movement, usually asymmetric, may be seen by an observant horsemaster who, with closer inspection may notice
    - a withdrawal of the narrow-pupilled eye deeper into the socket
    - a drooping of the upper eyelid
    - a protrusion of the third eyelid

which together form part of **Horners Syndrome**, which indicates some damage to the sympathetic nervous system (SNS) from

- tumour formation
- interference to cord tracts to the brain
- inflammation

whereby the nerves to the eyeball are disordered.

Peripheral Nerves

These are the paired nerve trunks carrying

- sensory and/or
- motor fibres and
- autonomic system motor fibres from the
    - brain – the cranial nerves (Cn I–XII)
    - spinal cord, the spinal nerves (C1–8, T1–18, L1–6, S1–5, Cy1–5) to all tissues of the body

By definition, these trunks, on leaving the protection of the bony cranium and spinal column, travel outwards to the extremities of the

- skull
- face
- jaw
- trunk
- limbs

invariably in the company of arteries and veins.

Some retain some protection by their position within muscle groups. Sooner or later they must surface

- en route
- at or near these extremities

and travel over bone and under skin with little protection against trauma.

The trauma can occur

• within the cranium or spinal column

but outwith the brain and cord tissues from

• skull and spinal column injury to nerve fibres
    • at the foraminae, from
        • direct trauma – concussion
        • pressure from
            • new bone formation possibly narrowing the opening
        • oedema
        • soft tissue swelling (muscle in particular)
        • acute but later with
            • fibrous (chronic) inflammation
            • vascular disorders
                • ischaemia
                • atrophy
                • degeneration
                • electrolytic imbalances in perineural fluid, usually oedematous
    • outwith the bony confines, the true peripheral trunks
    • at any point of the line of the trunk but especially where the nerve
        • traverses the surface of cranial/facial flat bones
        • curves round a long bone at a point thinly or not at all covered by muscle
        • passes over a joint promontory where it becomes exposed to
            • external contact trauma
            • parturition pressure
        • new bone (exotosis or neoplastic) pressures
    • stretch trauma as a result of exaggerated limb movement or accidental traction

In such circumstances a usually temporary interference with nerve message conduction occurs – temporary, i.e. provided the pressure or repetitive contact is removed. This trauma can be

• contusion with oedema

• compression with coincidental occlusion of related blood supply – progressive onset
• laceration in association with an open wound which is, by definition, much more serious

In all types the temporary condition may become more persistent even permanent, with degeneration and the necrosis of the nerve.

The trunk, as previously described, carries both sensory and motor nerve elements. Damage therefore causes

• altered input – loss of sensation
• altered output – loss of motor power
• 'break' in the reflex arc – loss of spinal or cranial reflexes
• interference with related autonomic control

In practice the primary clinical sign is

• paralysis of the innervated muscles with 'lameness', and when the associated area of skin distal to the injury is 'skin prick' tested
    • a variable loss of sensation

In fact the loss of sensation usually precedes the loss of muscle power but it is unlikely that testing for this will have been tried; muscle weakness therefore is invariably the first clue.

The autonomic nerve supply to the arterial smooth muscles of the locomotor area affected will also be disturbed: increased flow to begin then a decrease, with resultant rise then a fall in the tissue temperatures.

There is, in addition

• spontaneous contraction of some muscle fibres, a fasciculation
• loss of local reflexes
    • muscle atrophy
    • fibrosis
    • shrinkage of the muscles affected
• alteration to glandular function (the sweat glands) if the condition is protracted

The management and treatment is a veterinary matter.

Recovery, relative to the extent and degree of nerve injury, is invariably slow, months rather than weeks. If a nerve is severed the axon will regenerate and rejoin if the ends are not more than 2.5cm (1in) apart; growth rate is approximately 2.5cm (1in) per month. It will require 2 to 3 months for sensation to return and up to 9 months before function is restored.

Because of other wound complications in lacerations and severe contusions, the nerve ends or the trunk itself are often displaced and 'lost' in the soft tissue scarring. Neuro surgery is possible. Severe neuro damage has a poor prognosis.

Neuralgia

* pain along course of nerve trunk following
  * neuritis from
    * infection and/or
    * trauma

with hyperaemia of the nerve sheath followed by cellular infiltration of connective tissue.

The following nerve trunks from the spinal CNS are the most common, but even then, rarely affected. It was more common in draught horses falling on paved roads.

Suprascapular 'Shoulder Slip' or 'Sweeney'

This trunk is virtually unprotected as it passes around and over the spine of the scapula (shoulder blade)

* if the horse hits its shoulder when passing through a door or a gate the trauma can also damage the nerve
* at rest the affected horse stands with its shoulder bulging laterally and its foot medially inward because of the paralysis of the infraspinatus muscle, whereby it loses
  * lateral support of the shoulder, and
  * significant extension, and
  * adduction power for the limb
* at walk the inability to extend the leg requires the horse to swing (circumduct) it. The toe is dragged
* on weight bearing the shoulder bulges outwards – 'shoulder slip'; there is rapid atrophy of the infraspinatus and supraspinatus muscles – 'sweeney'

Radial Nerve 'Dropped Elbow'

This nerve supplies all the muscles which

* extend the elbow joint

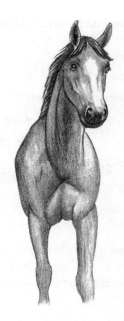

Suprascapular 'shoulder slip' – Sweeney.

* flex the 'knee'
* extend the 'knee' and distal phalanges

The apparent anomaly of a nerve which can 'inform' muscles of apparently different activity will be noted; the trunk carries fibres which do not all go to the same muscles and are programmed to 'fire' within a controlled pattern.

Exceptionally this nerve is well protected from its emergence in the brachial plexus in the axilla (arm pit) but because the foreleg has no clavicle it can be compressed onto the thorax. This was more likely to happen when restraint for surgery required the horse to be cast 'tied down' for some time; compression damage could then occur to the underlying limb. In similar situations forced restriction of this limb would add a stretch factor. With modern anaesthesia and sensible operating floors such trauma is rare

* accidental fractures of the first rib (racing falls, road traffic accidents) can involve the more proximal components of the trunk before they exit the brachial plexus
  * the paralysis is essentially an extensor paralysis of the foreleg
  * the horse at rest stands with
    * elbow, knee, fetlock, and phalanges flexed
    * toe of foot resting on the ground
    * the point of the elbow drops – 'dropped elbow'
* in forward motion

- the hind legs exaggeratedly try to propel the body forward
- the shoulder girdle tries to lift the affected limb but only a half stride length is effected
  - in less severe cases
    - the horse can extend its knee, fetlock and phalanges to advance the limb and take weight
    - but the shoulder 'jerks'
  - ironically the older causes of paralysis had a fair to good prognosis but that associated with rib fracture is poor

Post casting, the weakness can pass off in hours. In partial paralysis recovery takes 2 to 3 weeks. In full types, a slow recovery begins after 10 days but complete functioning can require 9 months.

Crural or Femoral Paralysis

This nerve innervates the extensors of the stifle. Like most hind leg nerves this is well protected by muscles but it can be involved following attacks of 'azoturia' especially when the deep pelvic muscles are involved.

Tumours and abscesses rarely can cause persisting pressure damage to it.

At rest the horse stands with the affected quarter lowered and the stifle (and hock) excessively flexed. Sensation is absent on the inside of the thigh.

Popliteal or Peroneal Paralysis

This nerve innervates the flexors of the hock. It is especially liable to be traumatised as it passes over the external condyle (knuckle) of the femur above the stifle.

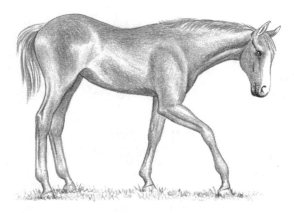

Injury to the right brachial plexus.

Here it is only protected by skin. Injury, however, is rare but can follow kicks or falls on the hard or when cast for some time especially on bare flooring

- the horse stands with the stifle and the hock extended and the fetlock, downwards, excessively flexed
- skin sensation is lost over the outside of the gaskin and the lateral and anterior aspects of the hock and the canon
- at walk the leg is jerked backwards and then forwards but comes to rest on the wall at the toe

Tibial Paralysis

- rarely traumatised because of good muscular protection but may be entrapped following bone and muscle damage to the area
- it supplies the flexor of the stifle and the extensors of the hock and digits
  - at rest the horse stands with the foot flat on the ground but with the hock excessively flexed and with the fetlock knuckled forward
  - at the walk there is a stringhalt-like action but with a more jerky foot placement

Distal Nerves to the Phalanges

- direct concussion trauma
- show jumping pole knock
- inelegant stride interference
- hit by polo ball or stick

The horse immediately goes on three legs as though the fourth was fractured low. Numbness quickly follows initial pain. Is comparatively short lasting.

The Compound Trigeminal Nerve Cn V

This is sensory from the head, including the **cornea**, yet the motor reactions when these areas are stimulated are

- rapid closure of eyelids
- twitching of the ears
- moving of head away

all motivated through the facial nerve Cn VII (digital pressure to the eyeballs causes a slowing of the heart!)

- damage to the motor elements of the trigeminal is

usually followed by profound disability to

- the muscles of mastication
  - inability to chew
  - to close mouth
  - loss of tone to the pharynx

usually from damage by

- trauma
- inflammation

Facial Nerve Cn VII

This nerve is vulnerable to trauma. It is the *most commonly affected*

- in the cranium by abscesses, tumours, oedema
- from middle and inner ear inflammation
- on the head from ill-fitting tack
- on the face by trauma where it curves round the posterior border of the ramus of the mandible
- on the lower face by too-tight nosebands

Signs

- drooping of an ear
- inability to close the eyelids and, when lower length only traumatised
- flaccid paralysis of the cheeks with inspiratory distension of them in the rostral area of the maxillae
- quidding

Vestibular Disease

In some human sports and pastimes involving fast rotating movement, the participants will stop and complain that 'my head is spinning', 'I'm dizzy', and will occasionally fall over – their vestibular apparatus, untrained for such accelerating unusual movement has failed to maintain a co-ordination of

- sensory input
- interpretation
- suitable motor output

Add to the movement a cacophony of sound, and the *'where am I?'* sensation can be worsened.

The cat, falling from a height, surprisingly seems able to land on its four feet, possibly painfully, but less seriously

than landing head first! Its ability to recognise where its head and body are in relation to its limbs at any moment during its tumbling fall, and its co-ordination at the vital time, are its safeguards.

The vestibular apparatus is the collective name for very complicated sensory receptors in the middle and inner ear which co-ordinate all the relevant information and forward it from there via the lower brain reflexes and efferent nerves to the various muscle systems, whereby the position of the eyes, head, neck, trunk, limbs, and their related movements are maintained.

The primary sensory receptors are in the three semi-circular canals within the bony labyrinth of the petrous temporal bone at the base of the ear. The afferent vestibular nerve is in the Cn VIII (acoustic) which also carries the cochlear nerve

- nostril fails to open on inspiration
- the sound side muscles appear to retract on that side, the affected side relaxes and droops to give a distorted muzzle

Horner's Syndrome may also accompany it, especially if the underlying cause is guttural pouch mycosis. In such a situation the Cn IX, X and XI may also be involved.

Acoustic Cn VII (See also Vestibular Disease)

Tests for hearing are very misleading in the horse, but

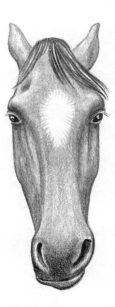

Vestibular disease.

unilateral deficit may be accompanied by greater use of head movement and the 'sound' ear to compensate. Degeneration of the tract occurs in the sensory ganglion. (The inherited coat-colour-associated deafness of cats and dogs has not been determined in the horse.)

The Vagus Cn IX and Glossopharyngeal Cn X

These are physiologically close, and dysfunction may be indicated by

- inability to swallow and a negative gag reflex when the throat is manually squeezed
- recurrent laryngeal paresis is a degenerative condition of a vagal branch, the recurrent laryngeal nerve. It may also be bilateral

In neuritis cauda equina it was emphasised that cranial nerves may also be involved in the polyneuritis with associated face, head and throat muscle paralysis. So too with EHV-1 infection and allergy when neuropathy produces cranial nerve lesions which are essentially central nuclei degenerations in origin.

Some Conditions Affecting the Nervous System

Condition	Breed	Sex	Age	Hereditable	Familial	Infectious
Cerebellar Atrophy	Arab horses	M	under 6 months	*		
Atlanto Occipital Malformation	Arab horses	M, F	from birth	*		
Cervical Vertebral Malformation (CSM)	Thoroughbreds Crosses	G	1–2 years		*	
Epilepsy (benign)	Arab horses	M, F	foals	*		
Narcolepsy	Shetlands	M, F	under 6 months	*		
	Suffolks	M, F	any age	*		
Night Blindness	Appaloosas	M, F	foals up	*		
Neuro Axonal Dystrophy	Morgans Standardbreds	M, F	young	*		
Degenerative Myloencephalopathy	Lightbreds Zebras	M, F		(*)		
Protozoal Degeneration (EPM)	older Standardbreds Thoroughbreds	M, F				*
Idiopathic Laryngeal Paralysis	Thoroughbreds Lightbreds	G	5 years and more (clinically)	(*)		
Shivering	Draught Breeds Crosses				(*)	

30 POISONS AND POISONING (TOXICOLOGY)

Poison – from the Old French *puison*, a 'potion': a dose of liquid, a draught, which has medicinal or, more commonly, a poisonous effect. Thus any substance which, when introduced to or absorbed by a living organism, usually in a relatively small quantity and, usually quickly, affects the well-being of that organism (cell, tissue, organ, body) up to its death; a morbid effect with a possible lethal outcome.

Toxin – a poisonous substance produced during the multiplication of a micro-organism. This substance is seen as having a toxic potential on body tissues with a variably lethal effect to cause a particular disease; for example, tetanus toxin. The micro-organism may or may not have pathogenic properties in its own right.

Toxic – from the Greek word *toxikon* meaning 'poison for arrowheads', from *toxa*, or 'arrows'. A substance capable of causing a poisoning effect; the state of having being poisoned; a disease resulting from the effects of a poison, generally from a poison, specifically from a toxin.

There is a seemingly confusing use of 'poison' and 'toxin'. For example: 'A horse has been poisoned ... a plant toxin is suspected', 'A horse has toxaemia' i.e. toxins in its blood and hence in its many tissues; 'A horse has blood poisoning', usually meaning a germ has entered the blood stream from a surface wound; 'certain chemicals are toxic' i.e. capable of causing tissue damage.

In specific medical conditions the vascular spread of **toxins** from bacterial multiplication, especially from the gastro-intestinal tract and the post-birth womb or from infected contused wounds, is more correctly spoken of as a **toxaemia**. Such toxins must be distinguished from **poisons**

of inorganic or organic origin, which can be sub-grouped as

- plant poisons
    - natural growth, or as
    - 'infected' growth of fungi on plants, especially their stored seed, with the production of **mycotoxins**. A special case is Ergot infection of growing grass and cereal plant 'flowers'
- chemical poisons
    - natural in the soil and drainage therefrom
    - compounded, as part of legitimate industrial, agricultural, and medicinal products

Poisoning in animals is usually a ***sporadically occurring event***. Some incidents may be prolonged through a failure to recognise the fact, and to deal with the cause.

Malicious poisoning occurs occasionally for recrimination, and perhaps more frequently for financial advantage; doping is the malicious use of drugs.

Accidental incidents of poisoning, far from being 'acts of God' as is often claimed, are more likely to be 'sins of omission or of commission' on the part of

- the owner responsible for
    - grazing
    - feeding
    - watering
    - health maintenance
    - disease prevention
- those directly involved in

- support activities such as
  - contract grassland management
  - building maintenance
  in, on or near an equine establishment
- other industrial businesses whose products, by-products and wastes could be hazardous via
  - wind drift and subsequent fall-out and
    - inhalation or
    - onto soil, grass etc., and ingestion
  - effluent into
    - direct water supplies
    - grazing
    - conserved feedstuff stores
  - direct access to their 'unsuitable' storage on or near equine used areas

It follows that the owner should

- be aware of the potential for poisoning incidents, however rare, which may be indigenous to their land
- employ a reputable firm, if not themselves qualified, to carry out seasonal 'agricultural' work which involves chemicals
- be alert to neighbouring activities which might be hazardous – industrial laws on this should be carefully implemented, but effluent into ditches and streams is always a possibility

Poisoning incidents are suspected when

- one or more horses in a communal situation are
  - found dead
  - unexpectedly or suddenly ill, with
    - nervous lesions: behavioural and locomotor changes
    - severe colic, especially with diarrhoea
    - diffuse skin lesions
  - inexplicably losing condition despite apparently good management
- there is circumstantial evidence of access to
  - poisonous plants
  - recent incorrect medication
  - new, doubtful, foodstuffs

- upwind spraying
- altered colour etc. of stream water
- dumped material onto grazing
  - waste
  - cuttings
- maintenance stores

There must be immediate co-operation between the
- owner
- veterinary surgeon, and a selected laboratory, eventually
- any third party, *invited in a friendly fashion* to effect a careful, clinical and environmental investigation – *thoughtless accusations only antagonise* and delay conclusions

Consult a veterinary surgeon immediately. Instant 'limiting' action at the time of the initial suspicion stage is vital.

If at grass
- 'stable' the sick
  - feed 'cut and carried' different grass, pending veterinary advice and possible treatment
- move any other, apparently healthy horses, to another field (not just the other side of the hedge) or into a yard or stables as above. Keep a careful hourly watch
  - search the field, hedges and 'new' dug ditches for any noxious weeds and their roots or tubers
  - investigate the possibility of some horses having 'got out'

If stabled
- if the fodder and forage are new (within one week's use) *stop but retain* (see Ragwort and Bracken). Change to a different supply or source for *all* the horses in consultation with suppliers
- if under treatment of any kind, stop; check the dosage and dilution rates being used
- check for possible external sources of contamination

Natural 'vegetable' accidental poisoning relates essentially to
- shortage of grass keep – and hence hunger, which 'overcomes' the unpalatability of toxic plants

- the horse being offered palatable but fungal spoiled corn
- the horse being allowed access to
  - a superabundance of fallen acorns
  - green, 'tasteless' yew
  - conserved hay with now tasteless toxic plants
  - only contaminated water

Accidental artificial poison is, as has been stressed, a reflection of stupidity on somebody's part. For example

- using a different animal species' food, usually a supplement, e.g. Monensin, a growth promoter for cattle, in horse feeds
- giving unadvised home treatment whilst the horse is on an incompatible or a synergistic drug
- allowing access to advertised toxic material camouflaged in a bait carrier attractive to horses, e.g. slug bait in bran, or Warfarin-type rodenticides in cereal feed
- giving incorrect dilution rates of additive or supplemental substances

There are antidotes to some poisons, but delay in diagnosis, and obtaining the correct antidote mitigates against success.

Self-preservation reactions minimise the risk of accidental natural poisoning. For example, the 'objectionable'

- taste
- smell
- texture

of growing toxic vegetation are perhaps the most protective.

Toxic natural inorganic materials which have concentrated in plants, or in water are not so readily recognised and avoided. The relevant substances are usually mineral salts. Horses do however fight shy of 'different' drinking water until thirst overcomes caution, by which time even an average horsemaster should be aware of behavioural changes.

Artificial toxic products vary in their 'warning' potential; markedly acidic or alkalinic substances are very 'off-putting'. Some lubricants, disinfectants and even, ironically, 'deterrents' and preservatives are conversely attractive to some horses.

Inquisitive gnawing could expose a horse to toxic wood preservative wrongly purchased for stable use.

Statistically the risk will relate to the

- level or degree of mistake
- toxicity of the substance
- amount and repetition
- susceptibility of the animal

From laboratory records it would appear that **plant poisoning is a bigger risk than chemical**. In the UK this may be a reflection of the prevalence of

- ragwort and bracken, and their
  - availability
  - masked presence of ragwort in hay
  - toxicity, both primary and secondary

Other factors are

- 'herd' application of insecticides involves all animals. 'Field' spraying of selective weedkillers exposes all grazers, but not all will consume the same amount of grass
- as most, if not all, such 'applications' are of tried and tested substances supplied with detailed instruction, the risk is almost entirely in the hands of the operator/manager
- the amount of 'dressing' per hectare is often such that the horse's average daily consumption (2.5% of body weight) of grass as dry matter (DM) limits the intake and so minimises any risk

Prevention

As part of good routine horsemastership look for, suspect, and have confirmed or otherwise, the presence of potentially toxic plants in

- field sources
  - hedgerow
  - sward, grazed and conserved
  do so in each season
  - spring and summer growth and flowering
  - autumn flowering and fruiting or seeding and fallen nuts and fruit
  - winter, as 'green' goes out of hedgerows, for fruit

assume that ditching could expose roots or tubers, certainly if the plant has been identified previously

- inspect fields especially for
  - dumping of garden refuse and other waste
- water
  - main supply should be satisfactory but
    - check if lead pipes or tanks are still in use
  - pond
    - static – fence off against consumption
    - draining through
      - beware blue/green algae in dry weather
      - have analysed especially for nitrates
  - stream
    - have analysed as above
    - beware changes in
      - quantity
      - colour
- bought-in feedstuffs
  - concentrates
  - supplements
  - additives

    should be satisfactory if from a respectable merchant
  - hay
  - bedding
  - shavings

should be obtained only from reputable vendors who warrant them free from poisonous plants and other 'toxins'. Store them, especially the grain and haylage, correctly. Do not buy bulk in excess of use

- cereals if ground/rolled   1 month
- hay, if under cover   1 year
- haylage, bag opened   1 week
- bedding: all must go under cover, or be wrapped

Toxicology

Clinical toxicology is the study and understanding of the adverse effects on health following exposure to substances which have poisonous toxic potential.

Most of the toxic effect of such substances is dose-related – *the larger the dose, the more pronounced the effect*. A sufficiently large dose is invariably lethal. Each

poison has its own low–high scale. Low doses can be sub-clinical in effect, or even 'ineffective'. When the substance has therapeutic or prophylactic uses the difference between 'safe' and 'damage' can be narrow. Likewise the safety margin of 'other use' contamination can also be small.

The toxicity of an active substance, including drugs, is described as the *mean lethal dose for 50 out of 100 test animals*. The amount is called **LD50**, and is by implication reasonably well above correct administration levels.

By definition, a poisoned animal has 'taken in' at least an LD50 amount. Survival will depend upon whether the animal's susceptibility level is above or below the average. *In practice, animals which show acute signs of toxic illness, will almost certainly die*.

The safety of insecticides, for example, is often dependent upon the fact that the host animal responds to the chemical differently to the parasite, thereby making its use a reasonable risk. This may not be so 'safe' when 'baited' toxicants against rodents and molluscs (slugs) become available to livestock which normally would not be exposed to the active ingredient on its own, or to certain weed control agents.

Some poisons are

- inimical to all animal species
- some more so to one species than another
- less toxic to some animals within a species
- susceptibility is influenced by age, health, use

In equine management

- *potentially* hazardous substances are *many*
- commonly *confirmed* substances are relatively *few*
- veterinary cases (of poisoning) are very low in comparison with other dis-ease causes

Indirect accidental poisoning can be

- calamitous
  - widespread, as in the
    - Chernobyl disaster's fall out
  - local, as in industrial escape of
    - toxic waste into water supplies
    - wrong ingredients used in compound feeds
- less dramatic
  - misuse of synthetic substances when applied

- medicinally
  - therapeutically or prophylactically
  - to the wrong animal (age, condition, other treatment)
  - to the wrong species
  - at the wrong strength at repeat intervals
- for related management purposes
  - without consideration to safety factors, for example a time lapse for treated grazing

Whether poisoning is natural or indirect, all animals exposed to it by

- ingestion
- inhalation
- contact
- injection

will be at risk.

Although a vet's case list does not have 'poisoning' as a regular item the prevalence may vary with

- geography
  - different soil compositions and structures encourage or discourage certain
    - grasses
    - plants
  - water supply level of
    - nitrates from fertiliser programmes over many years
    - arsenic from 'old' industrial waste
    - lead from 'old' mining and smelting and
    - pipes and storage tanks made of lead
  - active industrial fall out and effluent
- seasons/weather
  - growth rate of 'safe' herbage compared with
  - emergence of toxic plants and their persistence
- management systems
  - type of grazing
  - weed control
  - fertiliser application
- proximity of
  - industry including other agri-businesses

- urban development

The farmer and the veterinary surgeon, as well as, in the UK, ADAS and the NFU, will be aware of the risks inherent in the locality. ***The horsemaster new to the district should seek their advice.***

Apart from those poisons which cause 'surface' damage to the epidermal tissues of the mouth, feet and localise there, or have the indirect effect of loss of condition because the horse cannot readily get to sufficient grazing – severe lameness; cannot readily eat – mouth and tongue sores. ***The majority cause systemic illness.***

These frequently show ***signs similar to acute infectious disease*** and, broadly speaking are of the

- **inflammatory type**, in particular affecting the
  - gastro-enteric
  - cardio-vascular
  - neurologic (behaviour and locomotion) systems

and in the stages of

- hyperacute
  - usually fatal
- acute
  - possibly fatal eventually, or
  - variably regressive to
    - recovery or
    - staying progressive to a
- chronic state
  - irreversible organic dis-ease
    - clinical
    - sub-clinical
  - subsequent illness, invariably a fatal, acute dis-ease, due to further blood borne metabolite damage to distant organs

The lethal effects are the result of primary or secondary (usually via the liver) damage to the vital organs

- heart
- kidneys
- brain

In many cases these develop very rapidly following absorption through the digestive system, e.g.

- yew

- some hydro-carbon compounds

Others progress more slowly with signs of dis-ease of one or more systems, resulting in

- behavioural changes
  - somnolence
  - aimless wandering and ataxic gaits
  - convulsions
- colic, with eventual diarrhoea
- cardiac disorders
  - fast heart rate and irregularities
  - slow heart rate and/or
    - blood pressure changes
- respiratory
  - distress
    - anoxia

and many are eventually fatal, primarily or secondarily.

In general, whether plant or chemical, the toxic compounds are known or thought to *interfere with the enzyme activity* involved in maintaining cellular life.

At least some of the synthetic organic compounds act by

- over-stimulating the receptors of the autonomic nervous system
- inhibiting the enzymes responsible for controlling the duration of activity in the parasympathetic division
- stimulating the sympathetic division or mimicking the normal endocrine stimulators, e.g. the adrenergic effect

The morbidity is gross, as in chemical burning, acidic or alkalinic, following prehension, inhalation (more rarely) on skin contact.

The resultant stimulation of nociceptor nerve endings causes protective reflexes, resulting in

- rejection from the mouth, and protective salivation
- avoidance

In skin contact some material may be absorbed from the surface trauma to cause internal organ morbidity.
If ingestion does occur the gastro-intestinal tract is 'burned', often with serious consequences

- interference with cellular level activity

- interaction with vital processes involving
  - vitamins
  - electrolytes

Certain inorganic mineral elements are essential micro-nutrients (trace elements)

- copper
- zinc
- iron
- iodine
- selenium

A deficiency of these can induce metabolic disorder. **An excess can lead to toxicity.**
The essential level of copper for pigs, for example, is much higher than that for horses: a confusion in the use of compounded foods could be toxic to horses.

An acceptable and essential level of selenium could be exceeded with toxic effect by

- excessive supplementation
- access to certain grasses which, without damage to themselves, accumulate selenium to levels toxic for horses

Other non-essential elements such as arsenic, mercury and lead, which contaminate water or become available through access to dumped horticultural cuttings can be toxic at comparatively low levels.

Organo-chloride, organo-phosphate and organo-carbonate products used as pesticides have a *reasonably* wide margin of safety when used in animals. Their formulation is such that their lethal effect on the parasite is obtained by a

- lower relative dosage than is likely to affect the host
  and is
- effective through a different pathway than is possible in the animal

Constant unadvised or unprotected exposure of the operator is potentially dangerous.

Those designed to be rodenticide or molluscicide are directed at rodents and snails and are not intended for, in fact *must be kept away from*, other animals.

Whilst the dose available for the 'pest' is obviously

relatively small, repeat access by the domestic animal could lead to cumulative toxic levels.

The photosensitising agents 'gain entrance' by

- direct contact of unpigmented skin or

- by ingestion, then through the liver producing photo-dynamic substances carried to all tissues, but which become exposed to u/v radiation at unpigmented sites

Emergency Treatment

The horse cannot vomit or be made to vomit like man or dog, nor can his stomach or large intestine be easily and readily opened for removal of ingesta before digestion and absorption, as is possible with a cow's rumen.

Stomach lavage and subsequent siphoning off is possible. Treatment commonly recommended for bovine plant toxicity, apart from laparotomy, of dosing with copious strong boiled tea (tannin) requires intranasal stomach tubing in the horse followed by large amounts of liquid paraffin *after* attempts at gastric lavage. The veterinary surgeon will decide if toxin absorptive material such as charcoal and/or kaolin should be administered likewise

Supportive warmth, cardio-respiratory stimulants and central nervous system sedation may be necessary under veterinary advice, as well as neurogenic antidotes where relevant. There are few first-aid procedures available to an owner.

PLANT POISONS

A distinction can be drawn between

- recently (within the past 300 years) imported garden varieties, which equine evolution has not yet responded to!

- native flora which evolved and survived on land indigenous to horses, and to breeds within more local areas such as

  - mountain, moorland and heathland
  - fells and dales
  - downland
  - grassland

It has been argued that horses in their native environment were 'aware' of dangerous herbage; possibly an inherited awareness of

- bitterness or other taste factors
- repellent odour
- unpleasant muzzle and mouth sensation

acting as protective stimuli through the relevant sensory cranial nerves.

It could be argued that the plants 'used' these sensory outputs to protect their own species! Plants as 'rooted' living objects do not and cannot move to attack horses but, more importantly, are unable to 'run away' from 'predation' by them!

However, in all areas where they grew

- yew, an ubiquitous evergreen, was not unpalatable
- bracken, a more restricted partial evergreen, likewise

These are exceptions to the rule of indigenous plants.

The 'foreign' plants were not only evergreens and so colour attractive, but they were

- new, and therefore 'interesting'
- often tantalising by being within reach over the fence
- perhaps so differently unappetising not to fully dissuade cropping, but
- toxic in most cases to a variable degree

Despite nature's balancing acts for the protection of horse and plant, man, for obvious reasons had to assist with the

- manual removal of hedgerow toxic plants
- manual and chemical removal of herbage toxic plants
- chemical general weed eradication to maximise 'output' of herbage. As some of these weeds were also toxic, these farming activities minimised if not entirely eradicated the problem
- environmentally questionable destruction of hedgerows for cereal cropping – the advantage being that this also coincidentally removed many hazards of toxicity when rotation returned to hay cropping and, later, to grazing

Improved pastures require good swards for profitable grazing and for conserved crops. Apart from the deficits associated with 'narrow' (only one or two seed varieties used) seed mixtures such feedstuffs are usually toxic weed free. Ragwort is an occasional exception as it is resistant to herbicides; the seeds are readily dispensed and the plant emerges into flower in but a few days.

Permanent grass and its crops are seen as the ideal horse nutrient except that weed control is often less than satisfactory, especially regarding the ragworts. The crops 'taken' often include this toxic contaminant which loses its off-putting taste, especially in hay.

Meadowland and 'old' pastures

By definition such grazing is not that of 'improved pastures'. Drainage does improve its nutritional *quantity* per hectare, and by altering the soil structure to the disadvantage of coarse grasses and reeds gives an advantage to *more nutritious* species.

Where selective weedkillers and fertiliser top dressings have *not* been used, there is the likelihood of the survival of a wider range of grass varieties, as well as the maintenance of

- herbs, rich in trace elements
- wild flowers

Some of these however may be toxic at least seasonally.

Conservation of such meadow grass (meadow hay) has the same problems as other pasture crops, where there is

- no destruction of the toxic material, but
- destruction of the unpalatibility

The hedgerows (older and more 'natural') are more likely to have potentially poisonous plants than improved grazings. The most toxic should be known and are usually recognisable and easily removable manually. Many are geographically important, not present countrywide.

Grazing animals have 'lived' alongside these hazards for centuries. The safety factors are

- there is usually plenty of grass, quantitively at least
- the toxic plants are relatively few
  - except for seasonal crops of buttercups, daisies, etc., which are of limited toxicity
- most are extremely unpalatable

Where taste, smell and texture remain and continue to stimulate protective reflexes they must not be considered as absolute; they can be overridden by the higher brain centres of hunger induced by

- shortage of grass because of
  - overstocking and
  - dryness-restricted regrowth
    (in the UK drought is a rare single cause of severe grass deficiency, in terms of bulk at least)

- temporary obstruction to grazing – heavy snow, but a visible and accessible hedgerow!
- delayed spring grass growth in the presence of colour-attractive and growing hedgerow plants

The hunger encourages

- instinctive browsing (and barking)
- overcoming of distaste
- curiosity and opportunity
  - the green (shrubs) on the other side of the fence
  - the windfalls of fruit, nut and broken-off twigs with leaves
  - dumped cuttings
  - a newly opened ditch exposing roots and tubers which are often not as distasteful as the green plant

Poisonous plants can be catalogued according to the poisonous or toxic ingredients identifiable in them. These biotoxins are known as **active principals (AP)**; some of these plants are intrinsically capable of manufacturing their AP from normally absorbed minerals and trace elements under the influence of sunlight on their leaves' chlorophyll. Why they should inherit this ability is open to conjecture. The AP may be found in all parts, or selectively stored in a tuber, a stem, a leaf or a fruit (seed), throughout the plant's life, often more so at different times of the year.

Some plants only grow in certain soil structures, which are geographically restricted. Other plants can concentrate trace elements to a level which is injurious to the grazing animal but not to themselves. Selenium is the best example but this is rare in the UK. There are also plants, especially under the influence of abnormal, usually artificial conditions, which concentrate organic salts to a dangerous level; nitrate is a good example as are oxalates. Such AP can be described as extrinsic. The majority of poisonous plants, however, contain intrinsic AP. There is often more than one factor present. Analysing and determining the presence of AP is not difficult; deciding which is the prime factor is. The signs of the subsequent illness may be more diagnostic. It is also possible that the *ultimate AP is not yet scientifically known*. Most of them are alkaloids and glycosides which have numerous subgroups.

Some of these AP have medicinal properties. Although these were isolated only in the last 150 years the plant may well have been 'known' as a therapeutic herbal for much longer, for example, the foxglove and its AP digitalis.

The most important, in terms of toxicity, are the

- alkaloids
- cyanogenic and cardiac glycocides
- tannins
- photodynamic substances

Some 4,000 alkaloids have been identified and these are present in less than 10% of all plants, which make up 40% of all 'families'. The levels vary. Most mimic or block cholinergic transmitters and thereby cause parasympathetic upsets.

Plants most likely to cause immediate poisoning are

Yew

Cherry laurel

Linseed

Potato tubers (green)

Hemlock

Water dropwort

Buttercup (a local irritant)

Plants more ***likely to cause delayed poisoning*** are

Ragwort	– there is often no evidence of initial intake but usually of repetitive consumption, as from hay
Photosensitising Plants	– 1–2 weeks, and then only if in bright sunlight
Yew	– some situations

Systemic Clinical Signs of Poisoning

A series of charts on pages 378–381 list plants known to be poisonous and the most likely to be dangerous to horses. The AP are identified, and where appropriate, the main target system.

It must be assumed that many horses do consume toxic plants at some time, become mildly ill, which is missed or blamed on something else, or become sub-clinically affected. It is a matter of

- quality (toxicity)
- quantity

of the plant consumed

Key

Dr – diarrhoea; **C** – constipation; **GI** – gastro-intestinal (colic); **P** – photosensitisation; **CNS** – central nervous system derangement; **D** – found dead

	Dr	C	GI	P	CNS	D
Acorns		*	*			
Bog Ashfodel				*		
Box	*		*			
Foxglove						*
Hemlock	*		*		*	
Horsetail					*	
Laburnum					*	
Laurel (cherry)						*
Linseed	*	*	*			*
Nightshade					*	
Oak (young leaves)		*		*		
Oak (old leaves)				*	*	
Potato tubers	*		*		*	
Rye Grass	*		*	*	**	
Ragwort		*	*	*	*	
Rhododendron	*		*		*	
St John's Wort				*		
Water dropwort	*		*		*	*
Wild arum	*		*			
Yew						*

Whilst an animal's appetite for a particular substance, subsequent craving and access to that plant will influence the incidence and, to some extent the severity of any one toxicity the substance's level of toxicty, seasonal and/or distribution within the plant, available quantity and number of plants will affect the outcome.

These signs vary little, AP to AP (plant to plant). There is an overall similar pathogenesis involved whereby the

- gastro-enteric are primarily involved
- cardio-vascular and
- nervous systems

and, where secondary changes are allowed to occur, in time the

- hepatic/renal and
- encephalic sytems

are, usually lethally, involved.

Yew, therefore, can cause sudden death from direct heart

failure. Ragwort in slow cumulative fashion must first slowly overwhelm the liver from which metabolites lethally affect the brain and the kidney.

In the absence of an ability to vomit, poisoned horses which survive long enough will show

- salivation
- colic – severe
- diarrhoea – profuse

and directly or indirectly

- behavioural changes
- ataxia and weakness
- convulsions and death

The most important causes of plant poisoning are Ragwort, Bracken, Buttercups, Oak and Acorns, Water dropwort, Hemlock, Yew, Linseed and Cherry laurel.

Ragwort Poisoning – pyrrolizidine alkaloidal poisoning – seneciosis

The senecio genera of plants is one of the largest. Not all species are poisonous but the 'common ragwort', *Senecio jacobea*, and 'groundsel', *S. vulgaris*, are. The less common are the March and Oxford Ragworts. There are several significant features of ragwort. It is

- widespread
- a high seed producer, so 'spreads' rapidly
- very common on roadside verges and unattended grass-lands
- very drought resistant
- not very susceptible to weedkillers
- deep rooted: these must be *dug up and burned, cutting down is not the answer*
- unpalatable, but is often the only 'greenstuff' available in dry weather *and in overstocked pasture*
- the most common poison 'cut, carried and conserved' as in hay, where it is palatable, or at least unnoticed, but still toxic
- not usually a primary gastro-intestinal poison but when it is, as from 'necessary' eating of young green plants in

Common ragwort.

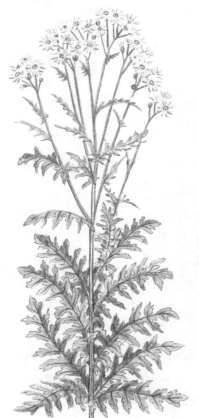

Height: 30–120cm (1–4ft) Ragwort has distinctive deeply cut leaves, and tall clusters of bright yellow flowers which appear (in the northern hemisphere) from June to October. Ragwort roots are tenacious, making the plant difficult to eradicate. Seeds are airborne, so spread easily.

In its early stages of growth, or if it has been grazed, ragwort appears in a rosette form.

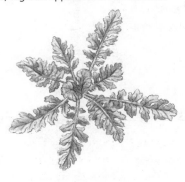

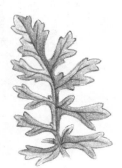

typical leaf

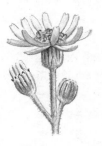

ragwort flower-head

Poisonous Wild Plants

Occurence	Plant	Poisonous Parts	Active Principal	Clinical Signs/System Affected
Very rare but lethal	**Deadly Nightshade** Woodland, scrubland, now uncommon	All, especially berries	Glyco-alkaloids, e.g. atropine and scopolamine	Dilated pupils, and inflamed mucous membranes of mouth and nose. Excited, inco-ordinated, not quickly lethal. CNS
Very rare	**Hemlock** Damp woodland, musty smell is very off-putting	All	Coniine, in hay	Paralysis, convulsions and asphyxia. CNS
	Horse Tails Contaminant of pastures and arable crops especially in damp conditions: widespread, gets into hay and straw, main source of toxicity	All, especially stem and leaf	Irritant salicylates, thiaminase (not destroyed in hay)	Signs of vitamin B_1 deficiency CNS. Mild colic with diarrhoea. GI. Delayed loss of condition in milder cases
	Linseed (seed of flax) Sold for feed supplement as seed or in prepared oil-seed cake or meal	–	Cyanogenic glyco-cides. Hydrocyanic acid liberated when cold water added or seed consumed whole	Interference with oxygen transport and so anoxia of CNS preceded by salivation, staggering, somnolence, gasping, convulsions and death
Common in dry years	**Oak (the tree)**	Young leaves in spring, acorns in Autumn	Tannins	Seasonal incidence
Most common cause of poisoning	**Ragwort** Widespread, waste land, verges, pasture		Pyrrolizidine alkaloids (not destroyed by curing or drying)	Acute cases rare, chronic secondary morbidity of liver and brain very common. CNS

Poisonous Wild Plants cont.

Occurence	Plant	Poisonous Parts	Active Principal	Clinical Signs/System Affected
Common	**St John's Wort**	Whole plant	Red fluorescent pigment 'hypericine', a derivative of naphthodianthrone. Some loss of toxicity on drying	Photosensitisation: permanent. Occasional debility, ataxia and coma. Secondary infection of skin lesions
Rare	**Wild Arum** Shady hedge banks, woodland	Whole plant	Irritant juice, a saponin, aronine	Reputedly causes abortion in mares and oral inflammation. 'Constipation' then scouring if large amounts consumed
Very common	**Woody Nightshade** Waste land and coastal shingle or in woods and hedges – 'a rambler'	Whole plant	Solanine, an alkaloidal glycocide	Salivation, colic, diarrhoea; inco-ordination. GI
Very very very uncommon	Foxglove Woods, heaths and hillsides. Early dominant plant in clearings	Whole plant	Cardiac glycocides, unaffected by drying	Diarrhoea, colic, irregular pulse: dullness, frequent urination. Tremors and convulsions. CNS

Potentially Poisonous Cultivated Plants

Plant	Occurence	Poisonous Parts	Active Principal	Clinical Signs/System Affected
Box	Rare to occasional	All	Alkaloids	Access to garden path bordered by box hedge. Colic, diarrhoea, inco-ordination, convulsions, coma and death. Gastro-intestinal (GI), CNS
Laburnum	Very rare	All, but particularly bark and seeds	Alkaloid (cystisine)	Accidental mixing of seeds and pods with dropped feed corn then fed, or when tied too close to a fence or to the tree itself. Ataxia, muscle tremors, colic, coma and death. CNS
Laurel (Cherry)	Very rare	Seed kernels especially	Cyanogenetic glyco-cide and amygdaline yield hydrocyanic acid (almond smell)	Inactivation of respiratory cell enzymes – oxygen starvation of the CNS. Death
Potato	Occasional	Green tubers and sproutings, especially if also infected with potato blight fungus (rotting tubers)	Solanines Alkaloids	Wrongly added to feed, or accidental access. Nervous signs, inco-ordination, coma, CNS, preceded by loss of appetite, salivation, constipation then diarrhoea. Mild colic, hyper-purgation
Rhododendron In woodlands as well as gardens	Very occasional	Leaves, flowers pollen and nectar	Diterpenoids – rhodatoxin, andromedotoxin (a glycocide)	Salivation, colic diarrhoea, perhaps constipation, trembling, difficult breathing recumbency. GI, CNS
Yew	Common	All parts except fleshy fruit. Most toxic in winter. Usually a single feed but repeated small intakes have been incriminated	Taxin a compound alkaloid mixture of volatile oils. Not negated by drying	Sudden death after access to windblown leaves and twigs. Less acute gives CNS signs – rapid, weak pulse, excitability, stupor and death

Poisonous Plants Found in Agriculture

Occurence	Plant	Poisonous Parts	Active Principal	Clinical Signs/System Affected
Rare	**Perennial Rye Grass** Hot dry weather with much dead plant material which becomes infected with fungi whose endotoxin is pathogenic	Leaf and stem	Neuro-toxin	CNS. 'Rye grass staggers', head and shoulder tremors. Ataxic, high stepping, collapse. Tetanic spasms
Rare	**Sweet Vernal Grass** A fungus is involved which parasitises in the hay. The ultimate toxin is an anticoagulant	Leaf and stem	Coumarin	'Sweet clover disease', acute, early death from internal haemorrhage
Variable	**Rye and other cereal grasses** The fungus is Ergot	Seed or corn grazed grasses leaf, stem and flower	Alkaloids and nitrogenous compounds 'Ergotamine' etc.	'Ergot of Rye' disease, mainly nowadays in wheat but also in pasture grasses. Vascular effect is called Ergotism

some quantity, there is an acute disease

Signs

- nervous excitement – violence
- anorexia
- rapid pulse and respiration
- colic
- weakness
- possible jaundice
- death in days or even weeks

Ragwort poisoning is most frequently a result of *eating contaminated hay over a period of time* to produce a chronic state – usually the only clue is **liver damage**, and then often sub-clinical and not especially diagnostic when overt. This damage is usually irreversible. Hepatic cirrhosis shows on autopsy.

The signs may be delayed for weeks to months after or during consumption

- possibly jaundice
- weight loss
- haematuria
- diarrhoea
- depressed appetite
- photosensitisation
- associated with an elevation of those metabolites (e.g. ammonia) which produce **CNS dysfunction**. Neurologic signs develop as an *acute condition*, an hepato encephalopathy, with
  - unawareness of surroundings
  - head pressing and yawning
  - lurching aimlessly – 'sleepy stagger'
  - diarrhoea
  - rapid weight loss
  - oedema

There is no cure. Beware hay bought cheap! Keep good watch and care in your own fields. In the UK ragwort is technically an illegal weed.

Bracken

(usually in mountain and moorland environments)

Bracken is the most common British fern. The AP is thiaminase, causing thiamine (vitamin B1) deficiency.

The green fronds are palatable and toxic when growing, and in bedding if cut when fronds were green and active.

Toxicity (**bracken staggers**) results from consuming small quantities each day over several weeks, as with bedding sources. Even then, signs often don't appear for up to 60 days afterwards. Sudden access to unchecked eating of the growing plant results in a sooner, more active illness.

The dis-ease in horses is markedly different from that in cows, where rumen digestion alters the ultimate metabolism. In the horse, the signs are

- muscular tremors
- inco-ordination
- staggering
- awkward stance, back arched
- head up and back – opisthotonos
- spasms
- recumbrancy
- coma
- death from heart failure

Responds to vitamin B1 at an early stage, injectable and oral; to compensate for the natural material destroyed by the action of the AP thiaminase.

Buttercups

Very acrid taste: selective grazing safety may be overcome by grass shortage and preponderance of the flower in grassland. It is now accepted that it is the pollen which contains the AP; the pollen 'dust' is tasteless or, at least not unpalatable, and is blown onto the surrounding edible grazing. The more plants, the more and more widely available the toxin.

Irritates mucosae of the mouth; this erythmea and swelling blocks outlet of parotid salivary glands which swell visibly (false mumps) from back pressure. Absence from plant by overnight stabling usually long enough to resolve condition.

Signs

- salivation
- parotid gland swellings
- inflamed mouth

- colic – rare
- inco-ordination – rare

Buttercups are **not** poisonous in hay; the AP becomes **inert**: there is no change in palatability.

Oak and Acorns

The common oak tree Quercus robur (AP is tannic acid)
- spring
  - young leaves; signs are delayed for several days after consumption (windy weather)

- autumn
  - old leaves, and acorns. Ripe normal fallen acorns in limited amounts throughout autumn weeks may cause mild colic and diarrhoea with inappetence. Gale-blown ripe, and especially unripe, nuts will offer large quantities of toxic material

Search fields with nearby oak trees especially if weather is very windy.

Signs
- dullness
- inappetence
- watery eyes, nose and mouth
- polyuria dark
- colic, often violent
- 'constipation' quickly followed by intense diarrhoea including blood
- death in convulsion

Water Dropwort

Grows in ditch banks, in wet areas especially. The roots are the most toxic **but** do not have distasteful characteristics as do the growing plant. Poisoning is most likely when a ditch is re-dug, so exposing the roots. About 1gm per kg of horse weight is toxic, AP is oenanthotoxin.

Signs
- salivation
- dilated pupils
- convulsions
- death quickly

Hemlock

AP, the alkaline coniine, does not survive in hay. Common on banks of streams, hedgerows, field borders. Smells of mice when crushed; the smell (and taste) limits likelihood of being eaten unless grass is very short. Possibly addictive. 1kg (2lb) of leaves will kill a horse. Nicotine action, first stimulates then depresses the autonomic ganglia – paralyses motor nerve endings.

Signs
- dilated pupils
- weakness
- staggering to loss of consciousness
- breathing paralysed
- death

Yew

AP is taxine, 2gm per kg of horse weight of the plant is toxic. Usually grown (in olden days, when the wood was used for bows) in churchyards. Drying does not lessen toxicity, which is greatest in leaves. Taxine is a heart poison. The heart **first** slows before **quickly** stopping. Other smooth muscles may also be depressed.

Signs
- sudden death – even whilst eating, but can be longer with
- trembling, dyspnoea, collapse, death

Linseed

Linseed is the product of the flax plant. It contains

- large quantities of relatively indigestible mucilage which is very water-absorbable as when cooked. This makes a non-irritant lubricating laxative. As such it is fed, for example with boiled barley
- high levels of phosphorus and vitamin B complex
- an enzyme, which when linseed is cold soaked, liberates hydrocyanic acid from a glucocide in the plant. This prussic acid is poisonous. Boiling destroys the enzyme: the safest way, or prolonged (12 hours) cold soaking, allows the hydrocyanic acid time to evaporate

Signs (of toxicity – develop quickly)
- excitement

- salivation
- dilated pupils
- laboured breathing
- convulsion
- coma
- death within one hour

There is a treatment by intravenous injection if seen soon enough by the veterinary surgeon.

Cherry Laurel

Of the rose family. Fruit stones or kernels of plum, cherry, peach, apricot and almond contain cyanogenic glycocide. The leaves of cherry laurel also do, and are thus a potential hazard because of the hydrocyanide. (See Linseed above)

OTHER SOURCES OF VEGETATIVE POISONOUS/TOXIC SUBSTANCES

Mycotoxicosis

When cereal crops are harvested, but because of bad weather are left over-long in the field and/or subsequently threshed and stored with higher than safe water content and/or in damp environments, there is a high risk of fungal mould development in the cereal. The grain (seed) stored as a feedstuff, whether whole or ground, is the most common site of mould growth. The generic name for the toxic substance in this mould is **aflatoxin**, which is a metabolite of the secondary metabolism of three main fungi **aspergillus**, **penicillium** (more important in poultry and pig feeds), and **fusarium**.

The toxin, once produced, is comparatively resistant to environmental factors such as heat, dryness, and pH variations. On absorption from the digestive tract it is not immunogenic, so there is no antibody formation response by the consuming animal. Conversely, the toxic effect is ultimately that of immuno-suppression in some toxin species.

Aflatoxicosis is primarily an acute toxicity which has a predilection for the liver. It is also carcinogenic. Acute toxicity is rare from contaminated feed stores which are usually obviously mouldy in parts, at least, and so unfit for use. Mistakes can arise, however, when there is failure to be aware and intentional or otherwise amateurish attempts

to mix samples and so dilute the risk. (Under strict commercial safeguards such dilution is permissible.)

Sub-acute toxicity is more common especially in young stock.

Signs

- ataxia
- jaundice
- dermatitis
- increased heart rate
- oedema
- hyper-production of oestrogen in mares (the fusarium species)
- greater susceptibility to infection and parasitism, these probably account for the reduced growth rate and unthriftiness which are significant .

Diagnosis

- absence of other causes of acute signs
- circumstantial evidence of suspected contaminated grain
- laboratory tests in these feeds

There is little excuse for these mycotoxicoses in horses; they are usually due to

- poor storage
- cheap cereals purchased
- bad horsemastership

There are EU regulations restricting the amount of permitted aflatoxin in any feed.

Ergot Toxicity

Ergot is the 'seed' or sclerotia of a fungus **claviceps purpurea** which parasitises various wild grasses and cereal grasses such as barley, rye and wheat. It attacks the flower head to replace the ovary, where it develops as a dark, tubular, slightly bent structure of 2–4cm (0.787"–1.575") length protruding from the flower head. No plant seed forms. Poisoning is from grazing affected pastures or eating contaminated grain.

Acute and chronic forms are seen, chronic being the most common.

In early Christian times the disease in man was called St Anthony's Fire, and was thought to signify a visitation from God. More recently it was thought to have been implicated in 'the witches of Salem'.

- toxic factors
    - alkaloids and other nitrogenous compounds, ergotamine and ergometrine
- morbidity – these damage the capillary lining and cause thrombosis with regional anoxia leading to dry gangrene
- region
    - peripheral areas – ears, tail, feet

Signs

- acute: not recorded in horses
- chronic
    - stiffness
    - lameness
    - peripheral coldness
    - coronary area dry gangrene, hoof separation
    - late abortion in mares

No treatment – if source removed, recovery usually follows.

CHEMICAL SUBSTANCES

In the UK there are strict COSSH and Health and Safety at Work regulations regarding the use, storage and disposal of these but the private/amateur horse owner is not always 'in the picture'. Disposal of unused and empty containers in line with official rules must be met. The merchant, chemist or veterinary surgeon who supplied them in the first instance will advise and be prepared to effect correct disposal for the 'small' owner.

Regulations require neighbours not to allow wind drift and water-carried waste to pollute your premises or land (especially where crops of any description are growing and/or being grazed) or stream water through your land. Good neighbourliness requires that you be advised if wind drift is likely to occur on any occasion, so that horses can be removed – as a precaution.

On your own premises, know or be advised how to use

- pesticides and insecticides
- herbicides
- preservatives

- actual risk
- possible risk. Direct and indirect
- duration of no access afterwards to
    - grazing
    - stables and fencing

Make certain you clearly understand

- dilution factors
- dosage rates
- method of administration
- contra indications of

Conform to correct procedures to protect yourself and employees, and be certain what substances you must not

- allow to enter River Authority drainage, directly or indirectly
- dispose of through local authority main drainage and or domestic refuse collection
- burn in the open

Contractors employed to carry out application of the numerous pesticides must pass an examination of competence and carry a certificate to that fact. Suppliers of chemicals must draw the purchaser's attention to the correct procedures and safety warnings, just as veterinary drug labels must display 'Warnings and Contra-indications' with regard to the use both in animals and to the user.

The following are potentially hazardous to horses, whether ingested, injected or applied especially if in excess, naturally or accidentally, or wrongly used

- drugs
    - topical
    - parenteral
    - oral
- herbicides
    - selective
    - defoliant
- pesticides
    - insecticides
    - anthelmintics
    - fungicides
        - vegetation

- woodwork etc.
- rodenticides
- molluscicides
- fertilisers
  - direct
  - indirect on herbage
  - long term residues
    - on site
    - via drainage
- geographically determined mineral levels in soil
  - nutritional errors regarding minerals and vitamins
- industrial contaminants
  - smelting fall out
  - effluents
- disinfectants
- detergents
- paint strippers
- insulating materials

Many compounds such as drugs, herbicides and pesticides have been shown to be also dangerous as

- direct poisons
- delayed poisons, usually affecting the CNS
- indirect in as much as they might be carcinogenic etc. especially to humans

Even the widely used Derris powder has been withdrawn. BHC, once seen as relatively harmless as an anti-skin parasite wash is no longer permitted in dog shampoo and is not 'data sheeted' for horse mange therapy. It is a chlorinated hydrocarbon.

Organo-phosphorous compounds used in sheep dips are now seen as potentially indirect poisons to the handler.

Fungicides on woodwork etc. are controlled. Many of those previously used in agricultural, horticultural and veterinary work for pesticides, weeds and drugs are now banned – for example arsenic, cyanide, copper, mercury and nitrate/nitrite inorganic compounds. Some still remain in private (amateur) hands.

ELEMENTAL AND SYNTHETIC CHEMICALS

The controversial use of the terms 'toxic' and 'poisonous' becomes clearer when the misuses of nutrients such as minerals, trace elements and vitamins are considered. As it has been remarked, a deficiency of one or the other of these substances at tissue level can cause dis-ease of these tissues and of the related body systems.

In some cases there is a deficiency in the diet, a reduced availability through chemical interaction in the digesta or an interference with their utilisation in the metabolic processes. There is the example of the effect of too much anti-enzyme, thiaminase, as found in some plants (see earlier), which destroys the essential vitamin B1, thiamine.

It is often forgotten that an excess of these essential nutrients can also be detrimental: their effects become toxic. The resultant dis-ease is called **intoxication**, whereby the body's use and tolerance of them is overwhelmed. In contrast, a poisonous substance is not normally one that is nutritionally required even at a lower dosage intake.

The relatively simple chemical formulation of inorganic minerals and trace elements differs markedly from that of organic biochemicals such as vitamins, but there is a close biological relationship between vitamins and trace elements, which act as co-enzymes.

Deficiencies of such minor as well as major mineral elements are important in their own right and in the efficiency of vitamin activity.

Although the horsemaster is rarely responsible for variations in the mineral/vitamin level of his home grown, and less in his bought in material, several factors are important

- imperfectly understood effects of fertiliser applications especially when crops specifically cultivated for dairy cows are used to feed horses. Young stock are particularly affected, liming with consequent excess molybdenum uptake and related reduction in clovers and trace elements
- over-zealous horse owners who overdose with mineral/trace elements and/or vitamin supplements

Dietary factors can affect the toxicity of normal levels of minerals

- ascorbic acid, amino acids and vitamin D all may enhance absorption and hence the toxicity of certain minerals
- phytate and oxalate can interfere with absorption of calcium which in turn can lead to calcium phosphorus imbalances

Intoxication by basic elements or their salts is therefore

related to

- excess to normal requirements of essential (for living)
  - major minerals
  - minor minerals (trace elements)
- excess of minerals which, though non-essential may be found in living tissues up to a safe level without detriment

Such excesses can be caused by

- above normal levels in the soil and therefore in the feedstuff
  - geographical peculiarity
  - local industrial contamination
  - fertiliser effect
    - present
    - residual and possibly cumulative
- accidentally too much in the diet from
  - incorrect use of supplements
  - contamination by the wrong supplement
  - addition of unwanted elements
  - access to other species of feedstuffs

It should be appreciated that many potentially hazardous minerals are in 'normal' feedstuffs as a reflection of their presence in the soil, whose produce is judged by the results of feeding it. Supplementation (and of vitamins) is usually made in the light of experience of the deficits in the animal's health known to be due to nutritional mineral imbalances and vitamin, seasonal deficiencies.

MINERAL/TRACE ELEMENT INTOXICATION

Aluminium

One of the few non-essential minerals, if consumed in excess through certain types of 'soil eating' or eating feedstuffs contaminated with such soil, will interfere with phosphorus absorption, a major mineral necessity.

Copper

A trace element, which plays a vital role in many enzyme actions, is said to be sub-optimal in most soils and so also in the crops. In cattle this becomes important in 'teart' pastures (those where the soil is high in molybdenum which 'locks up' the copper). Horses seem less susceptible. Copper intoxication is not common and, again, horses seem to contend with excess amounts.

The risk of dangerous excess copper comes from copper-containing fungicides as used in orchards, accidentally contaminating feedstuffs; pig and poultry supplemented feeds carried in horse feed bags or accidentally misfed; and from illegal contamination from smelting works.

There is some recent evidence that high performance horses require more than recommended normal levels of copper. Enhanced supplements are on the market, so extra care is required if two or more supplements are used.

Excess will lead conversely to reduced performance.

The signs of copper intoxication are not clear and cases of even chronic dis-ease are rare, unlike in sheep, where coffee coloured urine, bloody nasal discharge and jaundice are characteristic, along with anaemic weakness.

Fluorine

An essential constituent of bones and teeth. Long-term grazing on pasture (and hay from it) contaminated from 'fall out' from brick work smoke is a source of intoxication, especially in young stock, particularly cattle. In the UK Health and Safety regulations have curtailed this risk.

The source of phosphorous supplements determines its fluorine content but feed compounders and supplement manufacturers are well aware of this risk. Raw rock phosphate is the culprit. Unthriftiness and later lameness are signs. Dental scarring occurs in horses up to four years old.

Iodine and Iron

These rarely require feed supplementation but keen owners may see a need to do so based on human and porcine nutrition findings. An excess of either is most likely to be detrimental through a supplemented mare feed available to foals.

There is evidence of iodine deficiency and associated ineffective thyroid activity in foals.

Selenium

An essential micro (trace) element. Intoxication can be caused by

- excessive supplementation

- excessive uptake by certain plants, called indicators, growing in selenium-rich soils. Parts of Ireland are so recognised. Horses rarely have the opportunity to eat such plants so the risk in Britain is minimal
- injections of selenium as in suggested control of rhabdomyolysis must be used with care

Acute dis-ease
- respiratory distress
- diarrhoea
- death

Sub-acute or chronic – alkali disease –
- emaciation
- lameness – damage to the coronary band
- hoof sloughing
- loss of mane and tail hair

VITAMIN INTOXICATION

There have been no substantiated records of management overdosage of vitamins, and there is no vegetation used in horse feeds known to result in hypervitaminosis. A deficiency, especially of the fat-soluble vitamins A, D and E is possible and relates to the rations fed and to the duration of the storage of conserved fodder and grain, as well as to the individual plants involved.

Imbalances of vitamin intake can interfere with mineral metabolism. Excessive use of supplementary vitamin D can cause calcium disturbance in foals. Prolonged exposure of fat soluble vitamins, especially those which have not been commercially protected, can lead to oxidative reduction in their potency. This may lead to an interference with the digestion and metabolism of other vitamins especially of E.

SOME TOXIC AGENTS IN SIMPLE OR COMPOUND INORGANIC FORM AS DISTINCT FROM NUTRITIVE MINERALS

Arsenic

An active metalloid element present in the soil. In its soluble salt form it is absorbed by plants, usually at low parts per million.

It is concentrated by certain industries, for example ore smelting but waste, aerial or liquid, is rigorously controlled. It is synthesised in formulations used as drugs, pesticides, selective weedkillers, and particularly as lead arsenate herbage sprays (which can be absorbed through the sprayer's skin).

This made lawn mowings a danger not only in the untreated
- heated 'dumps' which, if consumed by horses, often caused fermentative colic, or as
- cold, spreadout, recently cut mowings which if eaten suddenly and copiously was a recipe for laminitis, but also
- if it is from recently 'sprayed' lawns then arsenic poisoning is possible as an additional hazard

Lethal doses are 1–25mg per kg of horse weight.

Signs
(as arsenic poisoning)
- colic – acute abdominal crisis type
- diarrhoea, often bloody
- weakness
- inco-ordination
- followed by collapse and death from myocardial degeneration

Mercury

In its synthetic organic form was used as an anti-fungal dressing of subsequent seed corn. Mistakes have been made whereby the corn is used in feedstuff. Pigs have been the usual victim mainly because the seed was often wheat, which is not a cereal commonly used as a 'straight' for horse feeding. Accidental access to 'dressed' stored seed wheat is a possibility.

Red mercurial blisters 'licked off' by the horse have been a source of poisoning.

Signs
Are severe, 'corrosive' gastro-enteric and later CNS toxicity. There is no treatment that can be given in time to horses. The poison is absorbed and becomes lethal quickly after signs appear.

A chronic form has been described as a straight central nervous system dis-ease. (The Mad Hatter of *Alice in Wonderland* was so affected from the mercury used in preserving the fur of top-hat manufacturing.)

Sodium Chlorate

A non-selective weedkiller. Through mis-identification from wrong marking and storing it has been mixed in feed such as bran, instead of Epsom salts. It is so unappetising that horses refuse it, but even a mouthful of a contaminated mash will severely irritate oral mucosae and the lips.

Mouth lavage with warm water and bicarbonate, 1.5litres (1 tbs/1 pint) confined to the lips and tongue will help clean and soothe. Do not squirt down the mouth. If, however, it has been swallowed in quantity, the conversion of haemoglobin to methaemoglobin occurs which, if not quickly treated, may lead to anoxia of the vital organs and death.

Lead

Average soil levels are 1.00mg/kg increasing in lead rich soil areas. It is an important industrial metal, poisonous to man and animals.

Toxicity arises from

- 'fall out' from lead rich ore smelting works and old dumps of smelted ore
- old lead paint – flaking off into feed, most common in young cattle with access to 'old doors'
- car batteries – breaking in field or pond
- putty, red lead, linoleum
- some lubricants – addictive taste to some horses
- old lead pipes and tanks (lead dissolves into drinking water) and subsequent water ingestion.

Signs

- acute merging into chronic or primarily chronic, then possibly 'flaring up' as a lethal acute phase
- peripheral motor nerve damage, with consequent
    - muscular weakness and paresis, staggering
    - bilateral laryngeal muscle weakness – 'roaring' – and aspiration pneumonia
- anorexia
- colic
- loss of weight

Veterinary treatment is possible if given soon enough or if the signs are mild, and confined to the neuro-muscular system.

Oxalates

An excess concentration of these salts is found in certain plants but is rare in the UK, or in plants dying from selective weedkiller application. Their presence in the upper digestive tract can interfere with calcium absorption. This imbalance in cases in the UK is so temporary as to be minimal in effect.

Organic Substances

In some situations horses will graze on treated pasture – before a safe period for reaccess – gain access to treated land and to stores.

In recent years the use of chemicals lethal to horses has been rigorously controlled, which has been emphasised several times in this chapter.

Herbicides

- selective weedkillers i.e. a field of grass or growing cereal crop can be treated without damage except to the weed element
- poisoning is unlikely to occur if correct procedures are followed and withdrawal times adhered to
- ragwort is one weed which is difficult to eradicate chemically

Pesticides

Those used in veterinary medicine are known as

- insecticides – against skin or ecto parasites – and by definition mean their application to the
    - skin for
        - direct effect on the 'insect'
        - indirect, after absorption and subsequent return to the insects' feeding habit via the blood
    - the systemic route by oral or parenteral administration
        - via the blood to the parasite

(The treatment to control internal parasites is by anthelmintic given orally or parentally. These are also synthetic organic compounds but none are in the same potentially dangerous category as insecticides.)

It is obvious that the risk of insecticidal toxicity is greater than plant pesticide sources in as much as the chemical is 'available' to the animal as well as to the 'pest'.

It is important to note that aerosol and fumigating anti-parasitics for buildings should not be applied to or allowed to contaminate animals eventually to be housed there. This mainly applies to sprays used in domestic flea control.

In other animal species dips, bands and tags do contain more dangerous ingredients and must not be used on horses unless they are data sheeted accordingly or 'cleared' by a veterinary surgeon. Likewise care must be taken not to augment their use with the same drug in a different formulation or with another insecticide of a different type.

It is impossible to list all the commercial preparations available. Your veterinary surgeon will advise or supply. It is also possible that in certain situations such as mange mite infestations the vet will prescribe from outside the data sheeted list.

Stable and livery-yard owners will already have the relevant Codes of Practice and Health and Safety directives. These are advised reading for anyone keeping horses and especially if they employ non-family help. (Health & Safety at work.) Insecticides may be toxic to horses (and other in contact animals) and the handlers. Care must be taken with the dosage and handling of the product.

Organo-Chlorides

These are no longer marketed, for example Dieldrin and Lindane. Left over (often concentrated with time) part used supplies are still to be found. They are insecticidal by interference with nervous system functioning. Poisoning through incorrect amounts of application or, more seriously, oral access, will present as central nervous system stimulation and convulsions in response to noise and light, then depression, coma and death. Some animals lie for long periods with persistent chewing action and salivation, and the temperature is very elevated.

Organo-Phosphates

These originally replaced chlorinated hydrocarbons and were used for both herbal and animal pests. They and the carbamate organic salt both inhibit activity in the insect of acetylcholinisterase whereby the neuro-transmitter acetylcholine in the autonomic ganglia accumulates to overstimulate to the point of paralysis of the target organs.

Different preparations have differing toxicity to animals varying from a few to hundreds of mg per kg. Label reference should be made if overdosage by application or accidental oral intake is suspected. The list changes year by year. Organo-phosphates may now be on the proscribed list. In the affected animal the nervous defects are

- excessive salivation and diarrhoea with colic and blood in faeces. Sweating, lacrimation, dyspnoea and contracted pupils are possible
- muscle twitching, stiffness, paresis and paralysis
- (if the particular drug can cross the blood–brain barrier) depression, broncho-constriction, coughing, oxygen interference, heart slowing and possible death. Immediate veterinary attention and the administration of atropine sulphate can often prove effective, along with special follow-up therapy

There is no indication and therefore no justifiable reason for using such organo-compounds on or in horses except under close veterinary supervision.

Weedkillers which may present a hazard through carelessness or stupidity are

- Bipyridylium agents
    - Paraquat
    - Diquat

These are extremely dangerous especially to man and to dogs. Once they 'hit the soil' they are inactivated; if sprayed onto static water and then drunk, poisoning will follow. The horse is *thought* not to be quite so susceptible, but mistaken feed addition will cause some morbidity, including

- oral and pharyngeal ulceration (salivation and swallowing difficulties)
- diarrhoea
- colic
- renal impairment
- pulmonary oedema and subsequent airway fibrosis

If suspected, even if not proven, get immediate veterinary help. There is no specific treatment.

Rodenticides

- ANTU – a thiourea derivative which fatally 'upsets' carbohydrate metabolism

- fluoroacetate – produces lethal lung dropsy (oedema)
- warfarin etc. – causes lethal internal haemorrhage usually in the pleural cavity

Toxicity is most likely to be from malicious attempts. Occasionally the carrier substance and the bait is inadvertently used in feed, or horses have access to it. Warfarin usually requires repeated daily intake for killing rats and mice, so accidental equine poisoning is rare, moreover the dose would need to be large. (It is also a therapeutic substance in horses as well as man.)

Signs include

- severe fasciculations of the muscles
- dilated pupils
- profuse sweating
- colic
- ataxia and paresis:
  - death in rodents

Poisoning by the warfarin family is susceptible to treatment, but poisoning by other rodenticides is not.

Metaldehyde Toxicity (slug killer)

This is more likely than rat poison toxicity. A 6% poison in 2.27kg (5lb) bran is recorded as killing 3 horses. 0.1mg per kg of horse weight has proved fatal.

Signs

- profuse sweating
- muscle fasciculations
- spasms
- inco-ordination
- heart and lung acceleration
- heart failure

There is no specific antidote.

Monensin Poisoning (rumensin supplement)

An antibiotic-like extract from certain bacterial growths. It is used as a growth stimulator in cattle, by stimulating propionic acid production in the rumen. The safety margin is said to be wide, but *horses are particularly sensitive*.

Usual toxicity results from access to cattle licks and field blocks. Affects the kidneys, liver and heart.

Signs

- anorexia, which is often the only sign, but in high intake there is
- ataxia and
- intermittent sweating, a fast heart and respiration
- colic
- reminiscent of azoturia (ER) signs, including blood enzyme changes but not creatinine kinase

Nitrates

In effect 'selected' weeds are stimulated to grow very rapidly. In the process their nitrate content increases and remains after the death of the plant. The dying and dead plant is appetising to stock given access too soon. It is the nitrate, not the weedkiller, which is toxic. It is converted to nitrite in the body and on absorption seriously interferes with cellular metabolism, especially the red blood cells.

Natural water sources such as springs, wells and streams may be abnormally high in nitrates. A chronic form of nitrate poisoning may result in anaemia, altered growth rates and reduced performance.

Phenol and Cresol

As in carbolic, tar, creosote and pitch, PCP wood preservative and some disinfectants by

- ingestion
- skin absorption

Signs

- inappetence
- thirst
- depression
- jaundice
- inco-ordination
- convulsions, coma, death

Treatment

Veterinary help is necessary in suspected cases.

Wood Shavings and Sawdust used as Bedding

A serious toxic effect can occur if the wood source has been 'preserved' with Pentachlorophenol. This fungicide is lethal in its own right but it is those contaminants found in commercial grades which seem to be most frequently implicated. **Dioxin** is the generic name. They not only cause severe skin irritation but are lethal following penetration of the skin and subsequent absorption.

Dioxin is thought to interfere with hormone activity but other features occur such as immune deficiencies. The dioxin can be isolated from the blood serum in acute cases. The common signs are wasting, with oedema, laminitis, colic and severe dermatitis with chronic skin thickening. The most severe cases have been recorded in the USA. *British commercial supplies of wood bedding must guarantee that treated wood is not used.*

There is some evidence that oils and gums from some woods may be an irritant to the skin and mucus membranes. Allergic lung conditions have been attributed to allergenic substances from milling or from dust when the material is too finely reduced. Badly stored and used shavings can be prone to fungal growth and resultant toxin production.

AUSTRALIA

In Australia more or less all the chemical and vegetable sources of poisoning reported in the UK are also seen as well as others, especially in the herbal side. There is a much wider range of mycotoxins particularly in farm animals, with fungal growths on stored feedstuffs.

Perhaps because of the climatic extremes and the wide-range grazing of many non-improved grasses native to the sub-continent there are seasonal occasions when these grasses wilt back to leave a decaying mat, which is ideal for fungal growth and toxin production.

Consideration is being given to these toxins as the cause of the neurotoxic signs previously attributed to the grasses themselves. Admittedly, there is still evidence for grass disease *per se*, especially when signs appear during the active growing phase. For example 'Phalaris staggers' is seen when Phalaris species are dominant in the pasture. 'Perennial Rye grass staggers' is seen in a dry autumn when the grass is hardly growing. The Rye Grass Staggers, as the name implies is a nervous syndrome – tremors and ataxia (stimulates an acute Wobbler disease) due to a primary vestibulo-cerebellar disorder. Given protection from falls, an affected horse 'self cures' when removed from an affected pasture. A liver damaging and photosensitising type of rye grass toxicity is associated with the growth of a parasitic fungus on the grass, Sporodesmium bakeri and its toxin phyllocrythrin.

Some of the toxic weeds not found in the UK are

Crotalaria (and USA)   Horsebrush
Tarweed (and USA)   Salvation Jane
Puncture vine (and USA)   Granksweed
Lantana   Jamia Sacahuiste

These are all capable of causing liver functioning deficits and secondary photosensitisation. Crotalaria species cause erosion of the gullet and the stomach lining. Affected animals cannot swallow; they die of starvation.

Cultivated toxic land weeds include
   Darling pea
   Romulea spp
   Poison vetch (selenium and a concentrating factor)
   Sneezeweed (and USA)
   Birdsvilla indigo
   Iceland poppy
   Gomphrena

All of the above cause neurologic signs.

USA

Forage Toxicity

Fescue poisoning – by substances present in the lush growth stages usually in the autumn rains following a dry summer and when other safer grasses are in short supply. In normal grazing conditions the unpalatability of fescue grass inhibits its consumption.

The toxicity is
- acute
  - high fever
  - accelerated heart rate
  - arched back
  - diarrhoea
- sub-acute
  - loss of condition
  - dull coat
  - 'cloudy' cornea

A particular feature of toxicity, especially when fescue grass is prominent in a pasture in early and late spring, is abortion in mares during the last two to three months.

Such at-risk animals should be removed during this period.

Prevention in all cases requires supplementary feeding if alternative grazing is not available.

'Alkali Disease'

Seen especially in the West, when plants have accumulated **selenium**, already high in the soil (up to 30mg per kg). Such soil is usually alkaline. If the final feed has greater than 5mg per kg then toxicity is likely.

The disease is seen in two types
- acute – rapid intake over a short period
  - 'blind staggers'
    - ataxia
    - depression
    - respiratory embarrassment with blue mucus membranes
    - blood-stained nasal froth
      - stumbling
      - prostration
      - death
- chronic – low level intake over a long period, 'Alkali disease'
  - loss of condition – emaciation
  - hair loss, especially that of the mane and tail (Bobtail disease)
  - cracks in hoof wall, laminar pain leading to
    - pronounced lameness
    - shedding of the hoof

Confirmation of cause is by analysis of hair or hoof parings.

Treatment
Remove from suspect pasture, feed a protein rich supplement (25%).

Prevention
Analyse feedstuffs and aim to feed at less than 2mg per kg of horse weight. Limit grazing per day on suspect pastures.

Locoweed Poisoning
(Milk vetch, legume family). (Seen also in Australia, Darling pea)

Some also accumulate selenium, but the main toxin is an alkaloid. The dangerous species grow in the high desert ranges of Western America and are most dangerous in the spring.

The plants are consumed over several weeks before the affected horses become 'loco' or mentally disturbed. Acute (usually only) form – nervous system morbidity
- excessive salivation
- 'roaring'
- aimless wandering
- staggering
- blind stumbling

If recognised early enough removal from the affected pastures may 'cure' the clinical signs but some form of neurologic deficit remains.

Sorghum Toxicity
(Milo, Sudangrass, Johnson grass)

Found in South West and Eastern America where such grasses are used as forage. The AP is hydrocyanic acid (HCN) and this is metabolised to cyanide. The level decreases with grass maturity and varies between the species mentioned, as does their palatability. Hay made from this is less toxic than the growing plant.

Cyanide affects the respiratory system and the resultant hypoxia causes CNS deficits
- acute
  - respiratory distress
  - flaring of the nostrils
  - staggering
  - involuntary urination and defecation
  - collapse
  - respiratory arrest
  - death (in a few hours)
- chronic ('Sorghum disease') following low level intakes
  - hind limb inco-ordination especially on turning and/or trotting – ataxia
  - bladder paralysis – cystitis
    - abortion in mares
    - deformed foals

Treatment
Even with treatment for bladder paralysis and associated cystitis the overall toxicity is incurable.

'Ryegrass and Dallis Grass Staggers'

A middle ear/cerebellar disease caused by a neurotoxin present in these grasses. The AP is thought to be a tremorgenic type; worldwide, most common in New Zealand. Occurs in late summer and the autumn when pastures are short-grazed and the grass is dry and stubble like. A functional transient neurologic disease. Onset is reasonably slow.

Signs

- tremors (possibly from a separate tremorgenic fungus in the mat)
- muscle spasm
- head nodding
- staggering gait, slow moving
- falling

Treatment

Change off the affected grazing, recovery is very slow but usually good.

Botulism

(see Chapter 20, DISEASE)

Yellow Star Thistle and Russian Knapweed
(Sunflower family)

These are problems in North California and elsewhere in the Pacific coast area. Found in the late summer and autumn in dry pastures in which the 'thistle' may be the only forage: it is palatable and possibly addictive. A neurotoxin (central nervous system) morbidity which permanently damages the cranial nerves involved in prehension and mastication, hence 'chewing' disease, the colloquial name for the toxicity.

Signs

- open mouth
- rigid facial muscles and eventual starvation (swallowing is not impaired)

There is no treatment. (Euthanasia on welfare grounds.)

Prevention

The weed can be eliminated by herbicidal application before seeding. Ploughing is similarly effective.

Hoary Alyssum
(Berteroa incana, of the mustard family)

Originally a European weed it is now found in the USA primarily in Minnesota but also in the northeast and other states in the midwest and in Canada.

Signs

In unexplained equine illness where the presenting signs are

- possible fever
- oedema of all four legs
- joint stiffness and reluctance to move
- short term diarrhoea
- pruritus (itchiness)
- premature foaling in pregnant mares

where alfalfa hay is being fed, Hoary alyssum toxicity should be suspected. The weed can be identified in the bales and manually removed. It grows in dry conditions particularly in gravelly and sandy soils. Where conditions decrease alfalfa growth the bales made may contain up to 50% of the weed; death is a possible consequence.

Early suspicion and removal of the weed is usually followed by recovery, although premature birth is still possible. Live births produce foals which are susceptible to indigenous infections.

Treatment

- flunixin meglumide
- remove suspect hay

Cantharadin Poisoning and Blister Beetle Consumption

The Blister Beetle is a member of the Meloidae family, especially the striped Epicauta species common in Southwest USA. An ingredient of the haemolymph, the body transport fluid, is Cantharadin, an intensely irritant substance. These beetles inhabit hay fields and become entrapped in alfalfa hay at harvest time.

Modern techniques of forage harvesting by which cutting and crimping are combined results in the immediate gathering of swarms of beetles, given no time to escape. They die during the 'making' stage and dry out to be compressed in massive numbers of isolated bales. The Cantharadin remains active.

Usually the morbidity of consumed beetles is relatively

high but the prevalence of illness in winter-fed horses is very variable, depending on chance access to contaminated bales.

Signs
Clinical signs vary with the numbers consumed
- high levels cause acute illness quickly leading to
  - profound shock
  - death
- lesser levels also cause acute signs of
  - general shock
  - gastro-intestinal irritation with colic and tenesmus (straining)
  - urinary tract irritation and kidney failure
  - synchronous diaphragmatic flutters (the 'thumps')
  - increased respiratory and cardiac rates
  - heart failure in three to six days
- low intake
  - less severe signs of the above
  - survival after seven days

Suspicion is based on
- absence of the other more usual causes of
  - colic
  - vague unwellness
  - urinary straining
  - feeding alfalfa hay (locally or imported from the southwest)
  - finding dead beetles
    - in the gut autopsy
    - in the hay
  - isolating Cantharadin from the urine

There is no specific treatment but
- general anti-shock therapy
- 'thumps' therapy of intravenous calcium borogluconate
- fluid replacement by intravenous route
- liquid paraffin by stomach tube

Plants that are Poisonous in Hay

Fiddleneck

Wild pea – Lathyrism, a sudden but usually transient paralysis of the larynx especially serious during exercise: lethal suffocation is possible.

Castor Bean

Yellow Star thistle

Ragwort

Oleander – cardiac dysfunction

Bracken fern

Horsetail

As advised for British horsemasters, poisoning is to be suspected if any otherwise unexplained illness of rapid or even abrupt onset is seen, especially when accompanied by
- CNS signs
- colic and diarrhoea
- sudden collapse
- quick death

Other poisonous plants of the hedgerow, ditch or garden (as dumped cuttings) are similar to those in Britain, plus: Choke cherry and Wild Black cherry (cyanide poisoning from the leaves of these trees which contain Prunasin) and Death Camas.

CHAPTER

31 SKIN DISEASES

INTRODUCTION

In general, skin disorders are spoken of as **dermatitis**, but since not all have a true inflammatory component, the more exact term used is **dermatoses**.

Usually, whenever damage to the skin occurs an inflammatory reaction follows: there is always a dermatitis. The degree, the acuteness, the varied secondary and/or associated skin/hair reaction, and the subsequent autolysis (self digestion) and immune responses, all make for many variations in the clinical appearance of the lesions. Conversely, many causative factors, other than direct physical trauma, can produce lesions which are sufficiently alike as to make differential clinical diagnosis difficult. Laboratory tests are frequently necessary to determine

- what specific treatment and management
- is it contagious?
- if a common factor is involved

The characteristic inflammatory changes always involve

- blood **capillaries** or larger vessels
- tissue **fluids**
- tissue **cells**

to produce the cardinal signs of

- **heat**
- **redness**
- **swelling**
- **pain**
- **loss of use**

Body tissue protection in all inflammatory situations is

through the immune responses which serve to curtail self - destruction. The skin is no exception. *The end aim is to restore body structure and functioning.*

Such responses may be

- too weak
    - lack of infection control
    - lack of toxin elimination
- too strong
    - lack of self-destruction control
    - excess inflammatory response
    - subsequent auto immune dis-ease development

Despite care, attention, and some knowledge and skill, the horsemaster cannot do more than

- appreciate that 'something is wrong' with a horse's skin's **A B C**, and be able to say that he can
    - see
    - feel

worrying changes in/on the skin, which are

- **itchy** (or not), or that
- the horse is behaving evasively or aggressively to these areas, especially when they are 'touched'

In practice, the horse's aberrant behaviour may well be the first indication of developing skin disease, e.g.

- a reaction to tack fitting, before a 'sore' becomes perceivable
- an itchiness, as the dis-ease process abnormally stimulates dermal and follicular nerve endings, before it erupts. Clinically there is
    - rubbing, leg on leg; body on wall

- head and neck rubbing on fences, with lice infestation; the abrasions are the main cause of the characteristic hair loss
- mane and dock rubbing on walls, with 'sweet-itch'
- leg stamping
- head shaking, usually to one side
- nibbling
- biting (but rarely licking as in the cow, dog and cat)

even to the extent of traumatic damage to other regions of the body and/or rapid worsening of the developing primary lesion in an attempt to ease the **pruritus**, the irritating itch!

If such warning signs are not presented, early awareness of skin disorders depends upon, in the working horse

- grooming – is a regular, not to be missed, opportunity to
  - *look*, to see
  - *touch*, to feel

(just as it is for many other aspects of good horsemaster-ship, in assessing the horse's **A** **B** **C**)

  - on unsaddling after exercise
  - on evening inspection

especially if the earlier work was in the rain or through mud and wet

  - at morning strapping
  - at tacking up

when

  - the eyes should scan the skin overall
  - the fingers should investigate any visual findings and explore tack areas, as routine even in the absence of clinical signs
  - around the girth area for a rash
  - under the saddle area for a gall

This is especially so in the early days of conditioning work when the connective tissues in general, and the skin in particular, are still 'soft' and have not yet gained their resilience to work stress. Be aware of

- a change in the normal lie of the coat in localised areas
- local unusual sweating or wet patches
- **lumps, bumps, soft swellings** and **'rashes'**
- 'sores' with or without oozing fluid
- reaction to digital pressure

At clipping

- exposure of subacute and chronic changes 'hidden' by the coat, e.g. subacute **rain scald** lesions
- during the next few days for flare up of **rashes**
- a little later, for specific signs, e.g. of **'ringworm'**

When rugging up watch for any 'reaction'

- from, for example, the rug's washing materials
- infectious, from rug's previous (or other) horse use

In the horse at grass full or part-time, rugged – beware

- rubbing *abrasion* of New Zealand rug
- infectious *reactions* where New Zealand, not properly cleaned, makes most contact
- skin *infections* associated with wet skin conditions induced by lack of care in rugging

Unrugged horses are not as likely to experience such traumas, but they are exposed in winter and at other times to

- long periods of being *rain-wet* (*see* **rain scald**)
- long periods of being in *mud* (*see* **mud fever**)
- *fly biting*
- plant contact reactions or by *'stings'* (nettles)
- various *pollens*
  - inhaled
  - ingested
  - contacted

all of which can cause skin lesions

- sun's *UV (ultra violet) rays* on 'pink' muzzle and heels
- *contact* with contaminated inanimate objects

all these can produce adverse effects which

- its coat may well hide
- long range, 'from the gate' inspection may well miss, or at least delay early recognition – field inspection should be more thorough
  - for 10 days or so after the introduction of a 'new' horse, with special concern for
  - contagions generally
  - aggressive behaviour leading to skin trauma or worse

The horsemaster should be aware that handling horses

with skin disease can be hazardous. Painful and/or severe pruritic lesions will cause the horse to

- stamp – without thought of where his feet are landing (**leg mange**, 'heel bug' infestations)
- rub – on walls and branches, irrespective of rider's wishes (**sweet itch**)
- roll – usually in mud or water when the skin is itchy, particularly when ridden (the various **urticarias**)
- become uncontrollable and markedly unsteady, will often roll and may refuse to get up, and when it does to 'bolt' (**nettle sting**)

Skin has an efficient ability to produce new, immediate local immunity which frequently effects a quick recovery without treatment or even slowly as with ringworm contagion.

The dermis, and particularly the germinative layer of the epidermis, has good regenerative capacity; quickly and efficiently in most cases this brings about satisfactory repair. Conversely, this self preservation may mislead owners regarding the severity of the conditions

- some dis-eases leave permanent full skin defects
- some are more likely to do so if early recognition is ignored or missed
  - wrong, sometimes unnecessary, treatment is given or applied

It is essential, especially in those diseases which are thought to be primary conditions but are in fact secondary infections or degenerations, that the importance of determining

- the *primary reason* and/or
- the trigger mechanism

is understood. It may be, for example

- structural damage from saddle pressure

predisposing to

  - an open wound, with or without
  - subsequent infection
- weather influences on the
  - three outer defenses of the integument
- regeneration of skin parasites

Fortunately, skin dis-ease is rarely lethal. It can, however, result in much economic loss, e.g. where the horse is laid off work because either it cannot be tacked or it is seen as a real or imaginary 'danger' to other people's horses.

Quick suspicion and early, accurate diagnosis favours minimal extension of the lesions and a quicker return to work.

The horsemaster must, as has already been emphasised, and will be further explained in later pages, be aware of what can develop in or on the skin

- *why?*
- *where?*
- *when?*
- *how?*

and appreciate the need to record

  - where it *started*
  - what the early lesion *looked like*
  - if it spread, was it as *single* or *multiple* lesions
  - if the horse was *itchy*
- what *management changes* might have been associated before the first signs

The horsemaster will want to know

- is it because of any fault on her part?
- is it contagious (selfishly – 'where did it come from?', unselfishly – 'where can it go next?')

Skin Susceptibility to Dis-ease

All body tissues have some forms of defence against micro-organisms. By its very position, skin is the most exposed. Its defences are good, but they too are open to many forms of breaching

- *abrasion*
- being too *wet* or too '*dry*'
- intercurrent *systemic disease* effects, via the blood supply
- *ectoparasitic* attacks
- various *allergic* reactions

It is the traumatic, often inflammatory, consequences of such assaults which are the first 'invaders'; the actual pathogenic germs, previously in passive mode, are actually secondary attackers.

Dormant or quiescent skin germs are no more likely to be pathogenic on one host than another. They may, given the right environment, rapidly become active and virulent. Conversely, contagion from an active situation will not *per se* induce a disease response in another animal of the same species if conditions are not suitable.

Such a distinction does not obtain in the ectoparasites such as mange where their life cycle, whether that includes a burrowing phase or not, seems to be independent of skin loopholes; malnutrition possibly plays a significant role.

It must be appreciated that

- *abrasions need only be minuscule* – a few broken hairs under the girth for ringworm to become active
- a wet coat, common in the English climate – for Dermatophilus to become effectively mobile
- sub-clinical illness can undermine general immunity whereby the primary trauma is not observed by the horsemaster. Consequently the infection, when developed, becomes an original clinical condition

This does **not** exonerate the horsemaster from being aware of the potential effects of

- the girth on the 'soft' skin of an unconditioned horse
- prolonged rain
- a horse 'due' for worming
- one worked with a mild fever or
- likely to have been exposed to
  - skin dis-ease elsewhere
  - muddy conditions cross-country

The horsemaster must always work in the belief that an undiagnosed skin dis-ease is a potential contagion and, for her own and the horse's sake, act accordingly. *This is particularly so with bacteria such as Dermatophilus, Staphylococcus, and ringworms generally.*

An abrasion can be inflicted on the human skin by a finger nail recently contaminated from an infection, and then used to scratch the nape of one's neck as one ponders the equine lesion!

There are many causes of skin morbidity. The various signs within these morbidities are often common to several entities. There are *many pathogens* and *many traumas* but *relatively few variations in the ultimate lesion*.

The signs are by no means diagnostic in all disease conditions. Even the signs of a primary skin dis-ease *per se*, as well as the predisposing traumatic type of lesions are modified and often markedly complicated or confused by further opportunist invaders. Some are characterised by pruritus (itchiness) which can stimulate self interference. Others are benign in this respect until compounded by secondary invaders.

Where and when inflammation is present, the cardinal sign of loss of use will be a **keratinisation defect**, producing

- **scale**
- **crust**
- **alopecia** (hair loss)

and the total disorder will or can go through three stages, of

- acute
- subacute
- chronic inflammation

Many are self-limiting to effect a cure or a standstill stage persistent at the subacute or chronic stage. All are related to the obvious fact that skin is 'on the outside'

- it touches all sorts of things
  - fauna
  - flora
  - inanimate objects
- micro-organisms are on it
- it is an organ or system dependent upon the internal blood supply which can deliver
  - noxious substances
  - by-products of infections
  - allergens which evince themselves in the dermis

Skin can be debilitated and so made less protective. It becomes susceptible to further assault. In the micro-climate of epidermis, hair, dander, sebum and sweat, many micro-organisms find shelter and nourishment. There they replicate, but cause neither harm nor irritation – live and let live! Species of small microscopic mites and non flying arthropods (invertebrates that have jointed legs) also live in and off these inert tissues and excretions.

Some larger ectoparasites are also programmed to eat debris and 'dander' on the surface

- their movement is usually irritating
- their 'mouth parts' may irritate still more

Others obtain nourishment by piercing the skin surface into the germination layer and the dermis. To this end they inject a keratolytic saliva which is chemically traumatic, so inflammatory and often allergenic (antigenic) and so hypersensitising.

In all such parasitisms there may also be the introduction of, or a 'paving the way' for, secondary bacterial invasion, transmission of viral infection, and subsequent antibody/antigen reactions. In some cases, the parasite's life cycle involves burrowing into the dermis with an inflammatory and hypersensitive response.

At certain seasons of the year and/or stages of their life cycle they will merely cause an irritation which induces the protective reflex action to dislodge them.

At other times they will stimulate more than a 'get off' reaction and create an inflammatory response. Now, 'there is something wrong'; the ecosystem becomes out of equilibrium and the possible first changes to encourage multiplication of germs into a pathogenic state begin.

When inflammatory or hypersensitive reactions are stimulated in the dermis (remember, inflammation can only develop where tissues are 'alive', i.e. have a capillary vascular and neuro-system at least) *then a dis-ease state is developed and can be perceived to a greater or lesser degree.*

Both physical and organic factors can, in addition
- prematurely loosen hair
- erode through the keratin layers

and create the right micro-climate for the
- multiplication of fungal spores, which
- create pathogenic changes in the germinative layer

It is not surprising, therefore, that the varying irritations cause the horse to
- stamp
- rub
- bite

and often more so when pathological reactions occur, causing
- self-mutilation of the abrasion
- erosion of the skin, thus weakening its defences and exposing it to
- secondary bacterial infection

Other Predisposing Factors

Indirectly from other system disease which, *inter alia*, causes
- fever
- dehydration
- loss of condition
- endocrine defects, as in equine Cushings disease and thyroid deficiency
- electrolyte and other nutritional imbalances of vitamins and minerals
- pathologically induced albumen deficiency

which 'reach' the dermis and the germinative layer via the blood, and are 'exhibited' on the surface as
- rough staring coat
- dry coat
- sticky coat
- localised sweating
- hair loss
- inelastic 'hide bound' skin
- 'thickened skin'

Directly from other system morbidity which extends to, or involves, the three dermal layers, as with
- infections
- systemic allergic reactions

Or, from being variably and/or continuously exposed to
- contact allergenic agents
- external factors causing
  - traumatic inflammatory morbidity
    - closed, bruising and/or
    - open wounds
  - irritation and ulceration by
    - chemical and
    - organo-chemical elements as in
      - detergents
      - leather dressings, with or without prior pressure trauma
    and as with
      - incorrect topical application of skin dressings
      - accidental chemical irritants
  - thermal extremes
    - dry and wet heat
    - solar irradiation
    - cryo (frost) applications and exposure

- radioactivity
- photosensitisation
- maceration from immersion in
  - water
  - mud
  - persistent abrasion of distal limbs, as from frozen mud in poached grazing areas
- pH changes, especially in the distal limbs' soil contacts
- periodic abrasion – when clipped
- ammoniacal contaminated bedding
- 'irritants' in wood and paper bedding

Viruses which invade direct are not common; the more common equine papovirus and bovine papillovirus may in fact depend upon insect vectors which 'implant' them. The virus of equine arteritis causes skin lesions as part of the extension lesions of the systemic disease. Equine herpes 3 (**coital exanthema**) is spread venereally; the predisposing damage need only be microscopic to the hairless skin and related mucosa during coitus.

Such invading germs are called **primary infections** in the context of skin disease.

Signs associated with skin dis-ease vary in the

- appearances of the lesions
- sites affected primarily
- rates of development
- tendencies to spread, and by
- complicating factors from
  - other illnesses
  - feeding
  - seasons of the year
  - weather

The horsemaster will see or feel signs as skin changes, e.g.

- swellings, small and large, with or without
- rashes, redness (difficult to see in hair covered areas), and excoriations
- weeping and sticky patches
- matted hair
- falling hair, with or without
  - scales and crusts
- itchiness

The veterinary surgeon will first describe these signs as typical of a known primary type lesion. These lesions are tabulated thus:

Macule – a round, flat, non-palpable area of colour change, level with the normal skin. Less than 1cm (½in) in diameter

- e.g. the blood spot in early Purpura, seen in hairless non-pigmented areas, such as the gums
- simple loss of pigment, as in older grey horses' muzzles

Patch – an area as above, but greater than 1cm (½in), e.g. the Welsh pony's muzzle's depigmentation, 'liver' patches in quarters and thighs.

Papule – a small, circumscribed soft to solid mass in the skin less than 1cm (½in) but raised, e.g.

- insect bite pruritic allergy
- non itchy granulomas

Nodule – a firm mass greater than 1cm (½in) diameter, usually raised and rounded: a more severe reaction than a papule as seen in

- melanoma
- nodular disease
- some allergies

Plaque – firm elevated flat-topped swelling, also greater than 1cm (½in). Can be irregular as well as circular, usually multiple

- allergic reaction to food and drugs

Tumour – any large mass, usually neoplastic, benign or malignant, in or on any area of the skin or its appendages

- sarcoid
- fibro sarcoma, etc

Vesicle – clear fluid filled, sharply defined, raised lesions up to 1cm (½in) in diameter

Bulla – a vesicle larger than 1cm (½in)

- they quickly rupture or are contact ruptured, to expose a reddish eroded under surface, e.g.
  - coital exanthema
  - Purpura haemorrhagica

- 'blistering' and burns

Pustule – a vesicle containing pus, e.g.

- later stages of bacterial infections and of
- coital exanthema

Weal – a sharply circumscribed, elevated, rounded or flat-topped, serum-filled area of skin, later with oedematous surround, e.g.

- food allergies
- whip trauma marks
- unknown factors

The hairs may be raised but, in the early stages at least, the epidermis appears intact.

Secondary lesions arise in or around the primaries, from auto-immune reaction to tissue damage and other allergic states, irritation from wound discharges, self-mutilation with secondary infection, by-products of the healing stage of acute or subacute primaries:

- **scale** – an accumulation of cast off epidermal fragments, larger and much more numerous than 'wear and tear' scurf, and localised to the primary lesion. White, grey, or 'coloured' by sebum and/or blood pigment
  - e.g. fine and flaky, as in **rain scald**
  - thick and adherent, as in **leg mange**

- **crust** – dried (inspissated) firm to hard and adherent mixture of exuded serum and/or blood and/or pus and sebum and of scale
  - e.g. **sweet itch**'s later stages, with possible secondary bacterial infection
  - **mange**
  - **wounds**, usually with secondary infection
  - **burns**

- **eschar** – a crust of sloughing tissue still partly attached
  - e.g. deep burns

- **erosion** – a non-penetrating skin defect showing as chronically inflamed alopecic areas
  - usually 'cause unknown'
  - possibly persistent mild abrasive rubbing or chafing – as in ill-fitting tack or harness

- **ulcer** – a more severe form of erosion into the dermis possibly resulting in scarring, but almost certainly resulting in white patches and white hairs

- **excoriation** – extension dermatitis from prolonged discharge onto the skin. May produce crusts and subsequent alopecia
  - e.g. discharging wound

- **scar** – the undifferentiated (i.e. no specialised skin cellular tissue) replacement fibrous infilling, following the chronic healing of a primary lesion which had penetrated to or finally ulcerated into the hypodermis
  - e.g. traumatic wounds

- **lichenification** – a chronic state of dermatitis
  - irregular alopecia
  - scaling
  - skin thickening and corrugating
    - e.g. sweet itch, persistent or repetitive attacks

- **fissures** – splits in the skin where the dermis has 'dried out' over mobile areas
  - e.g. cracked heels
  - dermatophilus lesions on 'flesh' muzzle
  - facial sunburn

- **pigmentary** changes – in epidermis and/or hair
  - increase in melanin – hyper-pigmentation
    - naturally present in patches
    - acquired as in
      - chronic inflammation
      - post-piercing insect bites
      - hormone imbalances
      - melanoma tumours
      - idiopathic (unknown origin)
  - decrease in melanin – hypo-pigmentation
    - complete in skin – leukoderma
    - complete in hair – leukotrichia
      - natural (congenital)
      - acquired
        - tack and other pressured areas, as in

saddle 'white marks'

- ill fitted bandages, as in leg 'white marks'
- freeze branding

- **alopecia** – complete loss, or absence of, hair from variable areas of 'coat'
  - permanent
    - trauma with scarring
    - idiopathic
  - temporary
    - post dermatitis e.g. rain scald

- **hypertrichosis** – increased growth and density of hair
  - natural, e.g. the Clydesdale's moustache

TYPES OF SKIN DISEASE

Developmental

There is uncertainty about genetic influences. Some apparently acquired conditions, usually without complications, are either delayed acquired or idiopathic (unknown but 'inner' causes).

Where there seems to be familial or genetic influence, there are several main types to consider

- pigmentation defects of skin and of hair
- cyst formation
- susceptibility to insect (and other) stings and bite reactions, whereas other animals in the same environment react less, or not at all, as the norm. This is an increased hypersensitivity
  - e.g. the atopic state 'permitting' sweet itch

Pigmentation Defect

- strong inherited influences, as in
  - Arabian 'pinky' or 'fading' syndrome around the eyes, lips and vulva lips

The condition appears to wax and wane. Also seen in Thoroughbreds.

Vitiligo

- irregular, variably sized areas often slowly increasing in number of depigmentation areas
  - idiopathic, in many pure breeds
    - macula, around the lips
    - papular
    - patches
- involves both skin and hair if naturally present. Possibly neurogenic and said to respond to tranquilliser therapy and vitamin/mineral supplements
- 'coloured' and 'spotted' horses are so marked because of the absence of melanocytes and so of melanin as in the 'white' areas. This affects both skin and hair
- the 'white marks' used as identification pointer may be
  - white hairs from pigmented skin
  - white hairs from unpigmented skin
  - sparse white hairs from 'flesh coloured'
  - unpigmented thin skin
  - showing hypodermal blood flow
  - acquired from low grade chronic inflammation

The lack of pigment is an inherited feature and contributes to decreased skin defenses.

True acquired disorders are

- leukoderma, and
- leukotrichia, following
  - trauma, such as wire cuts
  - freeze branding; the dermis proper is untouched, only the germinal layer's pigment producing cells are destroyed

Cysts

- on **head** area
  - **epidermoid**
    - nasal (in the false nostril) – atheroma (a fill-in or occlusion cyst)
    - conchal – a fistulous swelling on the edge of the ear flap (the pinna)
    - dentigerous – aberrant tooth nucleus in a bone cyst at the base of the ear
- on the **body**
  - **dermoid**
    - dorsum, on mid line of back, single, sometimes

multiple, containing coiled hairs in a cheesy material

The following types of skin disease are more commonly encountered.

Inflammatory

Traumatic
- physical
  - wounds
  - burns
  - scalds
  - 'scalding' by persistent spillage of body fluid over an area of skin distal to the origin of the flow
- photodynamic
- chemical – wrong strength and/or wrong use of
  - insecticides
  - antiseptics
  - disinfectants
  - blisters
  - others

Infectious

Viral
- **papillomatosis** – 'warty' growths due to host specific papovirus infection
- equine coital exanthema (**ECE**) – venereal
- equine **sarcoid**
- equine **herpes** infections (other than ECE), as blood transported effect
- equine viral arteritis (**EVA**), as blood transported effect

Bacterial ('on the back' of micro-traumas)
- **dermatophilosis**
  - rain scald
  - mud fever etc.
- secondary infections, usually
  - **folliculitis** (may appear to be primary)
  - **furunculosis**

- abscesses erupting onto skin surface
- sinus – purulent discharge, as from retained foreign body

These can 'spread' to deeper tissues.

Fungal
- **dermatophytosis**
  - superficial mycoses – **ringworms**
  - deep mycoses (rare in the UK), a subcutaneous type which breaks out to the surface

Parasitic
Roughly grouped as **arthropod** (segmented body, jointed limbs; as insects, spiders, crustaceans) invaders and 'attackers' that fly, and those that are more or less constant inhabitants of the epidermis and hair

- hypersensitivity, as induced by insects which fly in to 'attack' and bite or sting
  - usually seasonal, they are the most common cause of
  - **pruritus**, especially that caused by midges
    - types **i** and **iv** hypersensitivity reactions mainly to insect salivary antigens
- secondary bites, more reactive, as in sweet itch
  - midges
  - stable flies
  - gnats
  - horse flies

which may also, via their mouth parts and their feet, transmit
  - ringworm spores
  - papo virus, especially into the ear pinna (gnats)
  - onchocerca worms
  - other micro-organisms

They are mechanical vectors, unlike some infection-carrying blood suckers (arthropods) which 'inject' viruses and other germs into the host (or target animal) usually to become blood-borne therein.

- ectoparasitic irritant infestations – they are potentially 'on' the host
  - variably seasonal in their activity, usually winter
  - invariably pruritic

- lice – severity of irritation worsened by their species method of feeding

- manges – severe irritation

- ticks – painful irritation as the tick hooks in during relatively prolonged feeding

Further methods of grouping could be:

Pruritic diseases complicated by the secondary changes of self-mutilation leading to

- excoriation

- exudation

- scab formation, but primarily

- allergic reactions

- intolerances

- atopy

Generalised **secondary dermatitis**, which can further complicate these, is a syndrome, not a specific disease entity

- seborrhoea or greasy skin which can appear on its own i.e. be idiopathic or accompany parasitic dermatoses due to

  - helminth migration

  - ectoparasites

Pruritus with loss of hair
- lice

- mites

- ticks

Scaling and crusting disease, with
- pruritus, usually secondary

- non-pruritus as with the infections

Irritations, partly due to actual pressure touch, but also due to
- pain of bite

- pain of sting reaction

- hypersensitivity of, e.g.

  - diptera flies

  - hymenoptera

Evasive reactions, due to noise and/or visual presence
- 'blow', bot and warble flies

Papular lesions, which include
- macules

- papules

- plaques

Nodular – includes the papilloma which is viral 'warts' and aural 'plaques' and sarcoids.

In addition to the congenital cysts and to the now almost disappeared warble fly nodule, the important nodules, 'bumps' in UK horses are eosinophilic disorders or **nodular disease**.

Allergic

Such dis-ease presents as an **urticaria** and **angioedema** which are basically nodules and oedema. They can be immunological. Either will be **pruritic** and painful.

Auto Immune Dis-ease

Such are called **pemphigus**, lesions due to the formation of anti-bodies directed at keratin-producing cells.

They are primarily vesicles going onto pustules with seborrhoea, then crusts, leading to self mutilation. Epidemilogically most examples are related to food changes.

Metabolic

No primary lesions of this dis-ease type are clinically recognised, but

- malnutrition does have a dermal input, usually with

  - pigmental changes

  - atrophy of the dermis (**acanthosis**) and hypo-pigmentation or

    - excessive keratin production

    - see also 'urticaria'

Neurogenic

Little is known about these.

Autonomic Nervous System
- cholinergic sweating may lead to

- linear maceration and excoriation, possibly associated with
- a dermatitis
- scale
- crust
- alopecia
    - leukoderma
    - leukotrichia
    - the rare Pemphigus condition

These lesions may also be associated with auto-immune disorders of the skin.

Neoplasia or 'New' Growth

Neoplasia, tumours, '**cancers**' are relatively uncommon in the horse, but the list includes the following found on the skin.

- granulomata: chronic excessive granulation tissue
- sarcoids
- squamous cell carcinoma
- melanoma
- melano-sarcoma
- fibro-sarcoma
- lympho-sarcoma
- neurofibroma
- nodules – collagenolytic granuloma

Degenerative

True 'wear and tear' is unlikely to occur, because of the relatively thick inert epidermis and its 'expendable' layers and the marked dermal property of regeneration to maintain this.

Local lesions as seen in scars are the chronic stage of incomplete regeneration, reflecting the initial severity of the trauma and its penetration.

There are **dystrophic lesions** (failure to regenerate), as seen in the follicles of the mane and the tail, from not always known dis-ease. They are slow in onset and characterised by

- alopecia
- hyperkeratinosis, both tending to permanency

The wide variations in the relationship between a skin dis-ease and the development and final appearance as a lesion have made it more convenient, or often more explicit, to group the dermatosis more by the lesion than by a specific disease.

Obviously, in the final analysis, it is essential to have a diagnosis if

- specific treatment
- effective control, and
- ultimate prevention

are to be obtained.

The infections, the infestations (parasites) and the neoplasia are all capable of accurate diagnosis, even if sometimes only with laboratory help; treatment, if such drugs and topical applications are feasible and practicable, therefore should present no problems. The less identifiable urticarias, allergies and non specific lumps and rashes are more of a problem.

The dis-eases of the skin can be catalogued from a practising veterinary surgeon's point of view as

- conditions *usually requiring veterinary assistance*, and of relatively common occurrence
    - urticaria and other allergies
    - ringworm
    - rain scald
    - sarcoids
    - some manges and harvest mites
- conditions usually recognised and *managed by the experienced horsemaster* – perhaps because they are very common – but not always well managed
    - mud fever and cracked heels
    - sweet itch
    - melanoma – 'masterly inactivity', except to monitor 'fly blow'
    - lice infestation
- conditions *more rarely seen*, and therefore, not as well known
    - papillomata – 'warty' muzzle
    - various neoplasias other than sarcoids
    - chorioptic mange
    - drug related dermal eruptions

The description and management of these disorders is dealt with in some detail. Some are seen as separate conditions, when in fact they are sometimes two or more exhibitions of a common factor scientifically 'discovered', e.g. the name of the germ, long after apparently separate disorders were first recognised and given, often descriptively, a name of its own, as in 'rain scald' and 'mud fever'.

Little more will be said about developmental and inherited conditions other than the presumed inherent predisposition to hypersensitivity as in sweet itch for example. Enough has been said thus far about viral dermatitis to make the reader aware of, for example

- coital exanthema HV3
- EVA secondary effect
- Herpes virus 1 secondary effect

but more regard will be paid to the viral input as an infection, especially in Papillomata and Sarcoids, under neoplasias.

As already emphasised, the skin is most prone to external assault by

- physical and chemical trauma
- bacterial and other infections
- ectoparasitic infestation
- ectoparasitic 'flying' attack, and the
  - associated allergic reactions, urticarias and skin defects

These last four form a large part of this chapter.

THE DISEASES

Inflammatory

Infectious

In most horses the inert keratin rich layers of the epidermis and of the hairs are efficient barriers against invasion. Prolonged wetting will loosen these superficial layers and macerate others, with the physical loss of much of the barrier defence as well. The damaged area is now open to further environmental trauma as from

- wind driven rain
- heavy soaking rain
- repeated washing, as for show cosmetics and skin medications

- grooming tools
- protective clothing, especially if used dirty
- burrowing and biting insects (especially the stable and house fly)
- mud and other particularly abrasive materials

The last four mentioned traumatic 'vehicles' are common means of contagion – direct animal to animal. How important crusts, discarded onto bedding and grass, are as contagious fomites is not known but they are a possible danger to horses. If they are, then stables, yards and possibly fields, theoretically at least, are a continuing site for further infection.

It follows that when crusts and other debris from infected areas are deliberately removed from a patient they should be trapped or at least discarded onto concrete where they can be soaked in disinfectant and drained away. Suspected contaminated bedding is best burnt. Any recognised scratching and rubbing posts should be heavily creosoted.

Viral
(*see above*)

Bacterial
The hair (the coat) and the skin are continuously inhabited by potentially pathogenic organisms. Some, such as the bacterium Dermatophilus, especially its congolensis species, require this habitat for survival. It is an opportunist commensal. It has not yet been found as a soil saprophyte.

Other skin bacteria such as Staphylococci and Corynebacteria can exist on the animal and in the soil and vegetation.

Dermatophili
Pathogenic for man and all animal species, many of which can be reservoirs of infection. In some countries they have been recorded from mucosal epithelia with evidence of local pathogenicity. Much is still to be learnt about the life cycle.

There is no evidence that any horse is consistently invaded but there is reason to believe that all horses are at some time or other. These variable reservoirs of infection permit Dermatophilus to be always 'available' directly or indirectly.

As an actinomycite (a micro-organism that multiplies like certain fungi but requires light to do so) it basically lies in dormant mode as a zoospore, in scale and crust, quite firmly attached to hair shafts *where it can exist for 3 to 4 months even in these when fallen off the horse.*

If the skin and hair becomes wetted for some continuous time the crust softens and the zoospores are released to become

- activated – for germination
- mobile – to 'swim' through skin surface water

This mobile zoospore is chemotactically taken to carbon dioxide diffusions through the skin. These pinpoint faults in the epidermis are suitable for colonisation.

Within a follicle or microscopic fissure the spores containing hyphae germinate into filaments which ripen to release a new generation of spores and so on down into the dermis.

A feature of Dermatophilus is the quick inflammatory reaction its presence triggers. This is in the form of a massive white blood cell barrier formation which aims to stop deeper penetration. Surviving spores 'swim' away laterally with resultant lateral spread hence the rapid diffuse (usually relatively superficial) clinical signs.

The inflammatory response also produces a serous exudate and the production of scale and crust riding outwards on the seborrhoeic sticky discharge. It is dead and live germs, white blood cells and dermal debris which form these contagious deposits, becoming an ideal source of nourishment for the Dermatophilus.

If wet conditions continue, the life cycle does also; the clinical signs spread, and secondary commensal infections are possible. If dryness sets in, the surviving spores revert to the dormant mode.

Final healing appears to be due to the development of a 'delayed hypersensitivity' to the germ and the consequent destruction of it in the area affected. Provided the predisposing factors are brought under control and there is no serious secondary bacterial infection, the condition is self limiting in 3 to 4 weeks.

The basic reaction is an inflammation; the cardinal sign of 'loss of use' is a temporary deficiency in keratin and new hair.

Animals have a degree of natural immunity to Dermatophilus, presumably on a hereditary basis. This is substantiated in practice – not all horses become affected yet all in one stable are similarly exposed to contagion and to precipitating factors.

Some parts of the skin are more susceptible than others, e.g. white hairs, and especially white epidermis as in unpigmented regions.

Natural defence, apart from constitutional non-specific immunity, is dependent on the

- structure of the skin and the quantity and the quality of the sebum and other lipids, and the keratin
- nature of the coat, density, length and texture
- ability to mount a rapid local specific cellular immune response to invasion

There are specific differences in the two main Dermatophilic diseases, **rain scald** and **mud fever**, and their associated conditions. These reflect

- the environment of the horse
- whether it is in work or 'at grass'
- the source and the target on the animal of the required wetness
- the possibility of primary traumatising factors

but there are common initial lesions

- marked serous exudation
- matting of the hair into paint brush-like patches
- formation of crusts
- their eventual natural debridement (removal of infected tissue)
- retention of some infection in certain areas of hair
  - mane
  - tail

Pruritus is not a feature unless secondary, purulent infection occurs with

- itchiness
- tendency to self mutilation
- possibly a fever

Pain is also not a cardinal sign in rain scald unless there is secondary infection, or any crust is forcibly removed too soon. Mud fever lesions are, however, very painful on human handling.

Specific (humoral and cellular) immunity can be experimentally induced by vaccination. The need for such is important in countries where endemic hair and fleece disease is a serious economic herd and flock problem; there is a recognised breed susceptibility therein.

In unpigmented hair, and in those skin areas recognised as being most susceptible, the defensively important dermal Langerham's cells are now, from experimental work, known to be inactivated by the UV rays of sunlight (if the country is under a deficit ozone layer); so one defence is lost, even in Great Britain.

Natural immunity can also be lowered by malnutrition,

helminthiases and other coincidental diseases such as viral and fungal skin infections.

Epidemics in horses are however not a feature of either rain scald or of mud fever. Multiple cases in any one stable is more a reflection of a

- widespread presence of an initially dormant contamination, or ease of contagion as with free running groups
- prolonged predisposing factors, including seasonal ectoparasitism
- significant number of horses with
  - inheritable pigmentary deficits
  - genetically determined poor resistance
    - breeds 'out of' their indigenous environment
  - acquired deficits of resistance of a general nature
    - malnutrition
    - helminthiases

Winter Rain Scald
(Dermatophilosis or Streptothricosis)

This skin dis-ease can be listed as one of a group showing mats or clumps of hair followed by alopecia. Much of the epidemiology (how it arises) and the pathology (what happens) has been covered earlier.

Rain scald is a classic example of such a Dermatophilosis, an exudative dis-ease due to the inflammatory reaction to an invading bacterium D. congolensis. Because of the requirement for a wet skin environment it is a condition prevalent in periods of prolonged rainfall, and more so when hair is of 'aged' vitality as at the end of winter and before a new coat develops.

The cascade of events which can stimulate the dormant Dermatophilus are

- persistent wet coat
  - driving rain is traumatic to the skin especially as a horse naturally stands 'tail into the wind' – the wet is propelled against the lie of the hair
  - the saturation does not fully run off the coat along the drainage lines
  - the buttock, quarters, back and dorsal neck are worst affected – in that decreasing order
  - the sebum and other protective lipids are diluted and lose their waterproofing effect
- other traumatising factors
  - some out-wintered horses will be ridden. For this

they may be brought in and so allowed to dry to some extent; usually artificially with rough abrasive towels only on saddle and girth areas. The fact of riding can also have a traumatic abrasive effect

- if grooming is attempted further, abrasion will occur
- some unridden, grass kept horses will be New Zealand rugged; if this is not put on clean and inspected daily it will result in
  - rug abrasion
  - trapped moisture

to cause more trouble.

Generally speaking, the out-wintered horse is the one most likely to

- become affected
- have the early signs missed
  - they are not initially visible, even close to
  - they can be palpated, but obviously this means handling

otherwise the dis-ease can become well established before it is recognised.

Signs (winter type)

- the crusts can be felt as isolated small bumps under the coat
- the coat becomes matted, with serous discharge and diluted sebum into plaques or crusts of usually less than 2cm (3/4in) in diameter. They coalesce, and then lift the hair into a tessellated pattern
- if these are pulled it will hurt, but there is no pruritus
- when they loosen they fall off to reveal
  - a moist, pinkish, raw – sometimes bleeding – surface
  - the underside of the crust is concave with a sticky exudate, sometimes purulent
- older scabs are dry and the exposed skin is scaly and alopecic
- newer, intact lesions will be palpable under apparently normal coat
- eventual large areas of alopecia will follow the coat's original water shedding pattern
- in diffuse forms, especially over the rump and the loins, the clinical appearance is that of a mass of paint brush looking clusters of matted hair

- some cases will produce excess exudate to produce a seborrhoea
- lesions originating on unpigmented areas as in coloured horses will often laterally spread but, as a rule, the pigmented coat and skin must be wet

Summer Rain Scald
The signs differ because of the thinner, shorter coat
- the paint brushes are shorter and 'looser'
- they break away more quickly as crusts
- there is less late scab formation and
- quicker alopecia

Microsporum gypsum (ringworm) can produce similar crusts but these are usually wider apart.

Confirmation
Laboratory examination of fresh, carefully removed plaques.

Remember that untreated horses will rightly attract Welfare investigation
- get the horse into a dry environment
- expose the skin to the air, subject to protective clothing requirements
  - always use a daily clean undersheet if rugging is necessary for warmth. Remember – alopecia removes insulation
- consult your veterinary surgeon
  - well established acute cases will require veterinary treatment by
    - antibiotics, and possibly
    - antishock drugs, as well as
    - other supportive therapy
  - encourage drying of the affected areas
    - hair drier
    - heat lamp (with care when hair loss is marked, and if white skin is involved do not use UV lamps)

Management
- feed a supplemented, balanced diet including specific amino acids and trace elements (consult your feed compounder) for skin and hair regeneration; they do require a correct protein intake
- consider the need for anthelmintic treatment and

- beware secondary lice and mange (leg) infestation especially in young horses which were at grass as these two conditions can cause or be associated with a predisposing poor condition
- consult your veterinary surgeon for suitable antiseptic shampoos to help loosen the affected hair and the crusts
  - soften with good soap and warm water gently applied, rinse off
  - follow with antiseptic shampoo, leave on for ten minutes, rinse off and artificially dry. Do not rub dry
  - *do not* forcibly remove matted hair and crusts
- areas which remain weepy should be treated to hasten micro-climate drying with
  - lead lotion
  - witch hazel
  - calamine lotion
- *do not* tack again until
  - skin feels soft
  - hair has regrown

In less acute, less widespread attacks natural dryness usually is sufficient, but always
- shampoo loosening crusts off
- lead lotion will dry remaining moist areas from which crusts will more easily fall out
- remaining dry leathery patches will benefit from cod liver oil and lanolin creams

Prevention
This is very much a matter of good management
- horses at grass
  - beware the risk of endoparasitism during spring, summer and autumn, and lice in mid-winter
  - monitor availability of sufficient grazing
- unrugged
  - be aware of prolonged rainfall
    - especially during cold spells of spring and summer
    - if there are no natural windbreaks, consider
      - field shelters – more often used by horses against flies!
    - or if neither are used
      - periodically yard under cover during each

24 hours, to give horses a chance to dry out naturally if only for six to twelve hours

- clean, dry, straw bedding in a loose box (not in a yard) may encourage rolling which will
    - help drying
    - remove loose crusts

    (burn the bedding daily)
- watch for signs of persistent wetting along shedding lines
- antiseptic shampoo as a precaution – allow to dry off afterwards
- be aware of early signs as described earlier

- rugged
    - start off with a 'cleaned' rug
    - check skin before rugging, if necessary keep in until dry
    - check rug each day
        - inspect close contact areas
        - readjust fit

    if necessary, yard under cover as above, with rug off

- stabled, in work horses – rarely affected, unless management is poor
    - do not rug up immediately after work without
        - washing off and drying, using clean rugs, especially any under sheet
        - checking at evening stables that horse is dry and hasn't broken out
        - beware drips from roof and eaves

Unlike mud fever, rain scald is not a condition of working animals as a rule, unless kept and used in very sub-standard conditions.

Note 'Rain Rash'

An urticarial type of papule formation, which does not always develop into an acute Dermatophilus disease, and which also is not pruritic, is seen in some horses rugged up before being dry after exercise, or which 'break out' later in the evening without re-drying, it is thought to be urticarial and not primarily infectious. It may be related to rug detergents being 'washed' onto the skin. It goes down in two to three days provided care is taken to avoid on-going cause

Mud Fever

The fairly typical signs of a Dermatophilosis, of

- serous exudate
- crust formation
- erosion

usually first appear on the bulbs of the heels and then spread upwards onto the back (palmar/plantar) aspect of the pastern and sometimes onto the fetlock skin.

An almost consistent main predisposing factor is the wetting of these areas. The coincidental and contributory factors are

- unpigmented hair and epidermis in many horses' limbs – the condition does also affect 'whole' coloured animals – and the associated loss of melanin's protection
- mud contamination, which retains the wetness or prevents natural drying
- a possible coincidental inhibition of Langerham's cells due to UV (ultra violet) stimulation earlier in the summer
- the kinematics of limb action, which explains the presence more frequently in the hind than in the fore limbs

Fever is not an initial sign.

Although Dermatophilus infection is a regular bacterial invader in mud fever, often followed by Staphylococcal species, it is not such a prime inflammatory cause as it is in rain scald. It does seem to require, in addition to the wetness which here is not 'driven' or even just 'rained' onto the skin as with scald, the traumatic abrasive action of

- irritants
    - mud of varying pH and containing hard particle content
    - hoof oil splashes
    - 'wrong' dressings
    - heavily contaminated, dirty (as with dried dirt and grit as well as bacteria) over-reach and brushing boots
- seasonal ectoparasitism
    - mange (chorioptic and less frequently psoroptic) mites although these could be opportunist parasites

- 'chigger' mites
- soil and other sourced bacteria and fungi
- the stress on the skin of the constantly moving joints, especially the creasing at flexion and the following stretch of extension

There is often an on-going effect thus perpetuating the condition. Any Dermatophilus is quickly secondarily contaminated which compounds and complicates the dermatitis leading to

- deeper erosion with bleeding
  - more openings to primary and secondary germs
- delay in healing
- loss of dermal elasticity
- skin fissuring which is
  - painfully opened at the start of locomotion, giving a stringhalt like action to begin with
  - is painful to the touch – beware violent reaction!

Secondary, especially staphylococcal, invasion into the subcutaneous tissues will possibly produce

- suppuration
- cellulitis
- lymphangitis
  - aggravated pain and lameness
  - unwellness
  - systemic illness
- fever

These more variable contributory causes of mud fever produce a serum and altered sebum exudation which, in feathered fetlocks and coarse haired pasterns, appears as a seborrhoea, often called 'grease' or 'greasy heels', where the hair is wet, sticky and matted. In most cases, Dermatophilus also is involved despite the different descriptive name and so too the mange mites.

With insufficient management and less than adequate treatment, the acute condition will subside into the classical (winter) condition of cracked heels – a chronic dermatitis which develops sooner in the heel bulbs (for they are usually earlier acutely affected) and then on the pastern where it is erroneously called an eczema.

This chronic syndrome is really 'cracked heels and pastern'.

In the acute mud fever, when the underlying precipi-

tating factors are controlled and secondary invaders are cleared, the skin heals slowly but the lameness usually disappears quickly. A local cellular immunity quickly develops to finalise the healing process.

Subsequent re-infection may then produce an 'allergic' hypersensitivity reaction to the primary T cellular local immunity not unlike the original acute condition, but with less serous exudate.

If an immunity does not become 'solid', acute relapses are possible. In some post healing situations the weakened keratin, especially of the heel bulbs and related heel horn, is subject to fungal infection which can further erode into the frog and buttresses.

Diagnosis

- the characteristic signs
- the presence of predisposing conditions
  - differentially
    - photosensitisation (in the summer months)
    - chorioptic and psoroptic mange as a primary infection
- initially there is unusual sensitivity to hand and brush touch at routine inspections and grooming
  - the stickiness in the hair, especially if unclipped
  - serum spots on clipped skin, with
    - erythema (redness, with surface vessels gorged with blood) in white skin
    - heat in comparison with other leg
    - mild, first steps, lameness
  - later raw areas with scale and crust formation

Management

- stable or yard the horse out of the predisposing condition
- reduce feed where relevant
- if the lesion is severely acute i.e.
  - lameness for more than six steps
  - swelling
  - marked exudation
  - unpleasant odour

consult your veterinary surgeon for an examination and relevant treatment.

Meanwhile

- animalintex poultice, repeat about one hour later
- wash off with warm water and good quality toilet soap using discardable cotton wool swabs
- antiseptic shampoo, leave 10 minutes, wash off
- artificially dry
- clip hair as close as possible: avoid trauma, use scissors if easier. If too painful, await veterinary sedation
- bed on wheat straw or paper
- *do not* rub on or in any dressings
- follow veterinary surgeon's advice
  - be prepared for possible prolonged antibiotic therapy

If considered to be a 'do it yourself' case
- repeat poulticing twice daily for two to three days to continue softening of exudate
- repeat antiseptic shampoo daily; leave for 10 minutes, rinse, hair dryer dry
  - patiently but carefully attempt to remove crusts etc.
  - constantly consider advisability of veterinary antibiotics

If an extra irritation develops on the skin and under the coat, especially in adjacent areas splashed by the shampoo (or on handler who should of course, be gloved)
- wash off with soap and water, rinse and dry
- consult your veterinary surgeon (and doctor if relevant) – it *may* be a secondary or spreading infection and not a sensitivity reaction, but
- for safety, change the shampoo

Until all focal lesions have settled *do not rub in any ointments*; this could drive remaining infection deeper into the follicles and dermal faults. Afterwards, if the area is 'wet and weepy' apply copiously
- lead lotion
- witch hazel liquid or gel
- calamine lotion

If dry, hard and/or scaly, apply thin film sparingly of humescent/emollient **cream**, not an ointment, such as Dermobion (green).

If, on the other hand, there is a lack of response to 'do it yourself', and there is
- marked seborrhoea
- pus formation
- deep erosion, bleeding
- resistant scales and crust

then repeat poulticing and *get veterinary help*. The vet may advise
  - systemic antibiotics, and for how long
  - a change of antiseptic
  - suitable supportive topical treatment

Prevention
Wherever practicable try to avoid keeping the horse in potentially traumatising conditions
- do not daily graze unsuitable pastures
- do not turn out for part of the day just because it is good practice, particularly if the grazing is
  - rain soaked
  - muddy
    - or if the grazing is so scarce that it is not worth the risk anyway
    - where routine exercise is not possible or required, then hand exercise or
    - turn, one at a time, onto a prepared surface
    - exercise in hand on dry, non irritating surfaces e.g. roads

Where work must continue, as with hunters
- accept the fact that there are no known, effective, safe barrier dressings or even lavaging techniques which will **totally** prevent some
  - maceration from repeated and prolonged wet
  - abrasion from mud at work with consequent activation
  - contagion by bacteria at any time

The very nature of the work means that, to a greater or lesser degree, whatever is applied topically will be
- 'sweated' off
- washed off
- rubbed off and, of course

- antibiotics cannot be given 'for ever, just in case' during a winter season's work

Experience shows that prevention is very much a matter of assuming that each and every work in wet and mud will have contaminated even 'protected' skin with abrasive mud, potentially pathogenic bacteria. The horsemaster should therefore aim for a *thorough cleaning of the areas* after work.

The main advantage of a prework barrier is that it makes the cleaning easier – up to a point. The serious drawbacks are:

- they will shut in bacteria, even help drive them into the pores and follicles unless steps have been taken to 'disinfect' the area first of all; this is of course only possible to a degree
- they may, in the course of application break hairs and abraid the skin; it is very difficult not to have some grit left on the coat and/or in the grease especially
- they can be so messy after the work that some handlers fight shy of making a proper cleaning and leave dressing, mud and germ to be 'taken in' over night
- the decision to clip the distal palmar/plantar area of all four legs at the beginning of a potentially wet season is a difficult one – some think a 'Catch 22' situation

In the experience of most stables

- if feather and hair is left on, the susceptible horse will become affected despite the natural protection afforded by these and
  - early lesions will be more difficult to recognise
- if clipped out, there is a slightly greater risk from the abrasion and the wetting, but the very early signs will be obvious, but beware
  - clipping itself can traumatise
  - use human or dog 'fine' clipper or scissors
  - do not 'shave' too close
- it is a reasonable compromise especially in hunters

The second feature of prevention is

- get rid of the contaminants as soon as possible after work. There are several alternatives
- if a running stream is available walk in that until most if not all the mud is off
  - walk for about a mile to re-stimulate the

circulation and help dry the area
  - check suspect areas for early signs, or
- leave the mud on overnight
  - woollen bandage the legs (but this can pressure the contaminants in)
  - brush off next morning – pick off mud if necessary, but *get it all off*
  - do not use a stiff brush or a scraper, or
- hose down not forgetting the trunk areas (be very careful with pressure hosing, it is and seems more efficient, but can drive contaminants in)
  - again, be thorough
  - dry off legs, especially the pasterns
    - disposable paper towels
  - thoroughly inspect suspect areas for early signs
  - walk exercise on the dry for 10 minutes under required blankets
  - bed in deep straw
  - do not bandage the legs
  - follow as above

In the author's private stables the following protocol is followed

- the mud fever areas will have been clipped (but *not* down to skin level before hunting proper begins or earlier if necessary) and repeated when necessary
- in persistent wet weather and especially if *any* mud is likely to be encountered
  - exercise on the road, and/or in the school for faster work
  - carry on hunting, but be concerned that muddy conditions are also likely to cause
    - loss of shoe and its complications of
    - over reaches, treads and sole bruising

which are difficult to avoid, and any heel or pastern interferences can be an opening for Dermatophilus and other germs

- take extra precautions against possible mud fever
  - after exercise the day before hunting wash legs from fetlock down with half strength antiseptic scrub, leave for ten minutes, walk dry. Consider sponging ventral trunk areas similarly. This leaves some antiseptic barrier on the skin and hair
  - on return from mud contaminated exercise or

hunting, cold hose without pressure all over and especially the danger areas

- critically inspect these for
  - retained mud, which *must be completely got off* even by finger picking
  - any abrasions or interferences which could be a focal point for Dermatophilus
  - any early signs of mud fever
- antiseptic lavage the areas as previously

It has not been found necessary even in white legs to artificially dry off after routine management except walk exercise for fifteen minutes if weather is cold.

When lesions are seen

- soft soap and warm water to clean off even the smallest amount of exudate
- greater attention to antiseptic lavage – very soft nail-brush lathering – twice daily now
- antibiotic therapy right away, e.g.
  - potentiated sulphonamides, orally
  - penicillin (+ streptomycin), intra-muscularly

  both on veterinary prescription
- continue drug for 7 days at least or until activity is cleared
- topical antisepsis at intensive level until resolved
  - with hair dryer drying over affected limb area
  - clean towelling if trunk areas are affected

It is expected that this routine will prevent the dis-ease developing further, but should it 'get away' consideration will be given to

- swab testing for possible presence of infections other than and as well as Dermatophilus
- change of antibiotic if necessary
- use of supportive topical applications
  - lead lotion if very exudative
  - compound ointment/cream such as Dermobion if crusty and cracked
- where crusts are very adhesive, animalintex poulticing for two applications to soften and release these. *Do not forcibly remove*

An affected horse is advisedly not hunted until all exuda-

tive lesions have cleared and any fissures have healed. When work is resumed so too the preventative treatment as above.

The important understanding is that horsemasters must accept that

- the horse is a potential harbourer of dormant Dermatophili
- horses exposed to conditions as previously described will be predisposed to active infection variably likely relative to individual resistance, and that
- awareness of when the condition might develop is of prime importance in prevention

Hunting Dermatitis (Ventral Trunk Mud Fever)

In hunters and other winter cross-country horses working in wet, splashing mud, a skin condition of the ventral abdomen and inner forearms and inner thighs which is an hyperacute mud fever possibly of a hypersensitive type

- a very reactive primary soil particle contact irritant condition, with likely
- secondary Dermatophilosis, or possibly
- Staphylococcal infection

it is usually clinically active by the time the horse returns from hunting.

On the day – if very sore, stiff or dull, get veterinary attention. If not too bad

- antiseptic shampoo gently to remove mud as much as possible
- leave shampoo on, to dry
- hair dryer dry
- bed in deep straw
- reduce hard feed to nil

and then, next morning

- body brush off
- warm water wash with good quality soap to dissolve the sebum/oil exudate if necessary, and follow with
- antiseptic shampoo
- let dry on – hand or horse walker exercise if no discomfort
- if sore and/or sticky exudation continues or dull and off-food begins
  - get veterinary help for suitable oral antibiotic therapy

When back to free moving, much less tender, bright and eating

- slowly increase hard feed
- continue twice daily antiseptic shampoo for at least 5 days, usually longer
- leave to dry or do so artificially
- walk to dry further

Proceed to mud fever preventative measures.

Pastern Eczema

Distal plantar (and palmar) fetlock and pasterns and lateral hocks during 'at grass' periods can become excoriated by

- summer dried, hard clay soil particles as in old mud holes and rolling areas
- winter sharp frozen edges of ruts etc.

These parts of the limbs can then also become infected with saprophytic commensal organisms, e.g.

- dermatophilus to produce coagulating exudative crusts, followed by
- other bacteria, producing deep ulcerative dermatitis with or without pus

OTHER SKIN LESIONS ASSOCIATED WITH WET CONDITIONS

Galloping horses, especially, can so bespatter the anterior surface of their hind cannons that if Dermatophilus is present there, the wet conditions will be sufficient to activate them. The resultant lesion is like a less concentrated form of summer coat rain scald.

Susceptible horses also with unpigmented muzzles grazing in lush grass tend to get mild attacks. In summer this can be confused with sunburn and photosensitisation.

Young stock in wet yards can develop a scaly alopecia around the distal limbs following crusting seborrhoea. It is a variety of mud fever different because of the environment and the lack of exerting locomotory effects.

Cracked Heels

The condition is wrongly described; it may really refer to the pastern in its subacute or chronic stage and inherit the colloquial description 'heels'. The implication of 'cracked' to mean a chronic state is not fully accepted. Certainly the heel may move from the acute stage to the chronic one sooner than the pastern because

- it is an older site in terms of duration of the present dis-ease
- it is not stretched and folded as in the higher area
- if suitably bedded it will dry more readily than the pastern

If it is the pastern then the lesions may be

- a healing stage of mud fever 'kept going' by the functioning folding
- a primary stage of a condition not directly related to a typical mud fever, such as an
  - acute immune reaction
  - external contact allergy
    - leg mange on its own
    - photosensitisation (summer sun!)

In prolonged chronic states an exfoliative dermatitis spreads round the coronary band to give an irregularly rough, horny appearance.

Treatment

- if severe with lameness get veterinary help, otherwise in typical cases
  - treat as for mud fever
  - check elsewhere on leg for other early lesions
    - soothe and soften healed skin with humescent emollient cream
      - udder cream
      - Dermobion (green)
      - lanolin and cod liver oil
  - return to work out of the wet

Atypical Pastern/Cracked Heels

Whether allergic or photodynamic, there is likely to be some associated infection, especially when moist and purulent

- clean and dry softly
- pollen allergy should clear either by
  - changing from pasture to indoors and offering grass cut from elsewhere, or
  - waiting for pollen season to pass, and meanwhile, smearing with veterinary advised steroidal cream
- photosensitisation – consider possible causes

- liver metabolic genetic defect – consult veterinary surgeon
- change pasture or fence off recently dug ditch
- sunburn (has it been sunny?)
  - selective grazing hours
  - UV barrier cream, e.g. Surfer's barrier cream

Therapies for Dermatophilosis

The germ is easily susceptible to a wide variety of anti-septics (and antibiotics) when in the active stage of its invasion of the epidermis. The presence of serum, necrotic tissue, other non-susceptible germs and their pus, does interfere with the efficacy of some topical applications.

When in spore mode within scale and crust, the germ is not so readily got at by most applications, at least in concentrations which are not irritant or toxic to healthy tissue.

Fortunately skin, even dermatitic skin, is generally toxic resistant to, for example, half strength applications of chlorhexidine (which dilution could be toxic in open wounds especially joints).

In prevention management of mud fever, as has been emphasised, the essential aim is to thoroughly get rid of the mud; the methods of doing so have been discussed. A final lavage with a safe antiseptic which is allowed to dry on leaves the susceptible skin with a level of anti-micro-bial protection which goes someway to control subsequent invasion on a day-to-day basis.

In contrast to veneers of cream, ointment and other antibacterial salves, this liquid method avoids the risk of trauma to skin and hair associated with 'rubbing stuff on'.

There is always the chance that an individual horse may react to a liquid antiseptic in the form of a mild blistering of the skin, which would be counter productive in so far as this would 'open' the epidermis to invasion.

If this is experienced, the options are
- use the Hibiscrub in a more diluted form
- change the scrub to Pevidine scrub
- do not leave on to dry, wash off after 10 minutes
- avoid any antisepsis during the physical act of washing the mud off

During any unrelated subsequent need to use an antiseptic wash on this horse, do not forget to
- use it more dilute, say 1:10 not 1:1

- do not rub it in
- certainly do not apply with a stiff brush
- rinse off after 10 minutes soaking

In treatment, the rapidly produced acute stage inflamma-tory exudate, scale and crust must be removed twice daily. This seborrhoeic 'gunge' is sticky and oily, so requires warm water and good quality soap to emulsify and dissolve it for washing off. This cleansing even without antisepsis, is the basic essential

- it removes significant levels of infection
- it cleans the skin, the follicles and any fissures, to allow access for the follow-up antisepsis to the infected area
- the antiseptic recommended (follow your own veterinary's advice) is in the form of a detergent scrub which soon lathers up without excessive friction and finds its way into the skin and related openings and coats them
  - acts there and then
  - for longer unless washed off
- do not rub against the lie of the hair especially if the area is (wrongly) unclipped

Treatment must continue until *no further exudate* develops and *all sores have healed*; this may take a month or more especially if reinfection and further soil abrasion is continued.

The antiseptics suggested are
- Chlorhexidine, e.g. 'Hibiscrub', used 1:1 with water
- Povidone iodine, e.g. 'Pevidine Scrub', used 1:1 with water

These generic antiseptics are the least irritant to equine tissue.

Note, the word 'scrub' is a trade description emphasising the usefulness in 'scrubbing up' of hands and arms before gloving. In horsemastership such cleansing is advisable before dealing with wounds. *In mud fever do not scrub* – a sufficient lather can be obtained by hand and cloth rubbing.

Pevidine is however inactivated in the presence of 'gunge' but remains efficient if initial cleaning is carried out. It is more 'allergic' to the skin of horse and man (who should be wearing gloves anyway) so care is required. It can be a 'reserve' should germ resistance to chlorhexidine or skin irritation seems to be developing.

In those cases where there is evidence of severe acute lesions

• swelling

• heat

• lameness

• worsening despite topical treatment

and where a quick as possible return to work is required then veterinary advice as to systemic antibiotic therapy should be sought

> • the germ is susceptible to Penicillin and to potentiated sulphonamide. Some secondary invaders may require a different antibiotic
>
> • treatment must continue for several days after a clinical cure
>
>> • other topical treatments have been discussed in the earlier text

'Belt and braces' treatment plus hygiene will go a long way to prevent a contagious carrier state remaining quite apart from obtaining a faster acute lesion cure.

In rain scald cases most horse owners are glad when management with or without supporting therapy brings the horse to what appears to be a cure, i.e. areas of alopecia with some new hairs growing through and no further spread.

There is, however, an ongoing possibility of

• low grade activity in the mane and tail hairs which often look unaffected. This is because of a higher level of keratin in the shafts and related follicles, and the fact that most horses have pigmented skin there, together act as reasonably effective barriers against the development of inflammation

• it is in the coming weeks that a real dandruff, hair spiked crusts, can be seen deep near the skin, especially if a parting is made

• these are contagious to others in the usual ways

> • the dormant germ will reactivate when conditions get wet again and become re-invasive and more contagious when it 'swims' onto the shorter coat hairs

The crusts appear as variably sized scurf which does not readily brush off like normal dander or easily wash off. Where they fall are sources of reinfection.

It is important when managing rain scald that **the whole body, with mane and tail,** is involved in the antiseptic shampoos – working from the peripheries onto the lesions – and that after clinical cure these continue once a week for 4 to 6 weeks.

When the crusts are first discovered in a horse the shampooing should be done once daily for seven days during which time the crusts will soften and the spores will activate. Continue once weekly for 4 to 6 weeks to destroy the activated spores.

It is noteworthy that an outwintered pony or a cross is often 'hock deep' yet does not get mud fever; perhaps because

• white distal limbs are uncommon

• the coats (and feathers) are well developed and the sebum is rich and copious

• it isn't exposed to cosmetic washing clean each day

(do not start unless you mean to manage as for a hunter)

• what riding work it does is not usually severe, with consequential

> • over heating
>
> • repetitive friction of flexed skin surfaces as with fast and protracted exercise
>
> • concentrate feeding

It may be that they are (genetically) less susceptible or perhaps more accustomed to soil conditions of a steady pH.

Try to minimise muddy areas by changing field feeding areas daily; no sense in taking chances.

The hunter, on the other hand, is more likely to have one or more white distal limbs. Any feathers will have been removed and his lower limb hair barbered for appearance

• it is boxed except for exercise or work

• it is cleaned up often after work which cleaning is, by definition, usually arduous and painstaking

• it is on concentrate feeding

• its genetic history did not breed evolutionary resistance to mud

It is basically more susceptible and more occupationally hazarded to wet and mud. Hard or spikey bristle brushes must not be used.

Subsequent drying by

- exercise on the dry for one mile
- exercise on the horse walker

will not only dry but encourage

- warming blood to the extremity in a greater amount
- upwards massage of post exercise oedema which is one cause of swollen distal skin which is more susceptible to trauma
- bedding on wheat or oat straw (barley can irritate), paper but not shavings
- bandaging – a compromise decision – is often practised; 'loose' wrapping of mud-coated legs from hoof to knee and to hock in *clean* woollen stable bandages overnight will simplify brushing off the mud the next morning: subsequent antiseptic treatment as before

Irrespective of technique, always thoroughly inspect legs next morning. Do not turn out to suspect/poached grazing just because it is good general practice under other conditions. Daily exercise must of course be carried out.

In the process of grooming, the brushes etc. can become carriers. Hence the requirement for separate kits for each horse and regular disinfection and washing of brushes *and* curry combs used to clean the brushes.

FURTHER TYPES OF BACTERIAL INFECTIONS, USUALLY NON-PRURITIC DERMATOSES

Staphylococci

This behaves like any other coccal germ: it multiplies by cellular division. It also liberates a toxin and has the virulent property of

- producing pus
- entering, either itself or its tissue destructive toxin, into subdermal areas with resultant
  - cellulitis and possible
  - septicaemia
  - toxaemia

It and others like it often invade not only after physical micro traumas, as by excessive wetting, but also following

that caused by Dermatophilus active infection.

Folliculitis

- an infection and subsequent inflammation (a pyoderma) of the hair follicle by bacteria such as
  - **staphylococci**, and less frequently
  - streptococci
  - corynebacteria

  which are secondary to
- superficial cutaneous trauma
- other factors that compromise the skin's defensive barriers
  - prolonged warm, very humid weather, when there is also
  - excessive sweating when exercised
  - poor grooming and after care
  - worn, ill fitting tack including numnahs and leg protectors
  - unhygenic stable and yard conditions

Signs

- seen usually in spring and summer under tack, but not necessarily so, they show as
  - papules
  - pustules
  - crusted, tightly adherent scabs which, when removed, leave
  - pin-head 'spots' of alopecia
  - non-pruritic as a rule, but
  - painful to the touch, making saddling almost impossible

Furunculosis

- an extension of severe and persistent folliculitis, in which
  - the follicle ruptures into the dermis
  - under-runs, and then, in the surrounding area
  - erupts, to produce
  - secondary nodules
  - tracts draining pus
  - crusted ulcers – a more extensive pyoderma

Diagnosis

- by clinical signs
- laboratory determination of the causal germ

Differential

- dermatophilosis (especially mud fever and focal rain scald)
- dermatophytosis (the ringworms)
- can be part of mixed infections, especially on the
  - lower limbs
  - tail and mane, when pruritus is often present

Treatment

- sensitivity determined antibiotic, given preferably parenterally
- antiseptic shampoos
- elimination of any primary or predisposing factors

Fungal

Ringworm Dermatitis (RD) (Dermatomycosis)

This is probably the most common skin disease of working horses. It is caused by infection by a sporulating fungus

- a superficial fungal dermatitis affecting all keratinous portions of the skin
  - hair, especially the shaft, hence the constant associated focal alopecia
- epidermis of the skin
- hoof, especially heels and frog

In most cases, and especially in the earlier stages, there is no pruritus, so no itchy skin reactions, but it may develop in prolonged clinical cases and/or with secondary bacterial infections.

All species of the two main genus are contagious, but, surprisingly, not all by direct contact, horse to horse

- indirect routes are via fomites
  - tack
  - grooming kit
  - blankets
  - rider's boots and spurs
  - stable equipment
  - fencing
  - flying insects
  - mange mites

on all of which the diseases's morbidly produced scales and crusts containing spores can remain contagious.

The spores can persist off the animal for up to 10 years in a dark and slightly damp environment.

Pathogenicity

Ringworm is essentially a group of fungal invaded hair shafts on which the infection multiplies to

- destroy the hair
- descend into the follicle, where further multiplication occurs to
  - destroy the inert keratin to produce a surface papule from the serous exudate later becoming a
  - crusting lesion of less than ($\frac{1}{2}$cm ($\frac{1}{4}$in) diameter (sometimes wider, depending on species of ringworm) which raises the hair above the surrounding skin level
- as the hair shafts break and/or the roots loosen, the affected hair, now stuck to the loosening crust, falls out to expose a
  - flat ovoid to irregularly circular, grey moist, superficially exfoliated epidermal surface. This dries to a dull alopecia with a light scaling
- the periphery of the lesion is ringed with
  - newly formed, more marked, scale inside an
  - active perimeter which continues to expand
  - the outspreading, peripheral lesion develops as originally, but the hair fall is not so great as to be quickly obvious
  - some lesions coalesce with neighbouring ones

The original outbreak varies from one to several, occasionally many, individual sites dependent upon the mode of infection

- satellite, obviously newer, lesions indicate
  - new infection, or
  - direct spread from the originals

Ringworm produces a good skin immune response, thus a prevalence in animals of 4 years old and less. There is

- an eventual self-cure, with
- remission of existing lesions
- cessation of direct spread

* resistance to new infection

the immunity is, to all intents and purposes, solid and certainly for each species of fungus. Rarely is there reactivation of commensal infection or new infection.

Epidemiology
There are two main genus each with two or more species

* trichophytons
  * equinum – horse to horse by fomites (the most common infection)
  * verrucosum – from cattle, indirect through fences' and yard fittings' fomites
* microsporons
  * canis – from dogs and cats
  * gypseum – a soil saprophyte
  * equinum – weakly infectious, via rugs and tack, e.g. saddle pressure areas and insect bites

The horse is susceptible to them all.

Control methods do not involve identification, except for identifying source, but Microsporosis, which is mechanically vectored by fly bites, requires the difficult fly control techniques to aid recovery and stop further infection.

All species respond to treatment more or less equally, which again obviates need for identification. Diagnosis of the actual fact of fungal infection is of course essential from a zoonotic point of view.

A carrier, contagious non-clinical state does exist.

The spore is very resistant to extremes of weather, least so to bright strong sunlight.

Influential factors for prevalence and severity mainly occur in horses at the start of a new period of work

* in 'soft' skin conditions exposed to
  * contaminated tack, grooming kit and rugs (fomites)
* more often in winter time
  * low sunshine
  * damp conditions
* close contact with fomite transmitters
* microsporosis is more frequent during insect activity
* immunity status of exposed animals, and hypersensitive state
* overall health

Coalescence of varying aged lesions eventually present as
* irregular diffuse areas of
* crusts with hair
  * scaly hairless areas
  * dry alopecic areas which are the most diffuse

Spread between horses as well as on a horse is due, as a rule, to ill advised methods of
* grooming
* tacking
* rugging

All horses should have their own grooming kit (but see control, later). Tack is usually, but not always, restricted to one horse.

Sites
* these are related to
* genus of fungus and their mode of transmission
  * tack areas
    * girth ('girth itch')
    * perhaps the saddle, where the germ is readily 'spread' by skin movement under the tack to produce the typical follicular, papular, and crusting formations but with secondary erythema and seborrhoea
    * reins over sides of neck, from initial abrasion by the leather
  * insect vectors feeding areas
  * opportunity for 'horse to affected horse' contact and
  * contact with cattle fixtures, which it rubs with its
    * head
    * neck
    * quarters

in the course of normal bodily self-grooming activity.

Time factors
* incubation period 5 to 10 days
* hair and crust falls away 7 to 10 days after papule rises
* the hair is held longer, even not lost at all, depending on fungal species

- exposed epidermis 'dries' in 2 to 3 days after crust comes away
- lesion is active for up to 40 days, when peripheral scaling ceases
- new hairs extrude before this within the active periphery
- the new satellite papules are obviously distinct from active and inactive alopecic areas

Diagnosis

- the original raised hair papule
- the serial spread
- hair loss
- grey base of lesion
- variable crusting, peripheral scaling
- 'new' satellitic lesions related to
  - seasons of the equine year
    - different discipline horses recently in work in fly activity times
    - 'new' intake contamination from
      - equipment, and opportunity for
      - head to head communication
    - grazing cattle pastures – fences, gate posts etc.

Confirmation and identification

- veterinary opinion
- samples by *plucking* (not scraping) hair from lesion periphery or, less exact, of plaques and crusts, preferably with hair attached for
  - microscopic examination for spores and hyphae
  - culture, usually 20+ days before a negative finding is justified, and for genus/species identification
- laboratory confirmation of 'no activity' is often required for certifying a healed case 'safe' to mix with other horses within racing and other disciplines: a test open to 'mistake' if not done by a veterinary surgeon

Differential consideration

- rain scald (ringwormy hair is not matted)
- mud fever but ring worm is uncommon on limbs except hoof horn areas
  - other bacterial infections
    - folliculitis

- furunculosis
- urticarial lesions
- allergic reactions
- occult sarcoids

Management

- let deliberately spread in discipline's close season to produce immunity
- oral medications
  - the drug e.g. Griseofulvin, is transported via the blood to the germinal layer of the epidermis, where it enters the cells of the follicles, and then the new hair bulbs. Little is known about its excretion in the sebum, or in sweat or, for that matter, the minimal effective dose. The new cells then have to escalate to the respective levels of inert cells to be fungicidal 'on the surface'. A minimal course of 10 days is required. (In humans and dogs, it has been shown to require 6–8 weeks therapy to be effective.) Now thought to be of doubtful value in horses
- topical applications
  - tincture of iodine was an early recommendation, but it was destructive of tissue cells as well as fungi
  - twice weekly with diluted 'Imaverol' all over (apply via a household plant water sprayer) for 5 weeks
  - remove scabs with care and minimal trauma
  - 5% lime sulphur as a surface dressing, and
  - chlorhexidine etc. have been used

Because of the local effective immunity, lesions are usually self curative or 'regressive' and this can imply false positive value to any drug or dressing used

- carefully dispose of crusts, preferably by burning
- 'Virkon' for tack etc. disinfection
- spray buckets, walls, floors etc. disinfection. Rinse out buckets and feed bowls before re-use

It is advisable, however, to discuss with the veterinary surgeon how, and with what, treatment should be affected, to shorten the recovery period, to minimise satellite spread and contagiousness, to decrease the severity.

- identify animal and isolate, i.e. keep in own stable, use equipment only on it, protective clothing for handler who 'does' this horse, only, or at least, last

- disinfect equipment
- fresh protective clothing
- disinfect box
- treat as decided
- do not exercise *vis à vis* tack-affected areas
- see to nutritional supplements; greenfeed, reduction of hard feed
- if available, hand exercise in sunshine (beware of flies if microsporosis)
- monitor progress
- discuss feasibility and value of
  - whole yard medication
  - oral – of very doubtful use
  - topical – of little use if attention to indirect transmission materials is not done daily

Prevention

- careful daily inspection of all horses in the yard which have recently been in unusual/new contact circumstances e.g. temporary stables, or hunting
- care in avoiding such contacts where feasible and
- mix-up of grooming equipment and
- inter-use of tack with that of a new intake
- ignorance (e.g. handling of affected horse, even by offering titbits or giving a friendly pat)
- *isolate new horses for 21 days*
- keep their equipment separate
- disinfect all tack and equipment at beginning of new discipline season if new horses have been admitted
- beware sweating work in hot weather and concomitant tack abrasion on soft unconditioned skin

Photosensitisation

Tissues in a hypersensitive state to the effects of UV light.

Susceptible skin, by definition, has a light, pink dermis of unpigmented dermis and white hair. Usually thin in texture as found on the

- muzzle and face
- back of the pastern
- bulb of the heels

The sun's UV rays are strongest in the summer, less so in the spring and the autumn, and weak in the winter.

The sensitisation can occasionally be from contact with photodynamic plants such as the Trefoil clovers, rye grass etc. It may be a sensitivity to pollen in certain grasses rendering the area superficially sensitive to the photodynamic properties of the sun. It is more usually the result of a systemic hypersensitivity which is 'exposed' in unpigmented areas. These are subject to secondary infection.

The photosensitisation may be primary via the ingestion of photodynamic plants such as the ones mentioned above and St John's Wort.

It may be secondary to

- heredited ineffectiveness of the liver to detoxify the byproducts of chlorophyl digestion, an endogenous intestinal process. The phyloerythrin accumulates in the liver, does not escape via the bile but re-enters the circulation as a photodynamic substance. It stimulates inflammatory mediators which enter neighbouring dermal cells with photodynamic trauma. This is restricted to limb sensitivity
- certain plants and chemicals which give off photosensitive metabolites into the blood which cause liver damage with failure to detoxify

Signs

- erythema, oedema, necrosis, cracking and peeling
- in severe cases skin swelling, vesicles and weeping
- on the face and on the extremities

Treatment

- shelter from sun's rays (and remember that UV passes through glass)
- attempt to change from suspected pastures

If this is ineffective, suspect a liver pathology, acute or chronic. In some cases there are signs of hepato encephalopathy, a CNS disturbance.

The topical treatment is antibiotic and corticosteroid creams, palliative lotions and barrier creams of high intensity. Do not use antiseptics and dehydrating dressings.

It is *always worthwhile*, whatever type is suspected, to check for liver damage by laboratory examination of blood samples. Whilst a hepatic pathology is usually incurable, the other types are variably manageable as described; parenteral administration of

- thiamine
- choline
- glucose

can be supportive. Consult the veterinary surgeon.

A somewhat similar lesion develops in the pastern dermis as the result of a vasculitis and thrombosis of unknown origin in which an acutely painful weeping lesion develops in unpigmented distal limbs. This is distinct from acute mud fever and photosensitisation. Diagnosis is a specialised matter.

Differential Diagnosis

- old pastern injuries
- cracked heels from previous winter's mud fever
- straight sunburn on the face and muzzle of the light skinned (flesh marked) animals. The distal limbs are rarely involved in this

Ectoparasites and Related Disease

Ecto, 'outer'; *dermis*, 'the skin'.

Many species of arthropods 'use' animals, via the skin, as a
- habitat for all or certain stages in their
  - life cycle
    - on the surface
    - in the various depths of the
      - epidermis
      - dermis
- source of nourishment from 'eating' (biting)
  - hair
  - epidermal squames and the
  - sebum which 'coats' these, and from 'drinking' (sucking)
  - blood
  - serum, having 'pierced' into the dermis

Ectoparasites are seasonally intermittent in their prevalence or persistent. The host's response is
- irritation from the crawling or
- a traumatic effect from burrowing anthropods
- a hypersensitive effect from
  - toxins liberated by killed invaders (unusual)
  - toxins from the mouth parts of feeding parasites

- saliva required to make inert keratin 'soluble' in deeper tissues for piercing by the mouth 'parts'

resulting in a
- simple itch, a mild pruritus
- complicated by
  - mechanical excoriation by the host's
  - nibbling
  - rubbing, and further
    - secondary infection and/or further
    - compounded by the allergic hypersensitive reactions

The overall effect is a
- dermatitis of varying types and degree which is of
  - erythema in the early stages (not easily visible in a horse) with basically
  - dry lesions, but also
  - exudative, with
    - scaling
    - crusting
    - alopecia, and later
  - hyperkeratinisation and
  - lichenification

Some reactions are such as to classify the arthropod as a true pathogen, others as an irritating, disturbing pest which is rarer.

THE IMMUNE RESPONSES AS RELATED TO ECTOPARASITISM AND OTHER SKIN INFLAMMATIONS

There is much still to be learnt about these responses by an animal to the stimuli of 'non self' substances which gain entrance to their tissues; the **allergenic** or **hypersensitivity responses**.

It follows that there are still significant gaps in our ability to
- treat
- control
- prevent

such unwanted (wrong response) dis-eases of this nature, of which many, if not most, are exhibited *in, or on, the skin.*

The associated morbidity is loosely called 'allergic'. Since the tissue response falls within the group type Inflammatory, the standard almost empirical treatment is to shut down the cascade of inflammatory events which follow the basic disturbance of most cell disintegration by administering steroidal and other anti-inflammatory drugs. More specific therapy may, thereafter, be used if and when the precipitating cause is diagnosed.

Immunology is sometimes defined as the study of the mechanisms that an animal uses to

- preserve its biological identity
- recognise 'non self', and
- reject it, or
- attempt to limit its invasive effect, and to
- resolve the morbid damage
- 'remember', for future recognition and immediate counter action, the specific antigenic features of the invader

The mechanisms and the responses as exhibited by a reaction, are influenced by

- the animal's existing defence potential
    - genetic or acquired
- the antigen's potency to 'stimulate'

The memory is called **allergy**, or the state of being allergic. The animal is sensitised or programmed against subsequent specific antigenic (anti-allergic) stimuli. When the allergy is more or less fully protective, the animal is said to be immune. When the allergy is associated with cellular morbidity at subsequent stimulation (as distinct from primary dis-ease), the animal is said to have previously been made hypersensitive, not fully immune. It is, therefore, more scientifically correct, to call allergic disease a **hypersensitivity dis-ease**.

There is ever-increasing evidence that heredity does play a significant role in determining

- the degree of immunity (and 'memory') naturally attained
- the manner in which the allergy 'shows itself' or not, on subsequent challenge

Not all is as simple as even this! In skin reactions, there

are some which are not immune-related, at least in the first exhibition of the morbidity. Once again, however, there is a balance between the cellular toxic 'attacker' and the animal's tissue resistance or 'strength'. Some animals could be said to have tougher, more resilient, skin than others – or *vice versa*.

To make confusion worse confounded, some 'toxins', as prime irritants or traumatic factors, have a secondary allergenic component which not only leads to a hypersensitive state, but increases this with subsequent repetitive assaults.

At the first time, an anaphylactic reaction is potentially present. Its clinical effect with subsequent attacks is progressively more likely to cause this to the extent of being lethal e.g. the wasp sting progressive effect in repeated attacks in humans, which has not been recorded in equines. Massive single occasion assault, as with wasp swarm stings, can be immediately lethal from sting toxaemia and subsequent traumatic shock in horses: there is a hypersensitising possibility but no time to develop it.

Some animals have an hereditable predisposition greater than others to forming sensitising antibodies to

- environmental allergens (antigens) of
- the pollen of
- grasses
    - weeds
    - trees
    - mite dust

which can be

- (ingested)
- inhaled
- skin 'contaminated'

and the related hypersensitivity is then located

- indirectly via the blood onto the skin or
- directly onto the epithelial cells

This condition is called **atopy**, which when challenged in, or on, the skin, reacts with

- excoriations (with direct contact contamination)
- exudation in all cases, followed by
- exfoliation of the superficial epithelia
    - alopecia
    - pruritus

Secondary self-mutilation or repetitive challenge will produce

- scales
- crusts

and, if the dis-ease is prolonged

- hyperpigmentation
- lichenification

Atopy is primarily a Type 1 (immediate) immune response to mast cell degeneration, and active substance release.

A CLINICAL SUB-DIVISION OF IMMUNE RESPONSES, ALLERGIC SKIN DISEASE

Urticaria

Or 'hives' (from the Latin *urtica*, 'nettle) in man is almost always accompanied by pruritus; in equines the patient is often unaware of the condition

- it exhibits as characteristic weals arising from
  - vascular induced oedema in the dermis which
    - may arise suddenly as
    - a single swelling lasting 1 to 2 days
    - a waxing and waning swelling over a few days or be
    - long term (7 to 8 weeks) prolonged waxing and waning, variable in degree and in inter-mittency

Signs

- multiple weals
- ovoid or linear or mixed
- centrally depressed (doughnuts)
- soft, depressible, occasionally firm
- overlying skin is normal
- subcutaneous oedema may spread outwards
- the skin over this may exude serum
- there is no alopecia
- there is rarely pruritus

Causes

- immunological association
  - allergic

- atopy
- idiosyncratic intolerance to foodstuffs and drugs
- reaction to plant stings and other toxins
  - the nettle
  - insect saliva hypersensitivity
- insect bites

In most of these there is a marked

- hive formation
- with nettles, there is, in addition, a *very marked pruritus* with
  - frenzied behaviour, or conversely the fear or worry of the pain inducing a reluctance to move from a lying down position
- insect bites produce
  - papular lesions, limited hives, and rarely pruritus
- in association with, but not clearly explicably so
  - drugs and vaccines
  - infections
  - endoparasites
- dermatographism – pressure effects of
  - tack
  - whip strikes
- from contact with external applications
  - shampoos
  - antiseptics
  - insecticides

which may also be contact erosive irritants.

Sites

- head
  - eyelids
  - muzzle
- ventral abdomen
  - brisket
- extremities or
- wherever contact causes 'make contact'

A quite common condition variously described as

- 'heat' bumps
- 'food' rash
- itchy skin

showing as an urticarial reaction, but not always with typical weals, is very difficult to identify as to cause.

It could be from
- internal sources
  - food, especially some cereals
  - excess intake of molasses
  - new hay – immature amino acids
- external sources
  - change of bedding to
    - some treated wood shavings
    - barley straw
  - parasitic infestation

Most are associated with pruritus.

The 'bottom line' in the true urticarias is the triggering of mast cell degradation, with the liberation of active compounds, especially histamine, which specifically cause vascular leakage of plasma and consequent angio-oedema. In humans (and possibly in equines), these are recognised as

- exercise induced, increased body core temperature urticaria, often called a sweet itch, and so sometimes a pruritus with hives
- non-exercise-induced cholinergic hives, also with body core temperature rises, part of a dis-ease condition causing fever as part of the reaction
- psychogenic hives (This may be associated with [unknown] virus infection, a form of shingles)

Differential
- just possibly early ringworm
- other papular and nodular dis-eases

Management
- try to identify cause
- topical soothing agents
- parentral steroids – low dosage over longish term under strict veterinary control: may have to be Intravenous for a quick result. (Beware laminitis consequently in ponies)
- usually self cure but
  - stop suspected access and administration, or

wash off to get rid of all possible contaminants, natural or artificial

Control
- prevent exposure to known or suspected agents by horses suspected or known to be idiosyncratic

In certain intolerance suspected urticarias, there is doubt as to the involvement of allergy, but a mast cell degradation is clearly involved by the associated
- hives
- itch – often restricted to tail and mane rubbing, and so to a local alopecia there, or
- to an itch with rubbing and biting (flanking)
  - over ribs and flanks, with much self-mutilation

Most are short lived. Some are seasonal and possibly related to food intake changes.

The self mutilation types on mane, tail and flanks can persist as
- chronic crusting
- alopecia
- lichenification

Differential diagnosis
- sweet itch (as colloquially known in horses)
- pin worm infestation
- other causes of hives
- ectoparasites
- dermatophilosis (chronic carrier state, much less likely if any pruritus)

Intradermal immune reaction identifying tests can be considered as possible aids to diagnosis of skin disorders (and other systemic allergen associated dis-ease), particularly the atopies when skins presenting with

- papules and/or nodules and especially
- urticaria and/or
- pruritus

which cannot be identified and diagnosed clinically, and/or by the usual laboratory tests as
- infectious
- neoplastic

- degenerative
- traumatic
- physical contact
- irritant
- thermal
- photodynamic
- biochemical (ingested)
- poisons via blood to the dermis and so to the epidermis, e.g.
  - arsenic
  - mercury
- auto-immune

are then suspected as being allergenic hypersensitivities of immediate or delayed types, such as are the result of immune stimulation by

- biting insects
- free living mites
- food and drug idiosyncrasies
- inhaled antigens (to produce atopy)

the allergic state theoretically should be focally inducible in the skin by appropriate minute intradermal injection.

A series of different 'known' antigens covering the range of possible causes of the skin disorder in doubt are injected into the dermis of the patient.

The skin is observed at short intervals up to 12 hours, then twice daily for the next day and again (usually) on the 48th hour for signs of a typical papular enlargement.

Pruritus (scratch reflex) and circumferential weal formation are also looked for.

The induced lesions may simulate the original clinical ones, but a 'reaction' is the important clue, on which a diagnosis is confirmed. Treatment prescribed, if possible, and preventative measures taken, where practicable.

Research continues. This could also lead to the safe and practical application of desensitisation techniques. Sweet itch is a good example of a hypersensitivity much in need of this.

Recent work on the vascular permeability of the skin of insect hypersensitive ponies has clearly shown that histamine is involved in both early and late cases of a hypersensitive reaction.

Ectoparasites

There are several classes of the phylum Arthropoda, within which some genus are recognised as pathogenic, one way or another:

Class	Insecta	
Order	Anoplura	lice
	Hymenoptera	bees and wasps
	Diptera	flies

Class	Arachnida	
Order	Acarida	mites and ticks

Lice

Pediculosis is the name of infestation by these small, wingless insects, visible to the naked eye, variably yellowish-brown in colour

- the biting louse – Haematopinus asini
  - short legs and antennae
  - body flattened, dorso-ventrally
  - broad, flat, rounded head
    - prefers the finer, shorter hairs of the
    - head
    - dorso-lateral trunk

- the sucking louse – Damalinia equi – *larger* than the above so more visible
  - longer legs with 'claws'
  - body also flattened dorso-ventrally
  - bigger, sharper, pointed head (for obvious reasons)
    - prefers the coarser hairs of the
      - mane
      - tail and croup
      - lower limbs, and especially 'feathers' area of the fetlock

Both types are more active in the winter and early (cold) spring.

The housed horse is **less actively infested** because it is

- usually clipped out
- less in direct contact horse to horse, nevertheless,
- grooming and communal rugs are a source of contagion

The horse 'at grass' is more heavily and **more actively**

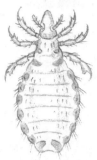

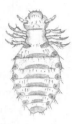

sucking louse   biting louse

infested, especially all over with the sucking louse, as it has a

- thicker coat which protects the lice
- ungroomed manually
- often 'huddles' with others
  - for warmth, and
  - in pairs for mutual, natural grooming, and so
    - contact or direct contagion is much more likely

On the horse, the adult louse travels over its predilection areas. Here eggs are deposited into the coat where they **adhere**, as nits, to the hairs; these are resistant to therapy before hatching in 10–14 days, to become larvae which moult 2–3 times during next 2–3 weeks to become adults, which depending upon their genus bite to ingest inert keratin and dried sebum or pierce the epidermis to suck blood and other fluids.

The two types are

- obligatory parasites: they cannot breed off the host, they die in 2–3 days after falling off involuntarily
- host specific – each species has its own louse species. Cross-over infestation to another animal species causes early death of the parasite

Pediculosis, being lice infested or 'lousy', is maintained year to year by some quiescent or inactive

- adults
- larvae
- nits (over the summer and autumn months)

with reactivation in mid winter, usually (northern hemisphere) *November to March*. All stages, except the nits, are susceptible to appropriate parasiticides.

In the absence of specific treatment pediculosis is self perpetuating.

The pathogenic effect of pediculosis is due to their respective activity

- running through the coat, and either
- gnawing at hair, follicle, and epidermal scale, or
- piercing the epidermis

which causes a pruritus of such a degree or intensity, that the resultant 'self mutilation' results in

- scurf formation
- extensive loss of hair – it doesn't fall out from the biting *per se* but from the rubbing against fences, walls etc.
- broken mane hairs
- 'rat' tail formation

In severe, uncontrolled infestations, there is also skin excoriation and deeper abrasions, self-inflicted with possible secondary infection

- coarse, broken, and sometimes matted coat
- large areas of alopecia
- dry scaly skin
- scurf from the rubbing
- restlessness and consequent
  - reduced feed intake
- possibly anaemia (with sucking lice)
- increased susceptibility to the effects of
  - internal parasites
  - intercurrent dis-ease – and *vice versa*. Such otherwise dis-ease animals are more prone to severe pediculosis

Diagnosis

- the persistent rubbing
- the increasing scurfiness
- alopecia with
- skin folds in prolonged untreated cases
- visualising the
  - adult in the coat, mane and tail
  - nits glued to the hairs: seen best in

- sunlight, or
  - focussed artificial light
- adults, fine combed out onto paper
- nits adherent to loose hairs, groomed out

Differential Diagnosis (rarely difficult)

- season – winter/early spring compare summer/early autumn of sweet itch, except for its chronic lesions of hypersensitivity on localised areas
- rain scald – more diffuse, less pruritus
- mange infestations – more *localised*, less hair loss from affected areas
- ringworm – more delineated lesions
- lice are *macroscopic*

Management

- topical insecticides – discuss up to date 'permissibles' with your veterinary surgeon
- beware, *some cattle preparations are irritant on equine skin*
- whatever is used should be repeated three times at 10-day intervals to 'catch' emergent larvae from the resistant nits. If done correctly this should effectively break the life cycle – on the treated animals. They will remain liable to contact reinfestation from untreated horses. There is no important or significant immunity development

Prevention

- three dressings at around 10-day intervals, especially of those horses at grass, in December and January (northern hemisphere), or begin earlier if weather cold
- beware rubbing and nibbling
- investigate
- treat appropriately
- maintain good winter nutrition
- maintain good worm control in the autumn especially

against hibernating small redworms

Ivermectin – (Eqvalan) dosed November and December (northern hemisphere) is reputed to be antilice, especially the sucking type but is not yet substantiated officially. Newer formulations are being developed to have a greater affinity for the epidermal germ layer, and possibly sebum, and so more lethal to the biting louse as well.

Hymenoptera – The Stinging Insects – Bees and Wasps

The 'sting' is usually a modified egg laying appendage and therefore is found only in the female. A bee has only 'one sting in it'; when used it dies after leaving the stinging organ in the animal stung. Wasps do not eject the sting, only the poison. Neither require the horse as a source of food or a breeding habitat.

They invariably sting in self defence, but this does not stop them alighting in the hope of foodstuff contaminating horse skin, *muzzle*, *lips*, and *eyes*, and hair anywhere, or when the horse nuzzles into a feed bin in which a wasp or bee is investigating. Occasionally, the inside of the lips are stung, but rarely further in. Reactions in the horse vary

- the buzz and touch irritation involve shaking or swishing off, which may trigger a sting but usually do not
- swarms are potentially dangerous and provoke more reaction from the horse – evasive galloping
- more stings – more risk of lethal shock
- individually and collectively, the sting poison causes toxic
  - erythema
  - papule formation with infiltration of lymphocytes
  - plaques
  - marked oedema, particularly around the eyes and, if a wasp or bee is swallowed, then mouth and throat will swell inwardly
  - oedema of the throat could be a possible asphyxiating reaction

There is little confirmed evidence of hyper-reactivity to intermittent serial stings, as recorded in humans.

Prevention

- nil

Management

- individual or few stings
  - if 'sting' is in site, do not pull out with fingers which may break the sting and leave a part behind – use tweezers and grip below the sting bag (of a bee). The horse is usually so pained that to do even that is difficult and dangerous to the handler
  - acid and alkaline dressings are useless, but
  - tepid water foments, followed by

- cooling lotions plus oatmeal paste; menthol and camphor, or thymol tinctures, can be applied
- swarm attacks
  - *get veterinary help* – don't wait 'to see how it will go'

The Flies (Diptera Insects) – The Biting Flies

This is the most numerous group of equine skin potential parasitic pathogens. Each species is seasonally numerous, some, like house flies and midges, particularly so. Some **bite through the skin** to obtain blood and in so doing are able to 'pick up' blood borne micro-parasites and 'transmit' them to other hosts. These flies are particularly likely to cause **skin reactions** by their piercing.

Some transmit as **mechanical carriers**, on their limbs and mouth parts, viruses, bacteria, fungi and helminth ova.

It is when large numbers of them, as with house flies, **feed off natural fluids**, eye tears, or unnatural fluids, wounds and other discharges, that they become particularly annoying and, even more importantly, inflammatory, directly or through the secondary contagion they carry.

In considering arthropods as direct causes of skin disease, it should not be forgotten that certainly amongst the Dipteras there are several which do not alight, let alone feed.

Their visual and audible presence is such however, as to trigger

- self preservation reactions
- skin twitch
- head tossing
- tail swishing
- stamping
- snorting
- kicking
- evasive running away

These are all behaviour changes. Some 'feeders' will stimulate such action but also clinical skin lesions when evasions have not been effective.

Horse owners are only too well aware of the nuisance value of flies when their presence, seen, heard and felt, causes disruption of grazing of horses at pasture and others in hand or when ridden.

In many cases, discomfort to themselves by skin irritation and painful bites is an added liability.

The flies are particularly annoying in late spring to autumn, even to the extent of making riding almost impossible during the day.

With the important exception of the midge, all horse related 'flies' are

- relatively large
- distinctly marked
- rarely arrive in swarms or large numbers, more often 'alone' (again, except the midge and the house fly)
- cause disproportionate un-ease

It is these characteristics perhaps, which make them seem particularly important in human minds. Perhaps, too, they have an understandable reputation of being 'dirty and horrid'.

Stable Fly – Stomoxys calcitrans

- a greyish, brown striped insect about the size of a house fly, perhaps bigger
- unlike the house fly, they sit head up, tail down, relative to the vertical elevation of resting places, and hold their wings divergent when resting
- up to 800 eggs may be laid in a lifetime, usually a month. These hatch in 1–4 days or longer in cold weather. The larvae feed on the vegetable matter and mature in 14–24 days of warm. Pupation takes place in drier material: it takes 6–9 days but much longer in the cold. A life cycle can be about 30 days
- they breed in faeces and and especially in rotting bedding (thus the need for good stable management) and other vegetable waste
- they prefer, and are most active, in bright sunlight
- there is a day-to-day variation in their presence
- they fly from late spring to autumn but only in short distances
- they feed intermittently, and usually go from one horse to another before being satiated with blood
- their bite is often marked by an escape of blood which attracts other flies, usually the house fly
- their saliva produces papules and weals (urticarial reaction)
  - up to 4mm (⅙in) in diameter, with

- erect hairs, and eventually a
- central crust
- the feeding sites are usually the
  - lower limbs
  - ventral abdomen
  - chest
  - back

The bite, as judged by equine reaction and human subjective description, is often painful at the time. When a hypersensitivity reaction follows soon after, it is invariably persistent for a while, hours or days.

Ridden and in-hand horses which, by definition, are not free to exercise their natural self defences, can become difficult, often very much so, when one or two flies attack.

The bite hole can be invaded by bacteria, fungi, especially Microspora gypseum, or at the original attack by protozoa and helminth ova.

Management (of the bite)

- rarely required
- the primary and secondary pruritic effect varies
- if, however, a horse is attacked by several flies at a time, the resultant pain and fear can lead to
  - excessive foot stamping
  - severe evasive action
    of such a nature that
- sedation may be required and supportive steroidal antipruritic therapy given

Less severe reactions will often respond to topical application of soothing/cooling agents

- witch hazel lotion or gel
- alum sulphate lotion
- 'lead' lotion
- bicarbonate of soda paste
- calamine lotion

Prevention (of attack)

- stable and muck heap management
- fly repellent dressings are available, but because of equine sweating they are quickly
  - diluted
  - evaporated
    some may prove to be contact irritants
- tags plaited into mane and tail 'show promise'
- house in bright sunshine if practicable
- provide grazing area shade
- horses will often voluntarily stand in the smoke of wood fires

The 'Horse Fly', 'Blind Fly', or 'Cleg' (in Scotland) – Tabanus Species

- large, brownish with longitudinal stripes
- up to 2cm (1in) long
- the eggs are laid in the vicinity of water, usually on plant leaves
- the larvae hatch after 4 to 7 days and drop into water to disappear into the mud. They are carnivorous, even cannabalistic, grow for 2 to 3 months, moulting several times, before pupating for about 2 weeks. Low temperatures may delay the life cycle from 4 months to a period of hibernation
- the adults fly in summer, especially in bright sunlight, particularly on hot humid days
- they feed on the
  - ventral abdomen near umbilicus
  - legs
  - neck and withers
  - muzzle
- they bite the one horse several times to reach blood

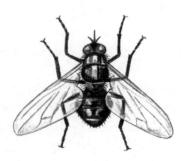

Stable fly (Stomoxys calcitrans).

repletion

- blood leaks from the site for a while and is consumed by house flies
- the bite is very painful and irritating, producing papules with a haemorrhagic central ulcer and later a scab
- they feed every 3 days and then shelter under leaves and stones

Management

As for Stomoxys for the bites.

Prevention (of attack)

- horses seem to get even more protection against Tabanoids by standing in smoke
- Oil of White Birch is commonly used by Scottish anglers against midges, clegs and mosquitoes. A few drops under a horse's belly and down the mane is helpful, when clegs become more than a usual nuisance
- restrict grazing in daylight away from pond etc. breeding and swarming/breeding sites
- stable horses where practicable when daytime conditions demand protection. Gauze doors will prevent access to flies (but not midges)
- in winter or cold weather, the adults often congregate in long clusters under eaves; these are easily brushed down and burned

Black Fly. Simulium Species, the Humped Back (Thorax) Fly. 'Gnat' in some Countries

- dark coloured
- relatively small
- eggs are laid on stones and plants just under water. Hatch in 4–12 days (temperature controlled)
- larvae moult several times in running water
- pupa develops in a water surface cocoon
- adult most active
  - early mornings
  - evenings
  - spring and summer
- do not enter buildings

Feeds on sites on the

- head
- ears
- ventral abdomen
- legs

The bite is very painful, a blood sucker. The saliva, in addition to antigens, releases a strong toxin causing

- increased capillary permeability
- epidermal papules and weals
- vesicles which erupt
  - haemorrhagic

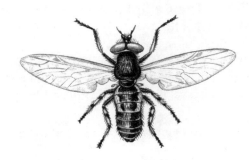

Horse fly (Haematopota pluvialis).

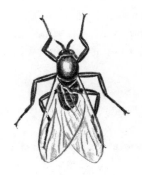

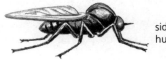

side view, showing humped thorax

Simulium equinum.

- necrotic sequelae
- said to transmit Papillomata virus onto muzzle and possibly the ear pinnae; healed lesions of the initial reaction and coincidental viral transmission onto the skin by the feeding gnat are
    - papillary acanthosis – **ear plaques**

The flies cause considerable annoyance and restlessness. Severe attacks lead to evasive behaviour. Swarm attacks: stampede group and multiple bitten animals are possibly liable to toxaemic death.

Management
As for other insect bites.

Prevention
is difficult

- adults have long flying time and range – 6km (4m)
- larvae are
    - under water
    - in running water
- *larvicidal treatment therefore would be pollution of river water*
- selective grazing 'away from water' is not effective
- repellent tags and sprays are a possibility

Other Flies

- the common house fly – **Musca domestica**
    - breeds in fresh manure preferably horse
    - the adult lives only a few weeks in summer, but during colder weather it 'slows down' to give a longer lifespan up to and including, occasionally, hibernation
- eggs hatch in 12 to 24 hours
- larva grows into maggot in 3 to 7 days which moult three times
- pupates in the ground for 3 to 30 days (temperature controlled)
- but the whole cycle *can* be completed in 12 days – so mass production of several generations in one summer
- the eggs, larvae and pupae, if protected, over-winter to produce next spring's crop (that's where the flies go in winter time!)
- the breeding and feeding habits make it a ready carrier

of bacteria and parasitic ova: its hairy legs pick them up as it wanders over faeces and rubbish

- it regurgitates to assist in further feeding, so that widespread contamination of human and animal feeds occur
- it often 'cashes in' on residual blood at the site of true blood sucking flies. It does not suck, it 'drinks' eye tears and wound exudates as well
- it is a worry to animals, causing restlessness and feeding interruptions
- it causes conjunctivitis with purulent tear flow which causes nasal gleet, a persistent nasal discharge with mucosal and epidermal changes at the nostrils. An overspill of this 'pussey' fluid will eventually excoriate the facial skin just below the medial canthus of the eye as well as the nasal signs
- it 'irritates' granulation tissue and *may* stimulate mutation therein to **sarcoid formation** and, of course, transmits secondary bacteria into wounds
- it transmits infections from animal to animal

Management
Since it does not suck blood directly, nor bite keratin, there is no direct skin lesion. The secondaries have to be treated as and if they develop.

Prevention and Control
These are aimed at the breeding grounds

- muck heaps: proper 'building' will create inimical heat to desiccate eggs and larvae
- discarded rotting feedstuffs, and
- unwashed utensils

Blow Flies – The Calliphorinae – Maggot Worm Flies

- the adult is 'bee' sized
- usually of a bright, metallic colour, green or blue, with brown or golden yellow markings; Green/Blue Bottle flies
- it flies (northern hemisphere) from April to September

A generation, subject to protein food and warm weather, can be as short as seven days. Several generations in one year are thus possible.

The flies breed by depositing their eggs in, and feeding from

- organic matter as it decomposes as in
  - dead animals
  - wounds in live animals
  - moist, rubbed-together surfaces – under tail root, between thighs

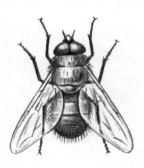

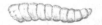
larva

Blow fly, Greenbottle (Lucilia caesar).

The larvae or maggots devour the tissues and drop off after a few days.

The resultant number of maggots and their activity is **myiasis**: parasitism by Dipterous (fly) larvae. The pupae live in the soil and their development is very temperature controlled; they may hibernate.

Myiasis is of greatest importance in sheep. In horses, the correct microclimate of

- wetness
- warmth is found in
- low grade bacterial activity e.g. necrotic heel and pastern wounds and
- in wounds which are
  - not wide open to the air, yet not fully closed, and in
  - lobulated melanomata in the perineal region, which become ulcerated
- paradoxically in myiasis the maggots
  - debride and
  - clean wounds to leave a healthy surface (if left too

long tissue erosion can become deep) and have been controllably used to do this.

Management

- all deep pockets, crevices and 'hidden' areas of wounds and ulcers must be
  - searched and
  - exposed when
  - maggots are readily
    - manually removed and/or flushed out
    - killed by insecticide (sheep dip, for example, but query permissible use)
- the wounds are then managed normally

Prevention

- monitoring and managing wounds being suitable traps
- regularly inspecting susceptible tumour masses
- in summer, especially in
  - hot, humid conditions, where necessary, applying
- insecticide at regular intervals

Culicoides – Midges (Associated Skin Disease is Sweet Itch)

In the UK the species of midge invariably involved is that

- active between late afternoon and dusk
- with preferential feeding sites
  - the long (coarse) hair of the mane at the wither end of the neck
  - occasionally more rostrally
  - occasionally the outside of the ear pinna
  - especially the dorsal root of the tail
- the consequential hypersensitivity to second and subsequent liberations of saliva onto the base of the hair, into the follicles and onto the epidermis, causes the most marked of skin hypersensitivity reactions
  - erythema (not readily seen)
  - congestion of the skin (can be felt) but especially
  - severe pruritus with consequent
    - nibbling

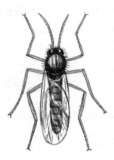

Culicoides.

- rubbing (often frantic) by the animal
- dermatitis
- excoriation open to
    - secondary infection

all incorporate the adjacent skin and hair areas
- the primary dermatitis is susceptible to the sun's rays, leading to
    - acute solar burn (photodynamic dermatitis)
    - increased pruritus
    - further infection

At the end of the midge season, the acute lesions 'die back' to leave
- alopecia
- broken hairs in and around the sites
- hyperkeratitis
- 'Buzzed mane' (USA)
- rat tail (UK)
  which worsen each year

The midge is reputed to be a mechanical transmitter of Onchocerca worm larvae.

There is strong evidence for a familial tendency or susceptibility to bite hypersensitivity, an Atopy. It is most common in ponies and pony crosses of all ages and of all sexes.

It is not surprising that a descriptive, disease name 'itch' is given, but why 'sweet'?

Diagnosis
Is based on

- late spring to early autumn acute attacks
- characteristic morbidity, producing more lesions from photosensitisation and/or secondary bacterial infection

Differential Diagnoses Include
- characteristic behaviour to effect rubbing of the affected areas: the pony will stop *whatever* it is doing to rub when the itch starts up
- seasons of the year compared to the less pruritic acute rain scald
- subacute and chronic lesions of
    - healing dermatophilosis
    - some manges
    - allergic tail 'eczema'
    - tail staphylococcal dermatitis

Management
- stable affected animals from
- 16.00hrs until dark, or overnight if more convenient
- install insect repellent strips to building interior

Note: the midge is smaller than a mosquito, and so can pass through mosquito netting, and so
- during bright sunshine keep in shade at shows etc. or
- fit a white (reflective sheet) over attack areas between classes or lessons if no shade available
- when at grass, bring in as suggested
- under veterinary supervision – at least at first, e.g.
    - short, quick acting injectable steroids (beware risk of laminitis and, to a lesser extent, predisposition to secondary infection)
    - midge repellent lotions mixed with organic oil, to prevent midge getting a foothold! (the slippery pole!)
    - Benzyl benzoate preparations are soothing and healing as well as insecticidal
    - antiseptic lavage if secondary infection is present

Prevention
- basically as for management, certainly for
- known subjects as judged from their
    - history and

- clinical signs of chronic lesions
- related animals
- precautionary anti-midge dressings on withers and dock areas
- where feasible, hogging of mane should reduce attractiveness for the midge

Long-acting injectable steroids have been used as a preventative of the allergenic or hypersensitivity response. The duration of their effectiveness is often less than anticipated, or advertised! 2 to 4 week intervals at most. They have been considered in the first year of signs, after resolution of the initial lesions, as a complement to management. But they are

- expensive
- hazardous *vis à vis* laminitis risk and bacterial infection
- often disappointing
- tend to be progressively more so

In ponies, and so ridden and/or handled by young children, the behaviour often over-rules control. The pony backs up against wall, or runs under low branches and 'brushes off' the rider

Gastrophilus Intestinalis (Bot) and Other Species

Inclusion of the next two Diptera species – the equine Bot fly and the bovine Warble fly – is justified in that they use the horse's hair for egg-laying.

The latter's development requires an escape route through the dorsal epidermis for its larvae, albeit, usually in vain. It is almost 'extinct' in the UK now that the bovine disease has been almost eliminated. The adults

- are not pathogenic
- they do not sting
- they do not bite or suck to feed
- their larvae are pathogenic
- their eggs are not susceptible to lethal applications; physical removal is difficult, even impracticable
- the live warble larva via its escape hole is exposed to lethal dressings – in horses, the bovine warble does not live to maturity
- the equine stomach bot is susceptible to medication, but unlike the warble with its obvious damage to

(bovine) hide and the economic need to eradicate it, the bot is not visible as a

- clinical entity, nor does it as a rule produce clinical illness, or at least, proven as such, except for subjective signs of general improvement in health after dosing against it
- specific dosing for helminths with Eqvalan or Equest should eliminate most bots

Most importantly, the presence of the flies of both these species attempting to deposit their eggs causes evasive action by the attacked animal. The warble fly is, not for nothing, called the **gad fly**, primarily in cattle, less so in the horse.

The bot fly certainly annoys the horse and in some cases will panic them .

- it flies during latter half of summer
- commonly called the bot fly, or because of its similar markings, but only one pair of wings, the Horse 'Bee'
- the adult lives only a few days
- it mates on the wing
- it does not alight, but hovers near the legs, and darts in to deposit and glue its many eggs onto the hairs from fetlock upwards
- the eggs are visible as whitish yellow elongated small objects
- the horse, no doubt slightly irritated through follicle nerve endings, rubs his leg with face and muzzle. The massaging effect hatches the eggs, and the larvae
- enter the mouth and mucosae therein
- penetrate the cheek and
- the tongue mucosa (causing ulceration)
- migrate to the oesophagus and
- travel down its wall to emerge through the
- stomach wall to attach to the stomach fundus
- little, if any, clinical signs appear from mouth and throat lesions. (It has been postulated that tongue and throat irritation could be a 'trigger' for 'crib biting')

Hypoderma bovis – The Cattle Warble Fly – The Gad Fly

Where the species still exists

- hairy insect, flies (northern hemisphere) in June and July

- it occasionally happens that the female mistakes her target and deposits her eggs with their clasps onto equine limb hairs
- maturation to hatching stage is as with the Bot egg, but the
- larvae crawl down the hairs and penetrate the limb skin, up under which they migrate to the oesophagal wall or the diaphragm, where they hibernate until end of winter
- re-activated, they proceed to the skin over the dorsum of the back
- a nodule is formed in which an escape hatch opens through which
- the mature larva, a warble, leaves to fall into the soil to pupate – usually the following January to March

In the horse, the unnatural or aberrant host, the nodule may or may not develop an opening. In most cases, the larva dies and is reabsorbed. Those which do proceed to maturity are invariably underdeveloped – the end of the road as far as the fly is concerned, but not of course for the equine host

- many types of nodules form in a horse's skin
- they are visible and palpable
- most are squeezed in the process of 'inquiring' fingers!

If, however, the nodule is that of the Warble fly larva and an opening is present, the squeezing is usually intensified – humans are very inquisitive! Then if the larva dead or alive, is ruptured in this process there is a release of toxic allergenic contents; there follows an intense anaphylactic response under the horse's skin – an acute inflammatory reaction with

- swelling
- oedematous lateral spread
- pain – if touched, let alone saddled
- spreading cellulitis
- possibly abscess formation at original site
- possibly systemic illness

Management
of the acute Warble reaction

- hot foments or poulticing
- steroid and antibiotics systemically may be necessary

- the horse is 'absent from work'
- subsequent saddle fitting requires care

A similar, but fortuitous crisis can follow saddling over an unnoticed warble nodule. Carefully feel and inspect routinely discovered suspicious nodules, usually isolated, in January to March (northern hemisphere) if typical signs of egg laying on legs were noticed the previous summer.

(Of historic interest: before systemically effective larvicides were available, cattle in the UK were dressed along their back every month for three months from January – under the Warble Fly Control Order – the lotion, usually of derris, entered the air hole and killed the warble larvae invariably without reaction.)

Diagnosis
in both cases – equine bot and bovine warble

- signs of eggs on limb and higher areas
- time of year
- presence of specific fly
- June and July for warble fly (now eradicated in the UK)
- late summer for bot fly
- development of warble nodule the following winter
- development of bot and the potential risk period
- known to be October to January (northern hemisphere) perhaps with
- suspected low-grade colic, possible loss of condition

Differential Diagnosis

- just possible lice eggs (nits) could mislead, but seasons are different
- in the case of warble aberrant nodule
    - usually only one or two – see nodular disease
- nodular sarcoid – (rare in the back) 10 or more and firm
- in the case of bots
    - any other cause of mild recurrent colic, e.g. tapeworm (this infestation can produce serious signs)
    - any other cause of low grade loss of condition – helminths, teeth etc.

Control

- Ivermectin in routine late winter/early spring worming

Mange mites.

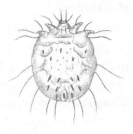 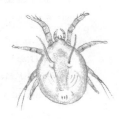 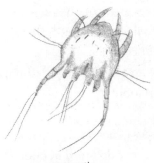

sarcoptes scabia   chorioptic   psoroptic

should be effective against warble larvae but by that time any damage by bots will have been done

Mites

The vast majority of this group of arthropods are free living. A few species are important in themselves as

- pathogenic parasites of man and animals and/or
- vectors of disease

Some free living types inhabit and feed on

- dust arising from disintegration of
- animal
- vegetable
- mineral debris

They are, like all members of the animal kingdom, **proteinacious.** These proteins are antigenic. In contact, especially with

- respiratory track epithelia and the
- epidermis generally

they can stimulate the production of antibodies. Subsequent further contact will trigger sensitivity reactions.

In this context, therefore, free living mites can cause illness albeit indirectly, e.g. the human asthmatic who is 'allergic' to household dust, is in fact allergic to dust mites, larvae and their faeces, as in the horse with COPD (heaves).

Acariasis (infestation by mites)

- skin infestation with mites including the **manges**, is relatively uncommon in the horse although the

Chorioptic type seems to have made a comeback recently

- most infestations would appear to be 'new'
- nevertheless, many are so much 'one off' cases in a yard or stable that they are either contagion from a
  - symptomless contagious carrier, or
  - a flare up of a carrier state in the same animal

Clinical disease usually occurs in association with

- malnutritional and
- helminthiasis poor conditions
- chronic intercurrent dis-ease, and in some types with
  - lowered vitality or altered micro-climate, as in leg dermatosis when chorioptic infestation may get a 'hold'

In all of these predisposing factors the epidermal and the dermal deeper defences would appear to have been weakened and/or immuno-compromised

- mange should however be seen as a primary contagious disease, characterised by
  - pruritus, often very marked
  - widespread from many focal infestations or
  - localised with peripheral spreading
- primary dermal lesions are
  - papules with
  - exudate
  - scale – limited
  - crust
  - alopecia with thickened skin

these are **all defects of keratinisation**, in the

burrowing type particularly

- secondary dermal lesions – bacterial especially
  - opportunist commensals
  - secondary invaders through self-imposed
    - excoriation

There are two types of acariases

- **manges** whose mites do breed in or on the equine skin
- **other mite** infestations, opportunists, temporary passengers with pathogenic properties which do not breed on the horse

All produce lesions which are basically similar. Moreover, certain other non-acarida skin invaders cause fairly similar signs with papules and keratinisation defects.

Laboratory diagnosis by sample examination is frequently required to

- identify acariasis from other pathogens and to
- identify which specific mite if acariasis is present

This identification is not only important from the point of view of treatment and control but also because one type of mange, Sarcoptic, communicable to other animals and to man (zoonotic) is notifiable in the UK.

The mites (adults) are invisible to the naked eye, except for one species, which can just be seen as very small white dots, especially in coarse hair areas such as the dock skin.

The life cycle is not completely known, but in general

- eggs are laid in burrows in the skin if the female is the burrowing type, or on the skin and thereafter at the edges of lesions
- larvae hatch in 3–7 days and
- after feeding, give rise to nymphs which develop in 2–3 weeks at the maximum, before moulting into adults. Gravid females then burrow, if that is their type behaviour, as in Sarcoptes. Others continue on the epidermal surface and in follicles

The genus causing mange in horses are four in number – **sarcoptic** mange, **psoroptic** mange, **chorioptic** mange, and **demodectic** mange.

Sarcoptic Mange (Scabies)

The adult female pierces skin to suck lymph and eat 'young' epidermal cells, causing marked pruritus and dermatitis. Her burrowing to lay eggs leaves a trail of production of

- an exudate which coagulates to form crusts
- excess keratinisation occurs with proliferation of connective tissue
  - the skin thickens and corrugates
- the hair falls out from lack of nourishment
- opportunist bacterial infection with suppuration may follow
- possible toxaemia from tissue damage absorption and/or secondary bacteria

The Sites

- fine or sparsely haired areas
- face and ears
- head and neck
  - spreads if untreated

The pathogenic results cause

- a constant itch
  - stamping
  - rubbing
  - nibbling
- **no** evasive action but the persistent itch causes
  - interference with feeding and rest
  - loss of condition
  - risk of self inflicted injury and secondary infection
    - purulent dermatitis

Psoroptic Mange

This genus is thought to have several species which parasitise specific host animals. An important example is 'sheep scab' (notifiable in the UK) because of its specific contagiousness and related welfare and economic effects in flocks.

There is a main and a subspecies in the horse

- adults live on the skin

- pierce skin to suck fluid and to eat 'young' epidermis
  - does not burrow

It can be highly contagious to direct and indirect in-contact horses.

Sites

- well haired, preferably coarser hair regions
- dorsal aspect of neck into mane
- base of tail
- unclipped regions, e.g. as in saddle clip
- the sub-variety localises in the ear – Otodectic mange

Lesions and Signs

- vesicles and
- pustules are formed at the bitten spots
  - serous exudate erupts onto skin surface
  - coagulates to form crusts
- hair falls out
- no marked thickening of skin
- the otitis variety produces a brown (ceruminous) exudate – otitis externa

The Pathogenic Results Cause

- head shaking
- rump rubbing
- general itchiness
- the ear lesions produce in addition to head shaking
  - drooping of one, sometimes both ears

Head handling becomes extremely difficult.

Chorioptic Mange, 'Foot Mange' or 'Itchy Leg'

- similar life cycle and feeding and breeding habits as Psoroptes, but does *not* pierce dermis. It feeds off epidermal debris
- can be present over lengthy periods, asymptomatically or intermittently active
- the usual lesions, but not as marked except for more scale and greater crusting. Neglected cases show lichenification and scaling, and itchiness which is

severe, and important because of sites

Sites

- pastern upwards, but not above knee or hock
- prefers long-haired areas, e.g. heavy draught and cob types
  - in feathers, and around and above fetlocks

Pathogenic Results

- marked stamping
- scratching
- biting
- rubbing the legs
- kicking, especially at night, is a characteristic
- self inflicted injuries
  - jarring
  - navicular bone fracture

It is said to predispose to 'greasy heel', or conversely to gain epidermal access because of it.

Demodectic Mange (out of an Arthropodean family, distinct from Sarcoptidae)

- adult mites (the cigar mite) are distinctly elongated in comparison with the other mites
- life cycle is not well understood
- adults apparently can survive for up to 3 weeks off the host, provided the environment is moist, possibly in un-dried grooming kit, or for a shorter time in tack
- directly contagious, but development of active mange in new host is dependent on that animal's state of (ill) health
- believed to be a persistent parasite with long periods of quiescence – asymptomatic. Any immuno compromised state will result in reactivation of the quiescent stages
- lives in the hair follicles and sebaceous glands
- eats epidermal debris

Sites

- anywhere, but especially
  - head, including
    - eyelids – and skin glands therein

- ear pinnae
- muzzle

Lesions and Signs

- variable pruritus
- loss of hair
- scale
- thickening and wrinkling of skin
- intermittent erythema
- occasional pustules – from secondary bacterial infection

Diagnosis of all pathogenic infestations

- in all 4 types, and especially with Demodectic infestation, can be initially suspected by
- sites described
- active/acute – marked pruritus
- chronic – marked scurfing, scaling, alopecia, some pruritus
- quiescent – perhaps alopecia and skin thickening from previous attack
- intermittent activity

Management

Suspicion of, and differential diagnosis from other keratinisation defects and actual diagnosis, are often slow to be investigated. Symptomatic treatment of the indeterminate superficial lesions can effect non-specific improvement without getting at the underlying cause. This obtains in several dermatoses.

Specific treatment must be rigorously applied and for long enough to cover the life cycle and to include a further period for residual (unsusceptible) eggs to hatch. Fortunately, the first three types are susceptible to most of the therapies. Demodectic is very recalcitrant

- *veterinary advice should be obtained for*
  - diagnosis
  - updated treatment
  - what drugs not permitted (in UK, EU regulations)
  - what drugs possibly toxic to horses
  - how to use
  - how long to use and at what intervals

It will possibly be (subject to own veterinary surgeon) the following

Systemic

- Ivermectin – full repeated dose – twice in two-week intervals
- especially against blood suckers
- possibly against other types

Topical

- whole or part body
- 5% lime sulphur and tar/sulphur compounds are 'old' remedies
- others as recommended 'permissibles', e.g. Cooper's mange dressing

Management and Control

- outbreaks of mange as were experienced in
  - cavalry and other army lines
  - stalled animals

are now rare; it is usually isolated cases.

Nevertheless, the mites are contagious so isolation of the affected animal during treatment, its equipment and burning of its bedding, disinfecting its tack and grooming equipment and stabling is desirable. Monitor, by laboratory samples, response to treatment.

Non-Mange Mites

- straw itch mites
  - these normally parasitise larvae of grain insects

Lesions

- when such larvae are few in number, the mites will infest, to obtain epidermal debris feed
  - man, when they are very pruritic
  - other animals, when pruritus is slight or absent
    - they do however induce
    - papular eruptions
    - crusts

Sites

- since the mites are transported by
  - hay
  - straw

and off

  - grazing

the sites vary, e.g. rack-fed horses will be infested

  - over head
  - along neck
  - on to withers

The lesions are self-limiting, management is not required.

Trombicula Autumnalis

- the Harvest Bug or mite, Red or Cherry Bugs, Chiggers
- both adults and larvae are reddish/orange
- adults are very large. They and the nymphs are free living and feed on plants and invertebrates
- the natural host of the larvae, which are blood suckers, is small rodents

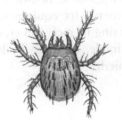

Trombicula.

The larvae, most plentiful in the autumn (hence Harvest Bug) can parasitise

- grazing animals
- man
- they suck blood for a few days then drop off, moult, and become nymphs

Sites

- head
- neck
- legs – around pasterns in Thoroughbreds, when it is called 'Heel Bug'

Lesions

- variable pruritus (some animals may become hypersensitive with increased itch following repeated attacks)
- eruption of watery exudate
- papules – larvae visible as orange dot in the centre
- crusts
- alopecia

Pathogenic Results

- itchiness
- stamping
- rubbing

Management

- rarely required as disease is self limiting
- if itchiness *severe*
  - steroids, but beware ponies and risk of laminitis
- if fresh lesions continue
  - change grazing and/or
  - dress daily with 5% lime sulphur
- avoid known infested grazings
- difficult to know which animals are, or will stay, free

Ticks

The true tick or Ixodes, is the genus of main concern to the larger, herbivores – cattle, sheep and horses. The hatched larvae ascend grass, gorse etc. and are rubbed onto the hair of the animal's head and legs as it passes or grazes near a 'nest' site.

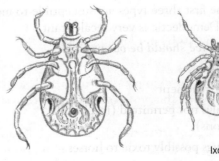

Dermacentor

Ixodes

Ticks (undersides shown).

It is a blood-sucking skin parasite, which buries its mouth parts deep into the dermis and 'locks' on until engorged with blood. It causes

- pruritus
- local hypersensitivity

both of which can be severe in situations where insecticides are not used. The larval, nymphal and adult stages all feed, but breeding usually, and egg laying and hatching, always takes place off the animal. The breeding cycle is complicated.

The tick requires warm weather for survival and multiplication, consequently, it is not a serious threat, in itself, to horses. The 'tick worry' syndrome, more common in subtropical countries, is rare in the UK. If it does develop, the usual signs of infestation and reaction appear especially in the summer. It is then often associated with hypersensitive reactions, and so increased pruritus and marked

- rubbing
- self biting
- stamping
- restlessness
- loss of condition
- papules, pustules and weals with subsequent
  - crusts, erosions and ulcers
- alopecia, mainly self-inflicted

Ticks are particularly important because their blood sucking makes them efficient insect-vectors of several infections, particularly in the warmer climates of Africa and America

- protozoan
- Rickettsial
- viral
- bacterial and
- Spirochaetal agents have all been confirmed

They are not common skin parasites in the UK except in the south west, when the protozoan cause of 'redwater' is well recognised.

Equine serological titre levels in the UK and in America have shown evidence of infection in horses with the spirochaete Borrelia burgdorferi.

In man, and in dogs in America, clinical signs of this lethal infection have been recorded. It was first confirmed in the USA town of **Lyme**, and this is the accepted name of the disease wherever found.

50% of ticks are estimated to be carriers in this USA district. In 1995, a clinical case was diagnosed in the UK, and confirmed by an intensive series of ante and post mortem tests. Despite serological evidence that there are horses in the UK which have been infected, the clinical cases so far have been restricted to this one and several suspected infections.

PREVENTION AND MANAGEMENT OF ECTOPARASITE DISEASE

Prevention aims at keeping the arthropod from

- becoming active in to life cycle at certain times of the year, e.g. **lice.** Applications which are insecticidal must be applied to kill the adults and larvae hatching from eggs already deposited on coat hairs. Since the eggs are not susceptible, the 'treatment' must be repeated, usually twice. **Mange mites** are dealt with similarly: there is no exact seasonal influence, these invariably require repeat treatments to get at the larvae and the adults to minimise tissue irritation. It is difficult to stop initial infestation other than by specifically treating all possible in-contact carriers. The midge, as with sweet itch, is a summer problem as a rule. The damage to the skin and coarse hair is from the keralytic effect of the saliva and the subsequent immune mediated urticaria. Management of the pony can be helpful.

- killing the fly when it lands to feed, eradicating breeding sites

- repellents aim to distract the flying insect from approaching and from landing

Repellents
Diethyl toluamide (DEET) Benzyl benzoate (in an oily base) applied as for sweet itch midge repulsion and to produce a slippery coarse hair and so incommode the insect!

Citronella oil and other volatiles such as lavender, rosemary, thyme, geranium, eucalyptus, tea tree oil, lime and juniper.

Insecticides
Pyrethrum (from a species of chrysanthemum), synthetic

pyrethroids (permethrin), peperonyl and its synthetic variations, selenium preparations, as a contact killer against flies, midges and lice.

Apply all these strictly according to manufacturers' instructions, especially as to dilutions and proximity to eyes.

Ectoparasitic Dressings or Applications

- beware 'snake hiss' noise of spray-on preparations. Once a horse becomes head or ear shy a problem will remain
- fly fringes and masks do help to protect eyes and ears. Any herb which contains garlic can produce a sweat which carries the repellent smell
- regular removal of bot eggs from limbs and muzzle
- keep horses away from fly breeding areas if possible

Lyme Disease

Lyme disease is multi-systemic; it develops and progresses over weeks to months. Temporary regression occurs in the earlier stages

- undulating pyrexia
- variable appetite, eventually to nil
  - synovitis
    - tendon sheath
    - joint (usually fetlock) lameness – intermittent and changing in character
  - acute inflammation in the eye
    - uveitis
    - blepharospasm
    - photophobia
    - ocular discharge

Lymphocytic mobilisation leading to renewed infiltration of
- synovial membranes of
- head and neck joints – difficulty in getting head down to graze
- epicardium, other membranes
- especially intra-cranium
  - meningo-encephalitis

Differential

- E. herpes virus 1 (and 4) and its secondary vasculitis

- toxoplasmosis
- brucellosis
- tuberculosis

Diagnosis

- geography
- clinical signs including tick infestation
- blood antibodies for Borrelia

Management

- veterinary help, diagnosis and for
- antibiotics which penetrate the blood brain barrier – prolonged treatment

This 'new' disease with its sequentially varied signs which can be individually confusing, does present difficulties.

Veterinary surgeons are, of course, aware that it can occur. Research workers are interested in its rarity as a clinical entity.

This is suggested as being due, in the UK, to the

- small numbers of ticks infesting any one animal
- small numbers of animals infested
- low pathogenicity of the Spirochaetie – so far
- other factors in the triple relationship

Prevention

Tick eradication is not easy. Control of infestation is mainly by using short grass grazing, avoiding gorse or furze, and other shrub areas.

A species of richettsia, Ehrlichia equi, is thought to be transmitted by ticks. The disease, Granulocytic ehrlichiosis, has been confirmed in the USA, Germany, Sweden and Switzerland. The signs are: high fever up to 41°C (107°F), anorexia and depression, lower limb oedema, a reluctance to move, and when movement is forced, there is ataxia.

In 1994 a case was confirmed in a Highland x Welsh Cob in Somerset (Quantock Hills – a well-known tick habitat). The germ was found in the cytoplasm of white blood cells, the neurophil. The pony responded to broad spectrum antibiotics. The closely related disease, **Potomac Fever** (USA) due to E. risticil, is usually fatal. The tick was believed to be the vector but there is recent strong evidence that fresh-water snails (parasitised by liver fluke larvae) play a transmission role. If this is so, prevention of

Potomac fever becomes possible. It occurs in late spring and early summer in temperate areas. The Potomac river was the site of the first confirmed case of this Rickettsia infection.

NEOPLASIA – TUMOURS

Out of a total disease/injury case load in an equine practice, 1–3% are tumours, 75% of these are of the skin, and of these 90% are sarcoid.

Sarcoids

Sarcoma-like. Previously wrongly called 'warts'

- a world-wide prevalence – no gender or breed susceptibility, except they are rare in Standardbreds
- a dermal/epidermal tumour
- well substantiated as of infectious origin, whereby the Bovine Papillomavirus interacts with the skin environment in certain horses of a possible genetic background

They exhibit or manifest themselves in six distinct forms.

Occult

In which the morbidity is restricted to the superficial epidermal layers, with

- lesions
    - slow developing
    - circular, or irregularly so, areas
    - grey, scaly surface of irregular pattern
    - hairless under and around the scales

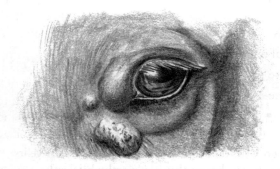

Sarcoids around the eye.

- common on hair-sparse areas
    - face – especially on
        - eyelids
        - base of ears
        - lips
        - neck
        - sheath (prepuce)
        - medial aspect of thighs
- less common elsewhere on body

Verrucose

Involving deeper epidermal layers, perhaps a mutated occult

- lesions
    - an irregular thickening of the affected skin, giving
        - a 'warty' appearance of hyperkeratosis
        - variable in size
        - indistinct outline
        - usually multiple lesions

Most common in the

- axillae
- groin

occasionally elsewhere

- face
- side of ear

Nodular

Usually in the hypoderma, i.e. subcutaneous tissue

- lesions – under a smooth shiny skin contour
    - variable size, up to 5cm (2in) in diameter, commonly in
        - groin
        - eyelid margins, with noticeable deformation
    - may ulcerate through to become fibroblastic

Fibroblastic

These look the most like a true 'cancer'; they grow rapidly

- lesions
    - ulcerated and often secondarily infected
    - liable to exacerbation by trauma
    - sometimes 'hanging' on a stalk (pedunculated)

- otherwise sessile (growing outwards) and growing by peripheral invasion

Common in most areas *except* the

- sides of chest
- neck
- back, *unless* 'primed' by skin injury

Commonly as complications of skin wounds, especially of limbs as a morbid mutation of granulation tissue thought to be stimulated by House fly irritation and possible virus inoculation vectored by the fly.

Mixed

A variable combination of two or more specific types to form, an irregular 'colony'

- lesions
  - commonly in
    - axillae
    - groin
    - around the face

Malevolent

A particularly invasive form of fibroblastic sarcoid which infiltrates lymphatic vessels with resultant cords or chains of secondary ulceration, even into the lymph nodes, (ulcerative lymphangitis). Very rare in the UK.

As will have been appreciated from the variety of sarcoid forms described above, the diagnosis of 'sarcoid', let alone of what sub-type, is not easy for the layman. As with other indistinct clues, it is better to see them as 'something wrong' and 'could be serious'. Call the veterinary surgeon sooner than later, especially for eyelid tumour-like swellings.

Sarcoids do not, in the accepted neoplastic sense, metastasise, but daughter or satellite lesions can appear around the site of an imperfectly eradicated primary.

Primary lesions can develop as contemporary groups.

Despite recognised viral input, they do not appear to be contagious to other horses. An insect vector is 'seen' as one route for transmission into granulation tissue of any sized area. *Suspected* outbreaks have, however, been recorded within a stable. The equine Papilloma virus has **never** been implicated.

It is unusual for a horse to have only one lesion. Duplication is, however, often slow

- experimental transmission by extracts has been effected; the transmissible agent has not been identified

- conversely, implantation of a surgically removed portion of a sarcoid subcutaneously (author's experience many years ago) was followed by a marked reduction in size of the others with eventual 'disappearance' of some: an immune response?
- some horses, if not all, may be (genetically?) more prone or susceptible
- Occult lesions are the most common in the UK. None spontaneously resolve
- all are 'dangerous' if only because of the risk of trauma from
  - tack
  - limb contact
  - external contact

which leads to

- haemorrhage
- secondary infection
  - bacterial
  - fungal
- exacerbation and/or into
- mutated forms

Management

- no one method has yet been found to be completely satisfactory in all types, nor even in a particular type

In ' safe' sites, and for small quiescent lesions, masterly inactivity is the order! Invasive or massive examples of other types are, on welfare and economic grounds, best euthanased. In the badly ulcerated types, fly strike is an additional risk. In medium sized lesions however the following have some good results.

Methods

- surgical removal, with consideration for
  - site
  - size
    - difficulty in defining deep limits which can create problems
- regrowths do occur, but may be delayed for years, but, in the horse, this is a 'worthwhile' risk. Nodular type is the 'easiest', but even here, secondary fibroblastic regrowth is a strong

possibility

- hot laser ablation
  - there are difficulties as mentioned above, as well as technical and cost problems

- cryosurgery – even with this there is a 50:50 chance of re-growth. It is often preceded by surgical
  - reduction in tumour size
  - excision where possible
  - if not, cryosurgery on its own is practicable – just. Lesions around the eye, or over joints are not suitable for this and other surgery

- immunity modulation
  - intra (and perilesional) inoculation of individual tumours with a BCG 'vaccine', repeated at several weekly intervals: useful in eyelid lesions. In the limb there is a risk of exacerbation. (The veterinary surgeon will take precautions regarding the concurrent risk of anaphylaxis)

- radiation therapy (Brachytherapy)
  - irradiated gold, radium, and iridium sources as implants; especially in peri-ocular lesions, and over joints, have given a high success rate

- chemotherapy
  - the topical application of cell destroying chemicals. The most recent, a mixture of heavy metal salts and substances which stop tumour cell division, shows promise. It causes necrosis and sloughing. The site is an important consideration; e.g. distal limb is usually 'out' since there is no muscle/fat subcutaneous cushioning

The importance during a pre-purchase veterinary examination, of sarcoids suspected as

- being present
- in their early stages
- having been present as judged by
- post treatment changes in skin and hair

can be appreciated.

Confirmatory diagnosis of a lesion being not only a sarcoid but also being malignant, i.e. liable to recur, demands biopsy for microscopy examination. Confirmation of suspected 'healed' lesions or surgical scars depends upon an honest declaration by the vendor, if asked!

The fact that the horse is a genetically potential subject for further lesions and that sarcoids can be at the very least, a nuisance, if not more serious, has to be reported and discussed very carefully especially at prepurchase veterinary examinations and, to a lesser extent, in assessing brood animals. Insurance cover is problematic. The veterinary surgeon must declare even suspicions in his certificate.

To euphemistically call sarcoids 'scars' or 'warts' is dangerous. To describe them as skin cancer, whilst not scientifically correct, does emphasise their seriousness, but can, to some, be scaremongering.

Squamous Cell Carcinoma (SCC)

A malignant tumour of the epithelial cells. It most frequently shows as an area of ulceration, without any visible underlying tumour mass.

In the common ocular lesions, they are often multiple as well as bilateral. Usually in 6+ year-old animals. Here they are on the

- conjunctival epidermal border and the cornea
- the third eyelid and
- the eyelids, and most frequently
- periorbital

They rarely metastasise from these sites.

A particularly serious but rare form arises in the gum epithelium of the upper molar arcade, or in the hard palate. It invades the para-nasal maxillary sinuses and nasal bones, producing

- facial swelling
- unilateral mucopurulent haemorrhagic nasal discharge
- severe URT necrosis

The primary site in the gum or palate is often very small. They are also found on the

- upper lip and nostrils, and here are confusing with 'grass warts' or papillomata (which are more sessile); *SCC do not bleed, as do carcinomata*
- external genitalia (coital bleeding)
  - male
    - glans or
    - body of the penis. May necessitate amputation
    - the prepuce
  - female

- skin line of lips of vulva
- clitoris

In these types, the ulcers are cupped or depressed from the pull of the involvement of the deeper layers of the dermis. Metastases are recorded usually into nearby bone by lymphatic spread, especially in face lesions.

Lymphosarcomas

These arise from the white blood cells, and most commonly affect the internal organs, where they become lethal.

Cutaneous lesions are seen

- bone ulcerating through the skin
- muscle ulcerating through the skin
- direct epithelial secondary lesions in external ocular tissues

Melanomas

Particularly a tumour of the grey horse, but not only. They are tumours of the skin pigment. They are mostly benign.

Common Sites

- under base of tail, where they are slow growing
- around anus and vulva (perineal)
- lips and eyelids, including third eyelid

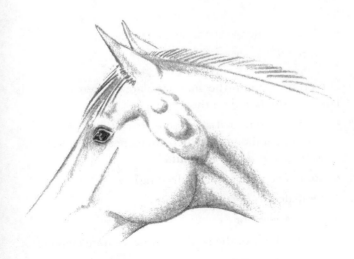

Melanomas on the parotid salivary gland.

- in the parotid region, where they tend to lie deep and stretch the overlying skin
- intra-abdominally, with implications for gut strangulation and nerve pressure – colic

A malignant form has been recorded, but rarely.

Papillomata

Warty-like outgrowths from the skin

- nose
- muzzle
- round the eyes
- occasionally elsewhere

It is a viral infection – papovirus (EPV)

- possibly picked up from grazings recently contaminated by other recently affected horses
- possibly dormant on the skin until that is sub-clinically traumatised by thistles, stemmy grasses, other factors
- produces a good dermal immunity, therefore, seen usually only
  - in yearlings
  - self limiting as immunity develops
  - host-specific to horses

Lesions can be

- fly struck
- secondarily infected
- traumatic to cornea if present on eyelids

Congenital lesions have been recorded on new-born foals and aborts. Can be seen inside ear pinna.

NODULAR DISEASE

The specific nodular disease refers to a condition which develops on the back area, usually under the 'saddle' which suggests a relationship to pressure with a secondary reaction in the dermis

- from dander being pushed into the follicles
- a response to tack dressing or other cleaning materials being forced into the skin
- a reaction to pressure-killed helminth, e.g. Onchocerca,

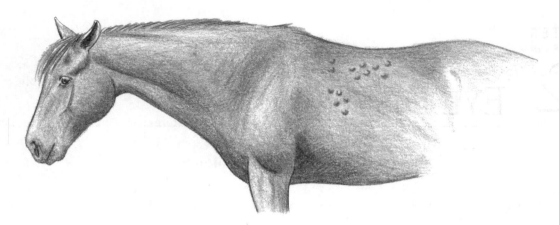

Nodular disease in the saddle area.

significantly this worm has been more or less eradicated by the use of the Ivermectins for routine worm control and the prevalence of nodular disease *appears* to have coincidentally dropped

There is no pruritus or pain to touch: the ridden horse is rarely inconvenienced. Most nodules disappear spontaneously, usually when the horse is rested.

Pathologically, the nodule is formed originally around necrotic collagen tissue in the skin (necrobiosis). Persistent lesion may become centrally calcified and this 'pea' can be pain inducing from pressure.

CHAPTER

32 EYE DISEASES

The eye is arguably the most important of the sensors. To some extent, however, to the horse, the loss of sight in one eye is not as important as it might at first appear. Man and beasts of prey are more dependent upon the focussing powers of binocular vision than the herbivores which, with mainly monocular vision as the norm, are more concerned with long range and initially unilateral recognition of potential danger, particularly by *awareness of movement*, rather than by exact identification.

It is in fact assumed, from practical experience, that a one-eyed horse is safer to ride than the horse which attempts to interpret incomplete information through a partially sighted eye. It may not, however, judge gate posts passed at speed sufficiently to prevent trauma to the rider's knee on the blind side! The horse may also be more likely to 'spook' at objects passing quickly from the blind side into the good field of vision.

The Blind Horse

Impaired vision in the horse is difficult to quantify, and it is not always easy to pin-point the source of the defect. In simple terms, any factor which reduces

- the penetration of visual light rays to the retina, the photo-sensitive cells at the back of the eyeball
- the conversion ability of the retina
- the transmission of that input to the brain
- the reception and interpretative powers of the visual centres in the brain

will reduce visual acuity, from

- impaired, to
- blind

The owner will be suspicious of defective vision if the horse develops

- uncertainty in the gaits – stumbling
- exaggerated steps – hypermetria
- poor awareness of objects
- jumping evasions
- an altered head carriage, as though using one eye more than the other
- increased 'listening' – exaggerated ear movement
- unexpected head shyness

The owner can try to test for vision by applying the **menace threat**. The hand should be brought slowly over the eye from behind the orbit at a range of about 15 cm (6 in). A reflex blink suggests that the horse 'sees'. (Note: any hand movement which causes air disturbance will cause a tactile positive reaction – this is not a visual reaction.)

The **fixation test** is more accurate. Blindfold one eye, and let the horse settle. Tease out wisps of cotton wool and let one float down over the eye at about 15 cm (6 in) range. If 'seen', the horse will fix on it and *follow it down*. Repeat with the other eye.

An obstacle course of irregularly placed straw bales, through which the horse is loosely led, first without a hood and then with the eyes alternately blindfolded, may produce evidence of a visual deficit.

It should be appreciated that such changes will have developed without signs of either one (or both) eyeball(s) and its surroundings being obviously dis-eased.

The veterinary surgeon will note these reported signs and then enquire whether there has been a recent history of

- virus infection
- bacterial infection
  - systemic

- regional, as with sinusitis or throat swellings
- local, in the eye region
- possible head trauma when the horse was
  - in use
  - in transit
  - grazed with 'new' horses

before he makes his own detailed inspection and tests.

Superficially, the veterinary surgeon will check for

- exaggerated eye lid reflexes
- corneal opacity, ulceration and an increased vascularisation of the sclera onto the corneal periphery

If the cornea(s) are normal, i.e. clear, he will be able to look ophthalmascopically through to examine the deeper structures which might be interfering with vision as the result of pathological changes therein. This 'work up' will include determining

- if the pupils are of equal size
- if they respond (contract) to bright light focussed through them, and that
- the consensual light reflex is active. (In the horse this is slow and often indeterminate, but if a light causes one pupil to constrict the other should eventually do so without direct stimulation. If it doesn't, it is suggestive of optic nerve damage – there is a 'cross over' of the sensory nerves)
- the iris is swollen
- the lens is translucent, allowing only a hazy view of the back of the eye
- there are cataracts present
- the view of the retina is clear or there are obstructions (floaters) in the vitreous chamber
- the state of the optic disc and the retina is normal

It is important to appreciate that a *recently noticed* or suspected visual impairment, in the absence of external signs of

- excessive tear flow and severe eyelid reflexes of
- photophobia and blepharospasm
- corneal opacity

is unlikely to be associated with an acute ocular dis-ease. It is more likely to be

- subacute from an earlier primary cause, which was

'missed' at grass or misunderstood as insignificant

- chronic, where it happened some time previously – perhaps in an earlier ownership, or forgotten about

by a new owner or a different rider, or made more 'active' by a new work programme or rider technique, as with 'periodic ophthalmia' disease changes.

Visual defects are relatively rare; in many suspect situations, what appears to be an eye problem is, in fact, more likely to be due to

- locomotor defects
- neurologic deficits with ataxia
- behaviour aberrations
- bitting, tack fit and rider problem

TYPES OF DIS-EASE

Developmental

Developmental dis-ease is invariably congenital

- inherited – only one dis-ease is definitely known to be due to a dominant gene
  - aniridia, or absence of the iris, usually with an associated cataract (there are others in man and dog)
- a possible genetic influence may be involved in, for example
  - anophthalmia – absence of an eye(s)
  - atresia – blockage of a tear duct
  - cataract
  - coloboma – a part missing in a structure
  - entropion
  - microphthalmia – small eye in a small eyelid aperture
  - dermoid cyst

By definition, these defects will be present in the new-born foal, but where blindness is a consequence

- that may be 'masked' by the foal's early chemotactic attraction to the dam's udder
- cataracts may not be diagnosed until a specific examination is made

• tear duct blockage may be 'slow' to show

At a conference on 'Genetics and Disease' as recently as 1994 defects of the eye with a possible hereditable cause were not mentioned, let alone discussed, thus indicating the rare incidence and relatively low economic importance of such.

It is recognised that in-utero damage to the developing foetus can arise from defects of the

• blood supply, with consequent mal-nutrition
• intercurrent dam dis-ease
  • toxins (bacterial)
  • viruses
  • vitamin deficiency
  • other diseases

and that congenital cataract is a typical example of the effect. It is then an acquired **embryonic** dis-ease.

Some breeds are thought to have an inherited susceptibility to cataracts which develop before or just after birth. For example

• Belgian Blacks
• Morgan horses
• Arabians (not English bred)
• Thoroughbreds

Inflammatory Dis-ease

Trauma

The equine head is a common site of contact injury but the eyes are set

• relatively high in the head at the junction of the face and the skull bones
• 'facing' more to the side than to the front
• lying mainly within the orbit; which cavity is demarcated by a ring of strong, prominent bone, particularly dorsally and caudally

Such anatomical features form a protective ring. Further protection is provided by the

• tough but flexible eyelids and the 'lashes' of the upper lid
• unique third eyelid, the membrana nictitans
• pad of fat behind the eyeball within the orbit

Reflex neuro-muscular mechanisms enhance protection

• the **menace blink**, an automatic closing of the eyelids when threatened – a visual reflex
• the eyeball withdrawal
  • if sudden external pressure is felt, a touch reflex when, in addition to the blink, the eyeball is retracted onto the yielding fat, thus
    • taking it inside the bony rim, and so
    • cushioning it to absorb undue pressure
  • the third eyelid is protracted across the eyeball under the lids proper, giving an extra defensive layer

Trauma may be an 'open' or a **'closed' inflammation**, the latter resulting in

• swelling of the skin and
• of the underlying tissues – bruising, and if severe
• fracture of the supra-orbital rim

causing

• pain
• closing of the eyelids, or at least a reflex induced inability or 'willingness' to fully open them
• distortion of the bony orbit if fractured

and, to the eyeball itself with non-infectious variable

• inflammation of the scleral and palpebral conjunctiva with associated excess tear flow
• congestive oedema of the cornea
• haemorrhage into the ocular cavities
• disruption of the uveal tract aqueous flow
• swelling of the eyeball
• possible subsequent partial collapse of the eyeball and, when the pain is severe
  • photophobia – dislike of (bright) light
  • blepharospasm – autonomic reflex tight closure of the eyelids

Infectious Inflammation

In the 'open' trauma of

• puncture wounds and/or
• lacerations of
  • the supra-orbital skin and/or the eyelids (by wire, thorns, nails, etc.) the resultant infection produces a greater inflammatory response and variably

greater pain with blepharospasm which cannot be overcome manually. Most eye problems due to trauma and/or infection will require local surface anaesthesia of the eyeball to accurately assess the seriousness. The tear flow is often purulent

Open trauma affecting the actual eyeball does happen, and the eyeball is invariably secondarily infected. It happens before the visual reflex operates. For instance

- superficial scratches across the cornea, with immediate
  - pain, blinking, or complete closure of the eyelids
  - clouding of the cornea
  - excessive tear formation with overspill
- laceration, the above signs plus
  - herniation of
    - deeper corneal layers or, if 'right through'
    - escape of aqueous fluid, and collapse of the anterior eyeball cavity
    - prolapse of part of the iris
    - possible penetration of the lens, and even
    - of the retina

A less serious but more common corneal conjunctival irritant inflammation is due to the lodging of foreign bodies such as grass seed, small twigs and straw under an eyelid or on the eyeball, as by an oat 'flight' which adheres to the surface. In the immediate situation there will be

Orbital discharge
- blinking, possibly some blepharospasm
- copious tear overspill becoming purulent in 12 hours
- attempts at rubbing the head on the foreleg to alleviate the irritation

Action in all eye traumas should be
- *send for the veterinary surgeon*

- *do not* probe or poke with tweezers or even cotton buds

- *do not* force medication between the eyelids

- double rack the horse in the corner of the box to obviate possible self damage by rubbing

- darken the box

In the treatment of eye conditions **under veterinary advice and prescription**, the necessary handling and restraint must be efficient, otherwise there is the risk of secondary damage to the eye – and primary damage to the handler(s)!

Do not medicate a horse with drops, or use ointment dispensers, previously used on another horse; one should finish medications or dispose of the remainder.

Do not apply any steroid preparation unless under strict veterinary advice, especially if the cornea is affected (when there is a risk of further degenerative change and ulceration).

In the case of eyelid laceration involving the edges, it is essential that good surgical repair is effected early to prevent eversion Ectropion of that lid with permanent conjunctival exposure, or inversion Entropion with corneal irritation.

When the eyeball is affected, medical dilation of the pupil to minimise the risk of internal adhesions is essential.

Conjunctiva

Conjunctivitis – a red or pink eye, with an increase in the diameter of the scleral (white of eye) blood vessels. It also affects the outer surface of the third eyelid, the nictitating membrane, and the inner surface of the lids. The eyelids as well as the conjunctiva are usually swollen with oedema.

When conjunctivitis appears in one eye only it is usually due to

- trauma, or a retained foreign body or to an
- antibody antigen reaction, as in periodic ophthalmia

When both eyes are affected it indicates
- conjunctival irritation by flies feeding off the tears
- systemic diseases such as

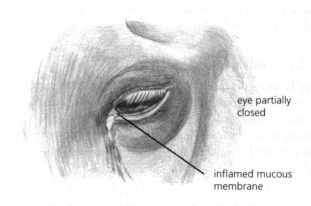

eye partially closed

inflamed mucous membrane

Conjunctivitis.

- strangles – with purulent eye discharge
- virus infections, especially that of
  - infectious viral arteritis ('pink eye') and to a lesser extent
  - influenza
  - herpes 1 and 4
  - adenovirus
- allergic reactions of a more general nature

Conjunctivitis is variably painful.

The Eyeball

Apparent enlargement of the eyeball with protrusion, causing

- difficulty in fully closing the eyelids, and
- the third eyelid to be partially protracted

is due to

- haemorrhage into the fat behind the eyeballs, as with trauma by
  - kicks and other blows
  - road traffic accident
- ascending infection from
  - maxillary and frontal sinuses – orbital cellulitis, a painful, fever producing, purulent condition
- neoplasia behind the eye, slow growing and painless at first
  - usually a carcinoma spreading posteriorly from the primary site on the third eyelid
- glaucoma

Sunken eye occurs when the bulbar fat is 'burnt up', as in malnourishment leading to emaciation.

Both eyes will be intermittently partly hidden

- in **Tetanus disease,** when the spasms of the eyeball muscles will snatch the globe back into the orbit causing the third eyelid to flick out of its recess and momentarily cover the eye surface. Diagnostically this spasm can be induced by lightly tapping the horse's chin
- one eyeball may recede, from atrophy following severe trauma, infection or tumour formation. Surgical removal may be necessary

Damage to the autonomic nerves in the cervical region from

- gutteral pouch mycosis
- deep laceration into the base of the neck bones
- accidental deposition of (especially irritating) fluid from through-puncture of the jugular vein by injection

causes **Horner's syndrome**, producing a usually unilateral

- constricted pupil
- droop of the upper eyelid
- retraction of the eyeball
- protrusion of the third eyelid

In the early stages there will also be unilateral upper neck sweating to cause marked wet staining of the skin. Recovery is possible.

The Cornea

Trauma, with or without secondary infection, has been described. Irritation from

- turned in eyelashes (entropion)
- sand, dust

will cause a rapid and marked blue clouding of the normally clear 'window' on the front of the eyeball; this is due to swelling (oedema) of the several layers of the cornea.

Pain with induced rubbing varies with the cause, as does

- lacrimation, excessive tear production and overspill
- eyelid closure

When due to a scratch abrasion, the pain is invariably marked.

In the more chronic stages the condition is called **keratitis**, producing a bluish white film over part or all of the cornea. It may be

- superficial, from external abrasion
- secondary, from internal
  - inflammation e.g. uveitis
  - pressure e.g. from glaucoma

An ulcerated cornea results from

- deep focal injury
- secondary infection of a less deep injury by

- bacteria, or
- fungi and

is often accompanied by vascularisation in-growing onto the cornea from the scleral blood vessels.

It is believed that an EHV-1 infection will produce a specific corneal ulcer, which will respond to specific antiviral medication. This is the only occasion in which a topical antiviral ointment is 'available' in the horse.

Uvea or Uveal Tract

Uveitis – inflammation – may be either

- direct, as part of
  - trauma, and subsequent
  - infection

  when the area including the iris and the peripheral structure is involved. This involves 'bruising', i.e. haemorrhage into the tissues, resulting in subsequent adhesions with
  - cataract formation

  and impaired vision
- indirect, as part of
  - systemic dis-ease
    - viral
    - bacterial – toxin or germ
    - allergic – antigen antibody reaction i.e. hyper-sensitivity; **periodic ophthalmia** is the most common

The signs are common to all causes, except for any obvious corneal penetrating lesions but especially in periodic ophthalmia. There is often marked

- photophobia
- blepharospasm

associated with the pain of the inflammation

- increased tear flow often becoming purulent

There is also, to a greater or lesser degree

- conjunctivitis
- corneal haze (oedema)
- redness within the anterior chamber and a later
- exudate of white blood cells behind the cornea
- constricted pupil, swollen iris

In addition to the lesions already mentioned there may later be

- glaucoma – from interference with aqueous drainage
- retinal degeneration
- optic neuritis

The outcome is variable, but the prognosis is poor in

- puncture-caused infections
- untreated hypersensitivity reactions, even in successfully treated cases; further signs indicate a 'further' case, a repeat allergenic attack
    - in the same eye
    - in the other eye

with increasingly poor prognosis with each attack

Vigorous treatment following a quick veterinary diagnosis is usually effective in hypersensitive uveitis, and variable in other causes. Delay in seeking veterinary help is often related to the owner's hope that it is no more than

- a 'cold' in the eye
- fly irritation
- a 'bit of a bang'

The absence of improvement within several days may be a dangerous delay even if professional help is sought then.

Periodic Ophthalmia

This is the commonest form of uveitis in the horse, but it is said to affect only 1% of horses in the UK. The causes are not yet accurately known, but suspected are

- infection with leptospira homona bacterium
- reinfection with leptospira homona and an associated hypersensitivity
- migration of microfilaria in the cornea or deeper tissues
- other viral infections in which arteriolar pathology is involved, e.g. HV-1 and 4

There was a high incidence of this uveitis in horses in the First World War, when contagion was a reasonable assumption, but otherwise present-day cases seem to be isolated.

The recurrent nature of this dis-ease can vary from weeks to more than 12 months and creates warranty difficulties if signs of previous dis-ease are seen, such as

- chronic changes in the iris and lens

- degenerative changes in the retina around the optic disc

at pre-purchase veterinary examination.

The need for quick veterinary attention in all cases of uveitis, especially in periodic ophthalmia, is the medicinal dilation (mydriasis) of the pupil to minimise the risk of adhesions forming between the iris, the lens and the cornea.

Iris

The tissue which forms the muscular mobile part involved in pupil size control is subject to the same dis-ease which affects the uvea, which is part of the iral periphery. Allergic and infectious inflammation is associated with paralysis of the dilatory pupillary muscles resulting in constriction of the pupil and the risk of adhesions, as described above. The unique equine corpora nigra can become grossly enlarged, which will then interfere with vision.

Cataract – a defect in the lens

A cataract is an opacity in the lens substance or its capsule either anterior or posterior.

A cataract can be a primary lesion arising with no associated signs of other dis-ease. It may be a secondary lesion resulting from other eye dis-ease or following a regional or systemic illness. It is clinically difficult to prove that primary cataracts are inherited. As such they are believed to be uncommon.

Even congenital cataracts can be secondary to embryonic dis-ease in which the blood supply to the developing eye is disturbed, usually resulting in malnutrition of its various parts. Some viral infections of the dam have been implicated.

The congenital condition may involve the whole lens or only focal areas. They are usually non-progressive and if deemed to interfere with vision, economic considerations apart, surgical removal of the lens before 6 months of age is feasible. A foal which is totally blind is, for obvious reasons, best euthanased.

Adaptation to 'no lens' is slower in a horse which has been ridden, even with impaired vision, and re-using is really re-training.

The ophthalmologist classifies cataracts in some detail but in practice those which are serious, in as much as they are progressive in size and density and eventually are vision impairing, are those which are **acquired**. In the earlier stages, particularly if only in one eye, the defect may not be noticed. Later, if in both eyes, the defect in seeing is exaggerated in poor light, as fewer rays are able to get through, as when moving from light to the darkness of a wood or at dusk.

Pupil size will increase with

- increasing lens opacity
- decreasing light and in some cases will be
- permanently dilated to reveal
  - the pearly white opacity of the lens

Acquired cataracts are usually the result of

- uveitis
- direct trauma
  - with corneal penetration and infection
  - without penetration but with haemorrhage into the posterior aqueous chamber or the vitreous chamber

Owner/riders are often unaware that their horse has cataracts. The degree of opacity varies considerably; not only is the horse apparently free of impaired vision but also the lesions cannot be detected by unaided inspection of the eyes; ophthalmascopy is required.

The congenital focal type, which is non-progressive is frequently of no consequence: the horse 'sees' round them. Acquired lesions can be of such a degree and location that vision is not impaired as far as the owner and veterinary surgeon can discern. Those which are subject to progression, as in periodic ophthalmia, will eventually become significant with repeated attacks.

More widespread, but still not impenetrably dense lesions, judged by an eye specialist as non-progressive, and not associated with periodic ophthalmia can leave the horse with acceptable vision. Such cases are often only discovered during a pre-purchase veterinary examination to the surprise of the vendor who, till then, had been unconcerned with the animal's performance. Hence the need for a specialist opinion – if only to satisfy the underwriters of an insurance cover.

Fortunately the horse does not require fine accommodation of focus. It can apparently cope with recognising shades and outlines rather than detail. However, when faced with a fallen log which could look like a crouching predator, the horse may well play safe. Its general, unpredictability can make such a reaction quite violent.

Metabolic Dis-ease

Little if anything is recorded, except for nutritional deficiencies of vitamins, especially

- vitamin A or its precursor, which is unlikely in a herbivore; theoretically this can
  - decrease night vision from retinal degeneration
  - cause corneal cloudiness
- riboflavin, causing
  - conjunctivitis
  - lacrimation
  - aversion to bright light – photophobia

The author cannot recollect ever being even suspicious of such conditions, certainly in the adult horse.

Parasitic Dis-ease

Such dis-ease is of minor importance

- the larvae of Habronema species are frequently deposited on the skin around the lower area of the periorbital skin and on the eyelids at the time the adult fly feeds off the tears
  - local swelling and irritation occurs, especially of the eyelids, with increasing tear flow
  - secondary bacterial conjunctivitis usually follows
- Onchocerca larvae occasionally migrate across the cornea to leave a keratitic white streak
  - this is usually painless
  - occasionally, when anthelmintic treatment causes larval death an acute, allergic uveitis flares up – a possible explanation for some cases of Periodic Ophthalmia

Swollen eyelids (puffy lids) as a separate entity

Signs

- soft to firm depressible oedema, usually on the upper lids

Cause

- reaction to
  - ringworm infection (differentiate from early sarcoid)
  - sarcoptic and other mange mites

- parasites – see above
- allergic reaction to ingesta

Degenerative Dis-ease

This is a rare category but

- optic nerve and cerebral 'centre' atrophy have been reported
- retinal degeneration with or without optic disc involvement is more common, as discussed under uveitis

Neoplastic Dis-ease

The eyelids and the nictitating membrane (third eyelid), the sclera and the cornea are epidermal tissues, and as such are susceptible to neoplasia as is the dermis and epidermis generally.

Eyelid (external surface)

- malignant melanoma (grey horses)
- sarcoids
- squamous cell carcinoma

The first two can be surgically dealt with, but tend to be recurrent.

Membrana Nictitans

- squamous cell carcinoma
- sarcoids (rarely)
- lympho sarcoma secondaries

Conjunctiva

Although the most commonly dis-eased of all the eye and adnexa tissues, it is rarely subject to neoplasia except where it covers the third eyelid

Cornea

Especially at the scleral junction at the lateral canthus

- squamous cell carcinoma

which will 'spread' over the related area of the cornea. It is more common in

- older horses; it does metastisise
  - by the lymphatic route to the neck and chest tissues

Iris

Very occasionally a tumour, possibly a melanoma, will develop in a corpus nigram.

Dermoid Cyst

A congenital growth near the corner of the cornea from which grow single or numerous hairs.

Blocked Tear Duct

Signs

- persistent overspill of tears at medial (nasal) corner/canthus
- flattening of hairs down the face
- occasional loss of facial hair along spillage track

The tears which moisten the cornea and have antibody properties to prevent ocular infection flow towards two ducts at the medial corner of the upper and lower lids. These unite to run down the naso-lacrimal duct underneath the bone of the face and nose. They open into the medial ventral aspect of the nostrils.

Cause

- obstruction anywhere, but usually at
  - the palpebral openings, from conjunctivitis
  - from trauma to the nasal bones
  - occasionally a conjunctival congenital fault – **atresia** of the duct

Veterinary diagnosis is confirmed by flooding the eye with fluorescin dye and looking for any drainage of it at the nostril. Fuller assessment requires 'searching' of the duct.

Treatment

Such as

- antibiotic therapy for conjunctivitis
- surgical drainage

is usually successful except in atresia.

Entropion

A turning in of the eyelid, especially the lower lid.

Signs

- corneal irritation
- lacrimation

Causes

- congenital, or first 'seen' in a foal a few days' old, will respond to simple intervention by subcutaneous filling to evert the lid
- acquired from laceration of the lid, top or bottom; at the time this requires careful suturing, or if delayed, somewhat more intensive surgical intervention

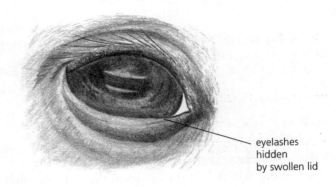

eyelashes hidden by swollen lid

Entropion.

Ectropion

A turning out of the lids to expose the conjunctiva.

Signs

- conjunctivitis
- lacrimation
- exposure of the conjunctiva

Causes

- rarely congenital
- acquired from lacerations, usually of the lower lid which droops

Treatment

Treatment is surgical.

LAMENESS: UNDERSTANDING AND DETECTING

DIS-EASE OF THE LOCOMOTOR SYSTEM

INTRODUCTION

The survival of the horse species during its evolution depended upon genetically programmed improvement in particular features of structure and functioning to suit its life in the wild and the essential 'fight or flight' behaviour in its changing environment.

The domesticated horse was then selectively bred for specific types of work in which these high performance systems were further improved – for speed, agility, stamina, ability and durability, relative to particular disciplines.

The continuing aim has been to produce individual winners within a breed or subtype that would

- go faster (there is, of course, a limit) or better, with more trainable skill, and to do so more
  - surefootedly, and to
  - go on doing so for more years
  and, by definition, with
  - greater freedom from dis-ease associated with occupational hazards, i.e. be more durable

If mistakes in selecting for structure and functioning did occur, and thereby produced a weakness in one or more of the high performance units as the result of

- conformation defects
- developmental orthopaedic disease (DOD)
- metabolic deficiencies
or they were exposed to
- work overload and/or
- insufficient training

then the tissue integrity and the durability of the locomotor system could be so compromised as to predispose to lameness.

The improvements were aimed at the structures and functionings already inherited to produce the biomechanical advantages of locomotion necessary for

- fright
- fight and especially for
- flight

The genetic influences (nature) enhanced, hopefully, by selective matings, were directed to the

- structure – the skeleton and the soft tissues which form the units of locomotion
  - axial – the vertebral column and its physical and **dynamic stability**
  - abaxial – the limbs, and especially their
    - **stay and suspensory apparatus**
    - limb columns of support, including alignment and proportions

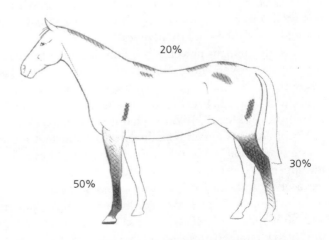

The percentages of damage in the locomotor system.

- **security of footfall and lift off**
- **integrity** of the related
  - joints
  - tendons and
  - neuro-vascular systems
- functioning
  - **muscle efficiency**
  - the back-up systems of digestion and metabolism
  - growth rates, bone density and maturation

Failures and/or aberrations in any one or more could have

- a deleterious knock-on effect on one or more of the others, with the possible outcome of
  - 'poor performance'
  - lameness

Various other 'nurture' inputs, e.g. malnourishment, ill health, unfitness and misuse could affect the **constitutional efficiency** derived from 'nature'.

It is not surprising that in work it is these special systems which are at greatest risk of overstress. Whilst these are mainly in the limbs the vertebral column is also important.

Breed and type identification is based on the overall 'picture' of that horse. This is primarily mapped out by its

- 'points'

to produce a pattern of

- bone lengths, and the angles of the joints between them

The resultant lever systems are motivated by the muscles whose geometry, length, width and volume, their force potential, reflect that of the area between the angles and extremities of the bones themselves.

Thus, the draught power of the Shire's bulkier musculature, with relatively shorter limbs and deeper trunk suggest strength rather than speed. The agility and the speed expected of the Thoroughbred is readily imagined from its more lithe outline. Each looks what it is meant to be.

Within a purebred animal, deviations from what is said to be the ideal conformation do occur. These may minimise athleticism or weaken strength, but by themselves do not directly cause locomotor dis-ease.

Cross breeding can make identification more difficult, and only time will tell how good the progeny, and its inherited characteristics, will be in a selected discipline.

Whatever the conformation of any horse, its usefulness will ultimately depend upon its own

- **balance** and propensity for self carriage – a well proportioned animal – and how that is compromised or complemented by the
- **rider's** ability

In the more obvious conformation aberrations, as seen in the abaxial skeleton

- an over-straight hind leg
- 'cow hocks'

and, in the axial

- an over-long neck

none of which are basically pathological let alone the actual cause of lameness, the predisposition to active disease is much greater. Thus the above examples could directly lead respectively to

- upward fixation of the patella (UFP) (this is disputed by some)
- degenerative joint disease (DJD) of the small intertarsal (hock) joints
- subluxation of certain malformed cervical vertebrae

all with clinical lameness.

Basically due to 'nature', but precipitated by 'nurture', the apportionment of 'blame' is not easy, thus, for example

- the stifle problem related to age and/or unfitness where a sub-optimal muscle power associated with a bio-mechanical, possibly temporary, fault in the essential 'locking' mechanism of that joint causes intermittent lameness. (Inflammatory changes may follow with an actual tissue morbidity in the joint cavity and so a persistent lameness)
- hock dyschondroplasia, an osteo-arthritis of the small tarsal bones and their joints, a morbid consequence of an inherited deficit in the weight-bearing conformation and function of these joints, an instability; it may be associated with structural collapse of the small tarsal bones and a subsequent angular limb deformity to the point of uselessness in the very young animal
- cervical vertebral malformation, a neck problem, a DOD of two vertebrae seen mainly in fast growing Thoroughbreds, whereby a subluxation occurs to produce a neck stiffness. The primary morbidity causes a variable compression of the spinal cord and a slowly progressive degeneration of sensory nerve tracts. A mild

ataxic locomotion follows. The primary disease can be precipitated into an acute clinical picture following a sudden whiplash injury to the neck, as from slipping over when galloping free. A rapidly worsening morbidity of these proprioceptor sensory nerve fibres follows with marked ataxia – a 'wobbler'

There may be an associated osteo-arthritis of the related facet joints in the less severe cases.

In broad terms lameness is more frequent in the foreleg in ridden horses and, conversely, the hind in draught animals. The distribution in any one type of animal is a reflection of the athletic discipline involved, including jumping

- speed and duration
- strength and stamina
- maturity and fitness
- ground surface

Most lamenesses are in one leg, but in conditions such as

- **tendinitis**, there may be low grade lesions in the contralateral tendon – especially in elite athletes
- **navicular** disease, the other leg's navicular area is usually also dis-eased if to a lesser degree. Closer investigation will show a bilateral, if asymmetric, shortening of the two legs' steps. Local anaesthesia of the more severe will 'allow' the other to 'become' more lame

Lameness producing morbidities in the posterior third region of the foot can simulate navicular disease in the early stages. Some of these lesions may also be bilateral – sometimes called 'navicular syndrome'.

Bilateral lameness is seen, for example, in

- laminitis, usually but not always only in the fore
- azoturia (ER) most frequently showing in the hind
- central nervous system lesions such as
  - tetanus, variably fore or hind but usually generalised
  - 'wobbler syndrome' may spread from the hind forward. The bilateralism is variably asymmetric
  - herpes viral endotheliolitis of the spinal cord, variably hind

Trauma, primary or secondary, direct or indirect, closed or open, sterile or infected is the basis of most locomotor disorders and the *fundamental purpose of the subsequent inflammation is to control the damage and to initiate repair*. This response produces, *inter alia*, pain and loss of use which to the horsemaster are *exhibited as lameness*.

Research continues to explain the pathology and, more importantly, the repair processes, the limitations of healing with regard to future athleticism, and the value of the various therapies.

The Distribution of Limb Conditions

The hind limb has the following features, as compared to similar areas of the forelimb

Hoof

- *less* susceptible to
  - solar bruising and punctures of the sole
  - concussion
  - compressive forces, especially in the posterior third, thus in work there is **usually** no
    - navicular disease
    - collapsing buttresses
    - falling-in heels
    - shoe creep with wall overgrowth growth – and so no corns
- however, the defensive hind leg kick can, if hoof contact with a wall is made, result in a fracture of the
  - pedal bone
  - navicular bone

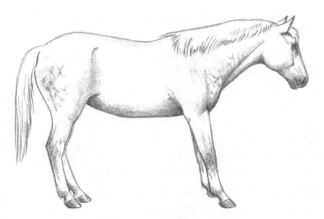

The stance of a pony with laminitis.

- laminitis is less likely, but not unknown
- other traumas, as in the fore foot, are less common except for medial coronary band interference

Fetlock

- *more* susceptible to
  - sprain
  - tendosynovitis (non-articular inflamed wind galls often with related deep digital flexor tendon (DDF) tendinitis in that area or lower
  - desmitis of the branches of the suspensory ligament
  - medial aspect 'brushing' interference

Cannon Region

- rarely affected with superficial flexor tendon (SDF) tendinitis
- less susceptible to splints
- equally, or in some disciplines more susceptible, to
  - sub-tarsal check ligament strain, more frequently with periosteal complications

Hock

- an anatomically and functionally different structure from the foreleg's 'knee' or carpus, and more susceptible to
  - acute strain of the true tibia-tarsal joint
  - DJD, chronic strain of the inter-tarsal joints leading to osteo-arthritis – **spavin**
  - strain of DDF tendon in the tarsal sheath with active **thoroughpin** formation and possible

Curb.

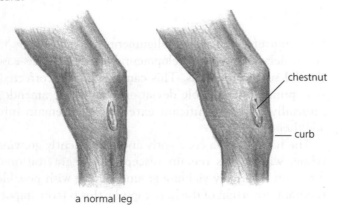

a normal leg

- periosteal reaction and permanent lameness
- strain of the plantar ligament – **curb**
- dislocation of the combined SDF and gastrocnemius tendons off the point of the hock
- rupture of the peroneus tertius tendinous attachment to the dorsal surface, thus 'unlocking' the reciprocal apparatus

Gaskin

- gastrocnemius tendinitis

Stifle

- variable sprain but usually only when the joint is markedly overstressed, with
  - possible complications in the associated
    - tibial proximal bone at the crest
    - the menisci
    - the cruciate ligaments
- **upper fixation of the patella** (UFP), and the less common conditions of
- lateral luxations of the patella
- exposed to external trauma from
  - mis-jumped obstacles
  - having been kicked, particularly in the proximal medial aspect of the shin bone

Persistent resting of *one* hind leg is significant; if some support is taken by the toe then suspect

- stifle injury, but do not overlook the severe, acute pain of
- navicular or pedal bone fracture, from
  - heavy landing on a small, round hard object on an unyielding surface
  - hind leg kick backwards against a wall, which will present similarly when toe support is minimal
- acute solar/white line abscess formation

Hip

- the joint itself is so well protected and secured by the extensive musculature that sprain is rare
- violent trauma, as from a fall or a road traffic accident, can cause
  - dislocation, but usually in association with

- pelvic fracture with very severe haemorrhage as a possible accompaniment if this injury is in a galloping horse which has fallen
  - pelvic stress fractures in the young (less than 4 year old) horse in fast work

Quarters

- muscle 'pull' (see myopathies) is possible and perhaps more common than is suspected

An average veterinary case list usually contains noticeably fewer hind problems than fore. The disciplines in which the horse is involved have a bearing on this. Where collection, elevation and extended gaits are expected, as in advanced dressage, there is an emphasis on hind leg overstress of the

- fetlock
- hock
- quarter muscles

Where jumping is carried out, whether cross-country or over show jumps, there is the risk of

- myopathies in the propulsive proximal muscles
- strain of the
  - sacro-iliac and other pelvic ligaments
  - vertebral ligaments, especially of the caudal thoracic and the lumbar regions

DISEASES

Developmental Disorders

- hereditable (the genotype)
  - congenital – bred 'into' the foal and present at birth
  - delayed (in clinical form at least), though genetically determined
- non-hereditable, i.e. acquired
  - congenital, i.e. acquired during foetal life and clinical at birth
  - delayed, i.e. acquired after birth to become (usually soon after) clinical

Hereditable Limb Alignment Deviations

Such sub-optimal conformation in the abaxial skeleton may also be congenital, but in many cases the malalignment is not recognisable until the foal is several weeks old. It is not yet known which parent is the more responsible for these malalignments. With the toed-in type there is much evidence that the stallion is responsible. He is said to 'throw the defect' in his progeny.

In many instances these deviations are most noticeable in the distal limb, producing the classical

- toed in, or toed out, stance with
- base narrow, or base wide, deviation from limb parallelism which begins proximally to the pastern, often at the fetlock and even higher

Deviation of the knee, fetlock and hock joints – medially, laterally, 'forward' and 'backward' – also occur.

Very few horses meet the idealistically correct specifications of limb alignment, with the associated flight paths and footfalls depicted in many text books. To recognise the variables from 'correct' to 'poor' or 'unacceptable', the horse, with correctly trimmed hooves, must be stood up square on a flat, level, hard surface. It should be viewed from in front of, or from behind, each leg; and from a central position between the fore and the hind legs from a little further back, and again 'opposite' each leg in turn.

A lateral profile impression is got from standing to the side of each limb. *It is particularly important to estimate hoof pastern axis from a low, horizontal viewing.*

Until all the long bones have matured (the last areas are in the distal radius and the tibia), there will be some two-way compression force on the 'soft' areas. This may subtly alter the inherited, congenital alignment, whether normal or not, especially if the foal is

- top heavy
- over-exercised, on hard ground with insufficient sward cover

Such 'nurture induced' malalignments are more likely to be the delayed type of developmental orthopaedic dis-ease (DOD) such as **physitis**. This can possibly be corrected. Any primary hereditable deviations cannot be amended surgically to any significant extent – they remain into adulthood.

The hoof, being a constantly and permanently growing tissue, will always remain susceptible to gravitational forces on a variably yielding ground surface with possible resultant distortion of the hoof capsule: this is more important if there is a tendency for the horse to be toed in or toed out so that more support is taken by one side of the hoof than the other.

Fortunately, these effects can be contained by good farriery which, conversely, should *never* aim for cosmetic correction at the expense of the hoof not being in line with the limb. Mild ground force reactions on the freely moving foal should naturally exert wear on the unshod foot to produce a more balanced footfall and way of going, to the benefit of total locomotor integrity – if there are no, more proximal, deformities or no overweight, this will indicate what is natural for that foal.

In hind leg evaluation the ideal depicted can be misleading. The imaginary plumb line does indeed bisect the thigh, point of hock, back of cannon and fetlock, but this does not emphasise the anatomical fact that *in a 'good' leg the plane projected forward from this line should be obliquely outwards* and not parallel to the mid line of the body as the printed diagrams suggest.

This *functionally* correct alignment is determined by
- the femur being hung slightly abducted (outwards) from the perpendicular, the
- stifles well apart from each other
- the femero-tibial articulation, the stifle joint, is tilted in such a direction that the hind limb in protraction and in retraction describes a forward and outward and an inward and backward flight path (the hind leg 'clears' the abdominal wall)
- the hock articulation is such as to have the front of that joint parallelling that of the stifle
- the point of the hocks thus come to face slightly inward, but they are *not* tilted to lean towards each other as in cow-hock formation

and so the
- cannon falls vertically to the fetlock, which also is slightly turned so as to move the pastern and hoof in this same slightly outward trajectory but, despite the slight toed-out stance, the hoof lands square to break over slightly off centre at lift off

If such a correct hind leg is manually flexed up through all the joints, it can be appreciated that the limb line is a zigzag or spiral, giving it a spring potential with built in kinetic force. It also enhances foot security and muscular power, features which are lost if the conformation tends to the absolute vertical and more so if to actual cow hock or, conversely, bow leg faults. In the former fault, undue strain

is imparted to the medial aspect of the hock with the risk of spavin. In the latter, the hocks bow out in the ground support phase, and a torque force is exerted on the hoof and on the distal joints; there is also a risk of interference during the swing phase.

It is important when assessing any one of the limb's overall alignment that the plane projection of the column of support is determined even when no subdeviation is seen. Is it facing fully forward, slightly out or slightly in? Whichever is the 'natural' for that horse, the hoof must follow that line and break over accordingly at lift off. Any attempt to alter the hoof cosmetically will adversely affect the other joints and detract from kinetic springiness.

Once it is confirmed in the weanling or younger animal that
- **neonatal** angular limb deformities are not present or have resolved and that
- **juvenile DOD** is not clinically present

any of the more common **hereditable** and (generally speaking) less serious limb malalignments can be assessed.

The hereditary limb alignment deviations are (incompletely) listed as follows
- **base narrow**, usually toed in as well; 'pigeon' toed
    - lands outside-in (even in the minority cases which are toed out)
    - weight is always taken on the outside hoof wall with

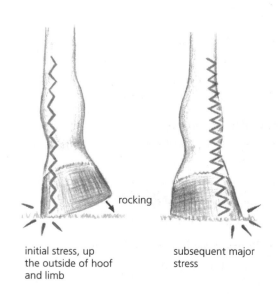

initial stress, up the outside of hoof and limb

rocking

subsequent major stress

A foot landing and rocking over onto full support.

- extra stress up the outside of the hoof and limb

It is now thought – from slow motion video studies – that as weight is increased at full stance position, the hoof which touched down outside in (or *vice versa*) **must further rock down to become flat on the ground** and it is here that this has most effect

- the inside (outside-in, toed-out cases) wall on contact is shunted upwards to predispose to heel collapse
- the stress is now directed up that side of the limb

- the swing phase of the action is described as 'paddling' or even 'plaiting'
- a potential, when 'work' adds to the innate design deficits of the deviated limb, for
  - articular windgalls
  - lateral ringbone
  - lateral sidebone
  - heel bruising and hoof capsule distortion

- **base wide** – usually toed out, 'splay' footed
  - lands inside-out – much more rare than the narrow stance
  - weight taken on medial hoof wall
  - extra stress up the inside of the limb, but subsequent rotation down to 'on the flat' changes the pressure to 'up the outside'
  - the action is described as **winging**, with
  - a potential for
    - limb interference even without the overstress of work, although muscle fatigue from work may make it more likely
    - hoof capsule distortion

The toed-in and toed-out deviations can occur on their own even in apparently parallel limbs, usually due to a slight fetlock or pastern deviation.

The base wide or narrow faults 'start' from the proximal joint levels. If from the knee or the hock there could be a lateral or medial deviation therein.

Lateral deviation of the
- carpal joint: **bow legged**, carpus varus
- hock joint: **bow legged**, tarsus varus

Medial deviation of the

- carpal joint: **knock kneed**, carpus valgus
- hock joint: **cow hocks**, tarsus valgus

Lateral deviation of the
- fetlock joint: **distal bow-leg**, fetlock varus

Medial deviation of the
- fetlock joint: **distal knock-leg**, fetlock valgus

These lateral/medial deviations cause
- overstress of the related joint areas
- a weak supporting limb
- a substandard action
- a potential for superimposed
  - DOD, e.g. physitis, which in turn may lead to further deviations of
  - DJD (degenerative joint disease) which if it develops in the young, open growth plate animal, is known as **juvenile DJD** (JDJD)

- palmar deviations of the carpal joints; calf kneed, 'back at the knee'
  - the ground force reaction is particularly diverted onto the
    - check ligaments, above and below the knee
    - dorsal aspect of the carpal bones, which become compressed with
    - potential of chip fractures (especially in young flat-racing horses)

- dorsal deviation of the carpal joint; goat or buck kneed, 'forward of the knee' and dependent upon the degree
  - with overstress onto the
    - superficial flexor tendon
    - suspensory ligament
    - sesamoid bones

The heritable malalignments are the consequence of genetically determined 'faults' in the geometry of articular surfaces anywhere up the limb, whereby planes of movement are altered, hence so too are the flight paths of the swing phase and the landing pattern of the support phase. Theoretically, the units of locomotion affected should have related structures, cartilage, joint capsule and ligaments, either genetically (or adaptively) formed so that the unit works in harmony. Where the distortion is not great the horse should move without difficulty and certainly not be lame; in other words, there is no pathological dis-ease in the uncomplicated mild cases.

The swing and support variations would be seen when action was viewed from in front or from behind, as a 'not straight' action.

It is advisable that continuing inspection of the growing foal is carried out to monitor the presence and/or worsening of any alignment deviation as compared to the diagrammatic ideal.

Neonatal Angular Limb Deformity

A **congenital** complex of limb malalignment which has doubtful or at most only an indirect genetic input. It is seen usually in the dysmature foal, i.e. one 'up to time' in terms of gestation period but not well developed or conditioned. It is weak in the legs but often lively and keen. Overdue foals also may, paradoxically, exhibit these limb weaknesses. In both types the foal is unable to press up into postural extension. It may walk on its 'knees' or on the back of its hind fetlocks; it may be markedly knock kneed in front or bow legged behind. Most, with common-sense management, recover.

There is much overlapping of direct and indirect causes of the juvenile development diseases of the locomotor system which are collectively known as **developmental orthopaedic disease (DOD)**. They 'belong' to text books on stud management, but they are discussed here primarily because affected youngstock which are nursed through the disorders can and do enter the 'market' at varying levels of usefulness, but still carry the associated weaknesses of

- acquired conformation limb disorders
- joint pathologies – juvenile degenerative joint disease **(JDJD)**, sub-clinical perhaps but likely to be physically stressed into clinical conditions

Up until comparatively recently there has been scientific dispute as to the true pathogenesis (explanation of the cause and the effect) and the subsequent incidence and prevalence of these development problems.

By definition, all are related to
- bone and its associated cartilages
  - articular
  - growth plate
- growth rates as they affect parallel development of
  - muscle and bone, especially in quick maturing types

- coincidentally compromised blood supply

and are limited to before the times of cessation of bone growth and maturation as determined by ossification of the cartilaginous centres, plates and foci of growth.

Thus seeds of future DOD are established at or soon after birth and certainly before 2 years of age. However, the clinical signs of some types may not recognisably appear until after that time. For example, the really serious manifestations of the 'bone cysts' and 'wobbler' syndrome require the stresses associated with the more mature horse. Conversely, bone cyst lesions may never progress to clinical levels; they are diagnosed fortuitously during radiography for other causes of lameness.

Many have a genetic basis – the risk is thought to be approximately 0.25%. Some are precipitated by trauma. Nutrition plays a variable role; it can affect the genetic ability of tissues to reach correct and synchronised growth and maturation especially in the quick maturing Thoroughbreds. Whilst rickets is not clinically recognised in horses, other calcium, phosphorus and possibly vitamin D imbalances in the diet associated with other hormonal influences do cause joint/bone disorders.

There are several sub-groups within DOD

- the **dyschondroplasias** – a failure of localised or focal cartilage/bone development. There is a breed determination as to which joints, and when clinical signs develop

  - **physitis** (epiphysitis) – growth cartilage plate deficit causing a compromised blood supply and bone mal-development of the distal radius and distal metacarpals and metatarsals, the columns of support, to cause acquired angular limb deformities

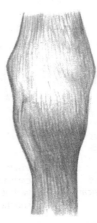

enlarged area above the knee

Physitis (left fore, from the front).

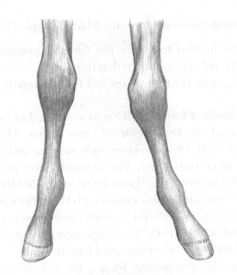

Angular limb deformity of the growing foal.

of the growing foal

- **osteochondrosis** – articular cartilage focal deficit, with
  - subsequent formation of **bone cysts**
- **osteochondritis dissecans** – avulsion of small areas of necrotic articular cartilage, with 'joint mice' (loose fragments of bone) formation
- **cervical lateral vertebral joint malformation** inducing the sub-luxation which causes specific

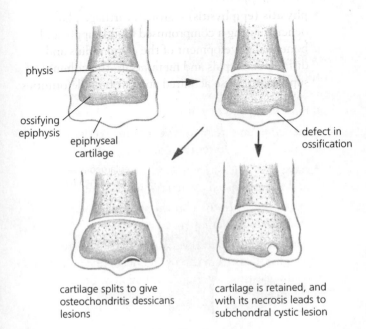

physis

ossifying epiphysis

epiphyseal cartilage

defect in ossification

cartilage splits to give osteochondritis dessicans lesions

cartilage is retained, and with its necrosis leads to subchondral cystic lesion

Osteochondrosis.

spinal cord sensory axon compression and a deficit in proprioception – the **wobbler syndrome**

- tissue growth imbalances
  - **rapid bone lengthening** as compared to parallel lengthening of related muscles causing, through tendon force, **flexural deformities** in weanlings and yearlings in which the associated upright hoof/pastern development is variably permanent
- tendency to obesity, and so to too much weight on immature and/or vascular compromised bones and joints in the columns of limb support, which may be already weakened through
  - conformation defects and associated uneven distribution of weight forces
  - any of the DOD
  - exposure to sudden, irregular, wrong surfaces at exercise

Abaxial dyschondroplasias are frequently slow in developing into DOD, and present as simple stiffness of gait. The epiphysitis of the rapidly growing foal can present as a lameness before the 'open' joint appearance of the bone disorder is obvious to the layman. Secondary limb distortion often follows if the initial condition is not quickly treated and will occur not only in the original area but in distal joints and in other limbs as well, as they come under abnormal loading. Effect on the hoof is often marked with pedal bone distortion and/or white line opening and subsequent infection to complicate matters.

The diagnosis, treatment and later management does not always result in a successful cure, particularly to meet the requirements of athleticism. Such animals, whether pure or cross bred, can often become pleasure horses whose prowess is not required until they are over 4 years old, so with time to compensate for it before their less exacting work starts.

In some cases, an affected animal will be left with low grade orthopaedic disorders which in themselves can present as ongoing risks of secondary joint arthroses, the DJD complexes. Others will have related, acquired deformities in the hooves, from the initial column of support abnormalities. Although such hoof faults can be rectified there is often an on going tendency to relapse to the originally induced hoof buttress weakness and collapsed heels.

Conformation defects of the hoof capsule can be an inherited feature in themselves; not only are they exposed to further change from any higher limb imbalances but they can, from footfall and lift off deficits, also exert reverse pathogenic effect on the units of locomotion up to and including the 'knee' and the hock before these areas' respective ossifications are complete.

On purchasing an adult 5 year-old horse or retaining a home bred specimen, previously treated or not, it is advisable that a careful assessment with expert farrier and veterinary help is made so that the situation becomes known at the start of work. Any possible corrections should be attempted and the possible risks appreciated or seen as not a worthwhile gamble considering the purchase price and/or later costs.

In the adult horse any DOD induced limb aberration is by definition a fixed feature, as are the genetic deviations. The bones are now mature. As already emphasised, the hoof wall is a growing tissue subject to many compressive forces. Any acquired changes in its conformation and in the wear of the shoe should be looked for at successive shoeings and be corrected by the farrier to obviate limb overstress and precipitation of DJD lesions. Where a hoof capsule fault is not recognised there can follow a blood flow disturbance and/or a distortion of the pedal bone and the coffin joint which is very slow to resolve even with special hoof care.

Certain discipline uses are more susceptible to the mal-effect of deviations; a horse may be a worthwhile purchase as a showjumper but not for use in dressage or eventing. A horse which has been in average work from 3 to 5 years and is acceptably level in action despite certain deviations, is unlikely to deteriorate unless the work load and type is drastically altered and/or farrier care is reduced.

The presence of self-corrected or contained DOD lesions and, of course, any evidence of DJD in the adult horse will amend the interpretation (prognosis) and therefore the value of such a horse with and, indeed without, heredited, basic limb conformation faults. Selection as a brood animal is another matter.

The horsemaster must appreciate that the basic effects of limb alignment disorders are

- insecurity of footfall and of lift-off in the
  - toe-in animal, and to a lesser extent in the
  - toe-out horse

At the faster gaits, the insecurity may be such that

- support gives way, so that a premature lift-off breaking over the quarter-wall will cause a stumble leading in some cases to sufficient acceleration forces to inflict a stress fracture **of the pastern** – usually base-wide, toed in
- interference during the flight phase by that limb

striking the other leg, as in the toed-out animal, bad enough to **wing** and **strike** – especially if base-narrow when 'brushing' may cause splints and sesamoid bruising

It is these traumatic risks as well as the decreased athletic ability of the poor actioned horse and the unpleasing appearance which devalues such (as yet lame-free) animals.

Attempting to alter alignment, even if recognised before bone maturity occurs, is often unsatisfactory (and especially so in the more proximal inherited types). It is effected by amending the conformation of the hoof and so its support phase induced pressures up the limb. More often than not the pressure rebounds, to the detriment of the hoof capsule and the related distal joints. To attempt it in the adult horse is useless, and the reverse pressures are even more detrimental.

Consideration of surgical techniques to control deviations associated with growth plates, although often successful, are outside the scope of this text.

Careful farrier trimming over several shoeings, in the mature horse, can slowly alter any hoof capsule geometry *per se*. It aims to

- return the hoof to the correct column of support line and maintain it there
- correct hoof wall flare with white line distortion and buttress collapse
- minimise interferences

If a limb deviation is unilateral, the adult horse

- may move, and always will have moved, in an unlevel fashion suggestive of lameness. This action is a physically induced, observable, functioning defect and not a morbidity *per se*, but it may
  - 'develop' unilateral muscle asymmetry, which visually exaggerates the unlevelness
  - have the basic unlevelness worsened because of any work induced overstress, with resultant DJD
  - develop DJD in the contra-lateral limb, or others, from persistent compensatory overuse
  - become affected in the axial skeleton due to the torque effects from the imbalanced abaxial action, or in 'resisting' the rider's attempts to obtain balance

In bilateral symmetric deviations which do not cause

imbalances of action, but which reduce the horse's freedom of action, secondary direct pathology is less likely.

In considering the predisposing causes of closed traumatic lesions which are not patently the result of a one-off accident, the following features are important

- hereditable conformation deviations
- DOD defects, i.e. acquired deviations in locomotion
- the inherited physiological or constitutional susceptibility to metabolic disorders leading to
  - muscle functioning deficit and early fatigue
- low grade, chronic, often bilateral but asymmetric lameness, such as arise from DJD

The other contributing, exacerbating factors to the predisposition to axial and abaxial potential trauma, both open and closed, are

- fast work before the horse is
  - conditioned – the 'toning' of the connective tissues
  - trained, i.e. fittened, for a known
    - distance
    - speed
    - stamina to prevent excessive work causing early flexor muscle fatigue and associated loss of flexor/extension balance
- work, when incidentally weakened
  - post injury
  - ill (fevered)
- work on 'dangerous', varying, unfamiliar surfaces
  - stony or other rough ground
  - pot-holed, burrowed, poached and now rutted
  - heavy and holding
  - slippery
  - ridge and furrow
  - extreme slopes
    - horizontal
    - vertical

These are all work load overstresses but which can slowly be trained for.

The phenotypical differences in horses bred to a genotypical line are not so well categorised as in man.

To breed for an 'obvious' phenotype, such as colour, is quite possible. To be able to 'fix' other visible characteris-

tics which are reflections of the total metabolic processes is not an exact science. Consider

- responsiveness to management and feeding
  - body fat/muscle, the 'condition' as in
    - a good doer
    - a bad doer
- training effects
  - athleticism
    - aerobic potential
    - anaerobic development
- keenness ('heart', 'guts')
- durability
- temperament
- fundamental attitudes and behaviour

All these may well be in the 'nature' of the horse but are variably responsive to all aspects of 'nurture'. They play a complementary role in the horse's athleticism and future susceptibility to trauma.

Inflammatory Disorders

A veterinary surgeon will acknowledge the inflammatory nature of the underlying morbidity which results in pain-induced lameness by using the suffix – 'itis' to the classic name for the tissue or the anatomical site, thus

- osteitis – inflammation of bone
- arthritis – of a joint, a range of inflammatory conditions usually implying a chronic state, but acute lesions with sudden signs do occur
- synovitis – of the synovia secreting lining, the synovial membrane, (the synovium) of a joint or a sheath or a bursa; the source of enzymes damaging to cartilage and associated with excess synovia production
- osteo-arthritis, or DJD – when bone is eventually involved, usually at the later stages
- carpitis – of the carpus (knee joint) but does not indicate which tissue within that joint or if it is soft tissue morbidity only
- septic arthritis – when the joint synovial lining is infected and the synovial fluid is purulent. Certain affected joints have a specific name when inflamed
  - spavin – the intertarsal joints
  - gonitis – the stifle joint
  - others must be content with

- arthritis of the shoulder joint or, more scientifically the scapulo-humeral joint
- myositis – of muscle
- tendinitis – of tendon, *not* within the sheaths
- tendo-synovitis – of tendon, within its sheath, which is also inflamed
- desmitis – of ligament
- neuritis – of nerve

The older descriptive terminology is still in use in everyday 'horsey' language, thus

- **sore shins** – a periostitis associated with micro fractures of the front of the (usually upper) metacarpal and metatarsal bone, the cannon
- **ringbone** – a chronic proliferative osteitis of the pastern bone resulting from a periostitis following direct trauma (a bruise) or a ligament attachment tear outside the joint area
- **articular ringbone** – when the bone within the joint capsular area is affected, as from an articular ligament attachment tear or, less usually, a controlled septic arthritis
- **splint** – the healed end point of a sprain or bruise of a periosteal interconnecting ligament, usually in a young adolescent horse's fore cannons, causing haemorrhage and
  subsequent new-bone bridging formation on the cannon and splint bone
- **sidebone** – the result of ossification of the lateral cartilage 'inflamed' by trauma

These colloquial names given to the local affected areas and the associated lameness have been handed down from one generation of horsemasters to the next. Many are still current language even though they were coined long before the underlying morbidity was known or understood.

It is important, however, for the horsemaster to know, even if she does not fully understand the why and the how, what the underlying inflammatory morbidity is and that it is, in the main

- common to all locomotor tissue dis-ease
  - there is no fundamental pathologic difference between, e.g.
    - a curb, an inflammation of the plantar ligament of the hock and
    - a 'bowed' tendon of the superficial flexor muscle

Traumatic

In locomotor system disorders trauma is a major factor:

- **internal** – overstress of one or more components of the units of locomotion, with no directly involved disruption of the skin; a 'closed' trauma and so not exposed to secondary infection
  - strain
  - sprain
  - concussion
  - compression
  - shearing or torque force including 'spontaneous' bone fractures

  related to abnormal forces generated *within* the limb, acute, subacute or chronic in effect and associated with accelerating forces producing jerk or whiplash and inelegant action, with resultant damage
- **external** trauma – the typical **bruise**
  - onto but not 'through' the skin, and from there variably onto deeper tissues even to the extent of bone fracture
  - open wound through the skin into variably deeper tissues thus exposed to infection as well as bruising into
    - non-vital areas
    - vital (synovial) areas

The associated variable lameness in both sub-types is the 'loss of use' sign of the inflammatory response to the trauma. It is a protective reaction stimulated by the cardinal sign of

- pain

and the other cardinal signs, variably perceivable

- swelling
- heat, and where applicable
  - vein engorgement
  - fuller arterial pulse
  - discoloration (present but rarely visible)

and, with open wounds, a subsequent

- discharge

In some conditions there is also a generalised unwellness, especially if the pain is severe, as in fractures and severe bilateral strain when there is

- anxiety, accelerated cardiac and respiratory rates
- fever, patchy sweating, inappetence

- reluctance to move at all

The hoof has a particular exposure risk; it is constantly and repetitively making and breaking contact with the upward ground force pressure, and with friction in axial and horizontal directions against the downward opposing force of gravity, i.e. the horse's (and rider's) 'mass x speed'. A fixed point, if only momentarily, it acts as a distal fulcrum around which all the body leverages are exerted; it is, after all, in ground contact for upwards of 25% of the time in locomotion.

It is these which can cause overstresses on the

- hoof wall
- coffin joint
    - its ligaments
    - navicular bone and its juxtaposition against the deep flexor tendon
    - arterio-venous shunt mechanism and the distal blood flow generally

Security of footfall, support and lift off depends on

- a strong, well conformed and buttressed hoof capsule
- an antero-posterior and latero medial balanced hoof
- an uncompromised blood flow

A well-conformed limb structure and functioning above the hoof can only be as efficient as the foundation support and its absorption of much of the opposing dynamic forces.

Infectious

- **primary**
    - **joint ill** in foals – septic arthritis
    - **brucellosis** (now rare) – desmitis
    - **tetanus** toxin – inhibitor, neuron-paralysis
    - **viral endotheliolitis** – indirect neuron-morbidity
    - ergot and other **toxicoses** – blood supply interference
- **secondary**
    - mud fever **dermatitis**
    - ventral trunk **rainscald** and **mud fever** dermatitis
    - **cellulitis** and **lymphangitis**
    - **clostridial toxin myositis** – blood borne

all interfering with movement, from

- pain and

- physical 'stiffness'
- tissue damage in some units of locomotion
- and sometimes associated systemic illness

Allergic Disorders

Lymphangitis – 'Monday morning leg', although designated as inflammation the cause is immune/allergic related. The resultant morbidity is inflammatory and is usually associated with a prior bacterial infection now 'lodged' in lymphoid tissue, hence lymphangitis.

Metabolic Disorders

- rhabdomyolysis (ER), azoturia
- laminitis – sequel to enteric and uterine toxicity, an endotoxaemia with morbidity of vascular tissue: here too the eventual result is an inflammation
- mineral imbalance induced osteoarthritis

Degenerative Disorders

As related to the locomotor system this mainly refers to the joints. It implies a slowly developing morbidity leading to a chronic state which, in the adult especially, is irreversible. At the very least it results in reduced useful-ness. There are, however, acute states with associated increases in pain which can arise as exacerbations at any stage, usually precipitated by sudden re-traumas: the lameness worsens.

The chronicity involves the

- synovial lining
- cartilage
- bone
    - centrally from the joint surfaces
    - peripherally at the capsule ligament attachments

The composite lesion is an osteoarthritis, and is categorised as a DJD. There is a basic inflammatory, sterile morbidity.

The various commonly affected articulations have collo-quial names

- hock (intertarsal bones) – **bone spavin**
- 'knee' (intercarpal bones) – **'knee' spavin**

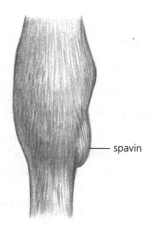

'Bone spavin' of the intertarsal bones of the hock.

- fetlock – **osselots**
- pastern and coffin – high and low **ringbone**

Not all, however, are confined to the abaxial skeleton, in which the lesions are most commonly distal where the joints have most overstress and minimal indirect muscle support. The axial skeleton, and especially the lateral articulations therein, are also common sites especially in the cervical and lumbar regions.

The abaxial lesion is invariably accompanied by an

- initial synovitis with effusion of excess synovia, hence a distention of the joint capsule gradually develops
    - articular **windgall** of the fetlock
    - **bog spavin** of the hock in some cases

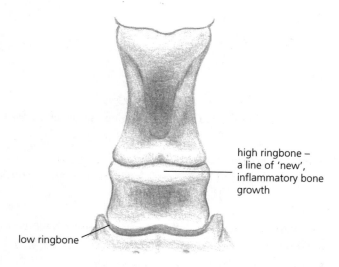

High and low ringbone of the pastern and coffin.

- low grade erosion and degeneration of cartilage
- osteitis and/or periostitis
- lameness

The precipitating factors are

- persistent overuse – wear and tear
- conformation defects associated with asymmetric weight loading as a sub-acute persistent condition
    - heredited
    - acquired
        - DOD
        - hoof imbalances
- acute sprain
- nutritional imbalances

A more chronic type of true joint sprain, especially in the hock and in the fetlock arises from persistent concussion, compression and 'shear' overstress.

The overall sequence of the traumatic-inflammatory events is

- synovitis – a release of chemicals which produce
- cartilage degeneration – a release of further chemicals which lead to
- erosion of the underlying bone (the main source of pain) and/or
    - thickening and degeneration of the synovial capsule
- subsequent inflammatory 'new' bone, as with
    - spur formation
    - periosteal proliferation
- reduced range of movement
- eventual ankylosis in some cases, e.g. spavin where the intertarsal (small) bones are involved as distinct from the true joint

Recent research indicates that with comprehensive early

- diagnosis
- therapy/surgery
- management
    - hoof rebalancing
    - nutrition correction where necessary
    - rehabilitation exercise

an affected horse can return to some level of work,

sometimes with continuing analgesic cover. This is known as regenerative joint dis-ease (RJD).

DJD can also be a sequel to
- primary bacterial infections, as from puncture wounds

or associated with
- vascular venous disturbances, as in the 'posterior third of the foot' syndrome

Muscles are also subject to degeneration changes
- atrophy through loss of use
  - paralysis
  - persistent spasm

- necrosis, as in some stages of rhabdomyolysis
- micro and macro overstress, and their repair scars

Neoplastic Disorders

Not of great significance as such but **sarcoids**, and to a lesser extent melanomata in locomotion areas, can be bruised, abraided and subsequently infected with resultant pain with lameness, direct from tack rubbing soreness or indirect as the horse attempts to move a limb away (abducts) from a painful site. The various **sarcomas** can, dependent on site and size, interfere with movement.

CHAPTER

34 DETECTION

INTRODUCTION

'Being level', 'sound in action', 'not lame', is defined as

- moving, in hand, under saddle or in harness, in the various gaits, in a visible and audible manner recognisable as the accepted normal way of going for a horse of that particular breed or type, subject to its level of fitness and training and to the discipline engaged in

- able to lie, get up and down, and to posture, in a normal manner

Being 'lame', 'unlevel', 'not sound in action', is defined as

- incapable of normal locomotion and/or stance, and so

- exhibiting signs of deviation, from the natural way of going in a gait or gaits and/or of posture, which suggest a dis-ease of the structure and/or functioning of the locomotor system

A lame horse may also show, in addition to the actual locomotor abnormality, a varying degree of

- resistance or evasion

- loss of balanced action

- inelegance when ridden or driven

Lameness is the visible and audible outcome of the horse's attempt to minimise the pain associated with the cause. In a few situations it is a biomechanical difficulty in performing normal limb flight and support, not necessarily associated with pain. In other situations the pain may also provoke generalised or systemic signs of unwellness.

However, it can also be sensed by the rider, who can appreciate the associated altered balance and rhythm of the horse 'through the seat of the breeches' and other contact areas – kinaesthesia.

It must be emphasised that the 'fact' as well as the 'where', 'why' or 'what' of lameness, fore or hind should, in this chapter, relate only to *new* conditions. Such newness is 'a first time occasion' with the implication that it is most likely to be traumatic in origin. The newness may be the clinical appearance of an unknown sub-clinical morbidity of variable duration, such as required progressive or sudden overstress to bring it out into a clinical activity which may now be subacute, as a

- slowly worsening action which attracts the attention of the rider and/or the horsemaster, or as a

- suddenly acute condition – an overt lameness

Perceivable conditions described as **chronic** had to start sometime; their presence should have been recorded and any subsequent flare up should be seen as a **new lameness**.

Remember, *it is the function of a daily routine inspection to detect lameness which is 'new' to the observer.* This is distinct from a prepurchase examination by a vet or adviser to detect undeclared lameness or chronic lesions likely to lead to lameness.

A suspected lame horse should be

- quickly detected as such

- methodically investigated to form an initial, even tentative, general assessment

- appropriately first-aided where relevant and/or given primary management

- more expertly/professionally investigated when deemed necessary

The horse meanwhile must be taken out of work and boxed or yarded, to prevent a worsening of the condition, in consideration of welfare and economics.

A horsemaster, to be worthy of his name, must appreciate that it is essentially more important to detect that something is **wrong** than to know the cause. His assessment must be based on the use of all his senses, including common sense. He will consider not only the lameness but also, in some situations

- the horse's conformation, sex, age and height
- its general appearance, behaviour and condition

He must know, as part of his essential skills, how to apply first aid and early management on basic and not heroic principles, yet be aware of his limitations and prepared 'if in doubt, to shout' for help.

He should, as a *potentially* proficient handler, learn about

- cause, effect and outcome of any morbidity
- the prognosis – the future usefulness after clinical recovery
- the reason for treatments professionally advised

Much of this latter information, the background knowledge, has to be learnt in theory and where possible in practice, but *the basic essential knowledge must be the ability to detect that lameness (and any associated injury) is present*.

The intention here is not to give an encyclopaedic list of all possible locomotor disorders; rather, the emphasis is on the *detection of a newly lame horse* and on the *underlying morbidities which are involved*.

In day-to-day management the horsemaster has the considerable benefit of knowing the horse

- its normal (usual) **A** **B** **C**, the presence of chronic lesions indicative of previous injury and when and why it was last lame, if at all
- the recent history of
  - the work done in terms of
    - speed
    - duration
    - complexity
    - terrain
      - hard
      - soft

- holding
- slippery
- on the flat
- cross country
- show jumping etc.
- when the lameness was first suspected
  - in which gait
  - if at a transition down, or a pulling up, or landing over a jump
  - shortly after the finish of work
  - later that day
  - was it quite obvious then?
  - did it get progressively worse, over what length of time?

A veterinary surgeon would ask these, especially if called to examine a sudden closed trauma type.

In the context of an owner's/horsemaster's detection of a lameness in a horse of which he has direct day-to-day knowledge the implication is that the lameness is either of

- sudden appearance, i.e. a 'new' condition or
- the clinical end point of an earlier reported deterioration in
  - action
  - performance
- an exacerbation of an old lesion

In any sudden lameness there is a strong suggestion of either a

- traumatic overstress, a 'closed type' *internal* injury
- traumatic wounding with skin involvement, the *external* type, closed or open (skin penetration)
- *metabolic* disorder – such as exertional rhabdomyolysis (ER)

External traumas are fortuitous and can happen in any phase of work (or at rest, where many horses are more prone to injury than when in work: a reflection of field management, perhaps!)

Overstress internal traumas are more likely near the end of the exertion, as with tendinitis. Conversely, an inelegant accelerating/decelerating stride could cause a primary overstress at any time during fast work.

Azoturia is a **functioning failure** in muscle metabolism,

usually during performance. Minor forms can develop after work as the horse 'warms down', or even in transit.

This will almost certainly still present signs the next day, but possibly in decreased form. If the original was a post exercise form and had been missed, the next day's signs could well be misleadingly mild and seen as stiffness. The acute stage can hardly be missed, the severe crippling hind leg's lameness and distress is very apparent.

Trauma of the open type including variably deep bruising, can of course occur when the horse is

- in stables, e.g. if it is cast
- at grass – when some disorders' early and critical stage can be missed

The use of colloquial names to describe or 'localise' the trauma are often misleading, in as much as they do not acknowledge that most traumas produce the same basic morbid changes. Consider 'sprain' and 'strain'. There is in both a closed, sterile **overstress** trauma, with associated

- bleeding under the skin and in the primary tissue involved
- disruption of tissue fibres
- interruption of the blood flow
- stimulation of the sensory nerves
- oedema around, and later below, the site

In a **sprain**, i.e. a trauma to a joint, there is specific damage to the *component*

- ligaments, both 'directing' and supporting
- joint capsule
- cartilage
- bone

and in a **strain**, the trauma is to the *tissues which move a joint*, the

- tendons
- muscles (in the form of a spasm or a tear)

The similar morbidity in these two areas of a unit of locomotion produces clinical signs typical of inflammation

- swelling
- heat
- pain, and associated
  - loss of use
  - lameness, the ultimate sign

Colloquially, a

- *joint* when **sprained** was referred to as 'blown up'
- *tendon* when **strained** was referred to as 'a leg'

and when severe to the point of rupture as 'broken down', thus describing a further, associated, anatomical defect.

Certain traumas were given more specific names relative to site

- 'curb' – strain damage to the ligament at the back of the hock
- 'a suspensory' – a strain to the ligament and/or its branches at the back of the cannon and the fetlock

'Strain' or 'Sprain'? It tells you 'tendon or suspensory ligament' or 'joint'.

Experienced older (and not necessarily tutored) horsemasters knew that galloping/jumping horses were prone to injury of the flexor tendons, most frequently of the forelegs, and that severe lameness was invariably the consequence. Many were aware that these were tendon traumas following the strain of overstress on them, particularly in the asymmetric gaits when one foreleg takes all the weight on landing and at lift off, particularly over a jump – usually the trailing foreleg.

They were also aware that the lameness was accompanied by marked swelling around the back and the sides of the cannon bone. The colloquial 'a leg' left no one in doubt as to 'what' and 'where', and bitter experience foretold a prolonged lay-off with a poor outlook. It did not determine if it was the superficial, or the deep tendon, or the suspensory ligament, but

- the horse was lame
- the swelling was in the back of the cannon, so
  - work was stopped
  - first aid and initial management applied

The more experienced horsemaster/trainer recognised that a horse which was a little 'short' in action, quite often both fore, showing a degree of puffiness and heat around the potential strain area, should be taken out of work, or 'let down' until the 'leg' went 'down' to normal and the stride length increased; the work load could then be increased *slowly*.

Such quick appreciation and action could prevent an actual severe strain; good horsemastership recognised the warning signs of a potential acute trauma.

Today, subsequent treatment and management

following high-tec diagnostic and prognostic tests of a possible or an actual strain will be based on a more scientific understanding of the pathology and the natural repair processes aided, perhaps even improved, but not noticeably speeded up, by electronic and other therapies.

Of course, recognition of 'a leg' can well be misleading unless the handler is aware of possible other anatomically close-by morbidities which have to be differentiated. Many, even experienced laymen, so dread the thought of tendinitis that any cannon swelling means a strain until proved otherwise.

Little harm will follow the optimal first-aid measure of cold water or ice applications, even if it is not a ligament or a tendon injury. Firm pressure bandaging, however, might well be contra-indicated, even damaging, and the subsequent management critically wrong, if the swelling is due to

- a local small wound with cellulitis, more so if it was
- 'sympathetic' inflammatory oedema up the leg, associated with pus in the foot, and disastrous if due to a
- septic windgall's purulent distension and inflammatory synovitis from a perforation, likewise a fetlock septic arthritis

Even when such a mistake in diagnosis is made, if the horsemaster is carrying out the second skill of management – 'is the horse responding to his treatment as he expects?' – the recognition of 'all *still* not being well' or at least not improving, might not be too late. It is the stubborn refusal to admit the possibility of error, that is so dangerous.

The majority of lamenesses require no more than reasonable horsemastership and common sense for detection and managing. It is their assessment which is more different but – important.

To find a horse lame when it wasn't lame yesterday (it is presumed that 'sound in action or not' is always looked for, as described below) will suggest a very recent traumatic incident

- an obvious wound
- 'picked up' objects in the hoof
- a history of a kick, or
- a reported entanglement in an obstacle
- a potential overstress related to
  - the type of athleticism
    - when fatigued or

- in which an 'inelegant' stride was witnessed

must suggest the need for

- inspection
- decision
- action

Such perception, aided perhaps by, for instance, *later discovered clues* associated with the **reactive inflammation**, should discourage concern about suspected, less common and often more chronic confusing lameness, for example

- navicular disease – when actually there is a stone lodged in the sole
- shoulder arthritis – when actually there is a thorn embedded in the forearm
- central nerve system damage ataxia – when actually there is bilateral high hind-leg mud fever

Always consider the whole limb and the horse's overall locomotion, even the whole horse, when evaluating a suspected lameness. Certainly *always examine the foot/shoe* even in more proximal dis-ease; both could be present

- sub-acute or chronic foot lameness can predispose to a new, higher limb trauma and clinical lameness
- a sudden foot lameness such as
  - penetrated sole
  - over-reach
  - clawed-off shoe with wall damage

can also precipitate a subsequent false stride, producing an

- interference higher in the limb or a
- strain or sprain

in the same or another limb which is 'seen' (and treated) as a primary condition, while the other, lower one, is overlooked or wrongly evaluated.

Impediments causing indirect lameness

- pain, from
  - primary pressures as in *ill-fitting tack*
  - secondary to dental/oral/biting problems
- training faults, leading to
  - imbalances and evasions, leading to

- interferences
- rider faults, causing the horse to attempt rebalancing the resultant reflex defects, with consequent trauma

can all be misleading

Less common, often less sudden, lamenesses do occur and their diagnosis, as distinct from the fact of a lameness, is not always a simple matter even for the veterinary surgeon.

For the horsemaster as well as the vet, the detection of lameness requires an ability to know what to look for in a normally moving horse in comparison with what is now perceived in an abnormally actioned one. Of course, to know it is lame is primarily important, and acknowledging that **the horse must stop work** is the first management decision, but it is often the fact of

- which leg?
- which area of that leg?
- what morbidity is present? (not always easily visualised)
- what caused it? (might never be accurately identified)
- what is to be done, and by whom?

that requires careful thought and often further help.

Many lamenesses at least begin as a subtle alteration in the way the horse 'goes', and this is not always easy to recognise, for example

- in hand at a walk on the hard it may not be seen
- in hand at the trot it might show, and even more so if
- ridden, but sometimes only if observed by someone on the ground
- it is often easier to see and hear on the hard if a concussive cause is involved
- action in the deep and the soft of a sand surface (not the soft of a slippery, heavy, muddy field) can conversely 'bring out' the sub-clinical 'joint', 'suspensory', or stay apparatus strain as the site of the lameness-provoking lesion exacerbated in the unusual going
- lungeing on 20-metre circles on a non-slip surface will also be a further test

The occasional refusal to jump is often put down to behaviour, and not to the horse 'telling' the rider that he is not so silly as to want to land on tender feet from a height, or with a painful 'back' lesion.

A disinclination to be ridden on one diagonal or in a particular lead is usually put down to rider technique error, especially if a better rider can 'encourage' the horse to accept his/her stronger aid, when in fact there is a pathology perhaps in the neck or the back if not in a leg.

A dressage judge's comments of unlevelness may be said by the rider to be a subjective error on the judge's part, when she may be telling you that the horse has 'told' her that it hurts somewhere.

Sooner or later all these may well, with continuing work, develop into clinical lameness, sometimes bilateral, but most frequently to a fulminating single limb condition due, for example, to

- an overstressed, mildly lame joint progressing into an acute inflammation – a **sprain**
- a tendon having been repetitively stressed, now causing an altered stride and support lameness from a finally overstressed tissue – an **acute strain**

It would have been better if the earlier signs had been recognised as warnings.

There are cases where there is no doubt that an altered way of going does exist, but the cause and often the exact location eludes the clinical expertise of a veterinary

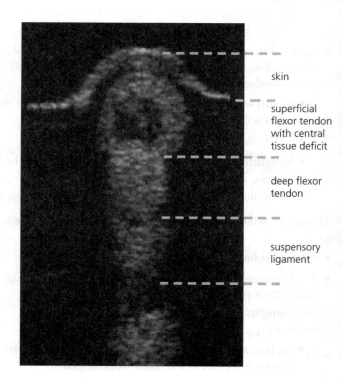

skin

superficial flexor tendon with central tissue deficit

deep flexor tendon

suspensory ligament

Ultrasonograph of a transverse section of the middle third of the metacarpus, the cannon of a foreleg.

surgeon who must then seek

- auxiliary aids such as
  - flexion tests
  - nerve blocking anaesthesia
  - intra-articular anaesthesia – to localise the morbidity, and
  - radiography
  - ultrasonography
  - thermography
  - scintigraphy

to identify the tissue(s) involved so that he can advise.

Observing the Lame Horse

The technique or skill in locomotor system inspection is basically the same as that for all systems

- perception used in a methodical manner
- the comprehensiveness will vary, for example
  - at grass, a horse will require inspection daily, certainly close-to, during the first week
  - after that time it will have settled with its field companions and got the explosiveness out of its system. Daily inspection need not be so close up
- a horse during conditioning road work at the walk will not be subjected to the athletic traumas possible in fast work, but the
  - mouth will continue to be delicate for 10 days or so, as will the
  - saddle and girth areas
  - limb interference and new concussive forces on the hooves, especially, will be possible hazards particularly if the horse is flighty or skittish

Thereafter attention can be directed, when trotting starts, to

- external trauma from extraneous objects
- slight internal traumas of tendons, joints and ligaments, especially if previously dis-eased, as it reacts to increasing work loads which can be adjusted down if necessary
  - each morning before another day's work, and more intensely as and when faster work begins
- more exact inspections now become essential, after work and particularly on the day after an increased work load or a competition, and as soon as possible after

- any possible traumatising incident, as from
  - a fall
  - hitting a fence, etc

and, of course, when

- *a change in its way of going* or *an obvious lameness* is seen or reported by the rider

From a locomotor system aspect, *check any alteration* in

- stance
- posture
- action, as in
  - moving over
  - turning in the box, and ultimately in
  - walk, trot, turn in hand, in the yard

are all primary indications of a disorder.

These initial clues compare with that of a dis-ease of the other systems' early warning, e.g.

- respiratory – a cough
- digestive – diarrhoea, or absence of faeces
- skin – a swelling, or a hairless patch

As with these basic examples, so too with seeing (and hearing) an altered action, the fact of a locomotor disorder is established. Further work may have to, even must, stop until more clinical information is obtained.

The various types of limb mal-alignment and foot-fall disorders, especially when unilateral, misleadingly suggest a lameness. They are *action defects* – functional, physically induced, gait deficits which, unless any predisposition to trauma materialises, will continue to be just that.

Mechanical difficulties have been mentioned; such dysfunctions must be, by definition, old, previously seen and, hopefully, already assessed.

A not uncommon, classical, mechanical lameness is that associated with intermittent, usually temporary, UFP (upward fixation of the patella) in the 'maturing' horse. Its newness may well relate to initial work although the predisposing conditions for it have been long established.

There are, however, physical interferences with a horse's action which do seem to cause unsuspected, new behaviour. Most have to do with tack becoming out of place. Fundamentally they then cause nerve stimulation not at all dissimilar in effect to pain sensation, but usually without marked primary inflammatory reaction and tissue damage. They can be quite dramatic, even dangerous, in the response of the horse, for example

- tack
  - the pinch of a girth
    - a shortened fore action as the horse tries to minimise the discomfort by not fully protracting the forelimbs. In some cases when mounted or ridden away, it humps its back, may even buck
  - the pinch of a saddle on the withers or pressure against the dorso-posterior shoulder blades when a new 'unfitted' saddle is used will provoke an unexpected
    - reduced stride, a reluctance to canter, and a refusal to jump
  - compare action in hand or bare-back without the suspected tack in place
- protective clothing, e.g.
  - the hind leg strap or fillet which breaks, permitting the other one to ride up the leg and there irritate the tender, hairless skin of the groin, to initiate either
    - refusal to move, or
    - violent attempts to break free
  - hind leg travelling boots (or wrongly applied hock dressing bandage) will create an initial strong, even violent reaction because the horse feels worryingly restricted
    - marked, rapid abduction
    - buck jumping forward

Whilst such altered action usually ceases when the offending tack is removed, as it would or should be as quickly as possible to relieve the situation (or the horse is progressively made accustomed to protective leggings by being hand-walked on the soft; or with bandages, hock particularly, gently hand-led around in the box to get it accustomed before being left.

Although its original presence and effect must have been seen by either the rider or the groom, an associated lameness at a subsequent inspection is unlikely; nevertheless, the areas in question should be inspected for skin galls, erosions or early mud fever lesions resulting from the initial abrasions or pressures.

It is the more usual types of occupational hazard-induced dis-ease which are more relevant to the routine inspection, where the associated lameness pain and the horse's attempt to alleviate the sensation of it, is exhibited at

- weight bearing (supporting leg lameness)
- limb flight (swinging leg lameness)
- or both

The horse could lie down 'to take the weight off its feet', but instinct 'warns' that this ultimate recourse is dangerous. Going down is one thing, getting up again quickly enough to escape predation is another! It is more likely to go down in bilateral lameness of the acute, severe types such as

- laminitis
- bilateral tendinitis

In severe unilateral, usually very obvious conditions such as

- long bone and (undisplaced) pelvic fracture
- acute joint trauma
- a nail into the sensitive hoof tissues

he will remain standing 'knowing' that he can at least try to escape 'on three legs and a swinger' or, indoors, be where he feels safe.

In displaced axial and pelvic fractures he may go down immediately and stay down. In foreleg injuries he will eventually feel confident in lying down and soon master the technique of getting up. In hind-leg pain, getting up and down is more difficult. In standing he has the advantage of a hind-leg 'locking mechanism' to help take the strain off the lame leg.

Patently, any acute lameness does not require much debate to decide that work must stop. It is with less severe traumas that recognition and assessment of a lameness is helped by an understanding of how a horse can move, yet minimise or alleviate the pain of doing so.

It is the less severe but reasonably obvious lamenesses which, if missed, could well lead to more serious consequences, that benefit from the routine inspection.

Some may not be recognised until the ultimate inspection – a ridden trot! At this stage it is worth pointing out that the comprehensiveness of the inspection will relate to the 'value' of the horse as a competitive athlete (not in money terms) and the degree of athleticism anticipated.

This does not mean that low-grade lameness should be ignored in the pleasure horse, but minor known unlevelnesses associated with age related wear and tear is not likely to be exposed to more than its usual stresses with which it has so far lived. *It is the new lameness, the effect of some incident 'yesterday', which is important.*

There are many adult horses which exhibit a morning stiffness but warm up easily and satisfactorily into a workable state; so, too, the day after a particularly exerting occasion – these are 'known' facts for that horse.

The horse instinctively needs to minimise pain by altering his body's balance or self carriage; he is freer to do this when not ridden or held close in-hand. Even when the weight of a rider is required to exaggerate the effect of gravity and so increase weight bearing for diagnosis, he must not be ridden 'collected' during such a lameness examination as this could mask the lame action. (There are exceptions but these are not usually a layman's concern).

The horse has particular structural and functioning facilities to effect the required alterations in the two phases of limb action

- the range of movement of the head on the neck together acting as a loaded beam whose displacement in two planes can alter the centre of gravity of the
  - whole body
  - parts of it

  to take more weight onto one area, and so lighten the affected one
  - move the centre of gravity more onto the forehand in bilateral hind-leg lameness, e.g. lumbar/pelvic pain
  - move the centre of gravity more onto the hindquarters in bilateral foreleg lameness, e.g. acute laminitis
  - onto one limb to off-load the affected contralateral one in its support phase, e.g. pus in the foot
  - a diagonal repositioning into three tracks locomotion, to alleviate support phase lameness
- the ability to stiffen the spine, reduce neck flexibility and reduce lumbo-sacral flexion, to minimise spinal swing and so guard painful areas therein
- the ability to rotate the pelvis with the lumbar vertebrae in decreasing range, to
  - off-load support from one hind leg, or
  - permit free swing of the contralateral if it is affected in a joint
- the ability to abduct or adduct a limb to reposition footfall from level to lateral or medial support
- *the absence of a collar bone*, whereby it can displace the thorax through unilateral lift on one side, thus freeing the painful contralateral
- transitioning into an asymmetric canter gait to ease the pain of trotting (recognition of lameness, unless of an extreme degree, is not possible at the canter and gallop)

Most signs of lameness are those of the above alterations to the way of going, i.e. action.

An ability to *assess* these is not immediately important for the layman provided he sees them as **different from the usual way of going** and seeks a more experienced opinion.

Where a suspected lameness remains doubtful at a routine trot up, the inspector can

- give the horse the benefit of the doubt *after* he has inspected the foot
  - work at the same level, but monitor it closely
    - during
    - immediately afterwards and
    - especially the next morning, or
- stop – don't take the risk – seek more experienced opinion

It will be remembered that the normal horse in the *support* phase has, if only momentarily

- the hoof level, toe to heel, side to side, on the ground
- the limb joints in their angle of maximal impaction or stability
- the limb in an extension, such as to take all the weight necessary without 'giving'

the *swing* phase will begin with lift off over the toe at the correct time so as, when judged bilaterally, to

- describe a flight which is equal in length from behind (caudal to) to in front (cranial to) the opposite limb's return to support, and in
- a symmetric gait, the suspension component, will be a replica in height and duration of that of the contralateral leg
  - that when viewed coming towards the observer, the
  - head and neck carriage will be correct for the gait and similar for each step
  - the points of the shoulder will come to the same level alternately
  - the knees and fetlocks will rise to the same level

- when viewed going away, the same balanced action and appearance will obtain in the hindquarters and limbs which will exhibit a vertical pumping movement **with the various 'points' reaching the same high and low levels** and **the shoe/sole showing the same angle of exposure** (especially at the trot)

This is more obvious at the trot when tail carriage is stationary, unlike at the walk when it swings with the stride.

Observation for limb levelness in support and in flight should be made from the side as the horse passes the observer.

In a shod horse on the hard surface advised for locomotion inspection, the hoof fall should be listened to. The percussion should ring true or equal for both fore feet and for both hind feet, and give the clear impression of a secure footfall, confident and unhesitating for the walk and the trot at which there should be little, if any, forward slide or lateral twist (the latter is more likely in the normal hind action).

In scientific studies of equine biodynamics, force plate sensors in the 'ground' are used to measure the 'pounds per square inch' of hoof contact. Variations between fore limbs and between hind limbs can be recorded and 'printed out' and the picture can play a part in monitoring the elite athlete particularly with regard to subclinical tendon stress **before** the trainer's eye and hand detects anything abnormal. In the eventer/show jumper, it will also warn of low grade pain in the all important posterior third of the hoof and in the check ligament areas.

When pain is present in a limb

- the normal, elegant reciprocal action alters, either in the
  - support phase, or
  - swing phase, or
  - both and
- the horse goes **unbalanced**, **different from normal**

Foreleg lameness

In a foreleg the deviations seen will be, for example

- less time will be spent in the support phase from pain anywhere in the total column of support, but generally with increasing evidence downwards and into the foot

- the contralateral limb will move more quickly and over a longer distance, to take on an earlier and longer support function to relieve the duration of pain in the affected leg when it is in support
- as the lame leg moves into its next support phase, the
  - head and neck will be lifted higher than usual, and certainly higher than in the 'sound' leg, and in some instances will be carried medially and away over the centre line. The head reaches its maximum height at lame leg support. The centre of gravity is thus swung away from the lame leg, so reducing the down thrust and therefore the concussion/compression pain
  - the percussion sound is reduced
- as it lifts off into the next swing phase, the
  - head/neck returns sideways and downwards, which latter movement gives the description of **'nodding down'** **as the sound leg bears weight**

Such obviously altered action is primarily seen in support phase lameness, but it can also relate to the swing phase disorders.

Dependent on the site and the type of the morbidity, all these deviations will be exaggerated on uphill or downhill surfaces and frequently in any site or type at downward transitions, i.e. at braking. They may be more noticeable in the first few steps or only after several, hence the need for a 30 metre lane. They may show better at a relatively slow pace and conversely become exaggerated when an increase in speed increases the concussive forces.

There are variations within the sequence of footfall which are more evident in less painful circumstances at slow pace, in either walk or trot; this gives the horse time to be more selective in pain evasion, but in principle

- pain in the toe area of the foot, and to a lesser extent in the dorsal aspect of the limb up to and including the knee, will encourage
  - heel first footfall and longer time on the posterior half of the hoof support
  - a quick break-over, and off the toe

and will eventually lead to
  - excessive shoe **heel** wear, which might start even before clinical lameness
- pain in the posterior third of the hoof
  - toe first, and reluctance to engage the heel
  - an inelegant shooting forward of the fetlock, and a jerky action

- excessive wear of the shoe toe area

Recent force-plate analyses and slow motion video studies suggest that in both sites the heel takes the weight eventually if not throughout.

- pain on one side of the hoof or the other from buttress forward
    - medial
        - the limb is adducted to permit the lateral web to land 'early' and take support longer under the column of support
    - lateral
        - the limb is abducted in flight for the converse landing
        - the shoe shows the expected wear of the outside or the inside web respectively

In practice, *support lameness is most likely to show when tissues with little room to escape from the effect of weight bearing are the site of the lesion*, for example

- sensitive tissues of the foot
    - the laminae and the corium of wall, sole and bars
- the coronary corium
- the lateral cartilages (questionable)
- the bones up the column which take the ultimate force
    - the related joint structures

When made to turn on the forehand the horse with low limb pain, especially in the joint areas, tries not to lift the foot off the ground to replace it further round, but aims to leave it in full contact, an established pressure, and to 'screw' round on it. This usually shows more when the affected leg is on the inside of the turn.

Some lamenesses induce this 'screw' when the affected leg is on the outside. In bilateral distal lameness, usually in the foot, the turn is not only stiff but the forelimbs are held forward of the vertical, and the feet tend to take more 'screw' weight on the heels.

A less obvious but similar action is seen in a horse ridden on a tight circle on the hard.

Pain in the stay ligaments, the flexor tendons and, to a lesser extent, the activating muscles which are in full tension at footfall and at lift off, will be exacerbated just as a joint is when it is compressed during the support phase; a lameness will result.

Swing phase lameness results from any attempt to reduce movement in a unit of locomotion where there is pain in a joint

- synovial lining
    - eroded bone
    - ligaments and related
        - tendons
        - muscles
- trauma to a ligament uniting two bones, as in early 'splint' formation. (This is more obviously seen as a later concussive support lameness when the periosteal reactions begin to consolidate)
- muscle pain *per se*

Such lesions will alter the

- outline of the swing's flight, and its
- duration

To compensate for this there are complementary changes in footfall pattern and duration, in

- the lame leg – often longer time on the ground
- the contralateral leg – often shorter time
- head and neck carriage which, along with the shoulder girdle 'on' the thorax, help to lift the whole limb over as much of the required flight distance as possible to make up for the forelegs' reduced flexion/extension duration
- there is a percussion sound change
- a tendency to
    - drag a toe
    - knuckle and trip
    - cause interference
- the sound leg sometimes exaggeratedly nods down

Fractures are seen as severe 'leg off the ground' lamenesses. When the pedal bone, and to a lesser extent the navicular bone, is fractured, the hoof capsule acts as a natural splinting, and thereby reduces the movement in the disrupted bone. When the initial traumatic inflammation subsides the lameness, especially on soft going as at 'grass', can be deceptively mild.

Hind-Leg Lameness

It is accepted that, for the layman especially, detection of hind-leg lameness is not easy unless the alterations in structure and functioning are severe and obvious clinically, therefore identification of 'Which leg?', 'Is it both?', 'Where in the leg?' and 'Why?', is even more difficult.

Clinical differential diagnosis is not easy for the veterinary surgeon, either. His expertise will include

- an eye for alterations in action
- an ability to analyse the subtle changes in the phases of the step (experience and practice!)
- use of 'ancillary aids'

all of which are described as 'doing a thorough work-up', if only to rule out the limb itself being the site of disorder causing an altered action, or 'Is it related to factors elsewhere?' Proximal hind limb lesions, less common than mid limb conditions, are more difficult to isolate and to confirm

The horsemaster's duty is primarily to **suspect** a new lameness behind. The suspicion may arise from the rider

- sensing it through his seat that the horse is showing a new evasion
    - persisting in one diagonal by 'throwing' the rider on to it
    - refusing to stay in a particular lead at the canter
- check the foot first
- walking in hand may confirm a suspected lameness. The lateral sway of the quarters, characteristic of the normal triangular foot fall, induces a swing of the tail in keeping with the rear end. **A possible hind leg/quarter/ back-sited pain will often show as more movement to one side than to the other and carrying the tail, unusually, to one side.** It is advisable to re-assess with the horse led from both sides alternately. The swing may be missing altogether
- trotting in hand on a firm to hard surface is best
- it may be necessary to exert the horse on a lunge, then return to a straight line trot. If still in doubt, rest for 30 minutes and repeat the trot
- work, straight or on a circle, in the soft may exacerbate a distal ligament or a joint pain – ride if thought advisable/necessary

When hind limb lameness is recognised, the 'way of going' is less diagnostic than in the fore, in deciding 'where' and 'why'. The reciprocal mechanism partially restricts isolated joint movement changes, especially from the hock proximally. Hind stride length, and 'use' of the hock(s), should however be scrutinised; invariably, however

- **the lame leg moves more in the two-way vertical plane than does the good leg, when in trot.** This must be judged by viewing from behind
- most frequently, the vertical excursion increase is **greater in the upward direction** but of shorter duration (this is difficult to assess)
- this visual difference can be made more obvious by attaching a coloured marker to both points of the hip. The observer fixes his gaze on these and compares
- less easily determined comparisons, even if marked, are the points of the hocks and the ergot area of the fetlock. The degree of exposure of the soles can also be gauged
- **the head of the tail may be seen to rise when the lame leg makes ground contact**; and it and the quarters may be pushed by the contralateral sound leg, or carried there through lack of abduction action in the lame leg to the affected side – with a resultant three track trot
- in moderate to severe cases **the head movement, as judged from in front, appears to nod down when the lame hind leg's opposite foreleg makes ground contact.** This suggests that it had been lifted up for the other foreleg's earlier contact; the impression is that the horse is lame on the same side fore as the suspected hind leg. Conversely
- a marked drop in a lame hind leg may diagonally influence the opposite fore into a head lift – remember that
    - more than one leg can be lame at any one time
    - quite frequently **an indeterminate hind leg imbalance develops following a lameness in the foreleg**

A shorter quarter rise, with a decreased period of rise, is seen in horses in pain during the swing phase as with hip region traumas.

In chronic lameness of a hind leg of more than 3 weeks duration, a less obvious clinical lesion in another limb may become more obvious when the first lameness is hidden by local anaesthesia, or when a more detailed investigation of the overall action and stance is made, hence the need for an all-round assessment by the horsemaster/ veterinary surgeon

- where confusion or indecision exists it is essential that veterinary help is obtained.
- stride length discrepancies can be judged from a side-on aspect by

- visual appraisal – at the walk and the trot
- stepping out in time with the horse's hind leg walk; the inequality in itself, is not diagnostic of 'why', and not always of 'which leg', but the shorter striding leg is usually the defective one

Any discrepancy could be due to the horse being led on too short a halter rope; loosen – with care – and walk well ahead with little contact on the head collar or halter. Compare by leading alternately on both sides.

Research work with slow-motion video recording of marked limbs in three planes of *clinically normal* horses has shown that there is a

- greater left to right discrepancy of flight paths and stance phases in the hind limbs, as compared to that in the same horse's forelegs, and that this
- is not uncommon

It is not yet known if these differences are

- an individual peculiarity of unknown cause
- evidence of
    - inherited or
    - acquired asymmetries from
        - development defects
        - trauma in the past
    - very low grade, sub-clinical inflammation and covert lameness

causing changes of pace within the gaits of walk and trot, some of which could worsen into clinical lameness with progressive and increasing workloads

It would seem however that horses have a greater scope behind for weight-loading transfer from one limb to another. The total hindquarter weight has to be apportioned somewhere, either transversely or diagonally; this apparently can be done without inducing original site overt lameness – up to a point. It remains uncertain if any associated neuro-muscular functioning and structural asymmetries at this level are the cause, the effect, or purely coincidental.

In overt bilateral hind leg lameness, the general impression is of

- stiffness
- altered support phase duration
- reduced swing phase length

all with

- ***failure to track up, at the trot***, and
- a rider's sensation of the horse being in 'two halves' from behind the seat

In hand

- walk
    - 5-metre circles
- trot
    - 10-metre circles slowly on a gritted or rough surface

may exaggerate either

- inside hind-leg lameness, or
- outside hind-leg lameness

the latter for spavin and UFP and some suspensory disorders, the former for more distal lesions generally.

On the lunge, on a school surface, or in a field

- the inside leg, if lame, drops to expose
- more of the outside leg croup – the gluteal muscles
- to ease discomfort the horse will break from a trot to a canter which, in bilateral conditions, will be a
- bunny hop because of reduced impulsion

Ridden

- at the trot
    - the horse feels 'dead', as if the hindquarters are being 'left behind', unconnected
    - evades
    - changes diagonal
    - pulls up jerkily
- at the canter
    - no impulsion, on one lead especially
    - refuses to go on any one lead, or disunites repeatedly

There are two syndromes which are most often seen in the hindquarters, although the forelegs can also be affected. They are usually neuro-muscular defects but this diagnosis and the associated, usually central nervous system pathology, is very much a veterinary problem. The signs for the horsemaster can be slow to develop but occasionally are 'seen suddenly'

- **weakness**, usually bilateral with hind leg
  - toe-dragging
  - stumbling
  - lowered swing phase
  - swinging gait – a pendulum-like lateral action of the limbs
  - line of movement easily pulled sideways when the tail is tugged to one side by the observer as he walks/runs alongside the quarters
  - difficulty in stepping up and over objects

- **ataxia**, usually bilateral
  - stands base wide – to gain a more secure balance
  - raised swing phase, high stepping
  - stiffness
  - inco-ordinated action, crosses limbs, treads on its hooves

Both weakness and ataxia are worsened by
- walking the horse in a tight circle
- turning it on the forehand
- backing it
- trotting in serpentines
- trotting up and down hill
- tail tugging, whilst turning in a tight circle on the fore hand, some or all of which may also induce unusual abduction or adduction
- blindfolding during the above movements

THE ROUTINE DAILY INSPECTION FOR LAMENESS

The extent of the inspection will vary with the work being done by the horse. The object is that *the horsemaster should be daily satisfied* that
- all is well with its action and stance and its general well being, or be quickly aware that
- something is wrong, all is not well, it is dis-eased somewhere in the locomotor and/or other systems
  - a possible structural or functioning change from normal which could be
    - an early indication of a potential, critical condition if work is continued

- e.g. a puffiness at the back of the cannon indicative of possible tendon overstress or something else in that region
- a kick-like wound in the skin over the non-fleshy part of the medial fore arm which could be related to a hair-line crack in the bone, not yet painful
- a sore under a saddle panel
- any systemic, intercurrent illness
- an actual lameness

In the course of the normal activities of horse-care, due consideration is necessary for
- teeth care and bitting
- saddle fitting
- hoof balancing and shoeing

any or all of which can influence the horse's way of going even to the extent of simulating and/or predisposing to a lameness.

A horsemaster must also know that
- the horse was ridden correctly
  - within its fitness and ability
  - on acceptable or known surfaces, and if
- an injury had occurred

The Handler

At a routine inspection with a known horse, its temperament and docility may be taken for granted with little risk, but
- a disorder causing lameness or other painful lesions can amend its behaviour
- an athletic horse is not a riding school plug!

It is advisable, both morally and legally, to protect helpers (staff), and sensible to look after oneself, wear, or have the handler wear, in and out of the stable
- stout shoes
- hard hat and gloves
- body protector, especially when dealing with youngsters
- no loose jewellery or flapping clothing
and make sure the handler knows exactly
- what to do
- how to do it

- for the handler's safety
- the horse's safety

The Horse

Statically

- if the horse is lying down
    - is this normal for this horse at this time?
    - is it refusing to try to get up, or can it not get up?
    - on getting up is it with difficulty?
        - one leg impediment or more?
- once up, is it
    - generally stiff?
    - how is it standing?
        - in resting posture for longer than normal?
        - are hoof placements normal?
        - is hind leg alternation normal?
        - is it showing
            - a leg completely non-supporting, or with only
            - a pointing of the toe
            - trembling in the proximal muscles
            - intermittently 'easing' of a heel in
                - one leg
                - both legs (fore or hind)
                - fidgeting from one foot to the other contralateral one
    - with a repositioning of body weight to concentrate gravity nearer the fore or the hind than usual?
    - will it stand 'four square' and hold that 'halt', or does it quickly rest a leg?

Now have it suitably haltered with a strong rope and a safe clip, free of all other tack and rugs. Relevant to the horse's temperament, it should be

- bitted with a Chifney, or
- bridle-snaffle bit secured with throat lash

The further static inspection may only require the horse to be tied up as customary; it can still be moved over then loosened for turning and leading out. One person can do this as a rule. Thereafter some of the hands-on skills will require the horse to be restrained by a handler, certainly for the 'trotting up'. Well experienced grooms can efficiently assess a horse's action whilst walking or running with it, but the perception range is limited.

Check all the previous day's tack contact areas (including mouth) for

- galls
- sores
- abrasions
- palpate along 'back' from withers to dock for soreness
- those particular areas most likely to have been traumatised by previous work
    - closed traumas – in tendons and ligament areas
    - external contacts and interferences, closed or open
    - puncture wounds
    - deep cuts
        - near vital areas or not
- embedded thorns
- 'mud fever' reactions in
    - usual areas and in
    - axillae, groins and ventral abdomen, especially in galloping horses in winter

It will be appreciated that some of this list would have been gone over the previous evening, and some even after the earlier cooling off period after exercise, especially if that had been strenuous and exacting.

It must not be forgotten, however, that there is often a delay in the development of a clinical inflammatory response to trauma recently experienced. Even a lameness may not have developed in some cases, even those which are later found to be due to quite severe strains or sprains. Early post exercise and/or injury, where the 'adrenalin is still flowing', the horse is still so keyed up that the pain is not yet dominant or, more likely, the swelling around the area is not yet sufficient to cause pressure pain; this is often the case at evening stables when a 'walk out' is not done, thus a developing lameness is missed until the next morning.

The inflammatory reaction to embedded foreign material from

- a thorn and its irritant content
- wooden splinters
- mud or dirt

may not yet be at its height; the bacteria have not multiplied sufficiently to produce a 'good going' infection and the wound, the point of infection, may be so small as to have escaped notice, by sight or touch, especially in unclipped limbs, at the evening inspection.

Dynamically (in the Stable or Outside)

* on being made to move over or turn round, or doing so voluntarily

    * is he moving freely and willingly?
    * reluctantly?
    * is he doing so stiffly or board-like – left or right – a loss of suppleness?
    * lifting a leg (snatch or slowly) off support?
    * hesitating to replace it?
    * screwing round on one or both fore feet?

* is there difficulty in passing the inside hind leg in front and beyond the other on a turn?

* is he swinging the outside hind leg out wide (circumduction) on the turn?

* is he showing unusual

    * resistance?
    * annoyance?
    * grunting?
    * distressed breathing?
    * marked respiratory movement?
    * marked pulse rate increase (when 'taken')?

* at the 'pick out feet' stage in this inspection

    * determine the state of the clenches and tightness of the shoes

        * if 'spread', or likely to be cast off
        * all studs removed, and certainly if unilateral, not only as potential causes of altered action but also as possible contributory factors to handling injury

    * examine coronet and other areas for open traumas

    * any unusual objection to having a leg lifted and held up?

    * is there heat or reactive pain when the coronary band and heels are handled?

* on being led out of box onto the yard, is the horse

    * reluctant to move?
    * generally stiff or especially so behind?
    * weak and swaying?
    * unsteady in front?

* stumbling in one or both forelegs with a knuckling or 'shooting forward' of the fetlocks, or tripping behind?

* will he stand when halted, or is he quickly

* resting a leg?

* displaying those signs described under 'Statically'?

The opportunity to enlarge on the findings made in the stable can now be taken in the daylight and with more room to look, when viewed standing back

* compare both aspects of fore and hindquarters and both sides and 'compare from memory'

* view over the quarters, loins, saddle and withers (stand on a stool if necessary, but beware!) for any *asymmetry due to swellings* (as distinct from atrophy which will develop only over several weeks or longer)

* unusual vertical displacement of the limbs

* unequal foot support positions – adducted or abducted limb

* displacement of head and/or neck and of tail, maintained whilst horse is held at the halt or which become obvious as he is allowed to relax and/or walk away again

From close in and again in a better light, with hand (fingers) and eye, *go over the limbs in detail* for

* any localised swellings

    * exactly where
    * their extent, contour, consistency and reaction to pressure

* any other **inflammatory** signs such as

    * heat, as judged by the back of one's hand and compared with the other leg
    * discoloration (of hairless, unpigmented areas as at heel bulbs)
    * discharge

        * *on* the skin, a dermatitis/cellulitis
        * *through* a skin-penetrating wound
        * from a natural orifice

It may be more convenient, even safer, because of the

* horse's temperament
* other yard activities
* weather

to do the above 'hands-on work' in the stable before the

horse is led out but

- there is less room
- light is restricted and/or throws deceptive shadows

Depending on these findings there may be no need to lead out to go further in the inspection. If lesions of trauma are discovered in the box or in the yard by this stage

- visually
- palpably
  - with inducible pain

it is reasonable to assume that

- lameness will be present or
- likely if exercise is engaged

The disorder has been **detected** and should now be **focally assessed**. It may however be necessary to inspect action to:

- help **quantify** the seriousness
- make sure there is **no other limb** more seriously traumatised without, so far, any clinical focal signs, but with greater lameness.

Specifications of a Trotting Area

Surface

- hard but not slippery, free from ruts, holes, stones, drainage channels unless at one edge or the other
- 30 metres long
- 2 metres wide to accommodate horse and handler safely
- slightly inclined lengthwise over at least half the distance
- level breadth wise
- free of dangerous objects or fittings on adjacent wall
- gratings or metal drain covers can be boarded and sanded over

Environment

- no close moving traffic or
- visible moving horses within distracting distance (an excited horse can 'forget' pain, especially if mild)
- secure against the horse that gets loose

Equipment

Usually it is better to see the horse move unencumbered by saddle and girth, rugs and protective bandages and/or leggings. In a young and/or excitable hot-blooded horse discretion must be used as to the need for knee pads, over-reach and brushing boots. A full bridle may be necessary, or a Chifney bit on a head collar. In 'difficult', especially young, horses a cavesson noseband and cheekpiece with a lunge line is the ideal tack. This will also allow a straight head carriage and minimal chance of 'halter/bridle lameness'.

The In-Hand Exercise Inspection

The handler is instructed

- to hold the lead rope (or where applicable, the unbuckled reins held as a lead rope) in the
- right hand for leading on the left or near side, and *vice versa*
- hold some 25cm (9 in) below the halter ring to give the horse a reasonably free head
- take up the slack in the left hand so as not to leave a dangerous loop or a long loose trailing end
- **not** to wind rope round the wrist or hand
- have a knot in the end of a rope and the individual reins

the handler will be asked to

- walk the horse over about 30 metres
- turn the horse away from the handler
- walk back to halt and then turn it **round** the handler, to another halt

Some observers prefer to have the horse trotted away and back without the walk, but this slight exercise could 'loosen' or 'warm up' a mild lameness, which then would not show at the subsequent walk. Others maintain that slight stiffness in one leg or both hind, for example, are seen best, or only seen, at an initial slow walk.

The horsemaster will take up a position about half way down the lane and about 2 metres out from the edge. Thereby she can view the horse coming to her, past her laterally, and away from her. A view directly behind or in front or from further away laterally can follow later if thought helpful. The rear action is the more likely to benefit from a tail-end-on observation. She must watch the horse carefully as it is slowed down and as it is turned.

The second turn will, because of the handler being on the inside, be more of a 'turn on the left forehand' around her. The exercise is now repeated at the trot or the walk as the decided sequence dictates. The turn at the end of the third run can then be tightened to an 'on the forehand to the right', the handler having changed sides for that but returning to the near side for the fourth (and final) run.

There are occasions (a horse going apparently slightly halter lame) when it would be an advantage to have it walked and trotted from the other side as well. Unfortunately few horses have been taught to do this; they tend to resist or try to move back to the 'correct' side, to the danger of the handler's heels or worse.

At both gaits the horse must be made to

- move out freely
- go in a straight line
- especially at the trot he should not be allowed, or encouraged, to slow up when only half way along the line

Safety Points

The handler should

- keep level with the horse's neck or shoulder
- distance herself laterally, by having the lead arm laterally extended
- not lag behind the horse to be level with the ribs, as this could encourage the horse to (playfully) kick out at what he now sees as a 'racing' opposition
- not have to drag the horse from in front

The horsemaster, if necessary, should

- demonstrate the above
- be prepared to carefully encourage the horse away – by voice, not by whip
- emphasise, as with other actions (such as turning), that the handler should be extra-careful of where her feet are, and that the walk and trot should be in a straight line

The hard walk/trot surface need not be concrete or tarmac, even though both these surfaces are usually ideal and do give a clear sound. Well-packed earth or rolled-in gravel can be hard enough to act as ground reaction surfaces sufficient to test for concussive/compression lameness. The effects of sand or other school surfaces are not ideal for these, but where

- extra 'let down' of the distal joints, and more exacting

lift-off are required, or when

- faster, more stretching tests are deemed necessary to 'bring out' strain lesions suspected during the walk and trot on the hand

then lungeing on a 20 metre circle in these gaits and then the canter on both reins **on the soft** is the method of choice. *Lungeing on the hard is not recommended for routine inspections by the layman.*

The continental assessment of Warmblood walk and trot is carried out in a triangle, a quick and satisfactory means of appreciating gait action (as distinct from concussive lameness, since facilities are usually in a school with a prepared surface).

The candidate is halter led at the walk along one walled or railed side for about 20–30 metres. It is turned inwards at 45° and led across the school for the same distance, turned back at an angle of 90°, and returned to the starting point. The walk is reversed and thereafter a trot is carried out on both reins. The observer stands at the start from where he can see the horse move away, go past and come to him, always with the handler on the 'inside'.

Other extra routine tests where lameness is suspected but not clinically clear are

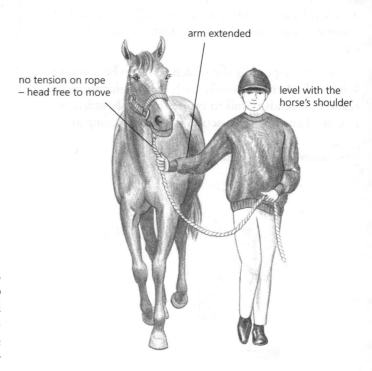

arm extended

no tension on rope – head free to move

level with the horse's shoulder

How the handler should be positioned and should hold the lead rope.

- trotting in-hand, with extra care, on both reins in a 12 metre diameter circle on a hard gravelly surface or a sand sprinkled concrete yard (knee booted), will exacerbate both fore and hind lamenesses

- trotting in-hand on a straight line with the horsemaster pulling on the tail will exacerbate lameness associated with hind-leg stiffness and/or weakness – tugging on alternate sides

- in-hand walking, increasing to a slow trot, on a 5-metre diameter circle, both directions, will make hind-leg disorders more apparent

  - upward fixation of the patella
  - wobbler circumduction

(But these tests are not usually necessary in the routine inspection; it would be unusual for them to be 'new' in a 'known' working horse)

- ridden, perhaps beginning at a 20 metre and tightening to a 12 metre on a school surface or in a field

  - both reins and changing diagonals within each 'rein' at the trot will show up disinclinations to use a particular leg, and pain under the saddle

- ridden on grass or firm artificial surface, in shallow serpentines at the trot, will often exacerbate distal foreleg pain and stiffness in the neck

- in hand and/or ridden, on firm up hill and down hill surfaces and across slopes, are further exacting tests

These tests, especially the ridden test, can be confusing to some onlookers especially with a young/or unbalanced horse who tends to fall in on the inside shoulder, suggestive of a lameness. This action is usually accompanied by

- the head and neck dropping with the supporting inside foreleg rather than rising up to drop (nod) when the contralateral takes support

- if in doubt assume the worst, especially if this 'way of going' is new

Flexion Tests

The controversial flexion tests will, if correctly applied, help to exacerbate a suspected injured joint which was insufficiently painful to produce a clear cut lameness. **It is not a beginners' technique**, and not one to be routinely applied, especially by a layman.

However, in explanation, the aim is slowly but firmly to move a joint or joints to the limit of flexion without applying more than a hand strength, and holding there for up to 2 minutes. The limb is then let go onto the ground for a count of three before having the horse trotted away.

A lame or lamer action for more than 6 strides is a pointer to a painful disorder in the joint being tested. The same area in the opposite limb should be tested for comparison. Some horses will go positive simply because of the unusual compression imposed upon their limb, hence the arbitrary 6-stride allowance. A similar positive reaction in the contralateral limb, especially if both were short lasting, could confirm such a *functional reaction* rather than a *pathological cause*. It could, however, indicate a bilateral if unequal lameness.

Flexion to the maximal range induced by minimal force is all that is required to induce extra tension and stretch, not a wrestling grip. Ideally, it would be more in keeping

How to pick up a near hind.

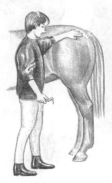

run the hand along the body and quarters

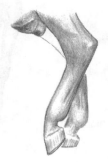

slide the hand around the inner side of the hock

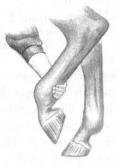

run the hand down the fetlock

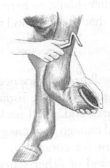

and pick up the foot

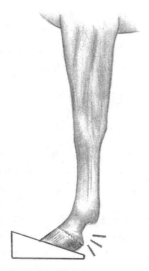

The flexion test for navicular – toe stretched out.

importantly, when the lesion is, for example, a fracture in a small bone or the condyle of a long bone in a joint region, such a test could inflict not only unnecessary pain but also serious complications

Compound flexion and abduction tests should not be attempted.

The horse should be correctly restrained during the flexing. For the handler's ego as well as for the horse's welfare, *first make sure that there is 'nothing in the foot'!*

No flexion test should be done on a mounted horse nor

with the locomotor dynamics if an extension could be effected, as it is in this position that the horse exerts maximum forces, but this is not practicable except for a complementary test for navicular disease when the horse is made to place weight on the suspect limb with the hoof on a 30° upward-sloping board to induce a toe extension with stretch pressure on the posterior coffin joint tissues, the posterior third of the foot.

The distal limb's three joints flexion test is one frequently employed, but it does involve all these joints – thus making interpretation imprecise.

Some points to remember

- when effecting a carpal (knee) flexion test do not direct the distal limb laterally but move the cannon to make contact with the posterior surface of the forearm; this is sufficient pressure

- the hock flexion, the **spavin** test, should be made so as to minimise the synchronised involvement of the stifle, otherwise a confusing result could be obtained. Most stifle lesions are associated with a clinical distension of that joint's capsule: a flexion test should not be necessary there other than to quantify the degree of pain. The horse may quickly and angrily 'advise you' of this without the need for a trot away – by a violent withdrawal and/or a marked, violent abduction of the limb

- where any joint area shows obvious inflammatory lesions there is no need for a layman to use a flexion test at all. It will be clinically lame anyway. More

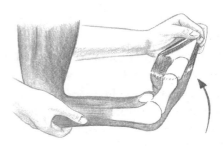

'three joints' flexion test – frequently employed, but interpretation between joints may be imprecise

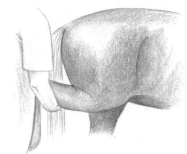

stifle flexion

Caution: to avoid a possible kick, the handler needs to stand at a safe distance, and not behind the horse

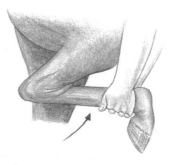

hock flexion

Three different flexion tests.

should mounting to ride away immediately follow a test. This is dangerous for all concerned; the horse might stumble, either from the exacerbated lameness or even from the functional 'numbing'.

Routine for a Detailed Hoof Inspection

Routine hoof inspection is an essential requirement for good horsemastership. The occasions for doing so can be summarised

- a daily inspection of the working horse, as described
- periodically (even daily) for a horse at grass
- on being brought in from grass at any time
- after work, even if on
  - a prepared surface
  - a hard road

It is assumed that a good relationship between a competent farrier and a knowledgeable owner is a 'must', not only for shoeing but also to minimise the risk of deterioration of the horny hoof and its angles with the pastern. Any changes are more likely to be a reflection of the horse's hoof growth altered by mistakes in trimming or by altered ground force reactions following more proximally induced imbalance

- altered angle of the walls with the ground
- flaring of the walls
- altered level of the coronary band, as seen at the heels
- contracted heels and loss of bars' line
- shearing of the bulb of the heels
- atrophy of the frog
- flattening of the sole

all resulting in

- imbalance of the foot support stance
  - antero-posterior with the pastern
  - medio-laterally
  - foot fall changes as seen at walk and/or at trot
    - outside in
    - inside out
      - disinclination to bear weight
        - at the toe
        - at the heels
        - one side (or web) or the other
- irregular wear of the shoe

- mainly toe
- mainly heels
- one side or the other along the web

It is appreciated that the above observations are **not sudden to be spotted on any one day**. These are more likely to be recognised by the farrier at shoeing or by the veterinary surgeon when examining for lameness.

The hoof must be thoroughly cleaned preparatory to being 'searched'

- if muddy, use a pressure hose on the
  - pastern/coronet
  - wall
  - heels
  - sole
  - frog
- if just dirty or dusty then use a stiff brush. The sole and frog may require washing to expose the surface horn clear of the 'use'-veneered surface
- pick out hoof (using a standard blunt-ended hoof pick)
  - under the shoe web especially near the heel ends (seats of corn)
  - into lateral and central clefts of frog – and if there is a deep inter-bulb cleft search this carefully with a small cloth 'pull-through' for grit, small stones and twigs or other debris: there is a thin tender horn on the sides and especially in the depth of this groove
  - surface of the sole with a wire brush or blunt hoof knife removing flaking horn, to reveal
    - bruising stains on the solar surface
    - splits in the horn
- cut away frog flakes or flaps and under-run areas
- inspect walls for
  - scuffs
  - cracks
  - splits
  - loose or missing clenches and check for missing nails from underneath on ground surface of shoe

and do not be satisfied just with removing a loosely embedded stone under the web thinking that only it was important. Conversely, concentration on a blatant strained tendon yet failing to detect a deeply embedded nail in the hoof, as from a spread shoe, is not good for horsemastership ego let alone the horse.

These inspections on a daily basis are to 'discover' clues which could foretell a possible future lameness.

If a lameness is seen in the absence of any perceivable lesions in the hoof capsule it should next be searched in more external detail. Using a light hammer and with the limb bearing weight (the contralateral limb may be lifted to accentuate this, preferably with the horse knee-booted and/or on a soft standing)

- tap each clench – look out for a snatch reaction, then
- with limb loosely suspended from back of knee and the hoof off the ground, repeat
- with hoof held as by a farrier, between or over one's legs (take care with hind legs)
  - tap each nail head
  - tap all round sole just inside inner edge of shoe
  - with hoof testers (if owned) or a blunt shoe puller (with delicacy!)
    - compress this same area at half-inch intervals; pay particular attention to seats of corn

If negative, carefully

- tap over whole area of the
  - sole
  - frog then
- with hoof testers
  - compress one side of frog with opposite side of the wall

Never hit or compress hard; a light or gentle squeeze can elicit a positive reaction. The frog area will require a little more. A hard squeeze especially onto the soles could result in sole penetration quite apart from a false reaction.

Any horse will react to a heavy bang with a hammer. Always compare an apparently positive site with that on the contralateral foot.

However slight the reaction, if such is not present in the other leg, consider it as suspicious. Do not work the horse without further advice. If a positive reaction does not indicate an area clear of the shoe but apparently under the web (or in a heel bulb) then the shoe must be removed.

If nails are to be drawn, do so on a bedding-free box or yard so that no nails are lost. If pain is present and likely to worsen with the inspection tests

- untie horse and have him held with
- knee pads fitted

Taking a shoe off in the customary farrier fashion, when done by a layman may cause

- excessive pain and
  - evasion with
    - danger to the handler
    - accident to the horse

In an emergency, household tools can be improvised in the absence of the correct ones. If in doubt call in the farrier or the vet. Whatever 'do it yourself' method is used, the skill is to

- loosen the clenches one at a time, even break them off when knocked up. Begin at one or other heel nail
- with pritchel, hoof pick or equivalent, loosen related nail head, and with hoof puller (or pliers or pincers) slowly withdraw nail, levering it back and forward a little way in the line of the nail heads or the fullering
- alternate inner and outer nails in sequence
- gently elevate freed shoe *from behind, forwards and inwards*
- watch for any escaping fluid or black pus from the
  - nail holes
  - white line, especially at the quarters and at the toe clip
  - seats of corn
  - with blunt shoeing knife or wire brush or both
    - scrape away black debris from white line and toe or quarter clip areas
    - over seat of corn
  - again, watch for
    - pus
    - blood from any area along this line, or blood staining

Repeat along a parallel line just inside the wall on the sole, and again look for staining

- red to brown in the sole is indicative of laminar bleeding. It will be crescent-shaped around the toe
- carefully scrape more out of seat of corn
- look for purple to red stain, or oozing blood
- apply thumb pressure to elicit pain reflex withdrawal

At all times beware of

- a sudden withdrawal of the leg being examined
- a stamp down with a foreleg, or a strike
- a kick from a hind leg

Provided there is no open ground-surface wound, severe staining, or badly broken white line in a horse where lameness is mild or just suspected, it may now be taken to a hard surface and there

- walked and then if necessary trotted slowly
- turned on the forehand

and assessed for any worsening of the lameness now that there is no protective shoe.

If positive, return to stable and seek help as soon as possible. If not worse, rest, but get eventual veterinary or farriery help: it is patently not an emergency!

IMPORTANT LOCOMOTOR INJURIES AND PROBLEMS AT SPECIFIC EVENTS

Locomotion implies activity; it is axiomatic that the more athletic the activity the greater the risk of occupational injurious hazards, both physical and physiological. These can affect the locomotor system directly and indirectly.

Horse Trials, Team Chases, Hunter Trials

The speed, stamina and agility required for these events decreases in the above order. Relative risk factors include

- the competitors are all mature
- the severity of the course, especially in horse trials, relates to the age (experience) of the horse and to the ability of the rider
- hunter trials attract a wide age range and range of rider ability, but generally a cross-bred, heavier, slower animal is involved

Strains

Tendinitis and desmitis (inflammation of a ligament) are common

- superficial digital flexor tendon (SDFT), usually in the foreleg
- deep digital flexor tendon (DDFT) accessory check

ligament in the older, heavier horse

- suspensory ligament (SL) desmitis branches, fore or hind legs; proximal area strain presents little clinical evidence, requires selective nerve blocking
- sacro-iliac and vertebral muscle and ligament strain from inelegant jumping

Achilles tendon dislocation, when the point of the hock area either

- hits back against a fixed fence or
- the leg is caught (at the hoof) and extraction force causes the tendon's cap to be displaced. The gastrocnemius tendon may be coincidentally strained

Wounds

- interferences (even with protective gear), often with deep bruising, sometimes onto bone
- lacerations, invariably heavily contaminated (beware vital areas)
- sole penetration, usually from flints and nails
- sole bruising, usually from blunt stones etc, or from generally 'hard going'
- stifle trauma, usually on fixed cross-country obstacles when the hind leg is 'dragged' over. The muscle-free anterior aspect including the patella is exposed to trauma. The bone(s) may be fractured
- fractures from
  - falls
    - shoulder
    - neck, back, pelvis, stifle area
      - neck is often fatal immediately
  - false strides
    - pastern

Metabolic

- exertional rhabdomyolysis (ER)

Showjumping

Strains

Much less common, but can occur during prolonged exertion, as with two clear rounds and a jump off against the clock

- superficial digital flexor tendon (SDFT) and suspensory ligament (SL)
- sacro-iliac strain (a repeat trauma)
- back syndrome

Both are low grade, usually exacerbated chronic lesions

- reluctance to perform
- noticeably stiff after jumping

but a really botched jump, with or without pole entanglement, could result in a new acute strain.

Wounds

Lower limb **fractures** are rare, but fatigue and mis-steps play a part, as does heavy impact with poles

Bruising

- self-inflicted from fore hoof (shoe and studs) impact on the under surface of the breast bone
- contact with fences
    - on the front of brisket
- interferences
- lacerations
    - splintered poles, jump cups
- exertional rhabdomyolysis (ER)

Endurance Rides

Except in long distance races, speed is not a prime factor. Fatigue of the horse (and of the rider) is. Fitness is relevant, as is the rider's awareness of changes in the going.

Strains

- uncommon, except of suspensory ligament (SL) branches and other distal ligaments associated with a 'twisted ankle'
- 'sore back'

Wounds

- concussion (bruising) of the soles; one-limb laminitis
- interferences, especially self-inflicted treads
- lacerations
- hind-leg lamenesses
    - muscle strain of the propulsion quarter and thigh groups especially if the course has steep inclines

- flexor area strain
- exertional rhabdomyolysis (ER)
- laminitis
    - often after the competition if a metabolic fatigue is present

Hunting, Orienteering and other Cross-Country Rides

All the disorders listed above under 'Endurance' may also arise in these activities. In fast hunting over grass (the Shires) and over moorland at fast gaits, but especially in the former with its associated jumping

- strain and sprain are common
    - superficial flexor tendon (SF) tendinitis
    - suspensory ligament (SL) desmitis
    - hind-leg myopathy
    - lumbar myopathy
    - exertional rhabdomyolysis (ER)
    - falls

Wounds

- interferences
    - more likely to 'be struck into' behind in hunting and some 'tear-away' rides
- lost shoe
    - wall damage at shoe wrench
    - nail penetration at the next foot fall onto twisted, spread shoe
    - solar concussion
    - wall damage if ridden on the hard
- lacerations
    - from extraneous items
        - wire
        - metal
        - stakes (beware vital areas in all such wounds)
- flints
- thorns
    - upper front of arm
    - back of elbow
    - pastern
    - coronet

- front of stifle and gaskin
- mud fever
- kick injuries
  - inside of forearm and gaskin with 'star' or actual fracture
  - lateral head of splint bone (closer encounter)
  - higher elsewhere
    - shoulder/elbow region
    - posterior rib cage
    - quarter muscles (longer range)
- exacerbation of low grade arthroses, especially after unaccustomed work on hills and/or in heavy going – may not show lameness until 'warmed down' and rested

Dressage

Usually from too rapid progression to

- advanced extensions in trot – foreleg distal ligament desmitis
- extreme collection gaits
- prolonged lateral work and turns
  - myopathic strain, in the hindquarters and lumbars
  - low-grade fetlock sprain, both fore and hind

- low-grade hock sprain
- gonitis (inflammation of the stifle or knee joint), especially from impulsion work
- acute foreleg fetlock capsule strain, as from using marked 'extensions'
- shoulder myopathy, likewise

Showing Classes

- athletic injuries are rare
  - more likely in working hunter classes
  - more common on hard going
    - 'sore heels', posterior third of hoof trauma syndrome
  - possible on wet, slippery surfaces
    - falls
    - inelegant strides
      - minor sprains distal limbs
      - interferences
- occasionally, exertional rhabdomyolysis (ER)

Colic can develop at any time during athletic work.

CHAPTER

35 SPECIFIC CONDITIONS

INTRODUCTION

It is presumed that the horsemaster has not only recognised that 'something is wrong', but also has a good idea of what part of the locomotor system is affected and, within the catalogue of dis-ease, what the pathology is. As emphasised earlier, the response should be to

• halt work

• assess the situation

• make decisions about
   • immediate action, including First Aid
   • the need for veterinary input

• initiate appropriate action

In dis-eases of the locomotor system, the abnormality is invariably that of

   • loss of functioning – **lameness**, and the associated
   • changes in structure

Much reference has been made to the macro-trauma, whereby the disorder becomes perceivable

   • visually
   • palpably
   • audibly

as an acute, even hyper-acute, condition, e.g. an

   • open wound, or a
   • closed trauma

best described as 'an accidental happening'.

It has been emphasised that the acute repetitive micro-damage from mechanical overstress, such as to tendons and some of the associated clues, short of active lameness, can be picked up by careful daily inspection – especially during periods when overstresses might be experienced as

• working on the unusually hard

• working in the very soft
   • at speed and/or other maximum levels
   • without correct 'warming up' (and 'warming down')

and, for example, failing to recognise the implication of stumbling

• the horse tripping forward off its support phase, in distal limb painful conditions, or

• tripping over its own foot at the beginning of lift-off, in proximal limb pain

which could be early warnings. Conversely, some such disorders can resolve unconfirmed, when suspicion has been followed by 'letting down' from the over-stressful levels.

Reference has been made previously to dis-ease of the axial column from atlas (C1) to tail (Cy3 or more); this chapter considers disease of the **back** – in correct terms the area from T1 to S1, which skeletal area includes the two major articulations in the thoraco-lumbar vertebral column

• C7 with T1 (sometimes referred to as 'T1 with T2')

• L6 with S1

The thoracic area from T8 (it varies breed/type to breed/type) encompasses the **seat**, hence is often called the **saddle**, to T18, correctly the most caudal extent for saddle contact.

L1 to L6 is the **loin** area (the coupling) between the thoracics cranially and the sacral area or croup caudally, inclusive of the Cy bones 1–3, 4 or 5.

The back is of course but the central area of the total vertebral column, and its structure and functioning interacts closely with the head and neck and the croup, and also – in a reciprocal fashion – with the abaxial skeleton, the limbs, and with the thorax. Its functioning is a reflection of the combined articulations of all these areas – a series of units of locomotion involved in posture, stance, and propulsion.

The back is seen as being
- structurally flexible
- functionally increasingly rigid from stance to the
  - symmetric gaits of walk and trot and then to
  - the asymetric canter and gallop (and jumping)

Movement is determined by the
- intervertebral articulation
- the directing and the restraining ligaments

and motivated by the
- epaxial muscles
- hypaxial dorsal muscles

which can act bilaterally or unilaterally, and the
- ventral musculature, including the
  - pectorals
  - ventral neck, and the
  - abdominals

all with paired bilateral or separate effect, as well as by the protraction and retraction of the limbs and counterbalanced by the neck with the head.

In the axial dorsals, and in the ventrals, the tendinous insertions are relatively short. The stresses are taken by the muscles themselves
- fascia origins
- special ligaments
- skeleton

Significant features are
- the 'spinal cord' within the vertebral column
- the paired spinal nerves exiting from between each successive pair of vertebrae
- part of the autonomic nerve system along the base of the column

Disease of the back will interfere with functioning
- intrinsically, including the nerve roots

- extrinsically
  - through nerve trauma
  - as the result of unbalanced lomotory effect on
    - posture
    - locomotion
      - secondary over-stresses
        - axially
        - abaxially
      - tertiary effect on the
        - saddle
        - rider

Recognition of back disease in specific terms of all the tissues possibly involved is not easy. Back diseases can be sudden or insidious in origin, and really amount to alterations in the way the horse
- goes
- behaves
- and, sooner or later, show as asymmetric muscle atrophy of reduced use

The composite functioning pathology is an interference with the integrity of the 'coil' principle of the vertebral biomechanics through the Centre of Motion (approximately T14) and influencing the Centre of Gravity. Athletic action should be balanced in the horse. The rider's position should be centred, and the saddle should fit.

The Diseases

Developmental
- the usually lethal neonatal structural spinal deformities
- those associated with Developmental Orthopaedic Disease (DOD), particularly of the C3 and C4 – the wobbler syndrome. Although not specifically 'back', the related neural deficits have a profound effect on the back and the locomotion

Inflammatory – trauma
- skin (hair)
  - pressure effects through ill-fitting saddle/girth, and unbalanced riding
  - epidermal and dermal disorders
    - ectoparasites
    - nodular disease
    - tumours

and mal-effects of saddling

- fascias and muscles
  - the dorsal area of the 'back' – pressures via the saddle, numnah and rugs
    - points and arch
    - stirrup bars
    - panels
      - flocking faults
      - gullet clearance
    - bindings
      - over withers
      - under cantle

Spasm

The most common malfunctioning of muscle not associated with a primary pathology *per se* is spasm. This is a protective persisting semi-contraction of one or more muscles, with consequent inability to relax. It is reflexly induced by a painful lesion in a related joint and associated tissues. It aims to guard against 'unwanted' further traumatising movement.

- local pain awareness control, as with
- para-vertebral tissue mobidity
  - strain of fascia and muscles
  - dorsal process traumas
    - over-riding of the dorsal spinous processes is common, especially between T12–T18. The underlying periostitis is associated with traumatic inflammation of the dorsal and the inter-process ligaments, following over ventri-flexion
  - supraspinal ligament strain
  - ventral vertebral ligament strain, resulting in
    - spondyolitis deformans
  - lateral articulation arthroses (DJD)
  - inter-vertebral foraminae occlusion
  all producing
- altered proprioception

Many myopathies result in secondary trauma in the related joints, and ultimately to footfall and support deficits.

Direct traumatic injury

- fall
  - impact
  - whiplash (usually cervical)
- slip – loses hind legs
  - tear of hind limb muscles
  - trauma to hind leg reciprocating muscles
  - vertebral ligament strain (including sacro-iliacs)
  - fascia tear

It is advisable when told by a rider that 'the horse did not go so well today (as it did yesterday)', to

- look at it, and to
- 'feel' the saddle and girth area
  - investigate further as required

However, it requires training and practice to

- interpret what is felt by **palpation** of the length of the thoracico-lumbar skin and, through it, the musculature
- assess a horse's reaction to manually applied stimuli to the 'back' and the ventral girth area

The horsemaster need only be able to assess the reactive ripple of muscle elasticity, in response to running the flat of his finger tips along the back, some 8–10cm (3–4in) lateral to the midline from the withers to the croup and compare left to right sides and to be aware of any

- tension
- altered tone
- evasion or resistance

to this touch – as compared with that of yesterday.

Bear in mind that horses' sensitivity varies; some are 'ticklish', others unresponsive or 'laid back', and yet again some are always on the defensive to such palpations, hence the need to 'know the horse' from the outset.

The horsemaster should realise that any horse will react to

- deep digital pressure
- hard squeezing, especially over the withers
- jabbing with the finger tip

and so give a false impression of 'pain in the back'.

In the absence of superficial lesions, the horsemaster faced with tacking and riding difficulties and new responses to manual stimuli would be wise **not to conclude** that the horse has a 'back' problem and that the back needs direct treatment. However, he can of course **suspect** a 'back' disorder, but must then seek a skilled examination and diagnosis of the whole locomotor system by a veterinary surgeon with, perhaps, the co-operation of a trained practitioner in a complementary discipline.

Even if sufficiently practised himself to be able to detect the palpable signs of

- deeper-seated pathologies in the
  - prominences of the dorsal processes
  - dorsal ligament
  - related muscle fascia

and capable of inspecting the saddle for ill-fit and assessing the rider for balance, he should know that these, except for a new rider, would be unlikely to appear as a sudden, new problem. Therefore, he must look elsewhere for the equitation difficulties which have been **now suddenly** reported.

The spinal prominens reflexes can be elicited by firmly running a hard blunt object, for example the blunt end of a pencil, along the midline over the supra spinous (dorsal) ligament, especially over the lumbar area, and then towards the dock from the croup, in a horse which has been encouraged and given time to settle to this 'new' inspection.

The response should be free and obvious. It is a reluctance, even an evasion to this involuntary response that is suggestive of pain, not the clear dorsi-ventral flexions. So too with oblique stimuli from the withers over the ribs and from the croup towards the buttock. The positive reaction is a reflex; *the negative reaction or guarding suggests that the conscious appreciation of pain has over-ridden the subconscious, automatic reflexes*.

Being cast or 'ditched' can cause both internal and external traumas, particularly if wrong techniques have been used to 'turn' or to extricate the horse. Major, often catastrophic traumas, do occur

- in National Hunt racing
- other cross-country events
- on the flat (less frequently)
- in serious road traffic accidents (RTA)

Any such injured horse either

- does not return home (fatal fractures, euthanasia) or
- does so in states of
  - locomotor weakness
  - ataxia, but

possibly so injured that it regresses into

- further ataxia or paralysis from
  - continuing intra-spinal (or cranial) haemorrhage
  - secondary falls during the convalescent, weak, period, with possible
  - displacement of the original vertebral fracture

with resultant further cord pressure, the last being lethal.

It is recognised that horses which recover from soft tissue injuries, even those resulting from severe traumas as mentioned above, do 'return home' following known accidents. Others, **without any proven history**, could have suffered traumatic overstress at any age, from

- falls at grass
- apparently harmless tumbles under the saddle
- attempts to accommodate peripheral induced imbalances in the locomotor system

and are, in fact, left with

- muscular
- ligamental
- vascular/neurogenic

weaknesses which could develop into, or predispose to, further deficits, from the stresses of further work.

It is then that horses with locomotor disorders, often unilateral, which cannot as yet be scientifically defined, develop

- dislike of being saddled
- unusual evasions and resistances
  - 'won't go well'
  - 'won't jump', etc.
- imbalances
  - neck stiffness ('won't bend')
  - 'three tracking'
  - loss of suspension
  - subtle lameness
  - poor performance generally

These are frequently not specifically diagnosed but just seen as 'something wrong' with the back. It is now that some owners see the see to seek help from complementary sources. Provided veterinary examination has ruled out or 'cured'

- any morbidity
  - in the 'back' region, which should respond to orthodox therapies (including saddle ill-fit correction)
  - elsewhere in the locomotor system (including attention to dental and bitting problems)

or has recognised any spinal lesions or residual deficits arising from earlier traumas and explained why some of these are

- incurable
- a risk if adjusted or mobilised
- a potential risk, *because some significant spinal bone lesions are not always confirmable* even with ancillary aids in the standing horse

then (unorthodox) complementary therapy is very often rewarding, though sometimes only temporarily so because the primary cause is neither exposed nor treated specifically.

It is believed that electrolyte imbalances associated with

- sub-acute sterile inflammation, and
- persisting local oedema and the physical pressure of slowly developing new bone production

on the connective tissues, muscle and ligament, close to and in the vertebral lateral joints, and therefore in juxtaposition to the emerging nerve roots, will interfere with nerve conduction and so trigger imbalancing reflexes.

To diagnose these 'scientifically', is almost impossible. However, the manipulative disciplines show that their therapy often relieves pain and releases spasm, allowing an automatic return to balance. Most other unorthodox disciplines, some even more difficult to comprehend, also do ameliorate pain, whatever else is claimed for them.

It is the welfare of the horse which is paramount and this, ultimately, is the responsibility of the owner. Some, even many, conditions still remain as a basic, pain producing lesion requiring *repetitive* treatment. It is these unorthodox techniques and disciplines which cannot be accepted by some orthodox practitioners because

- there is no 'black and white proof'
- there is no demonstrable evidence of the
  - underlying morbidity, or

- that it is the condition, as distinct from just its ill-effects, that is being treated

Increasing knowledge of biomechanics and how the kinematics alter with different morbidities directly or secondarily in the total vertebral column units of locomotion, is enabling all those interested to be better able to determine

- the areas affected
- the tissues involved
- the secondary effects 'referred' along the CNS

and to better decide which

- discipline
- modality

is best suited for attempted therapy.

Spinal locomotor system dis-ease can arise

- suddenly or
- insidiously

and the ultimate effect is to variably disturb the horse's balance.

Some sudden lamenesses of obvious direct cause may be identified and treated 'at home', some can not. Subtle lameness will present more difficulty. It is this which necessitates veterinary input and, *afterwards perhaps*, complementary help to alleviate the secondary effects.

The 'Bad Back Syndrome'

The various functional defects, often inter-reacting, which can produce behavioural and athletic performance changes collectively suggest to the horsemaster/rider that there is 'something wrong' with the horse's back.

They may develop slowly as part of a poor performance syndrome or, some at least, suddenly become clinical, to be 'new' conditions of lameness

- visible and/or palpable lesions over the neck, withers, saddle and the girth areas, loins and quarters
- alterations in the stride
  - shortening in the cranial phase
  - a subtle foreleg lameness, unilateral, or bilateral, but showing as unilateral on circles, with *negative* limb findings by both lay and professional examinations
  - similarly with the hind limbs

but are more likely to be seen as

- change of temperament
  - general bad temper
  - unusual behaviour at mounting
    - apprehension on seeing saddle being brought out
    - dislike of tacking up
    - unusual 'cold back' reaction
      - excessive and or sharp ventriflexion – hollowed back
      - excessive dorsal extension – humped back
        - violent action
      - continuing when ridden off
- reluctance to square up at halt and to stay standing
- poor engagement of hind legs
  - reduced impulsion
    - head up, back hollow, croup flat
- goes on three tracks
- evasions when jumping
  - dislike
  - refusals
  - failure to rise or to bascule
  - tail clamped down
- reluctance to lie down (fear of difficulty in rising)
- rests buttocks in stable
- inspection reveals
  - 'lumps', 'bumps', abrasions under saddle and girth area
  - loss of epaxial muscle tone
    - restricted spinal reflexes
    - reaction to vertebral palpation along
      - dorsal processes and ligaments
      - paraspinal fascia
      - epaxial and other related areas

Any or all of these are the consequence of pain, which *need not be apparently severe*, in the units of spinal locomotion, from

- micro-traumas of
  - spasm
  - strain
  - sprain

- fatigue
- skin, due to ill-fit saddle pressures, and the resultant
  - galls
  - sores from capillary flow obstruction
  - altered sensory inputs
- restricted paces from ancillary (gadget) tack mis-use, or bad bitting, or 'bad hands'
- inelegant, accelerated movements – minor whiplash and jerk
- over-extension of limb action especially in shoulder proximal muscles

Because the locomotor deficits and behaviour are often mild but occasionally progressive, the traumas are most unlikely to be of a major type.

The 'bad back syndrome' description is often misleading as it need not be the only axial or abaxial anatomical sites involved; the altered action and disturbed reflexes can have a detrimental effect both to the neck and to the pelvis *and*, by imbalanced ground force reactions, to the limbs. Conversely, morbidity in the neck and to a lesser extent in the sacro-iliac region can imbalance the 'back'. Moreover, a mouth discomfort or a limb lameness will imbalance the neck and the trunk, to possibly cause counter-balancing tensions. It can be a vicious circle needing skilled assessment.

The Neck Region

Can be micro-traumatised, by being

- persistently
  - over bent
  - bending at the 'wrong joint'
  - from the pain of a former
    - whiplash, or other
    - external traumas, such as
      - severe pull back on tied headcollar

The Withers Region

- saddle ill-fit, especially by the points
  - restricted scapular glide
  - pressure onto the scapula and its muscles
  - pressure into the scapular posterior muscles on landing over a jump
  - chronic low-grade ligament strain and bruising
- excessive extended trot strain of the proximal muscles

• trauma to the dorsal surface

The Saddle Region

• saddle ill-fit
  • wrong arch size, and points pressures
  • too narrow a gullet
  • stirrup bars pressure
  • girth abrasions
• incorrect riding

The Lumbar Region

• muscle fatigue
• low grade exertional rhabdomyolysis (ER)
• trauma from cantle panel's pressure, especially if during prolonged slow work
• repeated exaggerated (overstretched) jumping, and related muscular strain

The Sacro-Iliac Region

• the joint itself, but more correctly
• the associated ligaments
• the other sacro-pelvic ligaments from
  • traumatic strains

The Sacro-Iliac Joints Themselves

Acute trauma with clear-cut clinical signs does happen, but usually in the immature, unfit animal. Trotters and Pacers are most susceptible in their racing life, as are National Hunt and cross-country horses. The adult horse acute lesion may be an obvious new condition. A residual sub-acute or chronic weakness is seen but with minimal clinical signs except for, in some cases, a high hind-leg lameness which is difficult to pin-point clinically. Sub-acute, even acute, re-strains are possible.

The general appearance of this sub-acute condition and the usually apparent lame free state is

• asymmetry of the
  • points of the croup
  • quarter muscles
• reduced ability or performance from
  • reduced impulsion
  • fatigue sooner than expected

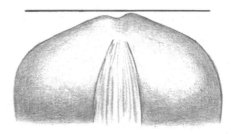

the tuber sacrale asymmetry and the associated unequal quarter muscles should be closely watched while the horse walks, indicating a problem in the sacro-iliac region

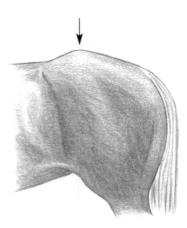

'Jumper's bump', the appearance of upward displacement of the tuber sacrale.

Exacerbations into lameness, as well as the possible cause of the original strain(s), result from

• disorganised take off
• severe one hind-leg slip
• falling with one hind leg extended into retraction
• falling back onto the haunches, all also possibly traumatising simultaneously, but they can occur separately, and traumatising also one or more of the
  • caudal hypaxial musculature
  • extensor muscles of the hip and the hock
  • epaxial muscles just in front of the croup, the caudal loins, whose loss of tone or mild atrophy exaggerates the appearance of the point(s) of the croup – the **jumper's bump**

Galls, Sores and Abrasions

By definition a

• **gall** is a minor pressure trauma of relatively small size, up to 6cm (2 1/2in) diameter, within the dermis following obstruction to the capillary flow of blood particularly on the venous side (lower blood pressure) which results in the exudation of serum to form a bulla or blister **without** a break in the epidermal surface

- **sore** is from greater focal pressure causing a dermal bruising; there is greater inducible pain from a further deeper swelling, but rarely any skin surface disruption. The skin texture is under increased tension and the hair is ruffled and may fall out

- **abrasion** comes more from friction; there is some bruising; the dermis is partially exposed and so is liable to infection

These are tack (especially saddle) induced traumas.

The conditioning of connective tissues such as the skin is part of horsemastership skill when bringing a horse back into work. The success or failure has a corollary in the human

- a sudden flurry of gardening with a spade, hoe or rake will quickly produce galls, rapidly becoming ruptured blisters on the palm unused to manual effort

- a too long walk, despite thick socks and hi-tec boots, will produce sores on unaccustomed heels, as will

- a rucksack on soft-skinned shoulders

Man can call a halt to such self-injury. The horse may show its early discomfort by evasion and reluctance, and even more dislike when next tacked up. In many instances the trauma is repeated, the gall becomes a sore or an abrasion and the open, albeit only skin deep, wound becomes infected – and the horse becomes a nappy ride even if treated amd protected locally.

Prevention

- have saddles *routinely checked by a qualified fitter*
- check daily common sites of trauma, especially in the early days after being at grass before conditioning is fully effected
- amend any questionable tack

Two practical features are important in prevention

- the conditioning horse is losing subcutaneous fat, and thus a degree of stress absorption; and at the same time, but more slowly, is
  - building muscle bulk
- a saddle which fitted the horse when it was at peak fitness and body tissue condition last year, **will not**

necessarily fit now in the grass fat state

- a saddle reflocked at the beginning of a new season will
  - bed down, but not necessarily in a way to accommodate the changed 'back'
  - not self-alter, to meet the structural changes in the fittening phase of work

The main areas of risk are

- the line of the points (and the arch)
- under the stirrup bars
- the panels generally, and gullet clearance

Management

Quickly recognised galls will soon resolve

- intra-epidermal oedema is absorbed
- the germinal layer rapidly replaces damaged cells
- thrombosed dermal capillaries give way to new capillary loops
- pain disappears

but the area remains more susceptible to further trauma for a week or so and thereafter always so until the overstress pressure is prevented.

Stop the cause until

- the lesion heals, and have
- the fault corrected before a return to work

Treat the affected area with astringents such as witch hazel. Monitor the abrasion for signs of infection. Re-condition the horse's back to the amended tack.

Action (after healing is complete)

- temporary
  - reduce causative pressure areas of the saddle
    - numnah: a soft but resilient material will ease pressure, but its softness can allow the metal/leather area to compress through it
    - seated-out felt which will not compress to nullify seated-out area
    - local reflocking
      - to form reduced pressure cavity
      - to lift the rest of the panel clear
- permanent reflocking
  - must be monitored at one month and again at 6 months

- a new saddle – *do not have the tree arch altered by force*

Azoturia (Equine Rhabdomyolysis)

For over a hundred years veterinary surgeons and horse-masters have recognised a specific syndrome of the muscles of horses which developed most commonly during work. Clinically it was a disorder in which the loins, quarters and thighs (and occasionally the shoulders)

- lost their propulsive power
- swelled up to become board-like
- the urine of such affected animals became discoloured

It was logical to assume these signs were related

- muscle rich in protein, when damaged, would surely lose protein into the blood, and thereafter
- be excreted in the urine

Protein was chemically recognised as 'nitrogen containing'. Therefore detectable 'excess nitrogen in the urine' must indicate muscle damage and be diagnostic for this disorder. Nitrogen, in early days, was given the Greek name *Azote* from *a*, 'not', and *zoo*, 'live', as it was well known that air deprived of oxygen but left with nitrogen could not support life. It therefore must have seemed quite reasonable to give the disorder the name 'Azoturia' – 'nitrogen in the urine'.

Muscle protein belongs to the functionally 'simple' group of proteins known as globins, hence **myoglobin**. When present in urine following myopathy it appears as a reddish brown soluble stain. The extent is roughly proportional to the severity of the dis-ease. In some cases its presence can obstruct renal function.

It is now known that the damaged muscle secretes high levels of enzymes temporarily detectable in the blood serum at variable levels indicative of the fact and the severity of the attack; their decrease in blood levels are converse signs of recovery from the active syndrome.

Further research into the muscle pathology not only showed that there was a

- **metabolic functional myopathy** – a muscle cell disorder, but also a
- **structural inflammation**, myositis, and a possible
- subsequent muscle fibre degeneration, a **lysis**

The clinical feature of the muscle stiffening to 'become like a rod' and the inflammatory reaction led to the syndrome being called

- equine rhabdomyolysis (ER), and because of its common association with locomotor muscle effort, it was qualified to
- **equine exertional rhabdomyolysis (EER)**

It seems to preferentially damage the Type II fast twitch muscle fibres. Since it is not a specific condition nor of a 'simple' cause it should not be called a disease *per se*, but a syndrome, and so warrants the amended acronym of **EERS**.

Since it can develop at the slower gaits of walk and trot, which are not necessarily exerting work, the adjective 'exertional' can be misleading. Most authorities now use **ERS** and refer to the history to define the level of work which seemed to precipitate the disorder.

Veterinary and medical (humans are also liable to metabolic myopathies) research is still not satisfied that it has anything like all the answers to the underlying faults in the functioning which produce the syndrome.

Over the years other variants of the original name have been used, which either indicated when the disorder was most common, or described the signs in terms of its result. For example

- Monday Morning disease (the original azoturia) seen in draught horses in the morning after a day without work
- Market Day disease – in cobs harnessed to carts taking 'Uncle Tom Cobbleigh and all' to market; their first real work for a week!
- Snow/Frost disease – in hunters after an enforced lay-off through bad weather; when they could go they were often over-fresh

Early in the twentieth century, when oats were scarce, the energy source was raw sugar. Later, in the second half of the century, it was shown that the condition could be induced by feeding 3kg (6½ lb) kilograms of molasses per day for a period and then exercising after a rest period of only one day. More recently a measured amount of soluble starch in the diet was found to be a potent trigger to increase the rate of muscle glycogen deposition and so precipitate the syndrome.

These three similar scenarios were *assumed* to be caused by too much energy feed with no work, and so too much stored muscle glycogen, i.e. carbohydrate overloading, which, with hard and/or fast work was metabolised anaerobically with the release of lactic acid, i.e. increased hydrogen ions, to produce an acidosis. This has never been proved scientifically.

The acidosis suggested the alkalising treatment and prevention with bicarbonate of soda, which was a standard therapy and management practice for many years. The fact that it was by no means always successful is now explicable. Further research into muscle cell morbidity may require a further rethink as there may be an inter/intracellular acidotic disturbance which does not show in blood samples.

The following three descriptions were also used in sports horses which became variably affected, and at differing times, in their work and which did not conform to the three classes above and did not have such clear-cut work features

- exertional myopathy, as in endurance horses further burdened with unaccustomed environmental excesses of heat and humidity
- tying up
  - the muscles 'knotted' into tensed areas; there is debate that this is a separate entity; it might in fact be just a milder form of ERS
- set fast
  - one of the signs when the pain and loss of functioning was severe enough to prevent movement
- cramp
  - what it *looked* like and possibly was, to some extent, *but* as seen in endurance cases, especially those shown to be in electrolyte imbalance, differed in as much as it is not just the Type II fibres which are affected

In many horses which fell into one or other of all these categories there was often, in the more than mild cases, a failure to pass urine, perhaps because

- of postural difficulty
- blockage of urine production due to the kidneys trying to cope with excess myoglobin

and when they did, it was often reddish brown stained as described earlier, hence one of the disorder's names based on a sign

- myoglobinuria (to replace the incorrect 'azoturia')

In some affected horses the overall condition was so severe that they became paraplegic and then recumbent; they had

- Paralytic myoglubinuria

In recent years American research has catalogued ER in racehorses and eventers, into

- sporadic ER – due to external factors which can affect the functional (and structural) integrity of muscle
  - strain
    - focal muscle groups – from overstress trauma, discipline related
    - general – over exertion
  - exhaustion syndrome, as in endurance horses
  - dietary induced
    - electrolyte imbalances
  all these can irregularly recur if they are not diagnosed and the cause eliminated and corrected. Even if they are, relapses, especially the dietary induced, do occur
- recurrent ER – due to intrinsic muscle deficits in functioning, at least two specific, and possibly hereditable, conditions have so far been identified. They are seen particularly in racing Standardbreds and in Quarter horses, etc. (similar aetiologies may exist in the United Kingdom). It is very likely that other explanations will be found, as these mentioned do **not** explain all the various cases seen
  - a non-soluble unavailable **polysaccharide storage myopathy** in which abnormal amounts of polysaccharides (PSSM) and glycogen accumulate in the muscles (especially the Type IIb fast twitch fibres), and the former certainly does not get, or cannot be, utilised when work starts. In this syndrome are seen
    - horses of calm demeanour
    - more in mares than in geldings
    - often
      - on the introduction to a high grain diet
      - in a recently purchased animal
      - one with concurrent disease
      - occasionally draught animals
    - usually exercise intolerant horses and/or
    - in some cases exhibiting muscle atrophy
    - muscle enzyme CK levels often persistently raised, even at rest, in blood samples

- **abnormal regulation of calcium** within the muscle cells, especially in Thoroughbreds
  - the disorder is more intermittent in comparison to the PSSM
  - occasionally recurrent
  - predominantly in young nervous fillies when first in training
  - episodes often occur
    - when particularly excited
    - after being off work for a week
    - after a change of environment
  - CK blood level increases are intermittent and unpredictably not always in accord with the clinical signs

These two sub-syndromes are the only types confirmable by laboratory histological examination of muscle biopsy samples.

It is recognised that in the UK

- the cause is multifactorial
- most cases are sporadic and individual, but recurrent episodes are certainly found
- where very probable explanations are available, e.g. the electrolyte imbalances, and in which correction is reasonably satisfying, it is not yet known
  - where the ultimate electrolyte levels have 'gone wrong' – between the 'manger and the bladder'!
- in most cases, despite cellular damage and lysis, recovered horses seem to perform well

Types and Times Affected

- the sports horse and pony – Thoroughbred and Thoroughbred-cross with many other breeds. The Thoroughbred influence in most 'sports' horses, hunters and hacks may explain the high incidence of this syndrome in them
  - the racehorse
    - there is no great sex difference except that young racing fillies are more prone
    - the age prevalence is otherwise wide
    - a genetic influence is suspected, especially in cases of *recurrent* metabolic upsets
    - it is seen in animals early in training for their discipline and it can also develop towards the peak or even afterwards in their fitness level

Current British research opinion is that there is an underlying but unknown individual predisposition to 'get azoturia' when 'wrong' management factors are triggered in that animal. The underlying predisposition as well as the triggering factors may differ between apparently similar groups of sufferers. They are not yet fully understood.

Signs of the 'Typical' Syndrome

These can develop at any time during exercise, even on off-loading, no doubt due to the physical effort and stress of transport

- gradual loss of gait impulsion from behind; this is usually more 'felt' by the rider than seen, in the early stages: the quarters feel as though they are 'dropping from under'
- variably rapid stiffening of the hindquarters
- sweating with marked pain evinced by
  - an anxious state
  - increased heart and respiratory rate
  - possibly a temperature rise
  - a reluctance (possibly inability) to move
    - a tendency to crouch or even go down if exercise is further enforced

It is, whatever the cause, essentially a metabolic disease closely associated with nutrient intake, intracellular energy storage (anabolism) and ultimate energy utilisation (catabolism) varying between and within individuals in the same and in subsequent seasons.

A veterinary surgeon should be called, even though many cases rapidly resolve, and urine, if and when it is passed, should be collected.

Differential Diagnosis

- the onset is very suggestive of colic – which dis-ease can *also* be a complication *any time in the episode*
- aorta-iliac thrombosis – quickly resolves immediately after work
- laminitis, especially in ponies – the initial stiffness, albeit usually in front, does produce a stilted, reluctant hind action
- a sequel to an earlier fall with developing spinal and other areas bruising effects

Sub-acute types of ERS do occur; they may be seen as a part of the poor performance syndrome rather than a specific rhabdomyolysis. The horse starts well but finishes badly, even stops: it appears fatigued. This is recognised in racehorses, eventers, showjumpers, dressage horses and show ponies and horses. Dressage and show ponies and horses may well fail to lengthen their stride, they cannot fully engage their hind legs. It is a very important consideration in the 'fading' endurance horse.

None of these necessarily go on to produce the classic signs but may do so on occasion (especially if work is continued); the horse's slowing down or stopping are perhaps self protective. When its performance does not improve with further training or proves impossible, then veterinary examination will show up the increase in blood levels of the muscle enzymes AST and CK which leak in significant quantities even from micro damaged muscles in such sub-clinical cases.

Many explanations as to the underlying cause or causes have been suggested; some have proved important, others not so. As with a lot of research, answers often lead to further questions. 'Tying up' is often the common denominator and so is used as the specific colloquial name, irrespective of

- 'when' and 'where' it occurs
- in which discipline or occasion
- what animal
- how often

when, in fact, this simple name may be descriptive of separate pathological conditions and perhaps specific to a discipline. It is even likely that the headings already listed will have to be subdivided into self contained disease entities with different explanations, treatments and management.

A comparatively recent discovery of a disease seen in resting horses at grass and, by inference, not given to exerting exercise nor on hard feed, is known as

- atypical, at grass, rhabdomyoglobinuria (**AER**)

here the syndrome can vary from

- sudden but severe stiffness to, and more commonly
- recumbency and death – both *without* any other systemic vital signs but usually with a myoglubinuria. Blood samples show a marked elevation of muscle enzymes

Early Management
When the acute case which develops in the exercising horse is suspected

- *stop work immediately*

- *do not* make the patient walk on
- cover quarters at least with rugs relative to ambient temperature and wind factor
- send for veterinary help to go to the selected *closest stables* to which the horse will be transported. A short journey is imperative for the average severity cases; even mild cases can readily worsen, as boxing requires considerable postural muscle effort. Although this posture effort involves slow twitch fibres whereas the dis-ease is mainly in Type II fibres, artificial postural muscle support is advisable, in the box or a trailer, to prevent the horse going down. *Drive slowly, especially on turns and bends.*
- if the case is very severe, and the horse is unable to move voluntarily
  - get a veterinary surgeon to the location
  - keep the horse on its feet
  - in cold weather try to obtain hot water bottles to go under rugs over the quarters and loins
  - offer a drink: *do not add electrolytes at this stage*
  - offer pulled grass
- if the patient is able to load, it is essential to take it to the
  - nearest stabling, and when off loaded
  - keep it quiet and well rugged especially if sweating, in which case do not apply artificial extra heat
  - do **not** offer high energy concentrates, even handfuls
- follow the vet's instructions carefully: he will give treatment to
  - ease the pain and muscle tension
  - alleviate the anxiety
  - limit further muscle damage
  and where relevant
  - intravenously inject rehydrating fluids
    - with added balanced electrolytes, especially in endurance ride cases affected by heat stress
and will give advice as to further management.

A blood sample to confirm raised levels of the muscle enzymes CK and AST is usually most helpful when taken after 24 hours.

The veterinary surgeon will instruct that the handler should monitor

- when urine is passed
- with what postural difficulty
- how much and
- what colour

As a rule, if none is passed within 4 hours or, at any time it is dark red from a high myoglobin content, he will return to give further intravenous injections to 'flush the kidneys'

- **do not give drugs that have not been prescribed** by the veterinary surgeon
- offer hay and water, plus
  - a 'slurry' of high-fibre, low energy cubes or meal, e.g. horse and pony nuts or coarse meal, broken up in water

Thereafter

- mild cases, even if acute to begin with, recover clinically in one to two days. The horse
  - is able to move freely and voluntarily in the stable
  - shows no sign of pain
  - has no reaction to muscle palpation
  - passes normal urine
  - is eating and drinking
- it can, if temporarily stabled, be transported home **preferably** by lorry, not a trailer, for ease of standing free

More protracted cases must stay where originally stabled until the above recovering clinical signs are established **and** both CK and AST levels in the blood are within a resting horse's level of normality as determined by the **same** laboratory.

During this recovery period the horse should be gradually introduced to

- carbohydrate, low-energy, high-fibre compound feed fed at low levels initially (consult with a recognised feedstuff compounder)

but **it is advisable to avoid**

- cereal grains and sugars
- bran

and continue feeding hay and allowing water at all times.

In a mild case which is alert and freely active **and** when the CK level is down to below twice the upper level of normality – usually in about 4 days – it can be turned out each day beginning at half hour periods and increasing

daily. This limited exercise should be available in

- a small field – avoid lush pasture
- an indoor school
  - sedated if temperament warrants, to prevent bursts of exuberance
  - avoid getting cold and/or wet
  - encourage 'gentle' exercise for short periods when out, in hand in straight lines

  do not lunge until both enzyme levels are normal; the effort of balancing will precipitate a relapse. Reduce or stop exercise if a viral infection is likely from in-contacts or even suspected. Stop exercise if clinical viral signs develop

The veterinary surgeon will decide as and when further tests are necessary including an estimation of electrolyte levels (by Fractional Electrolyte Excretion test) as part of a differential diagnosis of precipitating causes of ER in the particular horse, and later to monitor the benefit of any prescribed supplement feeding. This test is usually done after the patient has been on a trial diet for at least 2 weeks.

The timing of blood and urine sample collections is related to exercise and feeding; **this is important**.

Prevention (of relapses)

The horsemaster must continue to monitor the horse's

- action and demeanour when out and on slow in hand exercise
- urinary output (as best he can!) and
- appetite and thirst – slowly increase the amount of hay and horse and pony nuts

until the veterinary surgeon is satisfied that a return to work is feasible.

Future Work Management

This includes

- progressive increases in duration and intensity
- preceded by good warming up and
- followed by efficient warming down (cooling off)
- attention to the horse's behaviour patterns
  - is he better in company?
  - or on his own?

to avoid unnecessary agitation

- continuing the prescribed feeding

- adding corn oil, gradually up to 200ml (8 fl oz)) daily to compensate for the limited use of cereals or their total absence vis à vis
  - body condition
  - work anticipated: it is advisable to keep the 'feed behind the work'
- on planned days off, cut hard feed by half, from the evening before to the evening after that day off
- turn out to grass every day, even if only for a short while and certainly on a day off unless otherwise impracticable, when in-hand walking or freedom in a yard is advisable

A consensus among research workers indicates that a corrective and, more importantly, a preventative diet should have those feedstuffs containing soluble starches and sugars reduced considerably and the energy requirements regained by adding up to 200–400ml (8–16 fl oz) of corn vegetable oil daily.

In recurrent cases it might be essential to base the diet, corrected for balanced and adequate electrolytes and vitamins, on fibre, incorporating vegetable fat (oil) as the additional energy source.

The fibre should be maintained, with the emphasis on grass hay based on Timothy, and the ration should be correct for levels and ratios of calcium and potassium as well as the other electrolytes.

There is no guarantee that the suggested palliative diet will be effective on its own. Management with particular reference to stress and exercise must be looked at. Grazing or pasture exercise (in-hand exercise on grass) must only be on non-lush grass.

Aortic-Iliac Thrombosis (AIT)

A progressive vascular disease involving the aorta, just before it branches, or one of these, the iliac arteries or the femoral arteries, either uni or bilaterally.

The clinical manifestation is usually that of acute, severe, transient lameness in one (or occasionally) both hind legs at a variable time into intensive work due to insufficient blood getting through to the quarter, pelvic, and more distal muscles, thus depriving them of enough oxygen to meet the requirements for contraction.

Signs

- there is a rapid onset of a cramp-like stiffening of the leg
- swelling is not as marked as in equivalent lameness

from azoturia, but a hardness does develop
- lameness rapidly develops
- the horse's performance drops or ceases
- the affected area sweats profusely
- the signs rapidly disappear after work stops or is stopped
- the saphenous vein on the affected side is very much smaller in diameter than on the contralateral side, when the inner thighs are looked at and palpated
- veterinary rectal examination and ultrasonography will confirm. In the recovered animal the blocking remains, and can be identified by
  - rectal examination
  - rectal ultrasonographic inspection

Repeat attacks are certain. Euthanasia on humanitarian grounds is often the only answer.

A recent USA survey over a wide geographical area of 28 specialist veterinary centres was carried out. 8 veterinarians had not diagnosed a case in 15 years. 20 veterinarians recorded a total of 44 cases confirmed by rectal examination and ultrasonography per rectum. 20 stallions and 16 geldings were identified and only 8 mares. There was no particular breed dominance

- 15 thoroughbreds, 17 standardbreds, 12 others
- 17 were racehorses, 17 pleasure horses
- 9 were stud horses
- 9 were less than 5 years old, 19 between 5 and 10 years old
- 10 between 10 and 15 years old, and 6 of 15 years or older

The intervals between attacks also varied
- 7 for less than 7 days, several only a few hours before diagnosis
- 10 negative for one week up to one month
- 27 had a longer history of poor performance
- **29 _were treated_** with a multiple range of therapies over varying periods
- **3 _were left as controls_**
- 2 were 'clinically cured'
- 11 improved, but clinical signs continued
- 12 showed no response or deteriorated
- 4 were destroyed

the 3 untreated **_remained symptomatic if exercised_**.

A surgical technique is being developed to remove the clots. Their position and size, the duration of the previous results of medical treatment, are all variable factors for success.

The human disease is part of the atherosclerotic process which includes coronary heart disease and cerebral vascular crises – hardening of the arteries with subsequent thrombosis formation. Lower trunk vascular surgery has been successful, but required transplants.

Recent work suggested that what is thought to be a substance causing arthromata, **homocysteine**, is related to folic acid deficiency. Horses not on grass for more than 2 months are known to be possibly folic acid deficient.

In equine practice, for many years, the cause was attributed to migrating redworm larvae damage. Their access to the distal aorta and beyond was seen as *atypical*, but the proximity to the intestinal branch of the aorta and the typical thrombus formation at the T-junction couldn't be ignored.

This helminthic thrombosis and its associated colic is now very uncommon since the use of Ivermectin, as a relevant larvicidal anthelmintic, began in the early 80s.

There are, however, no statistics in the UK to relate this drug's use to the incidence of the aortic iliac disease (AIT), and only limited circumstantial evidence of successful use of it in therapy. One recent European veterinarian in stud and competition practice is on record as claiming more than circumstantial success.

The incidence in general practice is low in the list of lameness causes.

Management and Prevention
Action

- stop work
- keep moving gently at a slow walk when the horse does so willingly
- offer pulled grass or a handful of concentrate as a calming aid
- rug up
- box home unless the attack is in a school or manage
- do not exercise again until
- veterinary advice has been obtained for
  - differential diagnosis: it may be necessary to exercise to re-engage demand for a fuller blood flow to the quarters
  - prognosis
  - prescribed treatment

Upward Fixation of the Patella (UFP)

This mechanical lameness can be

- intermittent
- permanent, in as much as it cannot be reduced by human interference
- it is often bilateral but not necessarily symmetrically so

Anatomically, the patella is anchored to the antero-proximal tibia by 3 ligaments

- lateral
- middle
- medial, which is projected outwards by a cartilaginous flap origin before descending. This leaves a relatively wide gap between it and the middle ligament

Functionally, during the stance phase the 'gap' is positioned to override the medial trochlea (knuckle) of the femur, but is smoothly released by related muscle co-ordination in the normal horse if locomotion is required

- resting stance: the supporting limb hangs the patella onto the knuckle which brings the stifle/hock reciprocal mechanism into play, thus locking the limb with minimal postural muscle effort

In Affected Horses

- the limb stays locked when forward walk is required
- the hang-up is released somewhat later, and noticeably forcibly, by extra muscle effort – it 'goes off with a bang'!

Cause
The disorder is one of the maturing horse

- conformation
  - heredited 'straight hind limb', a wide stifle joint angle (recent research casts doubt on this)
  - relatively longer tibia than average
- constitutional
  - underdeveloped thigh muscles
    - youth
    - malnourishment
  - neuromuscular deficits, e.g.
    - spasm of the medial thigh muscles which insert onto the medial ligament
      - failure of co-ordinated action

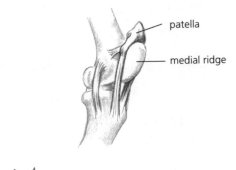

patella hooked over the medial ridge

— patella

— medial ridge

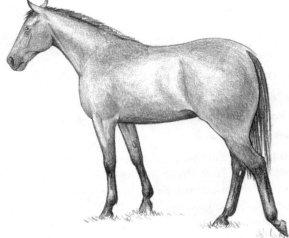

Upward fixation of the patella (UFP), the limb locked in extension.

Horses Affected

- usually light breeds and thoroughbreds
- usually 3 to 5 years old

may be bilateral, with one leg worse than the other

Signs

A horse may be found

- in the locked-limb position
  - with the limb extended backwards
  - the hock and the stifle cannot be flexed
  - the fetlock can be flexed – manually at least
- moves off with difficulty, and with an
  - explosive unlocking of the 'caught' patella
  - may continue normally until after the next rest
  - may intermittently lock for several strides with toe-drag during locomotion

- refuses to move, and is anxious
- lurches forward
- walks forward in an ungainly manner with encouragement
  - movement often releases the lock
- stays locked, and requires intervention as follows
  - approach cautiously, soothe the horse, apply a head collar and long line
  - do not handle hindquarters at this stage
  - beware of agitated lurching especially if in a box – keep the door shut
  - make sure there is clearance behind
  - encourage the horse to back up a short distance
  - lead it smartly forward
  - if there is no release, turn on a short circle or on the forehand first, towards the affected limb then the other way
  - back up again and lead forward
- if there is still no release
  - make the passage way outside the box non-slippery
  - pass a long rope to the handler outside
  - open the door and encourage out, the handler then
  - takes a closer hold, about 8–10cm (3–4in) of shank
  - leads the horse forward a length or two, then backs it up
  - horsemaster, with due warning,
    - smacks the horse on its quarter as it is again led forward
- it may be necessary to repeat this performance or, if still unsuccessful, call for veterinary help, Meanwhile
  - keep the horse walking and grazing
  - ***do not attempt manual release*** unless experienced

In less marked 'catching' cases, the signs can be better seen when

- the horse is turned in a short circle with the affected leg on the inside
- hand walked up a steepish slope; this may cause the horse, which is hesitant to extend its hind leg, to adopt a crouching action. Downhill, the action is jerky

The mild, more chronic condition

- a vague hind-leg(s) impediment, with occasional lame steps and/or a persistent deficit in hindquarter engagement

In all situations veterinary inspection and advice should be sought sooner or later. Farrier input may also be required.

Prevention

As discussed earlier this condition has some degree of genetic predisposition, especially the straight hind-leg conformed animal which should be seen as a suspect. Attention should be given to

- balanced energy/protein/ mineral nutrition
- consistent fittening for any faster work
  - reduction of both the above at the first signs of 'catching'
- discussion with the farrier about using long-heeled shoes to increase limb angles bilaterally

Management

In the early stages

- slow return to work *but no lay off*
- reduction of protein content of rations

In cases which do not respond to this, desmotomy (surgical cutting) of the medial ligament will be required.

THE DISTAL LIMBS, BELOW THE ELBOW AND STIFLE

'Big Leg' Syndrome

Signs

- a swelling of the cannon region, from the knee down
- to involve the proximal fetlock and, in some cases
  - the pastern area
    - mainly on the postero-medio-lateral aspects, posteriorly 'from the bone, back round to the bone'
  - of variable consistency and reaction to digital pressure
    - may pit on pressure, as with simple oedema – the filled leg

- mainly involve the tendon sheath only – non-articular windgall
- does *not* pit on pressure, is tense and sore, and with
  - variable systemic signs of inflammatory reaction
    - fever
    - inappetence
    - lameness

Conditions such as

- pus in the foot
- mud fever
- puncture wounds through the skin with cellulitis
- subcutaneous foreign bodies
- fractured splint bone
- other severe bruising

can all produce the 'Big Leg' syndrome.

The distension of the digital vein, bilateral below the fetlock and unilateral on the medial aspect up the cannon between the bone and deep digital flexor tendon (DDFT), is indicative of an inflammatory required increased blood flow to a distal region. Usually a severe bruise or an infection in the foot or pastern, although well delineated it is sometimes mistaken for 'a leg', particularly of a tendinitis or a main stem suspensory desmitis. A medial branch suspensory desmitis may also be wrongly suspected. The more important lesions of superficial flexor tendon (SF) tendinitis and suspensory ligament desmitis are considered later. A colloquial 'leg', an acute tendinitis or desmitis, is serious certainly in terms of recovery and duration of lay off.

The signs listed above often indicate serious disorders requiring accurate diagnosis and immediate treatment. Differential diagnosis must be rigorously carried out.

Consideration of recent activity will cover

- how did the horse finish, did it pull up?
- was it constantly changing lead before stopping?
- palpate both forelegs for
  - filling
  - swelling along the ligament or tendon
  - reaction to gentle pressure (remember: the suspensory is always more reactive than a tendon)

- see First Aid section
- later the same day
  - re-palpate
  - walk out and assess for lameness as well as local signs
- next morning repeat
  - if walk out seems normal consider
  - trotting in hand, if normal then
  - restarting work programme
  - *if there is any suggestion of lameness at any stage, stop work, get a veterinary surgeon*

If the horse develops, after work, a slight oedematous gumminess of the posterior cannon area; not non-articular windgalls, not a slight, quickly walked-off physiological distal oedema, but a distinctly unclean leg as judged by sight and feel even with the horse weight bearing on that leg, stop work, take further advice — because a 'leg', a strained tendon, *may not show severe lameness immediately*. A sprained ligament may appear sound in action at walk and in trot after a few days, but remain swollen. It is the asymmetric canter gait which 'fetches out' a clinical lameness which is obvious at the trot and even the walk, especially in the suspensory ligament and branches: *don't try it*, not at least until veterinary opinion, usually backed by ultrasonography, has been given.

Splints
Non-Infected Trauma

These can be defined as an ossifying periostitis of the second (MCll) and, less commonly, the fourth metacarpal (MCIV) or splint bones and the relevant side of the cannon bone (MClll). The word 'splint' is the colloquial name for the prominent new bone which forms at the site of the original strain of the binding inter-osseus ligament — an internal strain.

Once again, the early signs can develop reasonably quickly but are not sufficiently distinctive to be other than a

- slight to moderate lameness
- which worsens
  - with work, especially on hard surfaces

The lesion can develop in horses of all ages but is evident, primarily, between 3 and 6 years of age. It is usually unilateral but a similar lesion will often follow in the other leg.

In the absence of any foot problems the clinical picture of this lameness can be more or less confirmed by

- palpating for heat in the medial upper to mid cannon region
  - comparing with the other leg
- with the limb lifted, applying firm thumb pressure down over the 'splint' area between the cannon and the splint bone — a marked withdrawal reaction will be elicited
  - again compare
- there will be a soft diffuse swelling over the area
- later developing a hard deeper lesion

An atypical 'splint' condition is a

- bony lesion with
- related oedema, usually milder and firmer to the touch than in the more common type of splint, with associated inflammation and lameness

which can suddenly appear, 'that was not there yesterday' (it is claimed). That may be so, but it is difficult to believe, especially in the absence of an associated physical trauma.

Externally induced periosteal 'splint-like' lesions can occur from

- kicks — usually affecting the postero-lateral aspect of the cannon bone itself. A splint bone fracture may be inflicted as well with cannon bone star fracture
- a leg trapped between two hard objects can produce a fracture, usually of the head of the splint bone

There is severe lameness, in both cases.

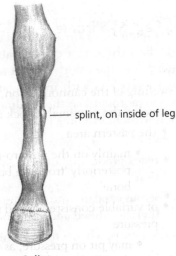

— splint, on inside of leg

Splint.

Synovial Enlargements
Non-Infected Trauma

Closed cavities related to the locomotor system are found in articulations, tendon sheaths and bursae. Essentially they consist of an outer fibrous cover, an inner secreting layer, and the synovial fluid or 'oil'. They serve to

- absorb concussion
- assist in the movement of
  - bone on bone, each with a cartilaginous surface, as in a joint where the synovia is a lubricant
  - a tendon moving over a joint through a sheath
  - protect soft tissue from bony promontory, as when a muscle or tendon passes over it

The amount of 'oil' is usually in the form of

- a thin film, as in the joint and sheath
- a thicker fluid cushion, as in a bursa

Their characteristic feature is that all are closed, not just shut away from the exterior, but the thin secreting or synovial layer is thick enough to form an avascular barrier between the 'oil' and the tougher vascular layer and its outer fibrous covering.

If this was not so the constant stress of compression and concussion would continuously risk microscopic leakage of blood into the 'oil', thus destroying its semi-viscous properties and functioning. Moreover, this isolation protects them from

- external infection, through superficial wounds
- blood-borne infection (the foal is more susceptible, e.g. 'joint ill' – a developmental associated infection)

If overstress does occur and the supporting tissues are acutely sprained, or the synovial layer is otherwise traumatised, then there is a considerable risk of macroscopic bleeding into the cavity, as well as the peripheral tissues. Milder overstress with inflammation is by far the most common morbidity, so the resultant closed, sterile inflammation without bleeding is a

- synovitis
  - reflex production of extra synovia (more protection)
  - serous exudate into the synovial fluid (which is thereby diluted and weakened)
- tenosynovitis, when a tendon sheath *per se* is involved
- bursitis

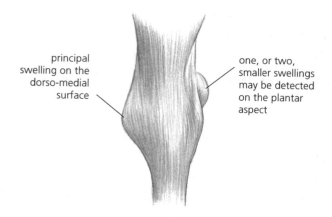

principal swelling on the dorso-medial surface

one, or two, smaller swellings may be detected on the plantar aspect

Bog spavin, the characteristic swellings on the hock joint.

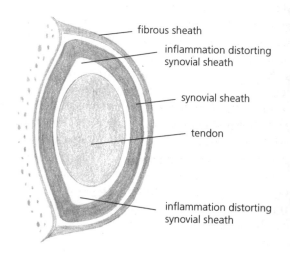

fibrous sheath

inflammation distorting synovial sheath

synovial sheath

tendon

inflammation distorting synovial sheath

Inflammation of the tendon sheath.

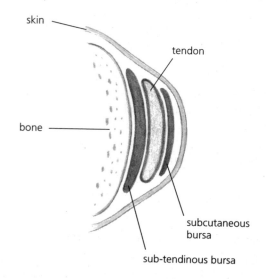

skin

tendon

bone

subcutaneous bursa

sub-tendinous bursa

A synovial bursa may be subcutaneous or sub-tendinous.

In all three situations there are the usual changes in the surrounding and/or supporting structures. The inflammation varies in degree, and may pass from the acute oedematous swelling into a chronic sometimes fibrosing state.

Most mild, one-off inflammations usually subside
- the 'old' synovia is absorbed and replaced with 'new' but
- the synovial capsule or sheath often remains distended, filled with excess synovia – there is a permanent variable enlargement
- any fibrosis tends to remain

The synovial sac or capsule can distend with excess synovia for apparently no reason and with no inflammatory peripheral change, especially in
- young maturing horses
- aged horses

This is called **idiopathic synovitis**. It could, however, be the result of insidious repetitive mild trauma, insufficient to cause
- inflammation, or at least a *clinically obvious reaction*
  - no pain on palpation of the adjacent tissues, or on flexion/extension passive movement
  - no interference with related functioning

This is common in
- the tarsal sheath of the deep digital flexor tendon DDFT (hind leg) – the colloquial name is **thoroughpin**
- the digital sheath of the fore, and more commonly the hind legs, is colloquially known as **non-articular windgall** and, scientifically, as digital flexor tenosynovitis
- the hock joint and **bog spavin**; in some cases associated with sub-clinical DOD
- the fetlock joint and **articular windgall** or windpuff

Occasionally they develop suddenly, to be recognised as a 'new' condition during a routine daily inspection. They are soft, compressible and painless to touch and are not associated with lameness.

Bursae do not, as a rule, experience idiopathic enlargement. When such an increase is size is recognised, it is usually due to external trauma; the reaction to the original trauma may not have been clinical on the skin surface
- as in **capped hock**

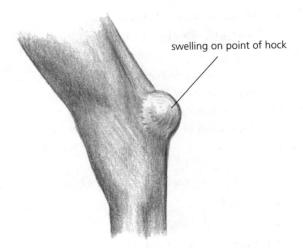

swelling on point of hock

Capped hock.

- related tendon trauma as in **extensor tendinitis** over the front of the fetlock joint – showjumpers in particular

They are usually
- mildly warm
- tense
- painful to touch, positive to flexion tests, and
  - show associated lameness with the inflamed other tissues involved

The joint capsules and the tendon sheath layers with their outer fibrous supports can become physically inflamed when a
- joint is sprained – **acute synovitis**
- a tendon is strained – **tenosynovitis**

The distended synovial capsule is tense, hot and painful to the touch or movement of the units of locomotion. Sometimes a joint capsule, such as in the fetlock, has its swelling masked by the surrounding inflammatory reaction – there is a lameness.

Infected Trauma

Synovial cavities can become infected by
- *internal blood spread*
  - the classic condition is **joint-ill** in foals, when a septicaemia from navel infection escapes into a joint coincidentally (microscopically) traumatised in its neonatal formative weeks.
  - brucellosis as a bacteraemia has a predilection for

connective tissues, especially of

- tendons, and so into their sheaths where relevant
- ligaments and related joints
- bursae, as at the poll and the withers, where it may form an abscess – **poll evil** (this is now rare; Brucellosis is more or less eliminated from its natural host, the bovine) from grazing following abortion in cattle

- *external invasion* from penetrating wounds direct into
  - joint capsule
    - by spread into tendon sheath
  - tendon sheath
  - bursa

This is by far the most serious of all synovial disorders, and apart from fractures and some tendinitis and desmitis cases, the greatest cause of loss of limb function, often of a permanent type.

Strained Tendon (Tendinitis)

The evolutionarily determined structure of the horse's limb has it standing on a horny-hoof covered third phalanx, i.e. on tip-toe of the only digit in each limb. The stance phase of a step is called unguligrade. The limb from carpus down (the manus, or hand), and from the tarsus down (the pes, or foot), is relatively long and there is no muscle tissue in these areas.

The force effecting tendons are those of the limbs' postural muscles

- a single extensor and
- two flexor tendons

It is the latter which experience the most stress
- the upward force of lift-off
- the downward stretch and hold of footfall and support
  - against the opposing forces of the give and take of the extensor muscle and
  - of gravity
  - relative to ground surface conditions

The jolting and compressive forces induced by ground reaction at footfall and support travel right up the limb to be dampened or absorbed by the extensive muscle support around the proximal upper joints and by the counter-poising of the lever system of the distal joints taken up by the tendons.

Further support is given by the check, suspensory and sesamoidian ligaments. Collectively they are the distal components of the overall stay and suspensory apparatus of the limbs.

These, coincidentally, generate a kinetic energy as they weight-bear; they release this force to assist the lift-off into the flight phase.

The tendons traversing the length of the cannon, especially the flexors, are particularly exposed to internal overstress during both stages of imposed muscular force

- the holding stress of 'let-down'
- the pulling up stress of lift-off

They lie between the skin and the bony cannon bone, unprotected by any other soft-tissue structures, and so are also exposed to external trauma, particularly from another limb's hoof and shoe interference. In the hind limb, this is most likely to come from that of another horse 'striking into' it. The force can reverberate through onto the

- superficial and deep flexor tendons
- suspensory ligament
- bone

as well as the initial skin contact, which can be complicated by penetration to

- lacerate as well as bruise the subcutaneous tissues
- introduce infection

It is the closed internal strain, or **overstress** which is the

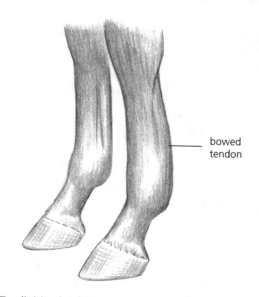

bowed
tendon

Tendinitis of the superficial flexor tendon.

most common and more serious condition. This is an occupational hazard of asymmetric gait speed, especially if jumping is also involved. Thus the incidence order is

- national hunt horses
- point to pointers
- team chasers
- eventers
- hunters

when most frequently it is the **superficial flexor tendon**, and usually that in a **foreleg**, is damaged.

It, especially, becomes narrower in cross-section in the mid-cannon area; consequently the forces are more concentrated in this sheath-free area. *It is the most common site of tendinitis or tendon strain.*

This tendon can also be strained at its insertions onto the periosteum of the latero and medio palmar aspects of the pastern bones, but much less commonly.

Deep flexor strain, conversely, is more likely to occur, where it is compressed as it rounds the flexion surface of a joint thus

- at the back of the fetlock between the sesamoid bones
- at its insertion onto the Plll

and is so more frequently in the hind limb, except

- on crossing the navicular bone at the coffin joint in the fore

The functional basis of fast gait (usually asymmetric) footfall or placement does explain the high susceptibility of the fore limb and its SF tendon, as compared to the DFT

- the heel makes contact first
- the fetlock begins to let down on it
- the superficial flexor tendon, *alone of the two*, takes the strain of the gravitational force
- only when the hoof is flat down and the fetlock is reaching maximum let, down does
- the deep flexor tendon take up its share of the stresses, helped by the
- suspensory ligament and so, often too late, saves the superficial flexor tendon from going beyond its 4% stretch safety margin

Tendon tissue is mainly collagen (type 1) protein, in the form of bundles of fibrils grouped as fibres within the whole, which is surrounded by a peritendinous 'skin' which runs along the vascular and neural systems to the tendon.

The fibrils are designed to have a helical or zig-zag crimp pattern which can pull out, thus allowing the whole tendon to lengthen (by about 3–4% in the foreleg superficial flexor tendon) and to recoil, giving an 'elasticity' to an otherwise almost inert tissue. This is also a stress-absorbing function and so helps maintain vitality and durability. The integrity of this elasticity is dependent upon

- the *crimp being conditioned to go to a 3–4% stretch* of its lax phase length over a progressive training period. The deformation of the crimp into a straight line will still re-form, even at this stress. If pulled beyond this, the recoil is lost and the debilitated tendon not only loses its elastic function, but is also exposed to

  - *complete overstress* – strain with peripheral and core tear or rupture

Conditioning and fittening work aims to physiologically stress the crimp stretch and recoil integrity progressively up to this four per cent. During the conditioning period microscopic overstress can occur at varying times and, later, during training work minor ones affect mainly the peritendineum, and the resultant

- capillary damage
- thrombosis
- anoxia

stimulates an inflammatory response which can be perceived by a diligent horsemaster in his routine 'feeling the legs' for

- a slight *puffiness* under the skin at the side and back of the cannon area
- a degree of pain when he palpates the tendon in the lax, off the ground position, and when weight bearing
- possible heat
- a degree of lameness

in comparison with the contralateral leg.

It is well recognised that both legs may be affected, one usually more than the other, to cause a shortening of the bilateral strides.

If a horse so affected is *immediately*

- let down in work
- given less hard feed
- given symptomatic treatment

the inflammation will quickly resolve and the

- fibrils will heal without chronic inflammatory

thickening (fibrosis)

- it will be able to return to progressive re-work within 14 days approximately

There are other conditions which can occur and which are difficult to differentiate clinically from the minor stress traumas

- the effect of **too tight bandaging**, especially if tape tying is used. This can cause vascular changes to the peritendineum, with puffiness and other signs of mild inflammation. Here, the skin will show more evidence of galling, even sores and necrosis
- minor interference trauma will present likewise, but the damage will show more as a distinct bruise, with or without superficial laceration

In any of these three situations, especially the micro trauma, repetitions (and especially if fast work is continued) may extend the damage to

- overstretch of the central (core) fibres
- degeneration of these
- vertical extension of this in both directions

usually one leg worse than the other.

A mature, 5-year-old chaser, hunter type in fast work experiences stress on the core fibres of the superficial flexor tendon, and thus overstress results in greater damage to the core than to the peripheral bundles. Such an injury **may** stand up to continuing work but eventually these outer fibres will go into a breakdown situation. When the peripheral fibres eventually strain as well there will develop a

- sub-acute tendinitis with
  - low grade lameness
  - thickening of the tendon, **or more usually**, an
- acute tendinitis with
  - marked inflammatory signs
  - severe lameness

Argument exists as to which fore limb is more susceptible to the acute lesion type of strain

- the leading fore
- the trailing fore in asymmetric gaits

i.e. which of these bears most overstress is at

- footfall and let down in the leading fore, or at

- lift off in the trailing fore

Acute Tendinitis

The pathological changes of an acute overstress or strain include

- damage to the peritendineum
- bleeding under the peritendineum and into the damaged tendon fibres and fibrils
- rupture of the fibres and further degenerative changes with consequent inflammatory signs
  - swelling of the limb from the
    - free blood
    - serous exudates from the damaged tissues
    - secondary oedema

    (the swelling may be a delayed feature, for up to 12 hours)
  - heat
  - loss of structural consistency – a soft mushy feel to the tendon
  - inducible pain
  - loss of function and so loss of use
    - lameness
    - further tendon damage to cause
      - partial or sometimes
      - complete rupture of the tendon

In external traumas the morbidity goes straight to

- **macro** damage
  - acute inflammation
    - rupture
      - physical laceration
      - subsequent tearing stress effect on the severely bruised tendon, partial or complete

Less violent traumas can precipitate the micro damage of

- capillary bleeding
- thrombosis
- anoxia – the components of a deep bruise

which can be the forerunner of sub-acute or acute strains in due course, or lead immediately to a severe rupture at the next footfall on this 'numbed' leg, or be indirectly responsible for a snap-action footfall in the contralateral overloaded leg. This is said to be an explanation of deep digital flexor tendon tendinitis within the fetlock canal.

The other interacting factors which predispose to direct strain are

- conformation
  - back at the knee – more likely to predispose to suspensory ligament and distal check ligament strain, but it does mean the let down could be interrupted into a jerk action
- hoof acquired deformities
  - weak low heels, long toes
  - abnormal bone angulations altering ideal tendon insertion lines
- unequal extensor/flexor give and take, resulting in
  - acceleration forces with third order joint acceleration and consequent jerk forces on the tendon
  - fatigue of the flexor muscles, thus leaving the tendon more and more on its own at let down
- unexpected passive overloading of the muscle/tendon – the false step
  - at let down onto sudden soft, to cause slipping into rigid leg protraction, with the hoof still on the ground after let down
    - holding of the hoof and
    - inelegant snatch lift-off, or
  - onto very firm – jarring, tendon vibration which if repeated may lead to
    - micro changes
- a trapped foot requiring extra forceful, sudden overstress, lift-off

To summarise, the wastage in National Hunt racing is said to be 30% due to strain. A tendon can only take

- so many micro strains
- so much stress on any one occasion

before overstress or strain occurs

- *an acute strain requires up to 14 months convalescence and rehabilitation*

Bramlage's healing periods for the stages of closed tendinitis are:

    acute (inflammatory), 0–48 hours, then to

sub-acute (fibrous deposition), 48 hours–4 weeks
maturation, 4–8 weeks
remodelling, 8–12 weeks
strengthening, 12 weeks for restabilisation and reorganisation of tendon fibres, then fittening – onto 12–13 *months* from date of injury

First Aid for Strains

First aid aims to minimise the capillary, arteriole and venule bleeding, by

- *application of cold freeze bandage* (over a gauge covering if necessary), or *cold hose* for 10 minutes, then remove or stop
- *application of pressure* evenly applied over gamgee, or by 'orthobandaging', *beginning at the coronary band and circling up to just below the knee*. Leave on for 1–2 hours, depending on initial severity
- reapply cold and pressure at 1–2 hour intervals, leave under pressure alone overnight – up to 6 hours
- if using cold water, grease heels and back of pastern
- always support-bandage other leg
- keep boxed. Get the help of the veterinary surgeon who will discuss ancillary diagnosis and treatment, such as analgesics and anti-inflammatories etc
- bed on *short* straw or other material
- remove all concentrate feed
- feed some cut or pulled grass, a little at a time, after each treatment, to keep the horse happy

The application of special splinting, e.g.

- the Robert Jones bandaging
  - with or without repositioning of the phalanges
  - the Monkey (or other type) boot which does reposition the pastern and toe

is a matter of decision by the veterinary surgeon, and these should be used only by experienced or by veterinary-supervised first aiders.

A temporary wedge under the heel area of the shoe is **not** beneficial, rather the reverse for superficial flexor tendon tendinitis, but when correctly applied does help with distal deep digital flexor tendon damage. Differential diagnosis is often outside the first aider's ability and responsibility. Thereafter veterinary advice is advisable.

In complicated tendinitis cases the struck-into limb, fore

or back, will result in either a

- non-penetrating trauma to the flexor tendons
  - possible complete breakdown of the superficial tendon or even deeper tissue (the first aid is the same as for the internal strain)
- penetrating trauma through the skin, with damage to the tendons (with infection) and possibly
  - complete laceration of the superficial tendon; the internal wound will be difficult to see or to feel when the horse is standing, even if not fully weight bearing; the tendon will have returned to its normal position relative to other juxtapositioned tissues and the wound in it will now be above the skin wound. In complete laceration there will be a gap in the superficial flexor tendon, **do not search**

This requires first aid as for any open trauma and, of course, **urgent veterinary help**.

Gastrocnemius Muscle Tendinitis

Also known as the 'gaskin' muscle, its tendon, in association with superficial flexor tendon, forms the Achilles tendon from the middle area of the leg bone (the tibia) to form a cap to the point of the hock. Although both these muscles function together as extensors of the hock, a strain of both together is rare. The gastrocnemius must either take more stress or come into play sooner than the superficial flexor tendon as it is the more frequently overstressed.

Signs

- enlargement of the Achilles tendon area
- distension of the bursa between the two tendons lying above the point of the hock and to a lesser extent just under, as
  - a 'false' capped hock
- lameness varies
  - in severe lameness there is
    - reduced hock flexion
    - altered arc of foot flight
    - comes off support more quickly than in contralateral limb

Rupture of both tendons does occur but it is rare. When it does, it is serious. It follows

- very severe strain

- laceration through both tendons

Signs (Both Tendons)

- the affected hock drops near or onto the ground – if the gastrocnemius alone ruptures, this drop is less
- the limb is protracted with difficulty, if at all
- the limb cannot support weight
- dislocation of the reciprocal apparatus; less than in peroneal tertius tear

In tendinitis of the gaskin muscle, overstress is the usual basic cause. Unusual or false functioning is involved. It is most common in elite athletic horses, for example

- show jumpers – 'jumping off the hocks'
- advanced eventers
- polo ponies – sudden stopping
- advanced dressage horses – elevated gaits

High power, rather than speed, is more likely to be the cause.

Apart from the structural differences in the muscles and their tendons which flex the distal joints of the fore and of the hind limbs these facts are also important

- in the fore, they pass through the carpal tunnel at the back of the 'knee', the carpus
- in the hind, they have attachments to the point of the hock

The functional stresses on them differ in as much as the

- fore foot has greater demands from foot fall and support, whereas the
- hind foot is more concerned with propulsion

Nevertheless tendinitis does occur, the gastrocnemius being the most susceptible in its primary role of extending the hock.

Suspensory Ligament Strain or Desmitis (SLD)

This ligament is anatomically a tendon, of a one-time muscle lost in evolution – a vestigial tendon. Although it does not act as a tendinous link between muscle force and a bone, it does function as a ligament, a very important part of the equine stay/suspensory apparatus; it is particularly vital as a support for

- 'let-down' and stance

and, from the kinetic force thereby engendered, it is also used in

• lift off

The entire structure

• the single origin of the ligament
• the single proximal third, the main part
• the paired branches

form several related functions

• supporting, to prevent over-extension (dorsal flexion) of the pastern
• limiting, to maintain alignment of the pastern by stabilising or holding the phalanges and, because of a degree of elasticity, a
• 'permitting' sling

which gives just so far in helping to control the distal limb's dynamics

They work in conjunction with the postural

• muscles and their tendons
• sesamoidean 'sling' ligaments and the
• separate joints' collateral ligaments

Their important biomechanical role exposes them to physical overstress which can cause a strain, (so called rather than a 'sprain' because of its tendon evolution, and because such trauma invariably occurs without any immediate associated joint lesions).

Whilst most common in the foreleg, the disorder occurs in the hind and can be bilateral in both fore or hind. Hind limb dis-ease has a poorer prognosis.

Strain of the origin of the ligament is not usually associated with marked thickening during the acute or the chronic stages. It is often associated with check ligament strain. In the hind leg there is frequently an associated periostitis, discernable by radiography, which has a poor prognosis.

Trauma occurs when

• flexor muscle/tendon function at 'let down' is disorganised usually when fatigue sets in, when
  • excessive support tension is exerted on the ligament
• the distal limb joints are exposed to accelerating forces
  • with whip lash overstress of the sling

Conformation defects which predispose are

• altered hoof/pastern balance
  • antero-posterior (broken back angle), with low heels and long toes, especially in the fore limb
    • breakover difficulties at speed
      • tripping
      • jerks
• toed in, toed out, with or without
  • fetlock varus and valgus deformity, with particular effect on one branch or the other – asymmetric overstress
• acquired medio-lateral imbalances, affecting footfall and support stability, again one branch
• 'back at the knee', with particular risk to the ligament proximally

Conditions affecting likelihood of occurrence

• suspensory ligament desmitis is usually associated with high velocity overstress
• the proximal, less common, main stem tears are particularly common in the
  • the young racehorse's forelimb
  • draught horse's hind leg, following
    • sudden effort or backward slip
  • traumatic interference – a blow –
    • on the cannon at the bifurcation level, the blow passing 'through' the also traumatised more posterior tissues
    • penetrating trauma, as with tendinitis
• one or other of the branches
  • overstress
    • acute
      • a combination of inelegant step and speed
    • sub-acute
      • an ongoing low grade overstress (micro traumas) usually associated with conformation defects – sudden acute tear may eventually develop

this insidious straining is common in the branches when ill advised

  • speed work, on
  • rough irregular going is involved
    • particularly in the unfit animal

Signs

- proximal area
  - acute
    - low grade inflammatory heat and swelling, not as marked as in tendinitis
  - chronic
    - no clinically discernible lesions
  - lameness is variable from
    - short lasting vague, to severe, to gait interference
    - negative at walk and trot, with possible
      - recurrence following faster work to produce lameness
    - when present, worse on soft going
      - especially on a circle
        - most noticeable with affected limb on the outside

In bilaterally affected limbs, chronic lameness especially is difficult to detect, and with the absence of focal inflammatory signs, a

- short striding gait and a disinclination to perform extended gaits
- diminished performance

are the only clues.

Mid-cannon area

- acute with marked signs and lameness is *usually* a closed strain, but occasionally from external trauma. If the ligament tears apart or is severed, the support function goes; the fetlock drops down and (if there is concomitant tendon severance) will fall to the ground
- a sub-acute or chronic form may develop in association with stress fracture of the splint bone. The 'new' disorder is the splint lameness
- the branches, usually *either* the medial *or* the lateral except in serious fetlock sprain trauma when bilateral branches and *other* related fetlock tissues are involved including possible displacement of the sesamoid bones. The hyper acute signs are of the total area sprain
  - acute
    - marked inflammatory reaction all round the fetlock, with swelling
    - inducible pain, concentrated on the affected ligament
      - lameness
  - sub-acute
    - less inflammatory reaction
    - swelling more localised to the suspensory ligament branch
    - inducible pain over it
    - lameness which can be severe
      - usually more noticeable on a circle
        - especially with affected leg on outside, but this varies with the branch involved

It should be appreciated that 'thumb and finger' pinching of the main body of this ligament will induce a withdrawal reaction more marked than from a tendon. This difference obtains even in the non-traumatised ligament: it is said that the early muscle tendon apparatus was associated with three- or four-toed equines where the muscle came below the carpus. Residual muscle nerves probably are still present in the ligament today.

Sprains

The acute closed disruption of the ligaments of a joint is relatively rare. The force necessary is more likely to damage the related tendons, but ligaments such as in and around the phalangeal joints and the fetlock can be 'sprung'. There is always the risk of an associated bone 'knuckle' fracture in any joint trauma. The possibility of an associated open wound must always be considered. The initial inflammatory signs can be confusing.

Be as sure as possible that there is no risk of infection, as from small puncture wounds and buried thorns which are difficult to discern. *If suspected, clip all round for better palpation and visualisation.* Therapy should be delayed until veterinary differential diagnosis is made, but a supporting bandage should be put on meanwhile.

First Aid

If satisfied that a closed sterile internal trauma is the injury, then 'cold' therapy is indicated

- as for strain and, if the area affected lends itself, to 'freeze' bandaging or to
- cold hosing and subsequent pressure bandaging, but not so tightly as to cause more pain or discomfort

In areas such as the 'knee' and the hock extra care is required for prominent points. The alternate cold and pressure periods, and the immediate management, are similar.

It is essential *always to seek veterinary input within 2 days at most* with sprains, before any further or different amateur treatment is effected; *if an open wound is discovered, or even just suspected, get veterinary help immediately*.

Management

The application of heat to sterile strains and sprains should not be started until after 24, preferably 36, hours. The intervals between cold applications can increase during this time

- after 12 hours increase to 3 hours at 5 times daily
- after 18 hours increase to 4 hours at 4 times daily. In these times the overnight interval can be extended both ways from midnight and 6 am.

Amateur or lay treatment for sprains for more than 24 hours is even more risky than with tendon strains; complications may be present, as described.

INTERNAL FOOT

Navicular Disease
Non-Infectious Trauma

Historical

Over two hundred years ago a German equerry described a particular lameness in riding horses as

- progressive
- incurable

with post-mortem findings which were

- confined to the 'small, shuttle-like bone in the foot'
- significantly similar in all cases

In 1816 an English veterinary surgeon noted a clinical locomotory picture in riding and light carriage horses of

- lameness in a forelimb which was
- progressive, to produce
- typical post-mortem findings, as recorded in Germany

He considered all these to be so consistent that they indicated a specific lameness disease. It took him 10 years to convince his colleagues!

Later in the century, Sir Frederick Smith, the senior veterinary officer in the Army Veterinary Corps who had devoted much of his time and energy to this common lameness associated with the navicular bone, came to the conclusion that it was a

- progressive degenerative disorder, causing
  - an increasing lameness in the forelimb
  - variably but usually bilateral
    - asymmetrically, so
- presenting clinically as a pain-induced posture and gait abnormality
  - at rest
    - a pointing of the foot, often intermittent and, in bilateral cases, alternating to 'take the weight off the posterior one-third of the foot – to ease the heels'
  - in locomotion, at walk and at trot
    - reduced stride and stance phases, with marked head lift
    - gradually improving with work, but
    - quickly recurring after even a short rest
    - signs worsening with the progressive nature of the disease until locomotory deficit was *always* present with *some* improvement when 'warmed up'
      - a tendency to land toe first at the trot, thereby minimising the duration of caudal heel support
      - an increasingly short stride, mainly in the anterior phase
      - developing, as the other leg worsened, into bilateral
        - shuffling, stilted gait
        - and, at rest, standing with the forelegs 'camped behind' the vertical
- with time (up to one and a half years or so) structural hoof wall and heel growth changes to produce a
  - blocky hoof appearance of upright walls, elongated at the heels, and narrowing between them, 'to ease heel pressure'
- a condition *which did not repair* despite, as seen on autopsy
  - a good blood supply

- the presence of new bone formation

He postulated that this inability, in fact the progressive nature of the disease, as judged by the

- customary worsening lameness
- the advanced nature of the post-mortem lesions relative to the duration of the lameness

was *because the primary causal factors persisted*.

Functionally, there was no way in which they could be effectively removed, except by laying the horse off to grass; even then it was most likely that the morbidity had 'gone too far'.

Smith recognised some of the possible causal factors but did not perhaps see them as significant enough to be part of an *escalating* picture.

His gross pathological post-mortem findings led him to state that the

- lesions begin in the bone's fibro-cartilage on the plantar tendinous surface
    - over the central sagittal ridge, or within a quarter of an inch (1cm) either side of it
- earliest changes are the formation of
    - brown stained patches on the surface of the cartilage
    - calcium deposits (specks) embedded in the cartilage

followed by

- ulceration of the fibro cartilage, then
- erosion onto and *just* into the sub-chondral bone

(this he called **osteoporosis**)

- engorgement of the related blood vessels in the cortical bone (which he described as an hyperaemia)
- thereafter the deep digital flexor tendon's subjacent dorsal surface showed
    - brown staining
    - superficial fibre splitting, and later a
        - tearing of the fibres across and off the deeper layers

eventually

- the formation of adhesions onto the exposed and ulcerated bone

Smith likened the condition to an **osteo-arthritis** as, later in the 1930s, did Oxspring *et al.*, and, perhaps because of the repetitive picture, they saw it as *a specific disease* and not a collection of lesions producing a lameness syndrome.

Smith also recognised other pathologies within and around the navicular bone which he considered need **not** be part of this disease

- new bone growths into the ligaments
    - from the dorsal border
    - from the dorsal extremities (later called **spurs,** by Pryor)

he did not consider them to be inflammatory and, unless so big as to interfere mechanically, not to be important

- vascular changes
    - areas of decreased bone density, an ischaemic necrosis which produced cyst-like lesions in variable depths of the bone and in variable positions; he assumed these to be painless unless they involved the synovium
    - changes in the size and the shape of the nutrient foraminae along the ventral border, a reflection of a required increased blood flow for
        - increasing age and increasing work load, a physiological process
        - pathological response to lesions such as
            - navicular disease, where they were the complementary effect but not the cause
            - other (inflammatory) disorders of the foot
- fractures
    - transverse from external trauma
    - 'chip' fractures on the lower border, possibly from distal ligament strain

Whatever the implications of these 'other' lesions, Smith was convinced that the basic osteo-arthritis was primarily associated with the functional as well as the structural juxtaposition of the deep digital flexor tendon and the plantar fibro-cartilage surface of the navicular bone – *an area of compression.*

It was not until the mid-thirties that the two RAVC officers, Pryor and Oxspring, had access to efficient radiographical equipment. Their findings on the three parameters

- clinical
- radiographic
- post mortem

now linked the signs of the disease into a more composite and plausible whole. They were aware that cartilage, tendon and bursa did not reveal morbid changes to x-rays, not at least to a critical or worthwhile degree. It was to be left to later workers to confirm their belief that the radiographically delineated bony lesions were by no means the earliest, but were nevertheless, historic clues. The disease, even now, had to be well advanced and, by definition, irreversible.

In post-war years it was realised that now 'seeing' such lesions was not in itself taking research into 'cause' much further. Radiography was but an ancillary aid.

Oxspring supported Smith's contentions that navicular disease was an

- osteo-arthritis due to
- compression stresses between the deep digital flexor tendon and the bone

Whilst the trio of parameters more or less confirmed navicular disease at clinical/radiographic level it was, in truth, just 'putting two and two together' and making a logical, reasonable 'four'.

Lameness was a sign of pain. Bone lesions almost certainly inferred pain but there was live evidence that some horses which were radiographically dis-eased did not evince lameness (routine x-raying of age and management related other conditions).

The converse also obtained; lameness, suspicious of navicular in the absence of radiographic lesions – perhaps not yet radiographically demonstrable? It was essential to determine if the sensory nerves to the navicular bone could be locally and specifically desensitised via the bursa, thus forming a fourth parameter.

If both left and right nerves in one foot are injected and the horse goes sound on it and, assuming a bilateral limb condition, now shows lameness in the second leg, then navicular or posterior third of the foot disease added to the implication of the x-ray findings is *pretty well a certain diagnosis*.

If only one nerve in one leg is injected (usually the medial), especially if some non-navicular disorder is suspected in the medial posterior one third of the foot and the horse goes sound, then it is *most unlikely* that navicular disease actively exists in that limb.

In horses, the sensory nerve from the bone can be traced and in most horses is a constant. It can be locally infil-

trated confidently in the knowledge that the bone (and its ligaments and possibly the related part of the tendon) will be temporarily anaesthetised. Even this is not enough since other tissues outside the navicular area will be desensitised at the same time.

The confusing fact that non-navicular lesions, suspected but not necessarily clinically accurately diagnosed, can be desensitised regionally via this peripheral nerve has encouraged specialist workers to attempt more definitive local anaesthesia by infiltrating into the bursa, by which only the navicular area is 'knocked out'. To be accurate this requires fluoroscopic remote guidance.

Such difficulties mean that general practitioners must still depend upon their clinical ability by comprehensively considering

- the progressive nature of the disease following an insidious start
- the typical gait and posture abnormalities
  - in one leg, likely but less advanced
  - in the contra-lateral, producing a
    - bilateral 'pottery' gait
- the results of selective but not truly specific regional anaesthesia
- the radiographic findings
- the ultimate changes in the hoof capsule

all of which *indicate the probability* of the disease, and

- the close grouping of the typical *post mortem findings confirm it* – later!

In one hundred years, many contradictory conclusions have been reached in many investigations. In the UK, available case material and, more seriously, available research funding have been limiting features.

Of course, controlled comparisons are also limited and double-blind trials of therapies, surgery and farriery are impracticable. Even with modern ancillary aids of thermography, scintigraphy, blood flow Doppler, ultrasonography, and CAT scans, in addition to radiography and local anaesthesia, there remain personal disparities in

- clinical evaluation and conclusion
- understanding the temporal order and the implication of the progression of pathologic events
- interpreting these various morbidities
- reaching opinion as to

- cause and effect
  - is it a disease?
  - or is it a syndrome, or even
  - several separate entities which are not necessarily related
  - which are the minimal criteria

It is now generally accepted that biomechanical **compression** stresses, perhaps also biomechanical **stretch** stresses, causing bone remodelling, associated with venous congestion (impaired venule outflow) and cartilage degeneration, are the principal pathological disturbances, which are seen as a

- syndrome, *not* a specific disease, based on the doubts which still remain – as to what morbidities are
  - the primary pathology
  - the secondary pathology

or are

  - the consequence, or merely
  - a coincidence

Most recent published projects give references to some fifty other researches. It is not a neglected equine problem. Until more is known, specific treatments, if any are to be found, must remain almost empirical. Prevention, it is almost certain, will depend upon conformation control, logical trimming and shoeing and sensibly restricted use of the susceptible horse type.

With hindsight we are sure that the eighteenth-century equerry had two basic parameters correct and these were confirmed in the early nineteenth-century work which pointed specifically at the navicular bone.

Smith, because of the lack of worthwhile radiography, was misled by his interpretation of the early discolorations. These are now known to be wear and tear marks, not superficial bleeding (pressure bruising) and *not* a significant navicular disease lesion.

Likewise, he saw gross soft-tissue lesions, as in the tendon and fibro-cartilage, as being earlier than bony lesions. It is now known that they are later. His negative bony lesions were surely a matter of 'hidden to the naked eye', even on histological – microscopic – examination post mortem.

His clinical acumen described a condition which is still accepted as a classic observation and reasoning, except that fibro-cartilage morbidity *must* have been preceded by

osseous changes.

His calcium deposits are now known to be mineral debris from ligament and bone degeneration which becomes embedded in the ligaments which themselves are radio-lucent.

Although he admitted to being less certain as to the causes of the disease and too emphatic as to how significant some were, his specificity of it being a disease and not a syndrome has **not** stood the test of time nor has Oxspring's similar belief when considered overall.

Predisposing Features

The members of the family Equidae of which Equus caballus, the present day horse, is one species, are further categorised as **solipedal ungulates** – in which each limb is a single column of bony support whose ground contact is by the pedal bone, the third phalanx, via the horny wall. This 'on tip-toe' is known as the

- **unguligrade stance** in which the pedal bone and its immediately related tissues are encased and protected in
- a horny capsule, the hoof

The resultant locomotor abaxial structure and functioning require a particularly efficient stay and suspensory apparatus. Conversely, these structures are exposed to a significant degree of functional stress.

As in the more proximal flexor tendons and suspensory ligament, so also in the distal podotrochlear (navicular) area, such stresses are more likely to become overstresses or strains in the athletic, lightweight breeds, for example, the Thoroughbred and its crosses. It is argued that crosses, bred to combine speed, stamina and strength with less 'excitability', can result in mismatching of the hereditable inputs of

- conformation
- metabolism, and
- ability

which could predispose to some of these overstresses directly and/or indirectly.

Predisposing Conformation Deficits
- too heavy a body for size of hoof
- inherited long-toed, low-heeled, flat-footed, but **not** actually with a broken back pastern hoof axis
- upright pastern
- 'broken forward' pastern hoof axis (less common), or

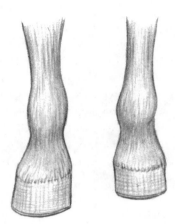

The contracted left foot, distinctive of navicular syndrome.

- 'broken backward' pastern hoof axis (most important and more common)

both acquired defects

- other defects throwing too much weight onto the forehand, e.g.
    - head and neck too big for the trunk
- angular limb and hoof deformities interfering with the column of support and limb balance generally

Predisposing Management Deficits

- selection of horses for work above their inherent ability
- irregular use – too much, too soon
- incorrect fittening
    - failure to keep exercised
    - unused-to terrain: too hard, too frequently
    - amateur riding
- failure to recognise these deficits, especially the acquired gradual hoof conformation regression
    - wrong farriery – not just the wrong farrier, but the wrong shoeing
    - possible nutritional imbalances, such as calcium/ phosphorus imbalances

A consideration of the physiology of the foot, as described by Sir F Smith in the early years of the last century, showed that, *on weight bearing*

- the coronary band, at the toe and at the anterior quarters, *contracts*

- the posterior coronary band, the related wall and the heels, *expand*
- the pedal bone descends, and so 'flattens' the sole

 all of which increases direct pressure on the podotrochlea, and in particular on the

- navicular bone
- deep digital flexor tendon
- bursa between these

Later work describes weight bearing as being a period of reduced blood flow via the arterio-venous 'shunt' mechanism.

The podotrochlea is a sub-unit of the coffin joint (Pll/Plll) with its relationship to the other tissues just proximal to and within the hoof capsule. It comprises the

- navicular bone
- plantar synovial bursa between it and
- that area of the deep digital flexor tendon's anterior, or dorsal, surface in opposition to the fibro-cartilage covered plantar surface of the navicular bone
- associated blood supply, especially that of the bone
- sensory nerve endings, in the
    - bone
    - tendon
    - synovial lining, and in the specific ligaments which are the
        - elastic (limited) bilateral proximal suspensory ligaments which arise from the distal lateral aspects of Pl and insert on the lateral and the medial dorsal extremities of the navicular bone. They then fan out along the bone's proximal border before they continue distally in association with the fascial connective tissue to insert on the medial aspect of the Plll's two wing cartilages, and also onto the wings themselves
        - the non-elastic, single, broad, distal suspensory or unpaired ligament which arises from the bone's ventral border and inserts onto the periphery of the Plll articulation surface. It acts to
            - maintain a firm association between the two bones, whereby they move as a single joint surface yet allow a degree of shock absorption 'give'

• support the palmar aspect of the coffin joint's synovial membrane

Although the navicular bone offers two articular surfaces, one to Pll and the other to Plll, these *per se* are not directly involved in this particular dis-ease of the navicular bone. What are involved are the related connective tissues, fascias and aponeuroses (attaching tissues) which blend with them and the collateral joint ligaments of Pl and Pll, and Pll and Plll, and the DDF tendon.

The interplay of these distal structures does not involve wide ranging flexion and extension, and literally no latero-medial displacement: much of it is in 'hold' mode, with the consequent tensions.

The deep flexor tendon, having exited its digital sheath, widens into the flat band which passes over the navicular bursa and the bone. Its excursion to and fro over it is not great, but its supportive function is extremely important within the podotrochlea, as the force line for action between the deep digital flexor muscle and the Plll.

At the area of contact of the tendon, its dorsal surface has a rudimentary fibro-cartilaginous covering. The synovial bursa is thus placed between the bone's and the tendon's fibro-cartilaginous surfaces.

The navicular bone, the distal sesamoid

• structurally acts as an enlargement of the coffin joint's articular surface, which it helps to stabilise. As mentioned, it and Plll move as one surface around the distal articular surface of Pll

• functionally it is a semi-roller like pulley under which (though technically 'over' which) passes the deep digital flexor tendon, *en route* to insert onto the semi-circular notch of Plll; more than just a fulcrum, it also maintains the tendon force line at a set angle for this insertion ***at all times*** – a standard line of action for this 'give and take' even though displacement of the limb through the fetlock deflects the line of the tendon proximal to the navicular bone over a range of 80–90° during locomotion. This function not only maximises a continuing tension onto the bone, but also minimises the possibility of third order acceleration and subsequent vibration between bone, cartilage, bursa and tendon

• along with its associated ligaments and the tendon, the navicular bone forms the major part of the **distal suspensory apparatus** of the limb, especially for the

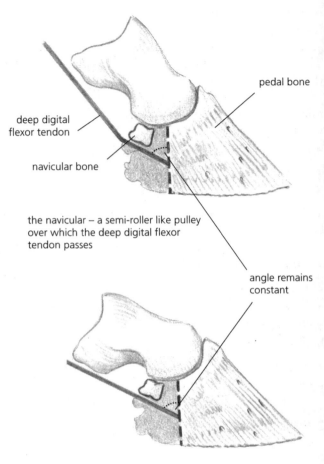

the navicular – a semi-roller like pulley over which the deep digital flexor tendon passes

regardless of the articulation of the pedal bone, the navicular ensures that insertion of the tendon remains always at a set angle

The function of the navicular bone.

coffin joint, by supporting it against over-extension induced by

• upward ground reaction force, and the
• downward force of gravity

In this function it is

• **concussed** indirectly relative to the pastern's degree of uprightness

• **compressed**, especially when the limb is weight bearing at stance, and especially during the support phase of locomotion

• **'stretched'** between the proximal and the distal supportive ligaments

Whatever triggers the overstress necessary to initiate navicular disease, ***it is these factors which are the basi*** *which predispose the horse to this very common forelimb lameness.*

The kinematics of the distal limb joints and particularly the three bone interactions of the coffin joint in its varied angular positions during the support phase, are not yet fully evaluated. In normal (for a breed) conformation at weight bearing the

- fetlock joint flexes and descends relative to the gait
- pastern joint tends to maintain a stable alignment
- coffin joint flexes to 'parallel' the fetlock

and they do so elegantly, rhythmically and smoothly – in balance, with the inherited morphology.

It is when this elegant 'give and take' balance is upset, and especially when footfall does not move smoothly 'over the fulcrum of support', or there are erratic joint directional changes, that overstress and strain develops.

The distal suspensory apparatus is particularly susceptible to

- **over stretch**
- **over compression**
- **vibration** following third order acceleration, but
- **concussion** seems to be of lesser importance

Stretch

Stretch by the tensions exerted on the suspensory ligaments

- the bilateral proximals which experience maximal loading when they are in vertical alignment as
  - just *before* break-over for lift-off

and minimal loading

  - just *after* break-over, until the next support phase

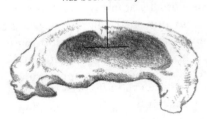

an extreme example – the normally opaque white fibro-cartilage of the bearing surface of the 'pulley' has been destroyed

The effect of navicular syndrome.

At maximal support they act as elastic springs to resist

- over extension of the coffin joint
- over flexion of the pastern joint, with excessive descent of the Pl, and thereby to help maintain the full benefit of the
  - flexor muscle's contraction force
  - kinetic force, induced in other tissues during 'let down' and support, for lift off

Compression

Compression across the short axis in the dorso-palmar direction, reflecting the pressure stress between the

- *upward* ground reaction force through Plll
- gravitational downward force through Pll

which together tend to move the pastern and coffin joints into extension and thereby 'push' the navicular bone backwards onto the

- bursa, and thus onto the
- deep digital flexor tendon, which then exerts an equal and opposite resisting force onto the bone via the bursa

Refined radiographic pictures of the bone clearly show that the trabeculae (bands of fibrous tissue) within the medullary cancellous bone are aligned to withstand this force, which is further loaded by

- increased weight, reflecting
  - additional rider
  - increasing speed

and exerted mainly during the

  - support phase, especially the caudal-heel-period
  - lift off

when the coffin joint is moving from flexion into extension during locomotion

- relative to
  - size of hoof capsule
  - hardness of hoof capsule

and their ground force input effects.

Vibration

Inelegant engagement could produce 'jerk' or third order acceleration. This is more likely to happen with

- an over-long hoof, weak heel, flat sole, conformation
- on hard going (especially if muscle fatigue coincides)
- false strides

- a return to work too soon following other types of distal limb trauma where there is residual pain and so an altered foot-fall, stance and lift-off

Concussion

Concussion, which differs from compression in as much as the stress is directed onto the navicular bone's articular surfaces

- it plays a minor role as the navicular bone
    - from its position out of a **direct** line between Plll and Pll
    - by the relatively thick hyaline cartilage coating its two articular surfaces
    - from the 'give' in its suspensory ligaments, it is well protected in the normal horse, but
        - on particularly hard going
        - over long periods, especially with an
        - upright pastern and high heel conformation

there could be a detrimental effect on

- elegant footfall, leading to jarring and vibration

and on

- blood circulation and the arteriolar venous shunt mechanism

It is also important to appreciate that, if and when pain arises from any of the above traumas, there will be an attempt by the horse to alter footfall and lift-off to reduce the pain; this may well influence these stresses for the worse, but it is believed that such alleviation is not directly possible in the full support period of footfall.

The associated clinical lameness is part of the navicular syndrome. In the absence of lameness, the over-stresses could be factors in the prodromal podotrochliosis.

The constantly growing hoof wall, and more so at the toe (unless it is trimmed correctly and when due) to maintain a balanced hoof, can lead to acquired conformation faults

- broken back hoof/pastern axis
- long toe, weak heels, under-run with distorted or bent, painful heel laminae
- buttress collapse, with solar corium pain
- flat soles, with reduced 'spring'

all of which further increase the podotrochlear compression factor. These acquired defects are more significant than the 'long toe, sloping heel' of inherited conformation

(which should be associated with growth and development of other related and balanced structures and functioning, with the result that the risk of overstress is minimised though not ruled out).

Recent force plate measurement research does suggest that such inherited conformation indicates a horse **more likely** to develop navicular syndrome and subsequent disease. Thus there is a marker for the disease being genetically programmed or inherent. Actual development would, of course, relate to a lack of control of this deterioration; such deterioration may be genetically predisposed to. The research has also shown that such horses have a tendency to 'go on the toe' even when the long toe conformation is not pronounced.

The very fact of shoeing somewhat reduces the natural physiological functions at footfall and at lift off, whereby the counter-pressures of bars, frog and sole are possibly disturbed to interfere with blood flows, especially the venous return.

To what extent, and with what detriment to the navicular bone, is not yet fully understood. If acquired hoof conformation defects and delayed inter-shoeing trimming obtains, then not only will vascular flow be at risk, but there will also be repositioning of the podotrochlea – and subsequent biomechanical, often radical, changes in compression and stretch.

Opinions differ as to the significance of latero-medial imbalances; navicular dis-ease is recognised in balanced feet – and vice versa. On its own, and especially if sheared heels are co-existent or in association with anterior/posterior imbalance, it must have some effect on the coffin joint's functioning. Vibration could be induced, thus leading to frictional disturbances in tendons, bursa and navicular fibro-cartilage, with coincidental heating – an acute bursitis, pain and lameness. There would also be unilateral overstretch on the supporting ligaments, and stimulation of their sensory nerves.

Some decades ago young Irish horses were imported as mounts for the Riding of the Marches in Scottish border towns each year. The same horses 'did' all the marches in any one year – usually at fast trot and, towards the end, at fast (possibly uncontrolled gallop) gait. It was claimed that many became 'navicular' cases. Unfortunately, there are no records of hoof conformation on arrival. Welfare interests intervened to obtain less spectacular, more sober events!

Third order acceleration forces develop in the coffin joint when it is 'made' to move into reverse rotation before coming to rest. From rest, any movement should start at zero acceleration. Without a momentary rest at footfall there is a jerking 'about turn' which causes vibration. Repeated vibration creates friction, initially in the tendon/fibrocartilage/bursal surfaces.

Overwork on the hard, at speed, will also predispose even in the well trimmed and shod horse.

All these defects will also interfere with natural movements of the coronary band, wall and heels at foot-fall with

- less contraction at the toe
- more expansion at the heels, whereby there is
- greater backwards and downwards movement of the bulbs

with resultant

- changes in coronary band and wall elasticity
- buttress weakness, heel shearing and subsequent
- interference with blood flow within the hoof capsule

It will be appreciated that mistakes in management involving inelegant movement will not suddenly induce pre-navicular bone changes, let alone the active syndrome. It is the *constant exposure* to their possible deleterious effects which is potentially dangerous.

The disease is rare in the hind feet where there is

- lower gravitational force (40% hind 60% fore, at rest)
- the ability of alternating weight bearing at rest; this minimises build-up of blood congestion within the capsule
- different functional requirements in locomotion biomechanics
  - propulsion off the whole hoof
  - rather than varying support at foot-fall and lift-off as in the fore

Collectively, the three main features when overstressed are most likely to produce an osteo-arthritic-like disorder of the podotrochlear elements, but not, *per se*, a dis-ease of the coffin joint itself. Other overstresses can precipitate degenerative joint (DJD) disease and related morbidities in the form of articular (and non-articular) low ringbone.

Over the years of research, two major schools have argued the pathogenesis superimposed upon the agreed compression factor

- a primary vascular disorder, with effect only within the
  - medulla, and possibly the
  - supportive ligaments

through an arteriolar/capillary morbidity arising from

- an obstruction to blood flow in some parts of the digital arteries outside the bone, but with direct effect on the bone's microscopic network, to cause
  - an ischaemic deprivation of oxygen
    - osteoporosis
    - soft tissue degeneration or necrosis
- capillary level changes, following
  - compression and the other overstresses

There is evidence of navicular bone hyperaemia associated with its remodelling in response to overstresses. Some authorities see this as a venous pressure congestion and certainly not an inflammatory reaction. The gaseous exchange of oxygen and carbon dioxide must be disturbed to some extent. The hyperaemia would definitely be a source of pain.

These openings in the lower border of the navicular bone are primarily for the arterial blood flow to the ventral and central parts of that bone. They coincidentally become recesses for the synovial membrane of the coffin joint. Increase in size and number (as judged radiographically in life) is evidence of

- physiological response, to meet the metabolic demands of
  - growth
  - continuing locomotion stress
    - living nomadically
    - working
- pathological response, engendered by
  - morbidly induced structural changes within the bone, presumably as the result of overstress compression and stretch

It is held by some authorities that their radiographic presence in a less than 4 year old horse is a poor prognostic finding. In older horses suspected of the pre-navicular syndrome a significantly marked increase in shape and number within a period of 2 to 3 months is also a poor prognosis – a secondary vascular disorder through a capillary/venule obstruction and subsequent back-flow vascular pressure following compression, etc.

Recent research points strongly to the scenario of initial biomechanical compression, with or without secondary venule obstruction. It refutes, on histopathological grounds, the primary arteriolar theory. It does acknowledge the variable presence of distal border foraminal number and shape changes which might be associated with navicular dis-ease, but classifies them as secondary to an already established bone pathology and associated remodelling.

The suggested scientific names for dis-ease of the podotrochlear area are

- **podotrochlosis** – a sub-clinical early morbidity
  - discernible only by post mortem histopathological investigation
  - suspected as a possibility when acquired hoof conformation changes are seen as typical forerunners of early abnormal loading of the distal suspensory region – a prodromal stage reflecting this suspicion
- **podotrochlitis** (chronica aseptica) – an established clinical syndrome (some will say disease) resulting from a chronic, degenerative *and* osseous productive disorder *not associated* with infection

The use of '-itis' is somewhat misleading; there is no actual primary inflammation. For all practical purposes the established syndrome is incurable, certainly after well established bone morbidity and positive response to anaesthetic blocking has been shown.

With the exception of foraminae at the ventral border of the bone showing radiographic changes in number and shape which *may* be significant for the disease in any one case, other specific navicular bony radiographic findings *usually* indicate a positive navicular disease or syndrome, with lameness as the rule. There will be soft tissue morbidity, albeit undemonstrable except by its pain response to local anaesthesia, of shorter duration.

Conversely, morbid lesions in the deep digital flexor tendon may be present but undetectable by presently available, practicable ancillary modalities before bone changes are radiographically discernible. This makes the disease difficult to interpret let alone to diagnose and give a prognosis. It is accepted that 40% loss of bone density must exist before the associated remodelling becomes radiographically apparent. Consequently, bone morbidity could still be present earlier but be undetectable; sophisticated CAT scanning and MRI techniques could well resolve these confusing signs.

However, it is believed that although the interrelationship between the autopsy findings, both gross and microscopic, and the changes thus shown in the bone's infrastructure are unclear as yet, it is indisputable that the primary disorder of navicular dis-ease is in the bone with secondary and/or concurrent degeneration of the adjacent soft structures of the podotrochlea.

It is a matter of research concern that the changes basic to navicular dis-ease in the medulla of the bone, its palmar cortex, fibro cartilage and the adjacent deep digital flexor tendon are diagnostically accessible only to a limited degree. The two most common lesions of significance in recent research programmes, partial thickness loss of palmar fibro cartilage and fibrillation of the deep digital flexor tendon, can be determined **only** on post mortem. Until techniques resolve this, the determination of a hopeless prognosis will remain based on positive radiographic findings, perhaps erroneously!

It is recognised that the principal factor in initiating podotrochliosis is the *onset and continuation of abnormal biomechanical patterns of loading*, transmitted through the forefoot, and that the main area taking most loading, normal and abnormal, is the distal half of the palmar surface of the bone, concentrated over and close on either side of the distal central sagittal ridge. The established, balanced 'give and take' of normal pressures between bone, bursa and tendon would seem to be areas primarily disturbed to produce the abnormalities in the bone.

These aberrant pressures cause the navicular bone to begin remodelling itself abnormally (as distinct from the normal morphological changes associated with maturity and 'normal' work loading). This remodelling can progress to a degenerative state or condition (DJD) possibly following venous return obstruction within the

- medulla
- palmar cortex

and then, and only then, leading to dis-ease of the

- fibrocartilage, and the adjacent
- deep digital flexor tendon

neither of which are radiographically discernible.

When pressure builds up in the bone (and/or in the bursa) there is pain and lameness. Wright suggests that the apparent clinical benefit of corrective hoof balancing and special shoeing does, to some extent at least, come from a repositioning of this load. But whether this is

- back to the 'ideal' original site, or
- to a new, less traumatised site in the tendon which 'presses' on a new more proximal, less damaged site on the bone

is not confirmed.

When disease has developed in the podotrochlear tissues they closely resemble the morbid changes of other equine DJD and are similar to human DJD (osteoarthritis). In both species, the milder forms of the associated changes can be attributed to age-related wear and tear, the more severe ones to pathological degeneration.

The recently demonstrated productive aspects of navicular dis-ease not only emphasise the non-ischaemic nature of it, but support the contention and the clinical assumptions that reduction in abnormal loading if effected soon enough, i.e. before positive radiography findings, could result in a clinical cure.

It will be obvious that navicular syndrome is not a sudden, one-off lameness as recognised at post-exercise or routine examinations. Nonetheless, it is a common progressive lameness. It is essential that the horsemaster, with farrier help, must aim for prevention particularly in 'conformationally risky' and force-plate foot-fall pattern identified animals.

With or without noticeable conformation faults, a working horse can evince gait changes from subtle to actual lameness. The causative pain is invariably in the posterior third of the foot and can be the result of

- ill-fitting shoes
- overdue shoeing
  - with pressure on the seat(s) of the corn
  - actual 'corn', usually medial
  - low grade bruising of the
    - sole
    - bulbs of heel(s)
    - over-reach interference
    - work on stony ground
    - underrunning of the heels
  - flaring of the walls
    - low grade localised laminitis (laminar strain)
    - early white-line 'dis-ease'
  - brushing interference
    - medial fetlock
    - medial/post coronary band
  - quarter (sand) cracks
  - inherited or acquired deep central sulcus of the frog extending up between the heel bulb – cloven hoofed predisposing to sheared heels
  - and, of course, navicular dis-ease!

Signs
- evasion especially on hard ground, particularly jumping

- refusal
- altered strides
- stumbling
- difficulty in lead changes
- lameness with increasing work at any one time
- postural changes – compare back pain and/or saddle ill-fit

In the absence of clues or signs other than the above, this syndrome is recognised as **posterior third of foot dis-ease**.

Diagnosis
- clinical evaluation and hoof 'search'
- unilateral nerve blocking; then, if necessary, the other side of the foot
- radiology
- further hoof search if necessary

In the absence of distinct evidence of a one sided disorder, including radiography of such traumas in a fore foot, it is advisable that a posterior third local anaesthesia is repeated in 24 to 36 hours, starting with the opposite side. *If both sides have to be blocked out* before action returns to normal, *then suspicion must suggest (early) navicular dis-ease*. This would be increased if the contralateral limb then evinced some gait deficit which could in turn be blocked out.

In the presence of the relevant hoof conformation defects, however slight, the suspicion of navicular syndrome would be even greater.

Whilst confirmatory diagnosis must depend upon
- intra bursal only anaesthesia, with
- repeat radiography in 6 to 8 weeks with especial references to
  - continuing foraminal changes
  - possible navicular bone changes

such suspicious, early findings would be the signals to instigate therapy at once.

This early navicular syndrome is often called **prodromal** or **pre-navicular dis-ease**. The earlier the horse's action is recognised as being significantly suspicious the better. This syndrome can continue for up to 18 months before podotrochlear changes develop, indicative of the degree of the hoof imbalances. Conversely, the effect of correction is not an overnight wonder.

The Pre-Navicular Period

As already discussed, the signs are those of posterior one third hoof pain, in association with possible conformation faults but in the absence of other pain producing lesions, as judged

- clinically
- radiographically, and by
- selective nerve blocks

Significant signs are

- intermittent lameness
  - unilateral
  - subsequently asymmetrically bilateral
- characteristically a head lift up on weight bearing
- more noticeable on the hard
  - straight line
    - under saddle
    - in hand
  - on circle (lunge) with suspect leg on the inside
- positive to
  - distal limb flexion test
  - forced extension of coffin joint on a block
- improves with work
- worsens following rest
- slowly progressive
- shortening of the stride, usually the cranial phase
- possible more landing on the toe (with shoe wear)
- pointing at stance (varies with individual cases and with softness of the bedding)
- easing of heels when bilateral (varies with individual cases and with softness of the bedding)

It is suggested that most of the pain in the early stages of this prodromal syndrome comes from stretching of the supportive ligaments, especially the distal impar, with stimulation of the incorporated sensory nerve endings leading to

- behavioural changes
  - temperamental deterioration
  - evasions and refusals

There is accumulating evidence that non-navicular posterior one-third foot lameness and/or eventual navicular disease can be related not only to fore limb(s) distal imbalances but also to **indirect** imbalancing – thus increasing the abnormal loading of one (and usually both) forelimbs' podotrochlea, e.g. from

- hind-limb defects
  - spavin, uni or bilateral
  - upper fixation of the patellar (UFP), uni- or bilateral
    - persistent, low grade muscular strain
    - conformation defects affecting action
  - sacro-iliac dis-ease
  - lumbo-sacral disorders
  - other 'back' disorders
  - ill-fitting tack – especially affecting the shoulder musculature
  - persistent bad riding
  - neck lesions
- foreleg conformation faults affecting action
  - flat-footed impact
  - varus and valgus limb deformities
  - over sloping pasterns

Signs of Navicular Disease

The signs are, fundamentally, a more marked evidence of pain originating from morbid changes in the

- cortical and
- medullary bone

presumably from venous vascular obstruction – pressure pain and coincidental ischaemic pain

- subchondral bone changes
- bursal inflammation, a synovitis
- tendon fibrillation and subsequent tearing
- mechanically induced stretch pain on the subsequent adhesions

The disease will certainly be bilateral

- the gait becomes shuffling and stilted
- this will ease off with warming up, to some extent
- posturally the horse may attempt to push bedding under its heels with the forelimbs 'camped' under body
- support its weight by propping its buttocks and/or a wide hind limb stance

There will be hoof wall changes ultimately

- an elongated heel
- more upright walls, especially posteriorly
- a shrunken frog
- the possibility of a ring-like groove all round the wall about one third the way down

There will be further disinclination to work – a clear anticipation of pain.

As has been explained, earlier research workers saw the advanced (radiographically confirmed) navicular disease as a true, complete disorder. More recent workers veer towards it being seen as a syndrome. In the author's view the classical, clinical signs with radiographical evidence and positive bursal anaesthesia indicate a complete picture, a disease and no longer a syndrome, if only because its lameness-producing morbidity causing pain is at the best

- only ameliorated (and then only for a limited period) by analgesics and corrective shoeing, and at the worst
- definitely incurable, warranting euthanasia on welfare grounds

Many horses do continue in work, and are made to continue, in work following amelioration subsequent to general treatment. The accurately correct diagnosis of true navicular disease must be suspect in some of these cases, or self-induced endorphin effect has produced a chronic acceptance of bilateral pain – in some horses.

Management

Not only is navicular disease a very common cause of lameness in Thoroughbred and Thoroughbred-cross horses; it is also a serious worry for a veterinary surgeon at a prepurchase examination.

It is the type of horse selected for use in a range of disciplines which causes the bulk of the case load for such examinations. A significant number, usually 5 or 6 year olds, are presented

- badly and/or overdue shod
- with unbalanced feet, especially in the anterior/-posterior plane
- not always well schooled into an overall balance
- showing unlevel steps on a 20m circle or less on the lunge or under the saddle on a firm surface
- arguably striding shorter than expected for their 'type'

(query saddle tree pressure, for example)

- flexion tests are inconclusive
- radiographs may show only foraminal changes
- blood sample tests for non-normal nutrients are negative

In fairness to all concerned, not least the horse, such subjects should be given corrective care and management over 8–12 weeks and then re-examined.

It is not surprising that all but the most perceptive of horsemasters miss the early stride and footfall abnormalities, which could indicate at least an early phase of the pre-navicular disease. The farrier may not have been encouraged (given the time at each shoeing and paid the related fee) to spot the hoof changes early on, and to deal with them.

The rider, especially working on the soft, could well miss the shortened gait, and all three the postural changes invoked by the 'easing the heel' stance.

It follows from this that management of a suspected case must aim at redressing any of the predisposing features, where feasible, in a horse already owned

- hoof balancing by a farrier, possibly with input from a veterinary surgeon
    - corrective shoeing for hoof and column of support alignment, e.g. egg-bar shoes
- setting back the work load
    - reducing body mass
    - better fittening
    - working on selective surfaces
    - slower progression through competitive levels
- veterinary advice
    - more specific diagnosis – nerve blocking, radiography, scintigraphy, and so more accurate prognosis
    - use of drugs, analgesics, blood flow improvers
    - surgery
        - wall grooving
        - desmotomy (the sooner the better)
        - neurectomy (not advisable)

Remember

- many posterior third of the hoof sourced lamenesses are not navicular disease
- if radiographic changes, apart from foraminals, are

negative the prognosis is reasonable *provided* the management is good, as listed above

- some suspected navicular disease cases, even with positive radiography (which are, after all, historical), may not be so. Specialised intra-bursal anaesthesia will help resolve

- doubtful cases will benefit from management of them as if they were early positives; further radiographs in 2 to 3 months which show no deterioration and provided any lameness is not worsening are good signs

When it is known that the signs, particularly the advanced signs, are progressively more likely to have a poor prognosis then it follows that prevention would have been infinitely better than management of the established condition.

In addition to these management factors, in particular the remedial trimming and shoeing (mainly to give a more evenly distributed weight bearing, as with egg bar and heart bar shoes), the medicinal therapy (subject to current research projects) is the use of blood-flow enhancers.

Surgically, the resection of the proximal navicular suspensory ligaments (which run from the anterior edge of the lateral cartilages to the dorso-lateral extremities of the navicular bone) has given encouraging results (J. M. Wright) with reasonable usefulness over a two-year period.

Prevention

This is mainly a matter of having the 'right' horse and keeping it so. Select preferably from

- a mature horse, i.e. over 5 years old, which has a proven record of reasonable work on good to hard going since first worked

- navicular disease-free parentage where possible

- a horse with good feet or feet which, given at least three shoeings, can be readily returned to this

- no history of lameness unassociated with external accidental trauma
    - the question of heredity is not yet resolved

- a horse whose skeletal structure does not suggest an animal that will mature into one with relatively too small hooves

- one free from signs of previous DOD (developmental orthopaedic disease) and DJD especially, but not only of the forelimbs, even though it is not actually lame now

Where doubt exists consult a veterinary surgeon and a remedial farrier. The pre-purchase examination will attempt to cover these aspects.

Laminitis
Non-Infected Trauma

A very common cause of disabling lameness, not only in ponies but also in cobs and other types in particular circumstances. The disease is usually the result of several contributory factors, not least of which is man's sins of omission and of commission. Statistically, the over-fat pony is the majority of patients. Its weight is detrimental in itself, but its obese state is usually complementary in effect on other factors.

In the dietary associated cases, generally it is

- over-consumption, especially of
- 'wrong' feedstuffs

which is mostly to blame.

These two features, together with obesity, can be disastrous if the horsemaster fails to

- know when the disease is likely to strike, and so
- misses the vital early signs, beyond which
- severe complications can arise

Mountain and Moorland ponies are naturally bred in an environment which requires them to diligently and daily nomadically seek out sufficient nutrients for their survival. They are not metabolically designed to live safely on

- cattle fattening pastures, even when that grass is permanent pasture

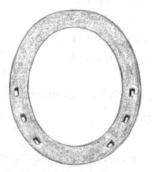
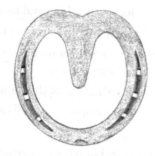

egg bar shoe   heart bar shoe

Remedial shoes increase the ground-bearing surface, and give support and stability.

• dairy cow improved pastures

nor do they require much in the way of supplementary fodder; their forage requirements are winter weather determined, when balancing vitamins and minerals with soluble fibre may be necessary especially for young stock. Good worming is equally important to prevent debilitation, but **over-feeding with high energy food-stuffs must be avoided**.

When crossed with light breeds of horses, their offspring are likely to be sold away from the indigenous grazing. Compound diets which meet both breed requirements must be carefully fed. Starch rich, high energy concentrates are contra indicated. **'Show condition' feeding can be dangerous**.

There are other precipitating causes
• mechanical (concussive/compression trauma)
    • prolonged and/or fast unconditioned road trotting
        • 'bolting' down a tar macadam road
    • prolonged athletic work, especially with jumping on hard ground
    • unshod work on excessively trimmed hooves
    • unilateral extra weight-bearing to ease contralateral limb lameness
• contra-indicated drugs
    • misuse of cortico steroids
• toxaemias
    • most species of animals, and especially the (better fed) domesticated ones, are at risk to toxic by-products originating from pathogenic bacterial proliferation in a body system
        • these may be disease pathogens
            • primary, as in strangles
            • secondary to virus infections
or opportunists which proliferate following disturbances to the normal defences of the body as by
            • overloading of the gut with starch-rich food (the second factor in the fat pony laminitis)
            • retention of organic dead material
                • retained afterbirth in the womb
• acute enteric disorders
    • colitis X
    • salmonellosis

• peritonitis
• pneumonia and pleurisy

These may be associated with other overstress factors of
• heat exhaustion
• fatigue
• travel 'sickness'
• electrolyte imbalances

During multiplication, the bacteria liberate an endotoxin which attacks the related systemic cell walls, which in turn liberate inflammatory chemicals. These toxins enter the bloodstream, a toxaemia, and eventually the blood vessel wall itself, where they affect the autonomic smooth muscles of the arteries. There, their vaso-active properties cause a
• **constriction of the vessel diameter** to
• **obstruct the flow rate and volume of the blood** with
• secondary **raised blood pressure**, a hypertension throughout the body

Hormonal imbalances can also predispose, e.g.
• prolonged oestrus
• hypothyroidism
• pituitary tumours – Cushings Disease of the older horse/pony – a corticosteroid imbalance
and precipitate the disorder.

In ungulates, this becomes particularly serious in the **delicately balanced blood supply to the tissues within the hoof capsule**, where there now develops
• micro-thrombosis of the hoof's laminar blood capillaries
• persisting arterio-venous shunting, with further flow reduction to the distal foot
• laminar oedema, from venous congestion and pain
• reduced perfusion and gas exchange through the capillaries with
    • ischaemia of the lamellae which have disintegrated
    • anoxia of their cells and tubules

It is now known that certain enzymes, Metallo-proteinase (MMP) are capable of lysing (destroying) components of normal lamellar wall. In those lamellae developing laminitis there is an increased production of this activated

MMP in response to trigger factors circulating in the blood. The MMP causes the lamella basement membrane (BM) to disappear and some to separate to form loose aggregates in adjoining connective tissue. The BM is the key bridging element of the hoof epidermis onto the Plll corium. This breakdown is the cause of the lamellar separation leading to

- necrosis of the vascular lamellae
  - loss of pedal bone support from the horny lamellae
    - the risk of pedal bone
      - rotation, or
      - sinking

all with considerable pain, there being no room within the more or less rigid hoof capsule to accommodate the swellings. The ongoing anoxia is painful in itself.

The horse species, specifically, is at particular risk

- as a soliped, it carries proportionately more weight per square unit of hoof ground force support, and more on its forelimbs. It is less able to cope with the laminar insults
- its small intestine is not functionally capable of digesting large quantities of starch, and is therefore
  - more susceptible to such overloading
- its large intestine and caecum, because of its convoluted structures is
  - more susceptible to neurogenic disorders

This predisposes to secondary bacterial proliferation and endo-toxin production.

The fat pony and cob, the most likely sufferers, are particularly likely to be affected in the

- spring
- autumn

when grass growth becomes lush, particularly if cold dry weather quickly gives way to warm, wet conditions. The flush of lush, rich young grass is more readily available and ingested. It is not unknown, however, for laminitis to develop on anything but rich pastures. *Susceptible ponies grazing what appears to be neglected, even horse-sick permanent pastures can, in the right environmental conditions, crop sufficient 'new' herbage to set up an overloading of the gut with soluble sugars in this grass.*

Stressed grass, pushed on quickly with possible trace

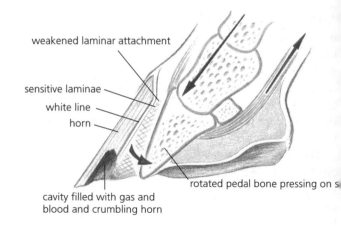

weakened laminar attachment

sensitive laminae
white line
horn

rotated pedal bone pressing on s

cavity filled with gas and blood and crumbling horn

Rotation of pedal bone resulting from laminitis and giving rise to seedy toe disease.

element and mineral soil deficiency, is now known to be extra-rich in fructose a form of glucose which cannot be enzymatically digested. It passes through into the large gut where it upsets the cellulose digesting micro-organisms as does overloads of starch.

When any of the predisposing factors are present or the predisposing other factors arise, there is usually some warning sufficient for a diligent, informed horsemaster to be aware of the *risk* of laminitis

- the flushing grass associated with weather changes
- suspicion or knowledge that a feed store has been 'burgled' by a horse, and not just by ponies
- overfeeding with cereals, particularly if the pony or cob was put on them too quickly. Any rich feed of more than 2–3 kg (4–6 lbs) in a stolen or accidentally given feed, when none has been fed recently, must be seen as sufficient warning to seek veterinary advice
- a mare has not cleansed within 4 hours of foaling
- a horse has an 'acute abdomen' such as colitis X or is recovering from colic surgery

There really is no excuse for precautionary steps not being taken. There is even less excuse for not recognising the very early signs of laminitis. If treated within 24 hours, and reasonably successfully within 48 hours, it can usually be halted before the serious sequel of pedal bone rotation occurs.

The fore feet (60% body weight support) are more frequently affected than the hind. All four may become laminitic, one hind foot alone when it is from contra-lateral weight bearing.

Signs

- first-time cases are usually
  - hyperacute with
    - considerable pain
    - reluctance to move or to have a leg lifted
    beware of the risk to the handler and patient of trying, let alone succeeding, in lifting one foreleg off the ground – the pony will collapse violently
    - locked fast to the ground
    - a characteristic stance
    - increase in the vital signs' level
      - heart rate of 100+bpm
      - fast shallow breathing
      - bounding digital pulse
      - variable hot hooves
      - coronary band hot, and painful when palpated
      - fever
      - mucous membranes injected (i.e. darker in colour)
      - *not* off food, if it is within easy reach
      - faeces reduced, from difficulty in posturing
  - acute, an improving situation or a less severe start
  - sub-acute, an improving situation or a relapse from an original acute or hyperacute condition
    - as judged by lessening of the pain signs, particularly an improved or less crippling mobility
    - stance remains altered for much longer

Early Management

- recognise the early signs
  - acute lameness, even refusal to move
  - postural changes
- *send for veterinary help immediately*
- onto both fore-feet, tape a four inch open weave bandage (still wrapped) along the frog area: leave the wall, bars and sole unencumbered
- slowly, with transport if and when necessary, move the patient to a loose box or a small covered yard (minimum 4m x 4m, 12ft x 12ft, for a pony, more for

cobs and horses)
- bed on deep, short straw, paper or peat
- let the horse lie down if it wishes **but**
- *beware of it being cast* or lying 'flat out' for more than 15 minutes at a time – *observe constantly until the vet arrives*

The first 3 days are critical. These 'days of grace' are, of course, only if the first signs of acute laminitis were seen and acted on. The vet may show that they were not and that radiography is immediately necessary. **Do not wait** 3 days in hope and **do not apply home remedies** other than the frog support. The vet will initiate

- control of the pain and the associated anxiety
- appropriate vascular amelioration
- appropriate shoeing in consultation with the farrier

Follow their instructions

- *do not* remove its shoes
- *do not* force exercise
- *do not* starve the animal, especially the
  - fat pony or cob
  - pregnant mare (consult a recognised feed compounder for a suitable diet – a hay balancer concentrate with minerals and vitamins)

Do understand that

- acute cases where the pedal bone rapidly sinks
- sub-acute cases which have sunk

whilst not incurable will take much time for you and your farrier, and consequent cost, to effect a recovery.

These are good reasons for, in the first place

- prevention
- early recognition – before sinking
- insurance cover

Prevention

It is important to know the susceptible

- horse or pony
- times of the year
- grazing conditions and sudden weather induced changes therein
  - manage accordingly
- beware the risk of

- stolen food
- sudden changes to high starch (energy) feedstuffs
- excessive (and fast) work on unaccustomed hard surfaces
- retained placenta
- acute digestive disorders especially severe diarrhoea
- act, with veterinary help, accordingly

Management
- veterinary advice and treatment, which should be carried out accurately
- with farrier help, based on
  - radiographic findings
    - pedal bone rotation or sinking and appropriate remedial shoeing
    - presence of a seedy toe, and its exposure by resection by rasping of the outer wall
  - supportive feeding relative to body weight, and required 'hoof'-specific amino acids and other vitamin/mineral supplements
  - progressive exercising

These require time, patience, diligence *and money*.

Seedy Toe Disease

This is a morbid condition of the laminae following the *focal* separation of the avascular from the vascular layers, as a sequel to laminitis in its chronic stage, i.e. after pedal bone rotation or sinking.

The subsequent disruption of the white line at the toe permits a secondary ascending infection into the necrosed, flaking laminae but with greater freedom to spread upwards and laterally with further destruction of the area which, as the name implies, is confined to the toe area of the wall, usually both sides of the line.

The hollow area is radiographically demonstrable. It can also be suspected by a change in percussion sound when tapped. Searching of the foot will reveal the dry mass of dead horn, which is also exposed when the outer wall is sectioned down through to the vascular (but sealed off) laminae. After removal there is a chance that the new wall will unite with the sensitive laminae *if* the pedal bone has been re-rotated to some extent.

Similarities can be noted with some of these foot disorders. They are not easily differentiated without profes-sional help

- the farrier for initial recognition of their existence before acute lameness develops
  - corns
  - white line disease
  - farrier errors
- the horsemaster's awareness of
  - sudden lameness, and his knowledge of any associated predisposing condition
    - punctured sole
    - laminitis

Pus In The Foot (Under-Run Sole)
Infected Trauma

This is a very common cause of lameness and may be sudden or gradual in onset. It is caused by bacteria entering into the sensitive (vascular) layer of the solar corium from

- a penetrating foreign body contaminated by dirt and so by bacteria, many of an anaerobic type
  - a picked-up nail or other sharp object
  - a displaced nail from a spread shoe which is stood on
  - a sharp-edged flint, tin, glass etc.
- infected faults in the white line to produce 'gravel'

Simple 'pus in the foot' implies that the penetrating object did not enter

- onto the pedal bone
- into the navicular bursa/coffin joint area

If restricted to the posterior quarter heel area, may produce signs of posterior third foot lameness but most unlikely to be bilateral in that foot.

Effect
The wound usually quickly becomes closed sufficiently to become 'short of oxygen'. The anaerobic germs rapidly multiply in such oxygen reduced situations. They are usually pus forming.

Result
The infection destroys sensitive horn which liquifies; the liquid causes pressure necrosis and further liquifaction of the insensitive horn. It takes several days for the infection to fully 'ripen'

- sensitive tissues become inflamed and
    - secrete serum which adds to the fluid volume
    - there is pain
        - from the inflammation
        - from the fluid's increasing pressure on the remaining sensitive tissues
- there is marked lameness of the weight bearing type
    - if toxins are produced and/or if bacteria gain entrance to other tissues
        - an oedematous swelling spreads above the hoof into the cannon area
        - there will be fever, increased respirations and heart rate
        - there may be systemic illness, a toxaemia or septicaemia, though these are rare
        - the digital vein on the same side pastern region and up the inside of the cannon, will dilate
        - the pulse will become *fuller* on the same side
        - vascular signs are greater in an **unshod limb** from both bilateral and unilateral inducing lesions, from the fetlock down; without shoe protection, the hoof is directly weight-bearing
    - the hoof wall will be warmer than the contralateral one

The infected purulent fluid can spread in two directions:
- up the inside of the wall in a narrow track to the coronary band, which develops an abscess swelling
- over the surface of the corium, close to the white line when it tracks towards the toe and beyond, and/or towards the heel. It may break out at the white line where there is any weakness

Occasionally horn necrosis will open through the sole to the surface with variable drainage.

Management
When an embedded nail or other sharp object is discovered it is important when withdrawing it to note
- where it entered
- what direction it went (the reverse of withdrawal direction)
- how deep it went – *draw a diagram immediately*
- was the buried part

- damp and blackish?
- blood stained?

    If in doubt about safety or ability to do these withdrawals, cover sole and frog with thick layer of gamgee to form collar/cuff round and over the protruding nail to remove risk of weight-bearing pushing nail further in. Tape on securely. Keep stabled on bedding till better help arrives. With splits in the horn, especially of the sole and if bleeding is suspected (brownish stain surrounding the hole) do not dig into, but cover and deal with as above

- let stand for one minute
    - assess temperature of the wall with the back of the hand, compare this with the contralateral foot. In some horses this will intermittently differ even in the absence of inflammation. If the suspect foot is hotter, assume that is significant
    - look for and feel for distension of the related digital vein on the inside of the cannon
    - feel pulse at postero-lateral aspects of the fetlock
    - compare both these with the other leg

A reactive first aid increase in blood flow should be brought about by the application of 'bearable' heat to the focal area of the foot using warm water, poulticing, or tubbing.

Warm Water
Warm cloths hand-held onto the area are of little value on a hoof, but of more use if fomenting the **skin** of the coronary band and/or heel bulb when a pus track has surfaced. The hot water can contain
- saturated Epsom salts
- ordinary salt – double 'normal' strength

but none of these *per se* are particularly useful. **It is heat that is required.** At least two towel cloths are used, one replacing the cooling one as required. There is no objection to using the same source of water but its temperature (elbow-bearable) must be kept up. These **fomentations**, as they are called, are usually maintained for about 10 minutes and repeated 3 or 4 times daily to 'draw' the area.

Poulticing
Less labour-intensive is the application of warm poultices. Always test the temperature against the back of the

hand or point of elbow; it should be just bearable.

Proprietory poultice compounds are available. Animalintex is so well known as to have become a colloquial substitute for 'poultice'. Instructions are issued with each packet. Such poultices, kaolin or Animalintex, are also used as the heat application vehicle to strained/sprained areas.

Poultices can be applied with the suspected area being targeted, rather than the whole of the wall, frog and sole. This will prevent softening more horn than necessary, which could necessitate a long recuperation time. The horn will stand, in fact needs, greater heat to penetrate to the corium and the vascular laminae. Care, therefore, must be taken to avoid scalding the more delicate coronary band and the bulbs of heel by either

• keeping these areas free of the application, or

• interposing gamgee between them and the hot material

Two or occasionally three poultices per day are used. The veterinarian or the farrier will normally re-examine after 3 to 4 days to detect the essential horn thinning which could indicate inflammatory 'pointing' and the possible need for surgical opening.

The application is insulated and held in place by 10cm (4in) wide masking tape. Where this engages the bulbs and the coronary band, for security it should be over a gamgee or other type of separating pad. Poultice boots, originally intended for the outmoded bran and epsom salts poultice, (cheaper, but messier and arguably less effective) are difficult to fit securely and without rubbing the heels.

'Tubbing'

The hoof and just above should be well cleaned before tubbing. Soiling of the salts solution will rapidly decrease the temperature.

Where there is an open wound of the skin, this method of heat application is absolutely contra-indicated. No matter how well cleaned the limb and even the addition of safe levels of antiseptic to the tub, the water will be quickly contaminated and the wound infected from its immersion. This particularly applies when the sole has been opened by poulticing or from the pressure of the pus – the abscess has burst. When *obviously still closed,* tubbing is permissible.

A form of hot fomenting, 'tubbing' is done by immersing the foot up to or just over the greased coronet, bulbs of the heel and back of the pastern, in saturated epsom salts solution.

A rubberised bucket is filled with 5cm (4in) of boiling water. Epsom salt crystals are stirred in until no more will dissolve – usually about 500g (1lb). By this time the temperature will have dropped to a bearable level, or even to a less than useful degree, hence the need for expedition

The limb is manually 'placed' in the bucket with the horse suitably restrained and/or distracted by hand feeding. *Do not leave tied up and unattended.* A 5 to 10 minute immersion repeated 2 or 3 times daily for 3 days, is an average programme. Where weather conditions accelerate cooling, a topping up or replacement of fresh hot solution may be required. *Do not pour boiling water into the bucket while the limb is immersed.* On removal of the foot, the distal hair covered limb and the bulbs of the heels *must be dried* to prevent maceration.

Cereals and their by-products, for example thick slices of bread 'buttered' with slivers of soap or bran with or without epsom salts and linseed, all hold the heat of boiling water sufficiently to act as emergency poultices. Here again, they should not be used for open wounds. The other poultices described should be used in such open wound cases.

It should be appreciated that poulticing and tubbing must be limited in duration and done to serve a need to overcome a primary disorder which, if not thus 'treated', could be, on balance, more damaging. Except in a corn 'piping' to the skin-covered heel bulb, judicious and *skilled* use of the hoof searching knife is to be preferred. In the UK, a farrier is legally permitted to do this; it is not seen as 'penetrating the vascular tissue'.

Do not administer antibiotics topically or parenterally without professional advice. Remember, however, that to be effective in preventing infection developing, they must be given within 12 hours of the puncture.

In pedal bone complications it is unusual for the infection *per se* to invade the bone unless the penetrating object has physically traumatised it and left infection there, causing

• bone necrosis from the trauma

• periosteal/pericorium abscess formation in several days

   • further necrosis of bone

• under-running of the sole

The pain is usually greater than when the bone is undamaged, especially after the first few days

• lameness is marked

• systemic signs are greater

• handling of the hoof becomes more difficult

Coffin joint/navicular area complications are usually the result of nail, needle or wire penetration. The pain is usually marked immediately after the trauma but it subsides quickly. If this suspected lesion is not quickly treated professionally suppuration sets in and an intense pain develops with

- systemic signs
- subcutaneous inflammatory oedema spreads up the leg
- the digital sheath may become infected and inflamed by spread from the navicular bursa
- treatment has to be intensive

EXTERNAL FOOT (HORNY HOOF CAPSULE)

All horn has a water content which varies upwards from

- frog to sole to wall
- is variable in the periople

This moisture is obtained by 'percolation' from the intercellular fluid (serum) of the respective coriums to the avascular keratinised tissues.

There is *scientific evidence* that *moisture does not*

- pass to the environment from the middle layer horn, or that
- the same horn layer absorbs any from wet grass or bedding or the atmosphere, in *healthy* feet except that
  - the periople does not have such an effective permeability barrier, and will exhibit moisture loading (as does human surface skin or finger nails if immersed for any length of time) – and this is seen around the coronet and the bulb of the heels over which the periople descends onto the wall for several millimetres
- the permeability barrier is a reflection of the fats and the other lipids particularly which impregnate the tubular horn
- 'hard' feet, as exemplified by the desert Arab and the mountain pony, as compared to the assumed 'softer' hooves of the lowland and fenland draught horses, are explained as evolutionary necessities *relative to ground reaction forces*

It is accepted that compression upwards from ground force reaction on the wall tubules (shod or unshod) will stimulate greater compaction in the distal areas upwards, and so produce a harder consistency and resistance to wear, as also judged by knife paring; it is certainly not a result of dehydration.

An unshod pony and cob, especially, will develop 'hard' foot horn if conditioned to do so by work on hard road surfaces, becoming capable of unshod work on a variety of surfaces.

It follows that the topical application of oils and greases will *not* penetrate healthy horn either to

- waterproof the hoof or to
- medicate it

They are cosmetics – wall surface 'beautifiers'.

Conversely, *it is known that persistent use of such topical applications will destroy the outer natural fats and lipids which protect the keratin*. Subsequent keratin destruction will lead to a weakening of the wall horn and that of the sole and frog, if they were also so dressed, and open up access to the non-keratinised horn and its corium for bacteria and, of course, unwanted moisture.

This is even more likely if the wall is already deeply traumatised, as from sandcrack and splits, or is deficient in essential nutrients such as calcium and essential amino acids, or disordered from food over-supplementation with selenium. White line disease infection is a good example. The *occasional* cosmetic use is unlikely to be harmful. Research continues for 'preservative' dressings for damaged or malnourished wall pending expedient treatment of any disorders which allow local loss of impermeability as well as a better understanding of 'balanced', protective feeding.

The use of dressings containing formalin, some up to 20% strength, cause increased cross-bonding of the superficial collagen content of the wall horn, and thus *'brittle' hooves will develop* with a reduction in natural protection.

Medication of the hair-covered skin of the coronet to stimulate horn growth – of the same (poor) quality – will not destroy the fats *provided* it is not allowed onto the periople. The sole and frog horn have less permeability resistance than the wall, but this discrepancy affects only the superficial outer layers. Nonetheless, destruction of what is there can be very detrimental; consider the possible causes of thrush in the frog and canker of the sole.

Deficits in horn quality are a matter for proper investigation, e.g. laboratory analysis of hoof parings and subsequent correct and nutritional supplementation, as well as farrier/vet co-operation to expose the usual secondary, often anaerobic, infection of the broached white line and between the two laminar layers, so too with the frog, and to appropriately treat them.

There is experimental evidence that horn strength is the same all around the hoof wall, and that this is related to pigmentation. However a black area is rather more resistant to abrasion than is white horn. Horn quality is said to reflect optimal levels of certain amino acids, methionine and cystine and of zinc. Low levels of calcium are related to some aspects of horn necrosis, as in white line disease.

Corns
Non-Infected Trauma, Becoming Infected

Corns are invariably a foreleg problem. They are not the same as those which afflict humans, but like them equine corns are also associated with pressure; in the horse it is onto the solar horn of the hoof at the 'seat of corn'. They are often bilateral.

Causes
Pressure from
- a stone wedged between the heel of the shoe and the solar horn, in the angle of the bar
- the heel of the shoe web, which with downward and forward growth of the wall is drawn off the buttress to lie in the angle of the bar, and there exerts pressure on the softer solar horn – too long an interval between shoeings
- broken back hoof/pastern axis
- overtrimming the heels, so that the shoe has no bar/wall support and immediately exerts pressure
- shoeing too tight at the heels (and too short) , which may cause other lameness producing morbidity as well as corns

Except for the wedged stone
- most corns occur on the medial heel area, but
- lateral corns will also develop in toed-in animals

Signs
- a slowly progressive lameness – worse on a circle. The early, mild lameness is often worse on turning tightly. Differentiate corns from early pre-navicular syndrome, or bad shoeing *per se*, and other posterior third of the hoof disorders
- a 'pottery' short stride pace, if the condition is bilateral
- attempts made to alter swing phase direction, to make

ground contact with the unaffected heel
- an intermittent easing of the heels off the ground whilst stabled

If the shoe(s) are removed at this stage and the 'seat of corn' is carefully pared, a brick-red staining of the exposed insensitive horn is discovered. This is pressure induced sensitive horn bleeding which has seeped down to the surface.

If the initial lameness has been missed or otherwise neglected, a pressure necrosis of the horn will develop
- the lameness will markedly worsen
- inflammatory signs will develop
  - the corn will open up under the shoe
  - infection will gain entrance
  - pus will form
    - this will track up into the sensitive tissue with
      - increased lameness and inflammatory signs
      - the bulb of the heel will swell and be painful to the touch
      - the abscess will ripen and burst to
        - produce a 'piped' corn
        - alleviate much of the pain
  - occasionally the pus will under-run forward

In some cases exercise on the hard will 'drive' the liquified horn necrosis into sensitive corium, with immediate lameness. In others, lameness is delayed until an abscess forms at the heel bulb.

Management
- suspect presence, then hoof tester pressure will pinpoint the area
- the farrier will remove the shoe, and
  - thin the horn over seat of the corn, to reveal a brick-red stain of a bruise
  - check for any black fluid (pus) in the area
  - if so seek veterinary help, to open the area for drainage (the farrier may do this to expedite matters)
    - if a piping corn is present, heat-ripen to 'burst' at the heel
    - flush into sole opening and, where relevant,

out through the heel with '10 vol' peroxide repeat daily until clear and clean

- have a seated out shoe fitted over corn area, with a suitable plug in the hole
- return to work progressively

Prevention

- attention to the potential causes as detailed above
- more conscientious picking out of the foot, with particular reference to stone or grit under the shoe web heel
- encouragement to farrier to trim according to alterable acquired hoof conformation faults and shoe wear
- acceptance that shoeing for hunting often needs a short, close-fitting shoe so the interval between shoeing should be kept to 4 to 5 weeks

White Line Disease
An Infection

As is implied above, this is a syndrome. It is sometimes confused with Seedy Toe disease but differs in the precipitating cause and the more widespread distribution around the total white line.

It is the consequence of a basic horn weakness lateral to the white line and is characterised by a progressive hoof wall separation between the laminar layer and the stratum medium layer of the wall, the highest water content in non-pigmented horn.

The area has a grey to black, dry, crumbly horn material that is easily picked out. The separation is progressive around the hoof, particularly at the toe and quarters. There are several names for it, e.g. dew poisoning, yeast infection, candida, hoof rot and onychomycosis. The actual cause remains unknown. The early stages, when a shoe is removed, show extensive, cheesy horn destruction with black pus formation.

It can be found in all four limbs, usually of the shod animal which has not been well managed – overfed; under exercised; feet not correctly picked out under the shoe web; shoes left on too long; excessive hoof washing; stood in wet bedding, or wet, lush pasture.

Hot, humid weather predisposes to the growth of bacteria and fungi, which gain entrance to the devitalised white line horn and so between the laminar layers. It can extend well up the wall with inter-laminar destruction.

There is lameness because the distal laminar support is decreased and the wall pulled away from the related sensitive laminae, rather than from the actual inflammation. The lameness can be confused with that of laminitis.

In earlier stages it is usually, and should be, recognised at shoeing, when extensive 'cheesy' destruction of horn is present with black pus formation in the necrotic debris.

This condition is closely related to horn quality. Ultra-microscopic examination of hoof parings will determine if there is a calcium deficit as distinct from the methionine, biotin and zinc deficiencies more usually connected with general hoof horn (keratin) dis-ease. Treatment by a vet is advisable.

Gravel
Infected Trauma

White line disease must be distinguished from **gravel**, which is an inflammation of the white line following a *focal* penetration of it from

- a deep wall split
- pressure from grit trapped under the shoe
- nail prick penetrating unusually low on sensitive wall, causing avascular wall damage and necrosis which, by working, is pushed through onto the vascular corium

The infection invariably travels up between the laminae along a very narrow line of least resistance to form an abscess at the coronet, where it ruptures and discharges. It is not a true 'pus in the foot', as the corium as such is not primarily penetrated.

Lameness is variable but is usually acute when the infection breaks through into the coronary band tissues.

Three factors are paramount in treatment

- remove all undermined hoof wall
- stabilise the remaining wall
- prevent further infection

Bruised Heels
Non-Infected Trauma

'Bruised heels' is a descriptive term for one type of post-third of the fore-hoof lameness. Bruised heels are often persistent and bilateral. It arises most frequently in horses with

- weak, under-run heels, whereby the fleshy bulb is brought nearer to the ground
- long-toed animals (often in conjunction with the above)

- those with a tendency to forge and/or overreach
- corns are a frequently related condition

The horse tries to go on its toes with a shortened step. In unilateral cases it shows as a distinct lameness, otherwise, if in both feet, as a hesitant, 'pottery', action especially when on the hard.

When one horn bulb is affected in either one or both feet, the horse attempts to off load the painful heel with – in time, the risk of uneven heel wear and subsequent sheared heels.

Splits or Low Cracks
Degenerative

Splits are not sudden conditions, particularly with regard to the inflammatory and lameness-making painful complications. Routine inspections, however, should appraise the horsemaster of the early signs. They are

- more common in unshod horses, especially on soft, wet grazing, often precipitated, and any lameness exacerbated, when the ground dries out and hardens
- work up the wall against the downward growth
- follow the line of the horn tubules
- can develop as fissures caused by nail splits in brittle horn, distinct from avulsions of superficial horn between old nail's clench holes as it grows out, or from the torn distal wall, as with wrenched off shoes; these are usually irregular in outline and *cross* the line of the tubules
- attract and hold dirt and debris and, when the fault penetrates to the corium, infection and pain develop

Sandcracks
Degenerative

These are more common in working horses, shod or unshod, as the result of

- a tread (injury caused by one foot treading on the other) in the fore or hind on the coronet, with a consequent deficit at a focal level of new tubule formation; from this a fault grows down the wall with the main wall growth
  - this may split ahead of the growth, and with movement the fault can
    - penetrate to the sensitive laminae
    - become widened as the two edges rub together or even overlap
    - develop painful laminar inflammation
- in the unshod, unrasped hoof, especially where there is a marked overgrowth of toe horn, particularly with medio-lateral imbalance, the torque effect of upward ground reaction forces will stress the horn and cause a coronary deficit
- a similar quarter fault in line with the area of heel expansion can also arise without a tread

Prevention

- routine rasping in unshod horses, especially after prolonged wet then sudden drying out of the field
- 'grass tip', a lightweight counter-sunk shoeing, in grazing horses on hard pasture land

Sandcracks are extremely difficult to treat once the wall is mobile either side of the crack. Veterinary/farrier input is essential

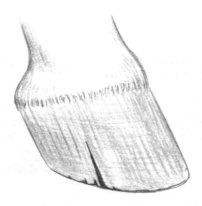

A split, or 'grasscrack' – a false sandcrack.

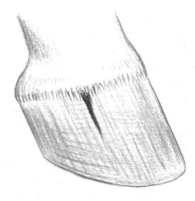

A sandcrack.

Over-reaches
Infected Traumas

Over-reaches are not not usually persistent, but are often repetitive.

The initial trauma is an
- open wound with
- severe bruising of the heel bulb
  - horn tissue only
  - coronet destruction
  - 'flesh' wound downwards onto the coronet

and there is invariably a
- secondary infection

They may be associated with a clawed-off shoe, with the further risk of a nail penetration of the sole or frog and/or a lacerated other limb.

The skin wound is usually in the shape of an inverted V attached at the base. Except in extensive injury up onto the pastern suturing is usually impracticable and ill-advised – the flap invariably dies. Proud flesh, a common complication of the skin, is a risk. Deficit in heel horn may also follow in associated coronary injury.

Management
- remove the flap?
  - it will eventually slough, but in the meantime can act as a
    - trap for germs
    - an irritant, stimulating more proud flesh
    - an obstruction to epithelialisation
  - removal is simple as it is no longer in nerve connection, but veterinary help may be required
- to bandage or not to bandage?
  - it is difficult to keep a heel dressing in place without skin and other heel bulb irritation, even to the extent of shutting off of its blood supply
  - the dressing becomes soiled and wet, and this is usually more complicating than leaving the wound exposed to the environment. Povidone antisepsis is an ideal lavage and Savlon spray, for example, will help to minimise proud flesh
  - laser treatment may be prescribed by the vet to help minimise scar formation which, if marked, is frequently re-traumatised because it protrudes

- exercise can usually continue, but preferably out of muddy conditions

If repetitive, consult a vet and/or a farrier, as there may be a deficit in stride length of a hind limb.

Shoeing Complications

This is very much 'in the hands of the farrier', who can only give a satisfactory service if allowed
- to decide the optimal interval between shoeing – adjusted, to some extent, to economically meet the mutual need to shoe as many horses in a yard at the one time as possible
- to carry out corrective trimming and/or remedial shoeing (at an acceptable but greater cost)
- the right environmental conditions
  - a dry box or yard with a non-slip floor, and so no need for bedding
  - good illumination
  - easy access to his equipment
  - a clean, dry horse especially with regard to the limbs
  - conveniently ready for him and brought to the tying up point by a helper which will minimise the farrier's 'time wasted' fees
- knowledge of the horse's immune status with regard to tetanus
- assurance that there is no active contagion in the yard and if so, facilities for the protection and washing afterwards. This applies especially to ringworm and strangles

The farrier will admit if he/she
- **pricks** a horse
- might have **nail bound** a horse

and will draw the owner's attention to evidence of
  - corns and white line disease
  - laminar and/or solar bruising and, in both situations, suggest why they have occurred and how they should be dealt with by the farrier
  - unacceptable or potentially worrying
    - changes in shoe wear
    - alterations in horn quality
    - acquired hoof conformation faults

- shearing
- collapsed heels
- bar bending
- buttress weakness

and what the farrier can do to help and/or if veterinary advice is needed.

Nail Bind
Non-Infected Trauma

A competent farrier will know when he has driven a nail too close. Prompt removal and repositioning should cause no future problem. He will however advise that particular attention be paid to a pre-work trot up for several days, to make sure that there is no inflammatory response.

Nail Prick
Infected Trauma

Basically, a nail driven wrongly by the farrier which is then a penetration of the sensitive laminae by a foreign body. The pricked horse will usually show immediate signs of the pain associated with the penetration into the quick. It will, by definition, **_not_** be near, let alone into, a vital site.

Ringbone
Degenerative

This is the colloquial name for **osteo-arthritis of the pastern joint** (high ringbone) or **coffin joint** (low ringbone), in which periosteal new bone develops on the articular edges as the result of supporting ligament overstress. The resultant tear, as with most short ligaments, usually occurs close to points of insertion and not in mid shaft. The arthritis is

- eventually chronic, with palpable and radiographically positive new bone formation
- an interference to movement
- persistently painful

The low lesion is within the hoof capsule and as such is not so common nor as productive of new bone but is more painful. The insertion of the extensor tendon onto the pyramidal process when overstressed can cause a fracture of that promontory. and an inflammatory enlargement of it, both of which are painful and lame-making and known as **Pyramidal dis-ease.**

Peripheral osteo-arthritis is associated with

- over-stress tear of the distal impar ligament from the ventral border of the navicular bone, and/or from
- strain of the insertions of the deep digital flexor tendon
- fracture of the navicular into the joint surface with displacement will lead to a chronic arthritis

Where a binding, supportive ligament which attaches **outside** the pastern bone's joint periphery occurs the resultant healing chronic new bone is known as non-arthritic ringbone. This, whilst remaining a palpable, radiographic lesion can settle to become painless. There is no interference with joint movement but it remains susceptible to further overstresses.

Sidebones
Non-Infected Trauma

This can be defined as ossification of the collateral cartilages, especially of the forefeet: a slow, chronic ossifying inflammatory response. It is not common in Thoroughbreds but is found frequently in horses with flat wide feet. Concussion from footfall on hard surfaces is the usual cause.

Base wide and base narrow stance respectively involve unilateral ossification or at least asymmetric bilateral formation. This is more likely when the unlevel footfall is acquired.

Lameness is not always present, and then usually at the start of the ossification which may begin away from the

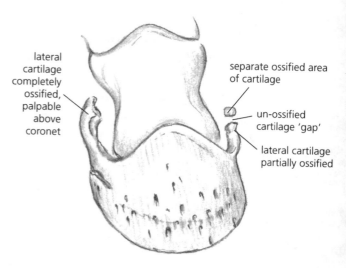

lateral cartilage completely ossified, palpable above coronet

separate ossified area of cartilage

un-ossified cartilage 'gap'

lateral cartilage partially ossified

Sidebones, as seen radiographically.

cartilages origin on the wings of the pedal bone. Eventually the side bones are palpable above the coronet or seen earlier by radiography. Massive formation may interfere with movement and there must be some interference with their functioning in the circulation of the hoof.

Pedal Osteitis
Non-Infected Trauma

Pedal osteitis remains an arguable condition. It is a sequel to tearing of the corium with the formation of fibro-osteotic chronic lesions and pressure between the bone and the hoof capsule. It can follow

- compression
- concussion

- stretch traumas associated with laminitis

resulting in osteoporosis and new bone formation, which is likely to be painful.

Wounds of the sole can penetrate into the bone to cause

- fracture of peripheral bone
- infectious osteitis with
    - abscess formation leading to a serious form of 'pus in the foot'
    - sloughing of bone
- fractures from
    - self-inflicted traumas, as from kicking a wall
    - weight bearing, at speed, on unyielding objects

PART 4

VETERINARY ASPECTS OF HORSE MANAGEMENT

FIRST AID AND WOUND MANAGEMENT

INTRODUCTION

A horsemaster's duties are usually routine. The horse is a 'beast of habit' and seems best satisfied with a steady timetable maintained by a conscientious handler.

A horse can also be unpredictable on occasions, thus adding a little excitement to the daily order. Such behaviour and, of course, the hazards of athletic employment, as well as the hazards of unemployment when 'at grass', can lead to sudden injury.

In most situations horsemastership, whether as an owner or as an employee, is the responsibility of one person. Success depends not only on the ability of that person on a day-to-day basis but also on her (in such situations it is usually female) awareness of the need, on special occasions, for

- extra help
- more skilled help and/or advice about management of injury

Horsemanship and equitation have only a passing reference in this book except that it must be appreciated that a rider's observations and opinion as to 'how the horse is going' or, more often, 'how it is no longer going as expected', are often the first clues to something being wrong with it.

Therefore, the essential day-to-day skills of the horsemaster, whether also horseman or not are

- recognition that 'all is well'
- awareness that 'all is *not* well', followed by
  - assessment
  - action

- first aid as relevant
- initial management
  - DIY management
  - professional input
    - veterinary surgeon
    - farrier
    - other
- nursing
- rehabilitation

In situations of injury and acute (suddenly clinical) disease the horsemaster must be skilled, or have access to someone who is skilled in

- first aid for the trauma
- initial management of the illness

thereafter it is a matter of decision whether she can go DIY for the

- management of the injury or for the illness

or, if professional help is called in, the subsequent management and/or nursing under supervision. Both situations involve varying degrees of nursing.

Legal Obligations under the Medicine's Act

These concern employers and employees in the UK, in equine work. Their duty is to ensure that the Medicine's Act is carried out in regard to the correct use of medicines

- for the welfare of the animal during its recovery from dis-ease or injury
- for the safety of the administrator
- for the prevention of contamination of the

environment by correct

- disposal of containers and 'giving' equipment, such as needles (sharps) and unused drugs

There are other legal requirements which are equally important

- Health and Safety at Work (HSWA)
- The Control of Substances Hazardous to Health Regulations (C of SSH Act)
- The Medicines (Restrictions on the Administration of Veterinary Medicinal Products) Regulations (no person is allowed to administer any veterinary medicinal, topical or parenteral product unless it has a **Product Licence**)
- Health and Safety Executive Veterinary Medicines: safe use by handlers
- The Reporting of Injuries, Diseases and Dangerous Occurrences Regulations (RIDDOR) – includes abnormal reactions in the patient and/or the handler
- Health and Safety (First Aid) Regulations (the care of workers injured or made ill in [equine] work)
- Disease of Animals and Approved Disinfectants Order

The private owner is not subject to all of the above. It is, however, sensible that he/she understands and applies them nonetheless.

The owner's veterinary surgeon has a responsibility in judging his client's competence in carrying out any related instructions, and certainly must carefully instruct on them as well as advising on 'safety first' requirements in the case of human contamination. An employer must satisfy the 'law' that an employee is competent – NVQ, or other exams or his own teaching – in working with them.

It is advisable that a private owner maintains a medical record for his own horses. Where other owners entrust their horse(s) to a third party and/or his employees it is essential that such information is maintained in a record book, i.e. 'what given, why, how much, when, how, and by whom'.

Categories of Veterinary Medicines

General Sales List (GSL)

Those medicines and other substances which are reputed to have a beneficial effect, without risk to the horse or to the handler, can be sold or supplied 'over the counter' by anyone from any place – for example, general purpose antiseptics and some antiparasitics (skin).

Pharmacy Merchants' List (PML)

A medicine which can be sold or supplied by

- a veterinary surgeon for *animals under his care*
- 'over the counter' by a pharmacist to anyone
- a registered agricultural merchant, only to *commercial* keepers of animals (e.g. a livery yard owner)

'Wormers' can also be sold by specifically trained farriers, saddlers, or a merchant, direct to horse owners or those having care of horses.

Pharmacy (P)

A medicine which can *only* be sold by a

- pharmacist
- veterinary surgeon for animals under his care

Prescription Only Medicine (POM)

A specific type of medicine which can only be sold or supplied by a

- veterinary surgeon
- pharmacist *on a veterinary surgeon's prescription*

Such medicines can *only* be administered by the veterinary surgeon or a horse owner/employee working under his direction and responsibility.

Controlled Drug (CD)

A medicine such as a narcotic or a habit forming drug controlled under the Misuse of Drugs Act and associated regulations. Their use on an animal is also regulated as for POM drugs.

All medicines and other chemicals must be safely stored with regard to safety (to children) and to the preservation of the drug against e.g. heat and sunlight.

Any medicine in whatever category *must* carry certain information on its package. For example, a tube of 'worm' paste must state its

- trade name and manufacturer, with an expiry date
- generic (chemical) name
- weight of active ingredient per unit of the total paste, e.g. mg/g
- what animal species it is for
- dosage rate (usually per kg body weight)
- method of administration and how frequently
- contra indications (e.g. 'do not give at the same time as drug x')

- danger, if any, to the administrator, e.g.
  - female
  - pregnant female
  - child under x years
    - by inhalation
    - ingestion
    - skin contact

and if gloves and/or mask should be worn

- preferred method of storage

The above information is usually printed in the form of a data sheet which also states that the medicine has a product licence for a particular animal species, as well as which of the categories it falls under.

When a veterinary surgeon supplies a medicine under the **Practice** label, he must attach or leave on the above information which he considers relevant for the owner/handler, *and* clearly names him/her and the animal as well as the prescribed details of administration.

The medicine *must not be given to any other animal*.

In the UK the horse is not classified as an agricultural animal, but this does *not* mean that it cannot be slaughtered for human consumption. As such, it must be certified as being **not** in receipt of certain medicines during the prescribed period known as a 'drug withdrawal time'.

This is somewhat similar (but for a considerably longer duration) to the Jockey Club rules for Non-Normal-Nutrient medication. An exact time is not known for some drugs; the onus is on the trainer.

In the case of Phenylbutazone ('Bute', to use the colloquial term), this time is quite short as far as the continuing effect on performance is concerned. However, it is considered that certain by-products of its metabolism will remain in the flesh for an unknown period. In the EU it is now a 'forbidden substance' for the treatment of *any* horse, because of the potential risk to consumers from its meat.

Temporary agreement has been reached for the UK whereby a horse can be claimed or said to be a 'sports animal' and *not* intended for slaughter. This must be certified by the owner (as from January 1998, no bute has been supplied without the veterinary surgeon receiving such a certificate). In order to permanently identify such a category, sports horses will eventually have to be 'microchipped'.

It is recommended that horse owners advise their veterinary surgeon of any **personal idiosyncrasy** they may have *vis à vis* medicines and other chemicals likely to be prescribed, e.g.

- general allergies
- skin sensitivities
- adverse response to
  - skin absorption
  - inhalation
  - ingestion

and, if female, if pregnant.

The veterinary surgeon will discuss these points as well as the general risks associated with, e.g. organophosphorus and phenol compounds, as found in disinfectants, herbicides and pesticides.

In general, any medicine to be given by mouth as a paste, a drench, or in the feed should have been prescribed, supplied, or administered by the veterinary surgeon who first diagnosed the dis-ease. The total amount supplied must be consumed by that animal. No supplies should be used for any other animal even of the same species.

A medicine for injection by whatever route – subcutaneous, intramuscular, or intravenous – must be supplied by the veterinary surgeon, or on his prescription, for a specific disorder diagnosed by him. It should be administered by that veterinary surgeon *or* by *the owner*.

Only under certain circumstances such as a training yard of horses, vouchsafed by the stables' veterinary surgeon, will such medicines be part of the stock contents of a medicine chest.

There are other exceptions

- anthelmintics to treat 'worm infestations'
- vitamin/mineral supplements
- other substances licensed for direct sale by an agricultural merchant or a pharmacist, but to commercial keepers of animals only

Many of the vast assortment of wound applications are directly available to the horsemaster. Their selection and correct use will determine their efficacy; this will relate to the trained ability of the owner, who should 'buy' with common sense or veterinary advice.

In many stables their storage and intermittent, often haphazard, use leaves much to be desired! On welfare and economic grounds it is advisable to discuss with one's veterinary surgeon, and so avoid unsuitable substances and uneconomically full shelves! Many 'skin' antibacterials inhibit healing, quite apart from others being toxic or destructive to vascular tissue. The 'crude' disinfectants should never be used on the coat and skin, let alone wounds. Hoof horn is a *possible* exception

The Protection of Animals Act can be important *vis à vis* 'home doctoring' of horses if cruelty, in its widest sense, is said to have been caused by ill-advised and/or inappropriate medication in any form.

First Aid

The initial action required for an *injured* horse, with the objective of *sustaining life* by

- careful, commonsense
  - inspection
  - assessment
  - action, which will require that the horse is caught, held (and restrained) so as to
    - facilitate the 'aid' with safety to the handler
    - prevent worsening of the injury before, during and after the 'aids' which are to *minimise*
      - **bleeding**
      - **infection**
      - **shock**
    - and, where and when practicable, by removing it to a safer place away from the risk of
      - further injury to itself, or incidentally to other animals and humans
  - help promote recovery by
    - deciding if professional help is required, and when
    - subsequent initial management

always with care for those assisting.

In the context of this book, injuries are those which arise from

- occupational hazards of work
- incidental hazards encountered in the
  - stable
  - yard
  - field
  - transit
  - road traffic accidents when led or ridden

The dramatic and often more serious incidents which are athletic, usually competition emergencies, such as

- recumbency following a fall, and the associated traumatic damage
- 'trapped' or 'ditched'
- cardio-respiratory crisis

are the responsibility of the 'on-course' veterinary team.

Similar incidents can occur in the hunting field and elsewhere, when there is not always a competent horsemaster, let alone a veterinary surgeon, on hand. For those who do come forward to help, the following points should be remembered

- winded (on immediate recovery), trapped and ditched horses will behave uncharacteristically in such frightening and/or unusual situations
  - *beware their explosive, erratic actions* (be careful of studded shoes)
    - get to the horse's head
      - if up, hold by the bridle
      - if down, sit on its head
      - await help
  - have someone attend to any bleeding
  - *do not* worry about a specific diagnosis
  - *do not* attempt to turn a fallen horse over (as a help for windedness) to further the assessment

Mistaking a winded horse for a spinal injured one can not only be wrong for the horse but also expensive for the person who gave the order!

Restraint and Protection

Injured horses usually find themselves in unusual, unaccustomed sites and situations. If lame, and so restricted in 'fight and flight', especially when trapped (as in wire), and even when not lame, the emotional disturbance can incite natural instincts of 'fright' with defensive 'fight' action. If such behavioural regression seems likely or has already begun, precautions must be taken.

Even when an injured, probably in pain, horse has been returned to its own stable there may remain a fear of confinement – 'no escape'.

From the handler's point of view it is better, where feasible, with general first aid (i.e. not emergency cases to

- inspect and act in the confines of a box (well lit) than in a yard or field – for obvious reasons

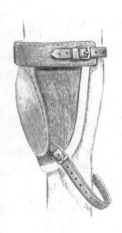

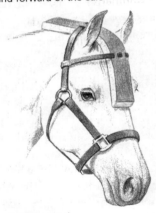

thick felt – behind, between, and forward of the ears

A knee pad.

A poll guard.

- short bedding will encourage foot-hold and will minimise other injury should the horse go down for any reason (fortunately most horses always want to stay on their feet), and wound hygiene is much easier. (Later on, long straw can be a nuisance to the lame horse as he will tend to entwine it on the lame leg)
- knee pads should be fitted where feasible
- so too, a poll guard, especially for a fractious animal
- handler and helper(s) should be dressed appropriately, particularly with regard to **head** and to **feet**

In the 'field' situation the tack, still fitted, will differ with circumstances. Whatever, the horse must have a bridle or a head collar on and, if possible, a chifney bit attached to the latter.

Assuming that the injury is associated with work and that the horse has been pulled up and dismounted (in other situations the horse may already be untacked down to a head collar) the restraint is but a matter of different detail

- have the horse held by its head
  - inspect briefly all over for obvious disorders
  - run up and secure stirrup irons – safer for the handler, and less worrying to the 'bouncy' horse
  - unbuckle the reins
  - remove from martingale rings
  - have both reins held close to the bit
  - remainder looped over same arm
- instruct handler to
  - gentle horse with other hand

- deal with bleeding: if necessary, apply further restraints (see below)
- if not bleeding badly, or bleeding is under control
  - loosen curb chain or noseband
  - remove saddle
  - cover back and quarters with a rug or a jacket
  - if feasible, remove 'leggings' and studs
- attend to other necessary first aid

The standing injured horse, by definition, will be conscious

- respiratory resuscitation will be unnecessary, but
- some horses will 'tongue swallow', especially if blowing hard. This can be alleviated, by drawing the tongue gently out from between the bars on one side
- a tendency to repetitive 'swallowing' should stop if the bridle is replaced by a halter
- walk the horse round, if not lame, to encourage it to
  - 'warm down'
  - protect against chilling as described above, and to
  - calm down (sometimes even a minor flow of blood will have so irritated the horse as to get it excited)

Further restraints are, progressively:

- offering feed or pulled grass
- grasping the fold of neck skin in front of shoulder line, or
- lifting the foreleg on the injured side, but not such as to offer the horse a different (human) prop (shown overleaf).
- encourage it to bear more weight on the other side, by pushing head and neck slightly away to that opposite side. This will facilitate lifting of the injured leg for

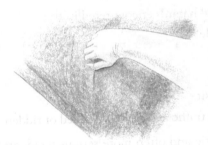

Grasping the fold of skin in front of the shoulder line.

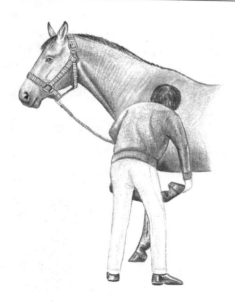

Lifting the foreleg on the injured side – but not so as to offer the horse a human prop.

then pass them to a (less experienced) helper/handler. Much better to have practised them in the course of other less urgent horse management cases, when such restraints are actually required, especially twitching, rather than try them in an emergency.

In some cases, first aid is still limited by the horse's excitement and/or temperament. Chemical restraint by the veterinary surgeon is then necessary. Meanwhile, the horse should be kept as quiet as possible, usually best obtained by offering feedstuff and *delaying* the specifically upsetting interferences.

The assessment of what is or is not 'serious' or 'freely' bleeding is based on the fact that most haemorrhaging is not life-threatening, nonetheless it is advisable to control it as soon as possible. To do so is usually more difficult, from a handling point of view, in limb injuries. Thin layers of cotton wool will invariably staunch the flow and can be reapplied repeatedly. Do not be heroic or expose helpers to stupid risks.

Transport of the Injured Horse

Any analgesia and sedation for travelling must be the responsibility of the veterinary surgeon, who will also have to certify, in cases of serious injury such as leg fracture and acute strain/sprain, or other injuries or disorders which could compromise the horse's welfare in transit, that it has been sufficiently well treated, prepared and managed for transit to a particular stable – the nearest when all circumstances have been considered. In the UK, *the driver must carry a copy of this certificate*.

inspection of the hoof. It may be necessary to reverse the loading to help restrain a leg for dressing and bandaging, if such weight bearing is not contra-indicated. Obviously, if a foreleg is injured the contra lateral one has to be lifted with due consideration for the seriousness of the wound and associated weight bearing on that leg

Ideally the handler must

- stand on the same side as the operator (unless lifting the contralateral foreleg, or if the injury is on a foreleg) *but* he must so restrain the horse that if it tries to turn, he controls it so as to turn the horse's quarters away from the operator. This is not so easy to do 'automatically' from the other side

- the free hand slowly squeezes and releases ('milks') the base of an ear, or

- if a halter is in place, the shank could be turned around the muzzle and passed through between the noseband and cheek piece where it can be engaged tightly and gently 'yanked' intermittently (the use of a chain length for this is not advised for inexperienced handlers, nor is the Indian lip gag), or

- a twitch is applied. It is better to do this 'too soon' rather than 'too late', onto an excited horse

Quite often the operator must initiate these restraints and

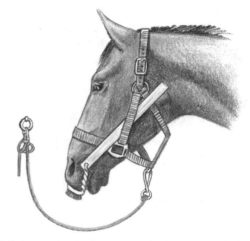

Twitch applied when restraint is required whilst, for example, bandaging (on your own). The shank can be passed through the cheek piece as shown.

The veterinary surgeon will be 'au fait' with the relevant Act, but there will be no excuse for anyone contravening it. All should read the requirements.

Preparation of the patient

- fit with head collar and rope shank, making sure that if a halter is used the shank cannot pull tight on the muzzle
- remove any shoe studs if possible
- support bandage the four limbs, including the specific dressing of the injured area if on a leg, as well as for other conditions
    - rug up over an insulating/sweat absorbing material – straw will do – especially if the patient is not yet cooled off, or if pain and/or shock is likely to produce subsequent sweating
    - fit head and limb protectors, if available, and as thought necessary
        - poll pad
        - hock point guards
        - knee pads
        - over-reach boots

Loading

- have patience! Coax with food and/or drive; **do not pull**
- use a low-load trailer, preferably with front exit
- a box with the ramp let down onto a convenient or contrived bank, or with a secure extension to give a lower incline
- sand etc. or straw should be spread on the ramp if not already fitted with anti-slip covering, and on the trailer or lorry floor if potentially slippery
- secure side-gates for guidance and restraint, or have vehicle stationed parallel with, and tight against, a wall or rails (which should be securely blocked with straw bales tied to the far side)

In Transit

A horse, as a rule, does not wish to lie down on the journey, nor does it readily give way to falling down.

In professionally, well supported limb injuries, i.e. with Robert Jones, or specific commercial boots, most will take some supporting weight with that affected leg. In first aid bandaging where the foot is left in the usual alignment, this is not so likely. Nevertheless, a three-leg stance

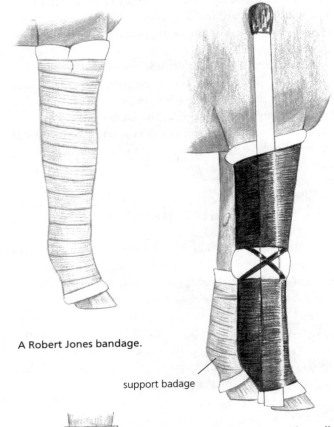

A Robert Jones bandage.

support badage

A Robert Jones, with a splint (usually applied by the vet).

A monkey boot.

by placing and mechanically restraining the hoof as shown, the column of bones from just below the 'knee' down is immobilised, especially through the fetlock, onto the platform; acute tendinitis and distal fracture cases can now weight-bear for transport

support is usually satisfactory, especially in a trailer where the partition or more usually the wall, can act as an additional support.

This partition should have a 10cm (4in) gap along the bottom and the horse should occupy the stall with the injured limb to the wall side. Thus the horse can spread its contralateral legs with the hooves into the gap to form a wider base but with the trunk still supported. A breast bar and a quick release head tie are important, the latter long enough **to allow sufficient freedom for head and neck counter-balancing**, but not to permit possible foreleg trapping.

A horse should be in the off-side compartment of a two-horse trailer. If the 'kerb' side is selected, the unused area can be counterbalanced to some extent with straw bales, the bottom one kept away from the central partition.

In a lorry, most cases will travel best when offered **total freedom** to allow them to take up their chosen position, usually diagonally with head to the rear. Leave head collar on, but unhook rope.

Make certain there are no dangerous projections or 'trappy' parts; these can be blocked off with securely lashed bales or with straw-filled sacks.

At all times, whether lorry or trailer is used, and especially on corners and particularly on roundabouts and coming out of them, **travel speed must be restricted and rapid braking or acceleration must be avoided.**

It is illegal for a person to travel in the same compartment as the animal, even on the other side of a trailer partition; better to stop and make periodic inspections.

If feed and water are necessary then offer at a stop, but leave neither with the patient.

Unloading

Again, ramps should be sanded or strawed, and the decline should be as minimal as is practicable. The landing and walk-away surfaces should also be made slip-proof especially for a seriously lame horse and/or a young and/or frightened patient.

Let the horse choose his own time, but maintain a secure rope/head collar hold. Young and/or excitable animals should be roped and handled on both sides, to restrain them from leaping off a ramp or attempting a later escape.

Recommended First Aid Kit

It is essential that there is a readily available and suitable first aid kit. There are strict legal requirements, as mentioned above, as to what drugs may be held 'just in case', even for emergency use, let alone for 'home' treatment of illnesses and injuries generally.

A suggested list of medicine chest contents is shown below. It is strongly advised that it is compiled, if not actually supplied, by your own veterinary surgeon. He will have experience of what is essential as well as how he prefers a patient to be treated with first aid before, if and when he is required professionally or not.

Key
* – obtain from your veterinary surgeon
** – ditto, but to his choice; he will advise on how and when to use

At the Stables
Hibiscrub 500ml x 2*
Pevidine scrub 500ml x 2*
Savlon spray or equivalent **
Sterile saline or isotonic fluid – 500ml in a plastic bag with nozzle x 6 *
60ml syringe (kept in sterile pack) x 6*
Cotton wool x 3 rolls
Animalintex x 10 or Kaolin paste
Intracite gel, 6 small tubs or KY Jelly 2 tubes **
Ice Tite or equivalent x 1 drum
Kool Pak or similar refrigerating material x 6
Gamgee (or equivalent synthetic) x 6 rolls (500g)
Orthobands 7cm wide x 30 *
Conforming bandages, e.g. Superflex or Vetrap (approx 10cm wide) x 20
Adhesive bandage, e.g. Equiplast (approx 10cm wide) x 10
Open weave bandages 8cm wide x 20
Medicated, non-adhesive, absorbent dressings **
Lead lotion 200 ml x 1*
Witch hazel lotion 200 ml x 1
Epsom salts 10kg (in damp-proof containers) x 2

Twitch
Thermometers x 2
Scissors
– half curved, blunt ended x 1
– straight, blunt ended x 1
J cloths or similar x 2 packs
Clean towel (wrapped)
Metal bowl 20cm diameter
Clean bucket, preferably stainless steel or enamel, kept for this use only
Disposable gloves x 2 packs
French chalk
Stable bandages
Hoof pick, simple shoe-removal kit including clench closer

In the Lorry
To be carried with, e.g. two horses competing in hunter trials, show jumping or endurance riding – in the 'team' vehicle

Pevidine scrub or Hibiscrub 500ml x 1

Sterile saline 500ml x 1

Plastic syringe 60 ml x 1

Cotton wool x 1 roll

Animalintex x 1 roll

Icebandages or packs, Ice-Tite or equivalent x 2

Gamgee x 1 roll

Orthobands x 10

Conforming bandages x 6

Adhesive bandages x 4

Leg bandages

Medicated dressings 10cm x 10cm x 5

Lead lotion or witch hazel 300ml x 1

Twitch x 1

Thermometer x 1

Scissors – half curved, blunt ended x 1

'J' cloths x 1 box

Metal bowl 20cm diameter

Clean bucket

Disposable gloves x 1 pack

Hoof pick, pincers and shoe-nail extractor

Clench closer

In a Hunt Coat or Endurance Pouch

Wrapped open weave bandages 10cm x 2

Hoof pick

Uses and Application

Cleansing

By definition, antiseptics are **disinfectants** which are 'kind', with limited toxicity, to living exposed tissue cells. Not all meet this criterion. Two which are acceptable, *if used correctly*, are Hibiscrub (Chlorhexidine) and Pevidine scrub (Povidone iodine). (Used at half strength, on wetted hands and arms, they act as efficient skin cleansers (non-irritant to most people) before touching a wound, instruments and dressings.)

- first, gross contamination should be hosed off – with a clean cloth held over the wound itself

- then wash hands in antiseptic scrub, and dry them on a clean paper towel

- put on disposable gloves

  - this is particularly essential under field conditions – even at the stables, and *especially* with wounds into areas of *tendons*, *joints* and *deep muscle*, it is advisable always to *wear disposable gloves*. To facilitate gloving-up, 'dried' hands can be powdered with French chalk

- the dilutions recommended are

  - Hibiscrub – 1:40

  - Pevidine – 1:7.5

  but both *must be kept out of the wound*, especially if it could involve a tendon, tendon sheath, or joint, or a penetrating flesh wound, and are used only to clean *around* the wound

- deep wounds should be lavaged with **cleansing fluid**, such as

  - isotonic 500ml – or home-made: 1 heaped teaspoon salt dissolved in 500ml (1 pint) of boiled, cooled water

  - normal saline sterile pack

  - Ringers or Hartman's solution

Other Cleansing Materials

Syringe 60ml *

Cotton wool (hospital quality) – used in the form of pledgets for applying liquids to a wound and subsequent wiping – once used, discard

'J' cloths or equivalent, or paper towels – general purpose domestic wipers

Savlon spray is a quick drying spray-on antiseptic for surface wounds and abrasions and in some cases for 'proud' flesh control

Dressings

Animalintex or Kaolin paste – a poultice mainly used hot to encourage the flow of blood to the area

- of a contaminated wound (under vet instruction)

- of a semi-closed wound to encourage more serum exudation with white blood cell extravasation, thus assisting cleansing and drainage

- to 'ripen' an abscess, especially in a hoof

- to encourage the flow of blood into a strained or sprained area, to increase vascular and lymph flow as well as increasing scavenging macrophage concentration

When used cold and dry the Animalintex, appropriately cut, makes a very efficient first aid wound covering under bandaging.

Intracite gel or KY jelly – these are lubricating, 'blocking' materials. The former may be used by the veterinary surgeon for subsequent treatment as a carrier or vehicle for specific antibiotics and chemo-therapeutic dressings. To the first aider their application quickly onto or into a wound will prevent secondary contamination whilst hair is removed and the area is being cleaned up.

They are easily lavaged or sponged out to permit deeper cleansing. Scissor-clipped hair is bound to fall into the adjacent wound. Getting it out is difficult, unless the wound is prepacked with gel or jelly.

Ice Tite – a post-exercise skin tensing application to minimise subsequent oedema. It also, through evaporation, acts as a low grade cooler.

Kool Pak or equivalent bandages – a handy means of applying cold. Some are re-coolable, others are 'once only'. Some require a gauze bandage under them to prevent skin 'burn' (read the instructions). Most will only give 15 minutes' worth of cooling.

Medicated, non adhesive dressings – assorted sizes

Gamgee – an essential pressure absorber between skin and plain bandage.

Orthobands – an expeditious way of bandaging-on a built-in pressure absorbing material over a dressing or a strained area in a controlled and evenly distributed fashion. (Somewhat more expensive than gamgee and bandages but, in first aid at least, a better choice.)

Conforming bandages, e.g. Superflex or Vetrap – non-adhesive, but good ones are cohesive/one turn on another. They wrap easily around the curves of the joints and hoof and can allow for the necessary pressure gap where necessary, as over the back of the knee (the accessory carpal bone) and the point of the hock.

Adhesive bandage, e.g. Equiplast – this sticks as it turns on the previous turn. (A good point to look for is ease of removal, rather than the need to be cut off, especially from a fractious horse.) As a fixer of dressings and conforming bandages, they need only be used at the extremities of the underlying materials, such as the conforming bandage. They can be used to exert further, but controlled, pressure as in the case of strains and sprains. In most situations a top stable bandage is used for added protection and to maintain cleanliness.

Open-weave bandages (wrapped).

Lead lotion – an astringent and cooling lotion. Can be applied liberally from saturated cotton wool for galls, mild strains and sprains, stings and nettle rash.

Witch hazel – as for lead lotion

Epsom salts (kept dry) – As a saturated solution, approximately 1kg (2lb) in 1l (2pt) boiling water in a black 'rubber' bucket, for 'foot' tubbing. Check water temperature on own elbow or back of hand before immersing the hoof. Liquid usually about 5cm (2in) deep should cover coronet and heels. Immerse for 10 minutes. The same strength solution, but cooler, can be used for lavaging open, contaminated wounds.

The salt, mixed into a thin paste with glycerine, makes an efficient cold poultice for hoof wounds, e.g. septic corn or subacute small areas of cellulitis.

First Aid Treatment for Occupational Hazards in Athletic Situations

Fractures

If suspected, *a veterinary surgeon must be consulted immediately*. Many minor splits in limb bone extremities and in the distal phalanges' shafts are not always immediately suspected or distinguishable from joint, and in the case of the fetlock, suspensory ligament strain trauma. However, their presence is not quite so threatening during the first few days provided the horse, because of its lameness and other signs of sterile trauma, has been boxed and veterinary advice sought.

Fracture surgery in such cases is rarely done during the first 4 days. Interpretation of radiographs is better when the initial swelling has subsided.

Fractures can follow closed sterile and open external traumas (blows), as well as torque and shear forces induced by third degree accelerations – internal overstress. Suspected shaft and joint extremity fractures, *especially in the proximal abaxial bones* are more serious and justify *immediate professional opinion*.

Other Acute Strains

The aim is to minimise swelling by hastening the clotting of the small blood vessels, usually by cold hosing at 1 to 2 hour intervals on day one, until veterinary help arrives or for the first 24 hours with an overnight break of 6 hours. Cooling pastes can be used overnight.

The need for veterinary help will vary with experience but it must always be remembered that a blow, especially from a kick or from strong contact with a fixed object onto an area free of muscle protection, e.g.

• inside the forearm

- inside the gaskin
- front of the cannon
- top of the cannon on the side, at head of splint bone

may cause a star crack in the bone. This remains susceptible to further jarring through ground support forces for up to 4 weeks, during which time a full fracture may be produced by inadvisable concussion on a hard surface.

In the absence of a fracture, the 'blow' trauma is treated as for a bruise, which is the associated pathology.

- where practicable, pressure bandaging is helpful
- if over a muscle area, beware subsequent haematoma

Haematoma

A **blood clot** will develop subcutaneously within 30–90 minutes following external trauma where there is limited or no muscle tissue to absorb the blow but where a small artery or vein has been ruptured, e.g. on the front of the knee.

Treatment

- box rest horse
- cold hose for 15 minutes every hour, for 4–5 hours
- pressure bandage where practicable, after each hosing

If swelling worsens, or if it doesn't begin to resolve in 3–4 days, **get veterinary help**.

When resolution begins, gradually re-start slow walking – 'hand graze'. If lameness is present, **seek professional help**.

When a big muscle group has been kicked or otherwise traumatised, box rest and begin cold hosing as above. The intramuscular bleeding will take several days to work to the surface to collect as a variably large, pendulous swelling

- **stop walking**
- seek profesional help

It is unlikely that haematomas will be lanced unless secondary infection is suspected. They will be re-absorbed over several weeks. A decision as to work will depend upon veterinary opinion. Cold hosing will continue twice daily for 15 minutes each time, for about 7 days. Any related skin wound should be treated as seems appropriate; the lesion, if any, is often above where the haematoma develops. The cold application is better kept away from the bruised skin.

OPEN WOUNDS

The injurious objects most likely to cause open wounds are

In the stable

- loose shoe nails – turned out clenches
- dropped shoe nail and other sharp pointed objects in bedding, e.g. plaiting needle, scissors, open knife 'lost' in the bedding
- wall foundation bolts
- door bolts
- splintered wood
- jagged and sheet metal
  - in walls etc
  - in feeding and watering 'furniture'

In the yard

- as for stables. plus
- implements (fork, rake etc.)
- other tools
- wire – loose
- gate bolts
- broken drain covers, and other hoof-trapping gulleys
- projecting metals from walls and rails
- glass
- trailing hose pipe and electric wires, which could ensnare and bring a horse down or cause evasive action

In the field

- wire fencing – whatever type should always be tense, **no barbed wire low down**, no broken ends or loose loops especially on the ground. If using mesh use pig rather than sheep with the smallest mesh, at ground level – which a pawing hoof will not get through or be caught on withdrawal
  - between heels and shoe
  - above the bulb of the heels, at the back of the pastern
  Note: **do not** leave feed stuffs on the far side of a fence, or feed just over a fence to other horses – the hungry horse will paw at the fence
- gates – the diagonal strap usually forms a 45° angle with the horizontal. Try to avoid this, but if unavoidable make sure horizontals at least are tubular and not

straight edged

- post and rails – rails must be watched for breakage, splintered ends and proud nails. Electric tape to prevent gnawing or crib-biting should be fixed just below the top edge of the top rail and should not be loose. Insulate near gates. When coming through a gate, have the bolt drawn back and secured; always lead horses through one by one and turn head back to the gate before releasing

- miscellaneous metal

- troughs – should have rounded edges, no gaps between the tank and a wall or an upright post that could trap a leg; there is no excuse for errors of omission over repairs

- stones, flints etc.

- kicks from other horses, especially if shod; there is no excuse for turning out two or more horses, shod behind – even friends

- state of the surface
  - wet, slippery and muddy
  - hard, dry

Cross-country

- stone walls
- fixed fences (closed bruising)
- kicks
- thorns
- spread shoes and loose nails
- interferences
- being struck into

Woodland

- stubs
- stakes
- wire
- machinery remnants

Roads

- slips – onto side (abrasions and bruises, but lacerations are possible)
- stumble – onto knees to cause 'broken knees'
- hit by a vehicle – RTA (road traffic accident)

Such contacts **will also cause varying depths of bruising,**

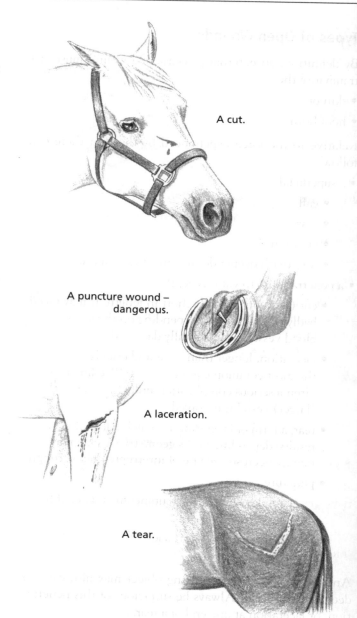

A cut.

A puncture wound – dangerous.

A laceration.

A tear.

as well as the varying types and depths of open wounds.

The foot (hoof) is most likely to be injured
- on the sole
- through the sole (and frog)
  - possibly into vital areas
- on the coronet
- on the heels
- by deep laceration of the hoof wall

and the pastern on the plantar aspect again including the vital parts of that area

Types of Open Wounds

By definition, an externally occasioned wound must first traumatise the

- skin or
- hoof horn

Relative to the force experienced by the skin there can follow

- a superficial
    - gall
    - graze
    - abrasion
    - sore (with deeper dermal bruising, as a rule)
- a penetration – to various depths
    - cut (incision), usually short in length. It may bleed badly or hardly at all depending on the size of the blood vessel coincidentally damaged
    - laceration, longer than a cut and usually jagged; the most common equine wound. Bleeding is not often a serious complication unless a superficial (larger) vessel is involved
    - tear, a form of laceration in which a flap of skin results; depending on its geometry the flap may rapidly necrose because of interrupted blood supply
    - puncture
        - simple, skin into subcutaneum and possibly into a vital area
        - deeper, into other tissues

An initial lacerating or cutting object may also cause a deeper penetration. Always be suspicious of this penetration, or laceration at one end of a tear.

All penetrating wounds will have **bleeding** to a greater or lesser extent, and will be accompanied by a varying amount of surrounding bruising, which tissue can be eventually infected by direct spread from the primary point of contamination.

Remember

- the initial **bruise** is a swelling due to the
    - escape of blood
        - the exudation of serum from the eventual clot
    - escape of serum from the traumatised tissue cells and intercellular fluid

- the secondary **swelling** is inflammatory (self defence) in nature, from the effusion of plasma from nearby undamaged small blood vessels

This reaction is produced by chemical 'mediators' which 'escape' from damaged cells, or are synthesised and released from blood and other healthy cells in response to the presence of such mediators. They induce

- **oedema**, attracting white blood cells
- and stimulate nociceptors, causing
    - pain

but these bioactive compounds are also eventually benefiting regulators of inflammation.

A penetrating wound can be

- open, and exposed to the air
- contused, partly closed and therefore variably exposed to air
- closed, the edges do not gape and the subcutaneous swelling further blocks off the deeper damaged tissues, or the keratinised epidermis (as in the hoof wall) does not tear or gape under tension

The 'successful' contaminating infection varies respectively from aerobic to semi or micro-aerobic and anaerobic. The associated germs are usually 'gram negative' (i.e. not susceptible to penicillin) in the last two situations.

All wounds, except

- bruises
- galls

will be contaminated by hair, dirt, etc. and so will be infected. If the horse continues to be moved, especially in the faster gaits after its skin has been penetrated, there is the likelihood of **suction aspiration** as the skin glides to and fro over the penetrated site, drawing in

- air, to cause subcutaneous emphysema
- germs, to cause subcutaneous infection

both of which, especially the air, can be further distributed well away from the entry site

- air can, for example, reach from a distal limb wound to the neck, shoulders and chest. Surprisingly, this is rarely contaminated and is as a rule slowly absorbed without complications
- germs will travel to the anular ligament area of the next joint, continuing the cellulitis – an under-

skin 'mud fever' type of inflammation
- the infection (whether aspirated or simply implanted) can go further to produce
  - lymphangitis
  - septicaemia
  - toxaemia

Contamination of the exposed dermis will produce a dermatitis. If taken under the dermis but 'kept' local, there develops the classical **septic wound** with, in a closed type, the possibility of **abscess** formation. This is a common sequel in, for example, the penetrated hoof.

Wounds can be in multiple positions. Open and closed traumas are likely in RTAs and jump entanglements.

Bleeding (Haemorrhaging)

- closed – subcutaneous or deeper
  - hidden – as so-called 'internal bleeding' (into a body cavity)
- open or external
  - through a natural orifice (not a first aid matter)
  - through a skin deficit
    - major, as from large vessels when it is
      - rapid
      - profuse with
        - quick loss of consciousness
        - death
    - less than major – **a first aid matter**

Action
Do not worry as to arterial or venous

- elbow and stifle, where there is no practicable way in which to bandage – use a hand held pressure pad
- over a muscled area with a shallow wound – use a hand held pressure pad, or for example on the neck use a pad bandaged on (but not so tight as to throttle!)
- in muscled areas with a gaping, deep wound – pack the hole with clean towelling

Where the bleeding is within an area which lends itself to bandaging, as in the limbs below the elbow and the stifle, the pad can be held in place by a simple bandage. This need not be so tight as to act as the more dangerous tourniquet. It is particularly required when the

- knee is opened or 'broken' anteriorly, with bleeding
- digital vein at the fetlock is punctured
- coronet and/or the heels are lacerated

Bleeding from such less-than-major vessels will often stop as the blood pressure drops, from

- reduction in excitement and/or fear
- cessation of movement and, in some cases, from a
- systemic fall in blood pressure from loss of blood

The lower pressures so induced slow the rate of flow and eventually allow a clot not only to form but to **stay put**, thus blocking the damaged vessel(s). It may take some

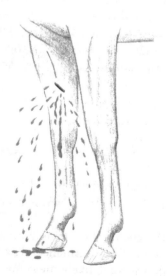

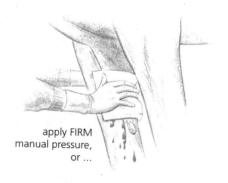

apply FIRM manual pressure, or ...

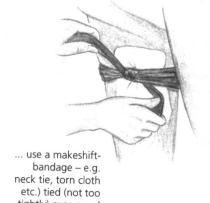

... use a makeshift-bandage – e.g. neck tie, torn cloth etc.) tied (not too tightly) over a pad

Immediate first aid to stop bleeding.

time and several pads or packs – *persevere until professional help arrives, if necessary.*

Bleeding is not only unpleasant to see but it also weakens the horse and so

- delays recovery
- reduces immune and other defensive powers

and therefore justifies expedient first aid control.

The wound can be treated to stop bleeding with no real need for concern for infection *in the first instance,* as in the hunting field or other extended cross-country events

- uncover one 10cm (4in) bandage, and apply it, still rolled, along the wound as a pad
- unwrap the second, and wind it quite tightly around the limb, over the pad
- some 25cm (10in) from the end, tear it down the middle
- 'half hitch' the two half widths
- use these to tie on the bandage
- if necessary, i.e. still oozing blood after 15 minutes, undo the first knot, but leave on, apply more pressure around the original dressings by means of a neck tie, stocking, torn cloth etc.

The 'Vital Sites'

In the 'unit of locomotion' the essential features *vis à vis* injuries are the

- joint capsule or synovium
- tendon sheath
- bursa

These are closed sacs containing synovial fluid which is secreted by the synovial sheath. This is basically avascular on its secretory inner surface.

Infection into such a cavity develops rapidly to produce *quasi* pus in the immediate absence of vascular tissue. Its secondary effect is to inflame the lining, and only when that has developed does a defensive action, inflammation, against the germs get into action via the exuding serum and white blood cells, with true pus formation.

By this time a septic synovitis has arisen, and the prognosis worsens by the hour – to involve cartilage and ligaments or associated tendons. Adhesions are then likely complications.

It is vital that, if a wound is suspected of having penetrated such a 'closed' area, the surface area (be it hoof sole or limb skin) is

- hosed or sponged clean, or
- antiseptically wiped clean if there is no running water, clean water or sterile lavage (see below)
- the area should be approached in such a manner that the water or the wipe always cleans *away from the entry point,* which should be *the last area to be cleaned off. Beware surface water running back over the opening*
- there is usually no requirement for bleeding control as the original laceration is usually small unless it is part of a more widespread tear involving a vein or an artery – treat the bleeding first
- the wound is covered by a clean, not necessarily sterile pad or cloth (as for a bleeding wound experienced cross-country). This is bandaged on over a pad of gamgee or orthoband, especially over a hoof solar wound
- *do not* try to plug or even dress the wound with *powder* or *ointment*
- transport is brought to the horse, or as close as possible
- the horse is taken to a pre-warned veterinary surgeon
- the veterinary surgeon will confirm (or refute) synovial penetration
- if 'yes', he will begin specialised lavage

This will vary incident to incident, but the basic aim is to flush out any contamination from the joint or sheath cavity before introducing a suitable antibiotic into it. It may require a general anaesthetic, and will almost certainly have to be repeated several times. Parenteral antibiotics will not get to the synovial sac until there is an active synovial hyperaemic inflammation, by which time often intractable damage may have developed as already mentioned. Supportive parenteral antibiotic therapy is, of course, necessary to back up the primary topical medication.

The fact that any wound, vital or otherwise, is or has been bleeding implies that some at least of the contaminating dirt, mud and dust which was inoculated by the damaging object will have been washed out. Nevertheless, all wounds should be seen as contaminated even if only from the germs 'innocently' living in the hair, and which is now turned into the wound. Here these germs become pathogenic.

The dirtier the wound the greater the contamination in terms of numbers, and eventually in virulence. The less open to the air, to its depth, the more likely the germs will proliferate, especially the anaerobes, until treatment is given.

As a rule of thumb, if first aid and especially appropriate veterinary antibiotic cover is effected within 3 hours, most infections can be kept under control. Vital sites require surgical lavage as well.

It is such quick attention which also augurs well for suturing wounds in other areas which can be safely closed either at the time or in 7 to 10 days after the acute inflammation has settled (i.e. the germs have been eliminated).

Cleaning and Dressing a Wound

It is not at all essential for a first aider to know, let alone try to find out, exactly what subcutaneous tissues have been traumatised *except* for

- being aware of the proximity and *possible* penetration of the anatomical sites of 'vital' importance
- it is important to have at least suspected if a wound may have entered a ligament, a tendon, or a tendon sheath, through a skin opening; the handler must not be tempted to be over-liberal with antiseptics and their concentration above the prescribed limits in such situations. Safer to use Hibiscrub (Chlorhexidine) as Povidone (as in Pevidine scrub) can be irritant to lacerated tendon and tendon sheath

As well as the synovium, tendons could be damaged by the wrong chemicals and the wrong strengths of correct ones;

The three areas of a wound site.

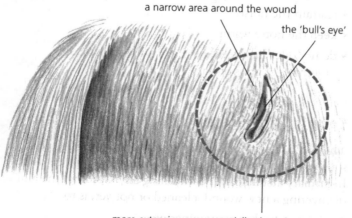

a narrow area around the wound

the 'bull's eye'

more extensive area, especially above but also below, from which 'fall out' or 'drip' can occur

so too with deep muscle wounds, where either chemical is acceptable at correct dilutions.

It is also essential to consider that what caused the wound might still be present, e.g.

- a flint partly embedded in the sole
- a piece of wire or a part of a nail
- a piece of wood projecting from the skin; all are obvious (if carefully looked for after thorough skin or hoof cleansing. Unless the handler is confident that he can retrieve all of it, it is better to pack the area so that the hoof, in particular, is protected against the object being pushed further in. Long bits of wood or wire can be cut short closer to the surface
- there still remains the possibility of **buried** material. *It is not advisable to go 'fishing'.* Simply treat and dress the wound as an external problem, and act accordingly – *but seek veterinary help*

Technique

In all limb wounds especially and, to a lesser extent, in those of the head, neck and trunk, particularly on the lower abdomen, it must be presumed that the skin and hair surrounding the wound is contaminated, not only by commensal skin bacteria but by soil saprophytes. Both, once they invade a wound, are potential pathogens.

The site should be seen as in three radii

- the wound, the 'bull's eye'
- a narrow, 5–8cm (2–3in) area around the wound
- a more extensive area, especially above but also below the wound, from which 'fall out' or 'drip' contamination can subsequently occur

Where mud is present cleansing becomes more difficult. In all cases scrub your own hands, rinse and dry. If the wound is suspiciously serious put on gloves.

Step 1   Assess the wound: with a pledget of cotton wool soaked in saline or water gently, pledget by pledget, expose the wound. Remove any gross contamination by further pledgets. **Do not rub in, wipe sideways and outwards.** Dab dry

Step 2   Introduce KY jelly or Intracite gel into the raw surface and under any over hanging flap

Step 3   Where possible, lightly bandage-on a dry pledget;

if this is not possible hold one in place as a protective, temporary cover

Step 4 A helper now cold hoses and/or scrapes off wetted leg from some 15cm (6in) above the level of the wound, down 15cm (6in) all round, until patently clean

Step 5 Shampoo on a half-strength solution of one or other recommended antiseptic, to work up a good cleansing lather on this area

Step 6 Rinse off and dry; use a hair-drier if coat is dense

Step 7 Clip hair off an area some 5–8cm (2–3in) around the wound

Step 8 Put on new gloves. Remove bandage (if one is used) and pledget

Step 9 Attempt to cut hair lashes off edges of wound, especially those now lying on wound opening. Cut, wipe scissors and clean repeatedly. Trim close over a 1cm (1/4–1/2in) around the wound

Step 10 Hose out the gel or jelly, then shampoo originally covered area with appropriate solution of antiseptic

Step 11 With appropriately *diluted* antiseptic-soaked pledgets of wool, one by discarded one, wipe gel or jelly out of the wound along with trapped cut hairs and other debris

Step 12 With further pledgets, cleanse the exposed wound, then the surrounding area for some 2–5cm (1–2in), with the wound covered by a hand held pledget this time

Step 13 If the wound is *shallow* and the base is apparent, pour in a little of the diluted antiseptic

If the wound is **deep** and its recesses not clearly delineated, load the 60ml syringe and squirt the antiseptic into the wound at all angles until all loose dirt and hair seems to have been flushed out. *Do not* try to penetrate deeper layers of tissue, and *do not probe* for holes in it
  • an initial lavaging with one or other

isotonic fluid can be used first but not after the antiseptic which should remain as a veneer

Step 14 *Do not* apply powder or ointments

Step 15 Dry off surrounding skin

Step 16 Cover and bandage if practicable

With deep open wounds

• *unless within a vital area*, lavage with normal saline (or Hartmans solution), direct or via the 60ml syringe until obviously clean

• squirt in a final dilute antiseptic solution via a syringe (the nozzle of this syringe need not touch the wound, and so can be re-used to re-fill out of the bulk antiseptic)

• with puncture wounds, whether over a vital area, or not
  • clean up the area as advised above
  • if sure it is clear of such a vital area lavage as above
  • swab or apply one or other antiseptic as above
  • cover and bandage

It is essential to get veterinary help with such a wound.

In the case of deep stake wounds into thick muscle areas or even suspected into a body cavity, the object is best left where it is but carefully reduced in length to leave some 15cm (6in) clear of the wound at both ends if completely penetrating through and through. If only one end is visible, reduce that end, otherwise, no heroics

• *send for veterinary surgeon immediately*

• restrain the horse

• keep the horse warm

• do not offer hard feed, but calm with occasional mouthfuls of grass or hay

Covering and Dressing Wounds

The kit list suggests that veterinary advice should be sought as to the appropriate material dressing to be used. In primary first aid, after controlling any bleeding, the aim of covering a new wound, cleaned or not yet, is to

• minimise further contamination

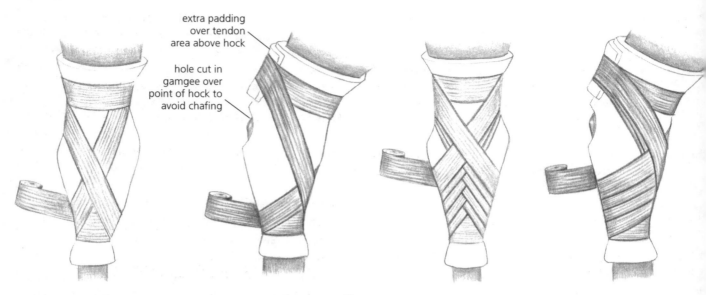

extra padding
over tendon
area above hock

hole cut in
gamgee over
point of hock to
avoid chafing

The stages of bandaging a hock.

- secure against abrasion
- continue haemostasis

There is only one consideration, therefore, for a simple covering, and that is *it should not stick to the raw surfaces* when the dressing is removed for veterinary attention.

Cold, dry Animalintex fits this requirement, and with the holding bandages, meets the other primary aim. A piece big enough to cover the wound by 5cm (2in) around the periphery is sufficient.

The more sophisticated, interactive, two or three layer wound coverings are used at progressive stages of the inflammation and ultimate healing. They are best prescribed by your veterinary surgeon. As a basic design they should have the ability to

- absorb excessive discharges, yet
- allow gaseous exchange
- keep the area warm and at high humidity, especially when granulation has begun

The type may be changed to suit the wound's progress. Replacement intervals are judged by the veterinary surgeon case by case and by state and stage of the healing

Bandaging

The aim is to

- give support to the damaged structures
- limit the movement over the wound itself

- give warmth
- prevent soiling and wetting of the wound and surrounding skin

Areas on the horse which lend themselves to simple bandaging, as distinct from

- Robert Jones support bandages
- casts, or
- strong, adhesive bandages which hold to the skin beyond the under-dressing

are mainly to the limbs from

- above the 'knee', down
- above the hock, down

There are now useful self-adhesive patches on the market for simple cuts on the head, neck and the limbs generally, but even such injuries necessitate

- keeping the horse away from mud and dirt, which could contaminate through even the best of dressings
- protective padding, if contact is likely with
    - other limbs
    - other objects

When the knee or the hock has to be bandaged there are several points to be observed

- support without complete immobilisation

- plan bandaging, to give
  - security, yet
  - allow some 'play', especially over the joint proper
  - *minimum pressure* over any bony promontory, such as
    - knee, at the back
    - over the point of the hock
    - here too, the Achilles tendon area must receive extra padding

In all but those simple wounds mentioned above, between the skin wound and the primary bandaging there must be a sufficient layer of pressure absorbing material, e.g.

- gamgee
- combined bandage and wool (orthobandage)

which serves to

- prevent undue pressure on the
  - wound, which could reduce circulation to and from the area including the regenerating skin edges
  - blood supply to the area and distal to it, and particularly proximal to it, to interfere with the venous return, the flow away from the wound
- allow sufficient tension on the bandaging to maintain position

In surgical bandaging of limb wounds, as distinct from stable bandaging, *the first turns must begin below the wound*, so that subsequent turns massage oedematous fluid up and away from the dependent areas and the wound. They should begin at the coronet and, unless necessary, stop just below the 'knee' or hock, and then return down to the coronet.

With conforming bandages the last two or three turns (each turn should cover two-thirds of the previous one) must be of less tension than the rest at the top, and to a lesser extent at the bottom, of the limb. The maximum tension should be set to the instructions on the wrapper or from the veterinary surgeon.

The top bandage, usually an adhesive type, is best used to retain the cohesive at the top and bottom and need not cover the whole area of the bandaged limb, especially if the dressings have to be changed at short intervals – ease of removal, economy of use! A stable bandage on top is advisable, *as is a support bandage on the contralateral leg*. All three limbs should be bandaged for warmth, in winter, and to minimise dependent filling.

It will be appreciated that the initial first aid bandage need not be more than a security for the wound cover. A leg bandage and a stable bandage over the gamgee, therefore, will be sufficient until the veterinary surgeon arrives that day, subject to the requirements of any special injury mentioned earlier.

At subsequent dressings of longer in between intervals when orthobandage or gamgee is used, the first conforming bandage can be dispensed with and the adhesive used over the whole area. Such dressings must be checked twice daily for slippage or, conversely. evidence of then becoming too tight.

It is good training to practise these bandaging techniques before necessity arises.

The Natural Progress of a Wound

A full thickness injury into the subcutaneous tissue or deeper.

Phase 1 – the inflammatory response

- formation of a clot
  - in the torn blood vessels – to stop bleeding
  - in the wound cavity and in surrounding traumatised (bruised) tissues from which arises primary pain
- this clot slowly contracts, and squeezes out
  - serum
- intact local arteriolar blood supply is temporarily reduced through reflex spasm of the vessel wall – the area feels colder
- a subsequent dilation follows, and the area feels warmer
  - a plasma-like fluid leaks from the capillaries and arterioles, and mixes with the serum to form further clotting which entraps bacterial contaminants and necrotised tissue cells

There is a variable degree of swelling in the tissues augmented by the production of **oedema**. The sero-fibrinous fluid exudes from the wound as a **discharge**.

Phase 2 – self-debridement, or cleaning out

- **white blood cells** are extravasated into the area, for
  - ingestion of bacteria
  - immune responses
- macrophages are extravasated, for further
  - ingestion of bacteria, dead white cells, tissue cell

debris, and to

- stimulate the attraction of fibroblasts into the clotted area
- release of **enzymes** and **other chemicals** which increase the inflammatory response
  - more blood to the area, with greater
    - swelling
    - heat
    - oedema
  - production of noxious stimuli
    - secondary pain

This phase usually begins at 6 hours plus after injury and continues for a variable time relative to wound size, bruising and infection. During this phase there is a period of bacterial multiplication, again relative to the degree of bruising and other trauma, but also to the presence of embedded foreign body (FB) or sloughed tissues too big for cellular digestion (hair lying in, or having fallen in after clipping, acts as a FB)

- the discharge may become purulent
- a peripheral, variably extensive cellulitis is likely, with
- subsequent increased vascularly
  - increased local heat
  - fuller pulse, distended (arteries and arterioles) veins
  - fever

The healing of a wound.

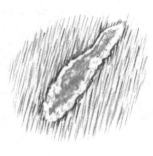

in-filled with blood and granulation tissue – but not above the edge of the wound; this contains new nerve endings and so is sensitive

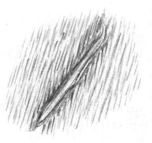

the skin then heals, growing horizontally over the filled wound; the edges meet and unite – this is called epithelialisation

An unhealed wound.

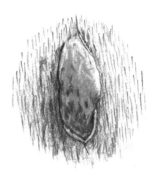

granulation tissue 'pushed out' to become proud flesh which is readily infected; it is relatively insensitive

- illness

all of which first aid and early management aims to prevent or at least minimise.

Phase 3 – repair

- myofibroblasts contract the skin surface of the wound
  - difficult in muscle-free areas – no compressible tissue to 'give' freedom to do so
  - impossible in hoof wall and sole
- **fibroblasts** proliferate in the subcutaneous area
  - **new capillaries** bud out in this
  - **granulation tissue** begins to form in the newly vascular residual clot
- the epithelium begins to grow in from the periphery, but it can be halted by the presence of
  - continuing discharge
  - an excess of granulation tissue which rises 'proud' of the new skin edges

Phase 4 – maturation

- the granulation tissue progresses to **fibrous tissue**
  - this fibrous (**collagen**) matrix mimics the basic material of the tissue(s) damaged – thus bone has bone cells which produce a soft then a hard callous, whereas tendon remains a 'soft' material. Here the collagen is often not 'as good' as the original
    - specific tissues are organised as near as possible to their ultimate functional requirements. Some, such as tendons, take months to do so
    - the epidermis closes the gap on the surface, sometimes not completely, so an undefined fibrous scar is left; occasionally, disorganised

granulation tissue (**proud flesh**) protrudes to form a raised hard irregular scar. The eventual pressure from this, especially in the pastern area, can cause lameness from the unyielding mass on deeper nerve endings

xuberant, infected granulation tissue *predisposes* to arcoid and other fibroblastic types of tumours, especially n limb wounds. It is essential to cooperate closely with the eterinary surgeon in minimising this proud flesh formaion. It is not easy, but he will advise, especially with egard to topical applications (especially those which nould *not* be used).

Vounds over the surface of a joint are more prone to roud' flesh formation

- no muscle to absorb pressure

- constant movement – unless immobilisation has been obtained

    - this stimulates *excess* granulation, and reduces epithelialisation closure

upplementary Observations on Wound Recovery

\s has been discussed in conjunction with disease in eneral and traumatic inflammation in particular, man and nimals have an inherent response capability which aims o preserve life, at least to the extent that the injured nimal will

- survive

- be mobile

- with sufficiently effective body systems be capable of reproducing the species

n some nomadic species, e.g. the horse, which depended ery much on the *flight* factor in survival (the precursor of he athletic animal) nature's purpose was not necessarily o completely restore such potential *maximal* ability, but ssentially to enable the recovering animal 'to keep up vith the herd'. Any resultant impediment to flight suffiient to prevent 'safety in numbers' exposed that animal to redators, and so to the 'law of the jungle' and the 'survival f the fittest'.

In domestication, such a partly recovered animal, if therwise suitable, could be retained and cared for as a

- companion for humans and as a 'nanny' for equine young stock

- brood animal, or perhaps an

- athlete at a lower level

    - all subject to welfare considerations

Acute illness and injury first aid and initial management aim to increase the chances of a surviving animal making a return to usefulness *beyond what nature herself could do*. It is an obligation of domestication and man's dominion over his animals.

If properly applied, they will further assist the natural responses by reducing the 'time lag' before repair and ultimate maturation of the healing tissues begins, primarily by speeding up

- control of bleeding, and related swelling and oedema

- cleansing (debridement) of the contaminated wound of both necrotic tissue and of infection

and by providing protection for the

- establishment and stability of the granulation tissue which will be the basis for new tissue

New tissue, however, has specific maturation times, as has been said:

- **connective tissue** and skin is relatively fast – a matter of weeks

- **bone** takes much longer to reach stability against normal stresses, and

- **tendon** even longer, measured in months

Such tissue-specific durations are more or less always the same when timed from the *start of repair* and not from the date of injury. Although the improvement in the initial 'lag' times can be effected, the difference, when seen particularly against bone and tendon repair times, is ultimately relatively little. It is thought, however, that good management including subsequent conditioning of connective tissue and the essential stresses and fittening, can make a significant difference to the *quality* of the healing, which leads to better *functional ability* and *durability*.

Conversely, healing which is delayed or disturbed will result in anything from poor functional capacity to frank scar tissue, an infilling with poor over-stress resistance: this is particularly so in ligaments and tendons, and to a lesser extent in muscle and skin and bone.

Scientists are constantly researching for treatments which will not only preclude this risk but actually *enhance the quality of healing*, especially of tendons and ligaments.

One such recent technique is the injection of 'Bapten' into a *repairing* strained tendon at around day 30 post injury, when fibrosis repair is established, and repeated twice. This has been shown to reduce the irregular geometry of new tendon fibres by interfering with the unwanted cross-linkage of the collagen, thus improving the degree of return of the all important 'crimp'.

A treated horse still requires 12 months plus before fast work, but it is believed that such a horse may have a significantly greater chance of withstanding the hazards of the further overstress of work (racing) than one not so treated, but such results need numbers and time to determine.

In the past, various orthopaedic interferences have been used after the acute inflammatory phase of, e.g. the tendinitis, has subsided

- daily massage of the tendon and its muscle
- stimulation of its muscle, to stretch the fibres into alignment, by
  - muscle stimulators
- implantation of carbon prostheses
- tendon 'splitting' with or without implants
- actual cautery in certain conditions
  - controlled, slow progressive work, but no turn out to grass to 'free' exercise

they have all had their protagonists and successes, usually based on being able to withstand more than 5 races or the equivalent in the discipline or sport in which the injury occurred. A reduced level of athletic strain, of course, gave better results, but all were relatively successful only if time was again given before asymmetric gaits were introduced.

It is with the many complementary disciplines and their exponents' claims of significant reductions in time required for 'useable' healing that debate exists. To date, the benefits are really only anecdotal and not backed by acceptable field trial studies. Nor are there proven records of subsequent durability which would reflect the belief that such therapies produce a better quality of maturation.

Reduction in the **inflammatory phase** of injury by complementary techniques is more demonstrable and understandable with particular regard to swelling and pain. The danger is that such clinical reduction may mask the actual repair situation with regard to a return to work especially in 'closed' traumas, and to cleansing and to repair in both open and closed cases.

Until the micro-biological activities of the modalities is better understood, **and** measurable, conventional practitioners can but accept that there are **possible** benefits

without the risk of adverse effects if applied by competent, trained personnel.

To these ends there must be co-operation – a benefit of the Veterinary Surgeons Act; so far this is not widely practised. Some complementary disciples have been more anxious to use the nuances of the English language to emphasise that they are not 'treating' disease or disorder but merely maintaining or improving an animal's medical and physical status quo, and that this does not require veterinary diagnosis. This lack of cooperation has prevented much useful collation of data.

Veterinary surgeons are fundamentally concerned with an animal's return to health and fitness **by whatever means**, provided these are not otherwise detrimental. Owners are often sceptical about this open-mindedness, human nature being what it is, but it does create unnecessary conflict.

The success of orthodox and complementary work depends very much on the subsequent management of the convalescent patient.

An *unsatisfactory outcome to nature's efforts* is generally due to

- uncontrollable, original haemorrhaging
- inability to combat infection
- weakness, predisposing to
  - other lethal complications and secondary infection
  - predation
    - and death (or variably short of this)

First aid aims to augment natural inflammatory responses by

- controlling bleeding more quickly
- reducing contamination
- preventing new infection

After-care or management aims at
  - creating the right environment both specifically
    - at the site of a wound, or the
    - primary site of an illness
  and generally, in terms of
    - protection against further trauma
    - nutrition, to encourage better healing
  i.e. nursing/management and retraining (or rehabilitation)

Patently, the sooner first aid is effected, the better. Simple procedures done within minutes are more effective than delaying until more sophisticated kit is available.

In summary, as emphasised earlier, the two *primary* aims are to

stop bleeding

• prevent further infection

and the one action, a bandaged-on or held-on pad, will effect both until the horse gets to, or help is brought to it, for more detailed efforts.

It is accepted that lavage is better than swabbing a wound; plain tap water is safe for initial 'DIY' cleansing, but it can result in oedema of healthy surrounding tissue if used for too long and too frequently, leading to maceration of deeper tissues *and* of the forming granulation bed. Veterinary advice should be available before this happens, but better an oedema than an infection!)

After a water lavage, a douching with normal saline (about 500ml, ½pt, relative to size and depth of the wound) or other isotonic solution, will 'balance' the fluids and the electrolytes in and around the cells. A final spray or douche (not a swabbing on) of appropriately diluted antiseptic solution (see first aid kit instruction) will form an antibacterial veneer. *Do not plug open wounds with powders, creams or ointments; nor spray with non-recommended solutions, especially antibiotics, unless the wound is superficial*, i.e. not right through the full skin thickness, and by definition, not a case for veterinary advice. Even then, antibiotic use is debatable and has wider zoonotic implications.

Where on-going DIY wound treatment is being given, it is advisable to use materials previously prescribed, or at least agreed to by the veterinary surgeon

• spraying with an antiseptic quick-drying agent is safer than swabbing on of liquid antiseptic, unless a once-only pledget is used

• a thick layer of ointment is uneconomical because

  • only the in-contact surface can be effective

  • the rest, unless of a clinging nature, will simply quickly melt and run off, or worse still

  • obstruct the outflow of exudate

There is accruing evidence that some herbal topical dressings have antibacterial properties. Owners who believe that such have worked well on themselves, quite understandably wish to give their horse similar advantages. It is advisable that discussion with one's veterinary surgeon is first done, in case of incompatibility with other drugs in use.

Some wounds progress better if left exposed to the air provided they are otherwise protected against further trauma or gross contamination. For example

• 'broken knees' where the joint synovium is not exposed

• deep abrasions and unsuturable lacerations which do not invade 'vital' areas

• 'gaping' flesh wounds

but keep the tail daily replaited where relevant, and anti-fly protection will be necessary in the summer.

Malnutrition and intercurrent disease, especially metabolic and endoparasitic, indirectly impair recovery. Septicaemia and/toxaemia delay the whole process, as do foreign bodies.

Any wound which discharges down over healthy skin will almost certainly produce a dermatitis. The potential track should be greased, especially into the back of the pastern and heels.

When a wound, usually due to a puncture, and its relatively small surface hole (which is invariably infected), closes over 'too quickly' – usually from oedematous swelling of the dermis – there can be a 'gathering' of fluid, fibrinous clot and cellular debris under the skin, now unable to discharge naturally.

The build-up of the retained inflammatory material is greater and quicker if there is a retained foreign body such as a thorn or a splinter of wood and/or necrotic tissue too

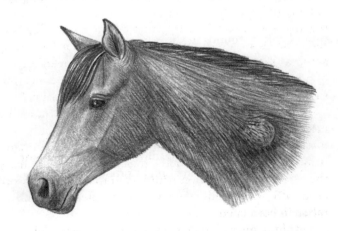

An abscess.

big for enzymatic liquefaction. The associated bacterial multiplication and associated white cell concentration along with dehydration by absorption of serum leads to a thickening of the material – making it even more difficult to exude through.

This purulent 'gathering' then develops into an **abscess** which is quickly 'walled off' by a thin fibrous lining to retain the contents and so prevent further spread into the surrounding tissues. Some abscesses will generate enough fluid pressure to break through the overlying skin: the abscess has ripened and burst out. Once the offending fluid has been discharged, the 'hole' heals in. The residual lining is dealt with naturally, but on occasions the 'hole' must be kept open.

Post First-Aid Decisions and Management

Should (after bleeding has been controlled, if possible) a veterinary surgeon be called? This will depend upon the

- nature and site of the injury
- experience of the first aider, and her
  - confidence in knowing what to do

There should be no hesitation in seeking professional on-site advice for

- suspected fractures
- **lacerated wounds**, especially if they involve
  - the axilla or the groin, where there are major vessels and nerves which could be subsequently traumatised
  - a horizontal or a spiralling track around more than a quarter of the circumference of a limb, thus probably involving related blood and nerve supply
  - apparently deeper structures
- **stab (stake) wounds** in the
  - axilla and groin
  - synovial 'vital' areas
  - chest, abdomen and throat
  - puncture wounds over, possibly into, or suspiciously close to, synovial 'vital' areas. Such injuries are often misleadingly small at the point of skin injury and, surprisingly, produce minimal bleeding

If there is associated

- marked **swelling**
- marked **pain on digital pressure**

- **lameness** or other signs of functional disturbance
- signs of **shock**

these should have encouraged an immediate call for on-site veterinary attendance (see first aid).

Paradoxically, experienced equine first aiders are more aware of how misleading the initial signs of an injury can be; they are more likely to work on the basis of 'one can never be too sure'. When such a doubt exists the situation should be at least discussed by telephone with the veterinary surgeon.

Legally, in the UK the non-veterinarian is prohibited from having and administering systemic antibiotics. Pain killers such as 'Bute' are also restricted.

All wounds must be regularly re-assessed over several days for complications, especially those which did not warrant initial veterinary attention or, of course, if not complying with his expectations. Such signs will include

- inflammatory swelling spreading from the original site
- stiffening of a limb or increasing frank lameness
- sweating, perhaps localised to the quarter area of that limb
- fever
- inappetence
- coldness (delayed shock) with rigors
- tetanus

Consideration for transport and the implications of the Transport of Injured Animals Act has already been emphasised. In this context closed injuries, the strains and sprains and the acutely incapacitating types of ER must be similarly managed.

Normally, an injured horse will be either

- at grass, and now has to be
  - confined in a stable away form its companions
  - fed different feedstuffs
- in varying, usually high level of work, now to be
  - confined in a stable, but still fit and full of energy
  - fed reduced feedstuffs, especially concentrates

Either of the above is a significantly different patient from one which is ill, possibly quite sick, dispirited and inappetent.

The injured horse will require attention to its tempera-nent as well as its wound or strain

- all stress factors should be minimised as far as possible
  - it should not be left on its own, or at least given the view of other stabled horses or another animal and human attention as other horses are taken out
  - be given the sound of quiet music
  - have its hay net topped more than usual (see dental disorders)
  - have extra 'comforting' attention given at grooming; and patience, tolerance and minimal restraint when dressings are changed
- in limb wounds, the muscles above should be massaged twice a day
- special attention should be paid to hoof cleanliness and overgrowth, and the state of shoes and nails if they have been left on
- the patient should be carefully monitored for worsening inflammatory signs in and beyond the injury
  - dullness
  - inappetence
  - fever with or without increased heart and respiratory rates
  - increased heat around the injury
  - worsening swelling
  - leg resting more than usual and lameness increasing

In the case of DIY managed wounds, the horsemaster must be satisfied that her care is resulting in

- progressive improvement, and not in
- a static situation, let alone a
- deterioration

and this judgement is based on recognising the appropriate signs of diminishing inflammation – or otherwise as in open wounds

- any original mistake in not recognising penetration of a vital area will have become apparent – there will be a marked regression. *Get help, it might not be too late*
- a secondary risk is the formation of excess granulation tissue and its intractable **proud flesh** development
  - this is *a common complication in DIY treatment*
  - it often surprisingly develops when the horsemaster considers that the wound is healing satisfactorily
  - earlier in the chapter it was pointed out that it is

more likely to occur in limb laceration wounds which were not sutured for one reason or another

- from the knee/hock down
- over joint surface areas

which have no muscle tissue underneath them to absorb the pressure of **healthy** granulation which is consequently 'pushed' outwards

- it develops mainly when the
  - control of secondary infection of the granulating in-filling has not been effective
  - the wound was not correctly covered or immobilised by dressings appropriate to the situation

The horsemaster must appreciate that any amateur attempt to reduce this mass can lead to more serious complications – take no chances.

Sooner or later she must expect to see the affected area return to its original size, shape (contour) and consistency, without asymmetric heat; remember, *a clipped out leg will feel warmer than the other one still with hair*. The structural improvement must be accompanied by a return to functional normality.

When a return to work is made it must be done gradually, not only for the underlying weakness but also from a general fitness level. The horse must be very carefully monitored and the slightest sign of a relapse paid attention to. Limbs with a distal wound from above the knee down are subject to lower cannon filling, but this will characteristically 'walk down' at least partially in the early days. There is a need for firm stable bandaging overnight.

Prevention of Injury

No horse, no matter how well cared for, can be guaranteed freedom from injury. The horse at grass and the horse in work are exposed to many hazards. Good horsemastership and field management minimise the risk for the full-time grazer. Similar attributes plus trained equitation will, to a lesser extent, reduce occupational hazards, but the fact of being in work is an obvious danger. This will vary with the discipline and the level practised.

There are basic principles of care for competition or work

- the horse – is it suitable?
  - conformation within a type
    - inherited
    - acquired, especially feet and lower limbs

- age
- condition
- fitness and temperament when fit
- previous experience or exposure to that work
- level of training reached for a particular stage of work
- freedom from intercurrent disease or chronic injury

The horsemaster must be
- capable of assessing states of fitness and of health
- prepared to expect injuries *vis à vis* circumstances of work and/or of 'resting' environment
- aware of them and of assessing them
- trained in first aid and early management
- aware of the law, as well as the techniques, particular to transporting an injured horse

A horse which is overstressed metabolically or constitutionally or compromised by other horsemasterhip mistake is much more likely to develop
- clinical illness from immunity suppression
- be injured because locomotor functioning is compromised by
    - early fatigue
    - weakness
  leading to
    - closed over-stress trauma
    - interferences

Reference should be made to Chapter 38, FITTENING and in particular the section on conditioning for preparation to a return to work.

INTRODUCTION

The domesticated horse should be managed in a manner as near to that of the wild, free living horse, as possible. The sick or injured horse is *suddenly* exposed to changes associated with

- changes in feeding and feedstuffs
- the restrictions of prolonged stabling
- decreased, even complete, lack of exercise
  - boredom
  - risk of developing stereotypical behaviourisms

All are possible stress factors, in addition to the primary factor. It is essential that the horsemaster has a constant picture of the ways and habits of the 'free' horse, as he cares for his patient, and in particular how he manages

- the reduced feed requirements
- the vital need for fresh air/ventilation
- consideration for the effects of boredom, loneliness and *inactivity*

as well as the particular nursing inputs of the illness involved.

'Nursing' is the application of particular and general skills to assist the horse's innate powers of recovery, and the veterinary help of medicine and surgery. *Nursing aims to improve the chances of recovery*.

In general stable work, economics, if nothing else, will see the on-going need for horsemasters, grooms in charge and owners to continue to be equine 'nurses' as **and when** required as distinct from full-time sick box attendants at clinics and hospitals run by equine veterinary surgeons.

Special Equipment for Sick Nursing

Tack room

- appropriate rugs, sweat sheets, stable/leg bandages; other 'protectors', e.g. head protector (as when a patient may become cast)
- twitch
- neck cradle
- muzzle
- complete (separate) grooming kit, including a strapping pad

Where and when necessary

- handler's protective clothing and boots
- disposable gloves
- disinfectants and antiseptics: separate buckets, soap, nail brush, disposable towels
- instruction list
- medical 'daily' chart or stable record book
- emergency telephone numbers

Medicine chest

- in addition to first aid kit, **specifically** veterinary-prescribed medicines and dressings

The Nurse

She must know her patient, i.e. its

- temperament
- idiosyncrasies

- **A B C**
- vital parameters
  - pulse rate
  - respiratory rate
  - temperature
- general history, as it was before nursing was required
- its medical history, and specific aspects thereof
  - dental care
  - shoeing
  - vaccination
  - worming when it was in health

and be able to relate these when relevant to the patient.

The handler in charge of a sick horse must be taught what is required of her, and be specifically instructed by the veterinary surgeon. She will require

- knowledge of drugs and dressings
- skill in applying these, and how to apply muzzle, twitch and cradle
- patience with the difficult horse
- willingness to give more than routine attention
- 'modesty' not to think she knows better (than the veterinary surgeon); but she will probably **know** the patient better than anyone

It is the nurse's particular responsibility to know from the veterinary surgeon what the feeding regime should be, i.e. solids, liquids; what it can have, when, how much, how often; what it cannot have – until when.

She must be able to recognise and to assess changes in appetite and drinking

- seemingly keen to eat, but will not do so from some receptacles
- positional alterations from that used to
  - on the floor, for respiratory troubles
  - at height suitable, for head and neck flexion difficulty
- sore mouth, 'teeth' and throat
  - cannot prehend, masticate, or swallow, as from
    - jaw injuries
    - strangles lymphadenitic swellings
  - does it quid and/or
  - hypersalivate?
- cannot posture to eat and drink, because of a locomotor

problem
- is it losing
  - bloom?
  - condition?
    - quickly, as with severe pain/fever
    - slowly, despite food intake
- signs of respiratory coincidental disorder
- signs of colic
- disinterested demeanour generally
- presently induced lameness, e.g. laminitis

The nurse must be aware of the importance of
- air hygiene
- ambient temperature
- body heat and its regulation, self and artificially
- correctly administering prescribed drugs
- controlling pain, under veterinary instruction
- minimising further or incidental traumas
- body care
- strict hygiene where contagion is present
- making much of the horse but not harassing it, and the value of
  - music (background)
  - visual companionship

Whenever an injury or an illness occurs, whether this necessitates a box rest or merely a short period off work, careful record of
- the date seen ill or injured
- the nature of the dis-ease
- if seen by the veterinary surgeon
  - his diagnosis and advice
- medication – as prescribed and directed by the veterinary surgeon, or DIY
- dressing – as prescribed and directed by the veterinary surgeon, or DIY

in all cases, especially if these include restricted medicin supplied by the veterinary surgeon.

It is important to know and to annotate the records as to
  - its susceptibility to
    - COPD and allergy to grooming 'dander'

- laminitis
- colic
- getting cast

These details will continue for the sick horse until pronounced 'recovered' by the veterinary surgeon, for the injured horse (i.e. open wound) until discharges cease, and for closed trauma until the acute sterile inflammatory signs have subsided. Further care and attention, management, is, of course, still necessary, with relevant observations or decisions being noted.

The Stable

The sick box should be at least 4m x 4m (12ft x 12ft), and

- have a split door, which opens outwards
- the bottom half must have a
  - top bolt
  - bottom kick-over fastener
  - middle safety bolt (against idle 'muzzle' on top one)
- the top half should have a grid for use, instead of the top door, when required – especially at night, to stop foreleg knocking and generally to stop weaving
- have one window which, in part, opens inwards; and the whole gridded off. An opposite ventilation outlet is essential.
- ideally the box should have

- a veranda roof, to protect
  - the horse, when allowed to look out
  - the handler and his equipment, when working there
- an anti-cast fitting around the box is an advantage

Lighting

This is usually poor in stables, especially for limb wound dressing

- a high source simply casts the shadow of the horse
- a bulkhead light is rarely powerful enough (it is essential in stables that the normal lighting is not a high heat emitter – otherwise it could become a fire hazard)
- a wandering guarded light from a nearby source is often necessary

Ventilation/Thermo-regulation

A horse stabled at any time should have fresh air without draughts. If boxed for a variable time as a patient this becomes even more important, and especially so if it is because of illness, particularly illness affecting the respiratory system.

Warmth must not be obtained at the expense of ventilation. Lightweight but thermally efficient clothing can be increased. Ear, head and neck covers can be added, and woollen leg bandages (essential for pressure against 'filling' legs) are also useful as heat retainers

- beware day and night environmental temperature changes
- monitor body comfort heat by feeling under the rugs at

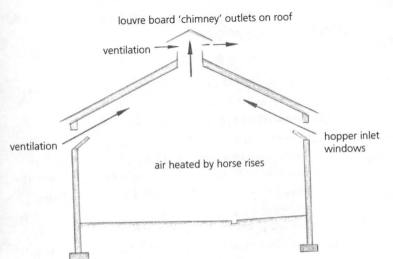

louvre board 'chimney' outlets on roof

ventilation

ventilation

air heated by horse rises

hopper inlet windows

Effective stable ventilation.

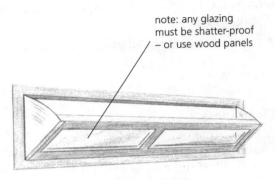

note: any glazing must be shatter-proof – or use wood panels

Hopper inlet 'window'.

Good ventilation in practice.

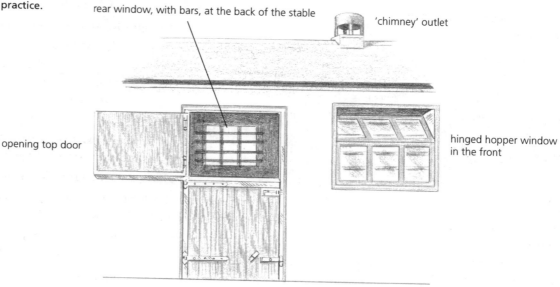

rear window, with bars, at the back of the stable

'chimney' outlet

opening top door

hinged hopper window in the front

the shoulder, rump and abdomen, and general warmth by feeling the ears. If the ears are cold, gentle massage of them should stimulate peripheral blood flow and bring up their and the rest of the body's skin temperature. Added clothing can be arranged accordingly

- a fevered animal and/or one in pain will periodically 'cold' sweat. This must be watched for; sponging down and drying off, followed by straw under the rugs, or a dry sweat sheet put on under fresh blankets, as required

- conversely, the over-warm animal will show discomfort, sometimes accelerated respiration, and will feel damp or unexpectedly warm to the touch. A reduction in clothing must be made with care against chilling. (Note, animals do not 'catch a chill'. They may **get chilled** with consequent reduction in natural defence against infection.)

- solar and radiant heat should be used under veterinary advice, and with particular reference to UV light and unpigmented skin areas

Cleanliness

Drainage
Beware blocking of outlets, especially if gridded, by bedding. A wet bed is

- discomforting for a patient lying down
- destructive to hoof horn, and is a source of ammonia which is

- particularly noxious and dangerous to respiratory patients
- irritating and possibly destructive of airway clearing mechanism to all

Faeces
These should be diligently removed for the same reasons. Remember the old adage

- one pile seen is acceptable
- two piles seen are reprehensible
- three or more warrant dismissal – of the stableman

It is easier to muck out fresh rather than trodden muck and is therefore more economical in bedding.

Bedding

- wheat straw is the ideal. For lame patients, the straw should be on the short side (as usually it is, with combine harvesting!)

- oat straw is more appetising but, subject to care over 5 to 7 days (use of a muzzle), most horses can be safely 'weaned' onto it with no ill effect. It certainly gives the bored patient a constant source of nuzzling and of 'chomping'

- barley straw – the same restriction applies, but it is not such a good draining bed

- paper also tends to get soggy and thereby requires greater attention

peat moss is ideal for foot lameness cases. It is expensive and carries criticism from nature conservers

Whatever is used must not be musty – there are brands sold as dust- and mould-spore free, but if eaten there is a risk of impaction worse than with sudden straw consumption. The bed should be well banked up around the walls, and well set at the doorway.

Stable Fittings for Food and Water

Have no metal projections, loose boards, or other objects, in the wall or floor. If a manger is present and has a space below, have this blocked up with bales, preferably sacked in plastic or, if uncovered, so placed that the strings do not present as a hoof catching object. It is advisable to block off (and remove) an automatic water bowl

- an unemployed horse will play with and overflow it, or sit on it, with possible flooding
- rubber bucket(s), handle removed, will allow estimation of water consumption

It is better that these are removable for daily cleaning. Water buckets can be refilled and put back. Utensils contaminated by

- saliva
- nasal discharge
- faecal droppings
- urine

are off-putting to any animal, but especially so to a sick patient.

Whilst contagion back to the donor is not an infection worry, any utensils brought outside should be *cleaned on site* to prevent the risk of being handled by others and used elsewhere, especially if there is a risk of contagion.

Very hot water and washing soda are efficient cleansers, and, by getting all grease etc. off, are reasonably good disinfectants. Any buckets so used must be swilled out with running water before re-use for food or drink.

Contagion and its Control

The veterinary surgeon will advise *and should be involved in relevant decisions* for the benefit of other horses in an outbreak, some of which could be in contact through thoughtless lack of care

- if there is an infectious agent involved
- if it is contagious
  - indirect aerosol, as with viruses

- contact nose to nose
  - nose to human arm or hand or clothes, and so to other horse
  - nose to inanimate objects, as with **strangles** (whose dried 'snot' or fomite can also be blown downwind)
  - horse to horse
  - horse to tack and grooming kit etc. and to other horses, as with **ringworm**

and will advise as to whether it is

- economically practicable to try to successfully prevent spread, or
- better to get the 'spread' over as quickly as possible

The horse which begins to cough could be a new contagious source (its temperature may have fallen to normal), or one showing an allergic (non-contagious) response.

It is better *for the horse's sake*, as well as for contagion control, that the cause is determined if possible.

If and when isolation for contagion control is decided on veterinary advice, it must be as near 'all-or-nothing' as possible

- a stable well down the prevailing wind!
- a separate handler using the horse's
  - own feed and water utensils
  - own grooming kit
  - hay, bedding and feed left nearby by another person – the handler should not personally take supplies from a communal source
- the handler should don
  - gum boots – disinfected before entering and after leaving the box
  - overalls, disposable or able to be hosed down – if soiled, hosed down in clean disinfectant, rinsed and let dry: preferably use waterproofs
  - disposable gloves, removed into a disposal bag, especially for
    - ringworm
    - strangles
- if the handler has no option but to help elsewhere in the yard, *he must service the isolated horse last*

Controlling contagion is not easy. If it can't be done even reasonably well, it is better, even with ringworm, to let the contagion take its course, under therapy, on its own. *Remember, ringworm is contagious to man.*

Those contagious diseases which develop in competition and racing yards present economic as well as welfare considerations. Some contagions are present but clinically, at least, inactive. A spread is therefore possible. Those which become clinically active must be considered in the light of 'what germ', the use of the horses, and the advice of the veterinary surgeon. Breeding premises are particular risks.

Grooming

Particular attention should be paid to sponging eyes, mouth, nostrils and the anal/vulval region once daily, the prepuce (sheath) once a week

- when an infection is present this sponging should be done by swabbing with pledgets of cotton wool soaked in warm water – one pledget for one wipe, then disposed of into a plastic bag

- in the case of an injury, such strict overall hygiene is not necessary – but is still advisable, even if to a limited extent. Sponges and cloths sooner or later get used on other animals, so are best avoided. Moreover, each horse should have its own grooming kit, as a general routine

If convalescence seems a lengthy business, then grooming must be reduced to avoid removing too much of the natural oils

- stain marks can be washed off
- the mane and tail regularly kept untangled
- the rest of the coat must be lightly body-brushed
- strong strapping is not necessary, but light strapping, hand massage or wisping of the major fore and hind quarter musculature and the proximal muscles of the limbs, especially those of any injured (lame) leg, is very beneficial
- the feet must be picked out twice daily. If the horse is to be boxed for more than three weeks, have all shoes removed, or sooner if wear and state of clenches makes this sensible
- any specific muscle stimulation will be prescribed by the veterinary surgeon, who will also determine
    - moving the patient to larger premises with room for exercise

- in-hand exercise during convalescence (beware exuberance!)

There are many examples of 6 months' total box res which have not appeared to be detrimental mentally o physically. Consideration will have to be made fo individual temperament; thoroughbreds and hot blood may be less accommodating!

A problem of prolonged stabling is the interferenc with foot circulation, particularly in cases of loss of on limb foot support. This deficit can affect not only the lam limb but also the contralateral persistent weight-bearin one. It may be necessary to build up the contra lateral foo to balance both limbs, when and if the injured one i therapeutically elevated by plaster dressings and splitting

In a loosebox, locomotion can be encouraged, and t some extent effected, by distributing hay, grass, concen trates and/or succulents in different corners. Veterinar advice will be given. This is especially important i patients with a previous history of

- DJD
    - arthrosis
    - navicular syndrome
- laminitis

Feeding

Not all sick or injured horses have necessarily come fron being in work and, therefore, on related hard feedstuffs Nevertheless, a change in diet is almost inevitable whatever the immediate past activity.

From grass to long feed is reasonably easy – cut and car the greenstuff; continuing to feed it is advisable for th horse's

- digestion
- contentment

but a complete change over, if it can not be avoided should be *gradual over 10 days at least*.

From working dry rations it is a matter of a rapid, *bu not suddenly total*, removal of the concentrates. If nc bedded on paper, the horse will make up for his appetite or straw with the risk of an impaction of the large gut. It i preferable to substitute a convalescent diet (e.g. gras balancer nuts, or convalescent diet) low in protein reduced in energy, and usually free of oats (check). Fee little and often even if only 500g (1lb), 4 times a day. Tr too, to increase the feed times for contentment, bu increase to appetite gradually.

Haylage products are useful and are also good stimulants to appetite, but they are 'richer' than hay; a low protein type should be used and gradually introduced over 3 to 4 days. If the horse is on haylage because of COPD, change to the lower protein value cut. Aim to have some long fibre available all the time.

Succulents such as carrot, apple and turnip are not only 'good' for the patient but if hand fed give an opportunity to 'make much' of the (lonely) patient. **Long sliced carrot and turnip are safer than chopped.** Apples are best fed halved.

Natural or near natural feedstuffs are usually the most tempting.

Beware
- feeding cut and carried **lush** (dairy cow) grass
- presence of poisonous plants such as **ragwort**, and lawn mowings
- **too much, too quickly** of anything different
- over use of **bran**

Consider
- palatability
- digestibility
- quality

In respiratory cases especially, shake out long feed away from the box, feed it and any concentrates from the floor. Otherwise the normal rules of feeding still apply, subject to veterinary advice.

The veterinary surgeon may advise special feeding and supplementation in the light of the diagnosis, the continuing signs and of laboratory tests – e.g. soya meal, cottage cheese, corn oil, amino acids/electrolytes and 'complan' casein, and probiotics by stomach tube if necessary.

Appetite stimulants are
- herbal blends of low energy leaf and stem plants
- alfalfa chaff – sometimes bitter for a horse's taste, but the change might be welcome
- cut and carried turf sods
- hydroponic 'grass'
- bran and linseed mashes and the other sloppy preparations
- hay 'tea'

NURSING SPECIFIC CONDITIONS

Respiratory Disease

Do not block ventilation in order to maintain box temperature. Do allow as much fresh air as possible. Turn out when and where practicable unless the horse is depressed, systemically ill or temperature is greater than 39.5°C (103°F). Control the duration of grazing *vis à vis* weather changes, especially if it rains. **Beware frosted grass** – in all circumstances. Use rugs when necessary for extra warmth and waterproofing. Do keep warm and use extra clothing in the stables as required.

If during a routine daily inspection there is a
- temperature rise
- cough
- nasal discharge

then suspect secondary respiratory infection.

Note: in some viral infections the temperature rises and falls within a matter of 4 days; during this time there is a dullness – if this is noticed, check the temperature.

Severe respiratory distress will necessitate veterinary help. The COPD patient will usually have a history of previous attack(s), but not always. The marked changes in respiratory rate and excursion of the respiratory embarrassment will be pointers.

Some coughs (a defensive reaction) are related to inhalation of allergens: pollen, mould spores, and other physical irritants. These are rarely associated with a fever (but remember the short period fever mentioned above), or rapid 'spread' to other horses. Check
- respiratory rate and excursions, and temperature
- presence of a new batch of hay (or bedding)
- a musty bale of hay or straw

An allergic horse may 'react' to these new exposures
- a first time
- as a flare-up or recrudescence

Equine Influenza

The virus responsible and its various strains makes this the most highly contagious respiratory disease. It spreads rapidly within a few days in unvaccinated yards, by direct contact as well as the aerosol route. Vaccinated animals will respond variably to invasion.

A significant number of newly infected animals will show no clinical signs despite having a sub-clinical viraemia, but in the unvaccinated or previously unexposed horse a new infection will usually show typically with

- acute onset fever of up to 40°C (104°F)
- harsh dry cough
- copious serous, becoming mucopurulent, nasal discharge
- marked depression

In the partially immune, previously exposed horse the clinical signs are much reduced, to

- slight or absent fever
- a nasal discharge rapidly developing in other similar horses
- some coughing at exercise

The virus can be shed for up to 10 days in the first category above and proportionately shorter in the other two. Since the viral strains are highly immunogenic, long-term carriers do not occur.

Veterinary advice is essential re return to work.

Equine Herpes Virus Respiratory Disease (1 and 4)

Clinically, in primary or in recrudescent cases there can be

- acute onset of nasal discharge
- slight fever of up to 39.2°C (102.5°F), even sometimes higher
- soft cough (**not** now thought to be the common cause of sub-acute 'stable' cough in young horses)
- possible non-septic sub-mandibular lymphadenitis

Respiratory excretion of the viral strain usually stops after 14 days. Some animals can go longer, even weeks. From a practical point of view, especially due to its latency tendency, all horses should be seen as probable carriers: spread to susceptible other horses, especially when stressed, is an ongoing hazard.

The rate of spread varies (aerosol spread is limited, usually direct or indirect, by fomites and other physical means). Recrudescence does occur, with nasal shedding of the virus, particularly after stressing, such as by transit and mixing of groups.

Equine Viral Arteritis

Spread

- nasal direct contact, but it is slow
- venereal is quick, as mating is the 'vehicle'

The diagnosis of the **lesser viral LRT infections**, and **primary bacterial pneumonitis** are a matter for veterinary input. The viral coughing form is usually of short duration and any lymphadenitis is not abscess producing. The primary bacterial infections may cause prolonged coughing periods and reduced performance. They are now thought to be what racing yard and other Thoroughbred units used to call 'the virus'!

Stop stud work: see Code of Practice with special reference to abortion and to paresis cases, especially with herpes infection.

In all viral respiratory outbreak situations

- try not to let the germ spread outside the affected premises, or
  - take even apparently normal horses away from that yard to communal gatherings
- monitor all carefully
  - take any with a fever of 0.5°C (1°F) rise or more, out of work
  - in competition yards it is often cost effective to
    - move suspect cases to a separate yard – down wind or afar
  - use separate staff and separate equipment
  - monitor those carefully
  - monitor those left *particularly for temperature rise*
  - do not mix either suspect or 'clean' with other horses in other situations, or especially

- where horses are due to run within 14 days
  - move them upwind to separate stables
  - separate staff and equipment
  - monitor temperature twice daily

- compete if clinically normal
  - especially careful monitoring for exercise overstress

Do not 'run' any horse which has a temperature rise of greater than a quarter of a degree C (half a degree F). *There is a risk of cardio-vascular/muscular overstress from associated inflammation of these tissues.*

Do not medicate without veterinary advice
- there is no practicable anti-virus drug
- the wrong drug could
  - delay recovery
  - encourage resistance to bacterial secondaries
  - infringe discipline rules over long periods with some drugs

Strangles

A bacterial contagious, technically not a respiratory disease but affects the rostral area of the upper respiratory tract in the primary condition.

The signs are reasonably characteristic once the submandibular lymph glands become inflamed, enlarged and painful to the touch. The nasal discharge which comes after the gland swelling is more rapidly purulent than in virus cases, but the early signs of depression, inappetence (more significantly a disinclination to masticate and swallow) can be misleading. Fever is invariably higher than in the viraemias.

In mild cases some animals which did not form abscesses in the lymph nodes will later (2 to 4 weeks) produce signs of purpura haemorrhagica.

In many yards it is usually considered that the hygienic standards required to control an outbreak are too high for satisfactory implementation. (Confirmed non-Thoroughbred outbreaks should be notified to the Welfare Department of the BHS.) It is often thought best to let an outbreak run its course rather than isolate and/or treat with antibiotics, but discuss with veterinary surgeon.

Nursing of Strangles Cases

The bacterial inflammation in the naso-pharyngeal area not only makes mastication and deglutition painful and difficult but it also diminishes sensory inputs of taste and smell.

It is essential to 'symptomatically' treat these
- decongestive 'steaming' of nostrils with 'Vick'
- hot foments of the throat
- poulticing of any glandular enlargement
- regular removal of pus from the nostrils by wiping with disposable swabs
- feeding
  - gruels
  - grass

at suitable heights above ground level, to minimise postural difficulties, but always as low as possible.

Colic

Management (it is hardly 'nursing') aims at minimising self-injury by the horse when going down and when down and rolling. This requires

- constant awareness of safety for the helper(s) – the fewer the better in the box at any one time
- fitting a strong headcollar and rope shank (double the usual length)
- if there is time between bouts fit
  - a poll guard
  - knee pads
  - fore-tendon boots (if shod behind)
  - add extra bedding, well heaped-up round walls
  - block off spaces under a manger
  - remove all loose 'furniture'

It is **not** essential to keep the horse on its feet to prevent going down and then rolling onto its back/side, usually with the limbs acting as a prop on the adjacent wall. It can lie there for many minutes without embarrassment to the respiratory system or from pressure on the back and quarters.

It is helpful if
- when it is down
  - the head is pulled away from wall contact, until extra straw is dropped into that area (control of violent rolling is difficult)
- when it gets up
  - leverage on the halter rope aims to steady it and to minimise violent activity. (Do not be heroic!)

In less violent cases, when there is

- occasional striking (stamping, scraping in fore)
- staring at flank
- some sweating
- crouching/stretching/lifting and kicking with hind

it is helpful if the horse is led out onto grass or sand or into a school, to be gently led round for 10 minute periods and offered pulled grass in the intervals. After some 3 sessions the horse can be taken back into its box and allowed down if it wishes; or kept in the field or school – but not let loose – and allowed down if it must.

During these times observe for passing of wind, faeces, urine.

Monitor the pulse at 15 minute intervals, observe respirations, and take the temperature reading if deemed safe to do so.

Post-Colic Management

The veterinary surgeon will advise; he may decide to stay with the horse until all acute signs have settled or until pulse is steady and under 50bpm. He may leave the horsemaster to monitor the less than settled case with special regard to the pulse (if he is satisfied that the carer can take it accurately).

In impacted colics the usual stomach tubing will not

- quickly produce satisfactory defaecation, but it is essential to know 'what was passed' and 'when'
- prevent some recurrent pain, for which eventuality the veterinary surgeon may leave a painkiller injection with the carer under prior instruction

and he will advise on feeding and watering.

In acute abdominal crisis cases which require surgery, very strict instructions will be given for post-operative care. Here, as in most colics, the horsemaster will be advised to **look out for loose faeces developing towards diarrhoea**, a forewarning of possible endotoxaemic shock or, conversely, failure to defaecate after a 4 hour or so interval. This too can indicate a 'shock' situation, but the patient will show also other signs such as faster, shallower breathing, patchy sweating, and a deterioration in general demeanour and interest. The veterinary surgeon will instruct as to when, if at all, a case can be left unattended and if so for how long.

Convalescence will be a composite nursing/management matter under professional advice

- feeding
    - hand grazing – when and how often
    - hay
    - 'convalescent' diet
    - mashes
    - access to water
- clothing, warmth is essential
    - blankets
    - leg bandages
- exercise
    - in-hand several short times each day, with an opportunity to graze
- grooming, including cleaning of orifices

Laminitis

Do

- *manage laminitis as an emergency*
- *get veterinary help as soon as possible*
- provide a deep bed, and let the patient go down
- fix frog support on both fore feet
- offer water *ad lib*
- small quantities of old pasture grass – a handful every hour, unless advised not to by veterinary surgeon on his arrival

Do not

- force exercise (get the horse home by transport)
- remove the shoes
- force it to walk round its box, let alone outside

Do not starve a laminitic case. In a fat pony this could be dangerous because of the risk of hyperlipaemia. In all case there is an on-going need for the **correct** nutrients at the right amount.

Always get the vet's advice on

- management
- feeding
- drugs – this must be accurately followed

Equine Rhabdomyolysis (ER)

In recent research, emphasis has been placed on the following points regarding post-recovery management

- the ration should not contain oats
- the horse must be exercised slowly **each day** and/or have access to exercise grazing, **no lungeing**
- precautions must be taken to prevent chilling
    - in frosty weather
    - in cold, wet weather

by suitable clothing, not by cancelling time out at exercise or free grazing, to avoid the cold.

As work increases, the extra energy intake should come from alfalfa hay or chop, and/or from vegetable oil.

Where electrolyte imbalances have been diagnosed, regular laboratory check-ups to monitor the required supplementation must be made, especially in those cases shown to involve calcium.

Once again, veterinary supervision must be obtained.

Lameness

The early and subsequent management of acute/severe lameness will depend upon the diagnosis. On the assumption that box rest is necessary, the following points should be noted

- the bedding must be deep and soft enough to make standing as comfortable as possible; yet if straw is used, it should not be so deep or consist of long straw as to make it likely that the lame (difficult to lift and protract) leg (in some cases the contralateral leg) will get wrapped around and so trapped by the straw
    - wood-shavings or paper bedding are ideal for boxing up to one month, but they will require extra-careful management as to mucking out
    - peat moss is better for longer term stabling, especially for pedal bone fractures
- the legs must be support-bandaged, and these changed twice daily. This is particularly important for the contralateral limb in unilateral lameness
- the feet will require regular picking out and inspecting – shoes removed on veterinary instructions, and not longer on than 4 weeks
- grooming to improve postural muscle tone should be augmented by strapping or massage. The muscles of the lame leg must be monitored for 'atrophy of disuse' and professional advice sought if necessary

- feeding will be for maintenance, but some convalescent diet may be required

Pay extra attention to the quality and the quantity of the excreta

- reduction
- dryness, or
- increase in moisture content and possible diarrhoea. Either should be reported

Clothing – rugs must be removed once daily and re-adjusted twice daily, paying attention to any skin lumps, bumps, or rashes.

The Acute Eye

The corneal/scleral damage will cause a residual photophobia and blepharospasm, which could encourage self-mutilation unless protected against. Keep the stable darkened, not at the expense of good ventilation but certainly protected against direct sunlight.

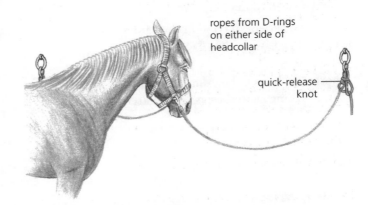

ropes from D-rings on either side of headcollar

quick-release knot

Double racking prevents the horse from rubbing its head, particularly on its foreleg.

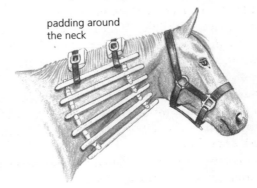

padding around the neck

A neck cradle.

Restraint aims at preventing the horse from rubbing its head on a foreleg or door post. The ideal method is double racking from one wall across the corner to the wall on the adjacent side. Ropes run from the side 'Ds' of the headcollar, which should also have a throat lash, to rings in the walls at the height of the eyes when the horse is standing at the halt. They should allow head movement to and fro from the haynet and water supply, but not sufficient as to get lower than the 'knees'.

In some occasions a neck cradle is necessary. The horse should be let down twice a day and led out to hand graze if no bright sunlight.

Choke

Many chokes, especially on compounded feedstuffs, are self-curing. Most which remain clinically affected have choked at the distal end of the neck length of the oesophagus – a swelling may be seen on the left hand side in front of the forequarters.

Do

- *remove all feedstuffs*
- *send for veterinary surgeon*
- walk the patient in hand in the yard for 10 to 15 minutes, with 10 minute intervals in the box
- if symptoms clear, do not stop the veterinary visit. The horse will have to be examined sooner or later for predisposing factors, especially teeth faults

Do not

- try to massage this 'swelling' up or downwards
- 'drench' with any liquid
- attempt to pass a stomach tube

When pronounced clear, let free in box with **no straw bedding** and offer clean water, and hand-held pulled grass. When this is easily consumed, hand graze for 15 minutes at half-hour intervals, 4 times. Return slowly to restricted diet, on veterinary advice. Monitor carefully for several days, for early signs of re-choking.

Collapse

With fits or convulsive-like, uncontrolled movement

- loosen girth, if saddled, remove when feasible
- replace bridle by head collar
- **send for veterinary surgeon**
- put down a thick bed, and work under the horse as well as possible
- do not restrain, but rather support at any attempt to rise
- keep the horse quiet
- beware horse's impulsive movements, on getting up especially
- prepare box as for colic cases

CHAPTER

38 FITTENING

INTRODUCTION

Definitions of 'Fit'

Legally: 'well adapted or suitable for a declared purpose', e.g. riding or driving, and 'competent to do so'. Physiologically and structurally: 'in good athletic condition and healthy, able and willing'.

'Fittening' is a progressive application of how to get the horse up from rest, then to condition it by increasing slow work and, *only* subsequently, exercise it so that it will in due course do what is expected with 'no sweat, no strain'.

Whatever level of fitness and use is aimed at the horsemaster has the responsibility of

- knowing horses as a species – and the particular horse
- recognising its health, readiness and willingness and its limitations
- being quickly aware of any deviation from these
- able to correctly apply a training programme
- capable of monitoring the results of this
- using common sense to stop, think and re-assess rather than push on regardless – a week off now is infinitely better than a complete breakdown later

Fitness

To be 'fit for work' implies a physical and physiological (structural and functional) level of readiness and willingness to perform

- at a particular level of work within a particular athletic requirement
- to go on doing so towards a prescribed level and,

when there

- to go on doing so for a prescribed period without becoming stale (going 'over the top')
- with minimum risks of injury or illness attributable to the stresses of that work

Being 'got fit' results from a continuing response to graded increases in the natural stresses of planned, progressive intensity.

The desired level of fitness is attained through broad stages over a related time schedule beginning with a primary, significant *change in management at the end of a period of rest* of one or more months, usually at grass.

The four stages are distinct in theory but overlap in practice. For descriptive purposes they are

1. **Management change**
2. **Conditioning**
3. **Fittening**
4. Skill or ability **'learning'** and refining – often part of 'doing' or competing

1, 2 and 3 are basic to all forms of work; 4 is, to a great extent, discipline orientated. In all types of riding (and driving) flatwork skills and responses to the aids are necessary attributes of future success and safety. In stage 2 these are taught to the young horse, or they are given again as a 'refresher course' at the start of each subsequent return to work. Fortunately the horse has an excellent memory, but proprioceptor retraining or retuning is important initially (see later). The skills of more advanced work such as show and cross-country jumping, dressage as a discipline, 'showing' and of such sports as endurance riding, gymkhana and polo are introduced during the fittening stages 3 and 4, eventually perfected and ultimately 'polished' in actual doing or competing. In elite situations, more than discipline training may be necessary – frequently one for the horse and another for the rider.

All stages fall within the general term 'training'. A trainer, however, is seen as one who specifically deals with a particular, usually competitive, discipline and does so with horse and rider as a unit.

Horses are intrinsically athletic and, unlike many humans, tend to remain so because of their life-style. Individually and in groups, horses free in the wild or loose in a field still practise the required techniques of survival: defence, agility, bursts of speed and, to a lesser extent, endurance. A nomadic existence for routine grazing behaviour also kept the wild horse on the move. They 'ate on the hoof' and became and remained physically fit – up to a certain level sufficient for the requirements of survival and reproduction.

This exercise maintains a base line of fitness on which, after a management change, man builds a training programme. At the very least, the freedom to be reasonably 'natural' on safe, not over-fattening grazing, keeps the vital systems exercised and toned. In particular it maintains the important circulation to the feet and venous and lymphatic drainage upwards in the limbs; it allows normal feeding posture, i.e. head and neck down for coincidental 'drainage' from the airways – a 'fresh air' life and a natural, grazed diet.

An individual horse is usually selected on its

- genotype – the breed or its crosses' particular, known forte

- phenotype – the breed or its crosses' overall shape, its conformation; but 'handsome is as handsome does' is a reasonable truism. A subjectively assessed good or faulty conformation remains just an opinion until time and use prove it one way or the other. There are, however, certain (usually limb faults), congenital or acquired, which fundamentally hazard the horse's athletic ability to work in a particular discipline and/or to remain capable of doing so

- character and temperament – the unqualifiable, subjective assessment of determination or willingness for the job. Training and using may, one way or the other, affect these attributes, which are perceivable only when the horse is actively engaged in its particular discipline. One feature of temperament associated with a desire to win was often described as 'heart' or 'guts'.

('Stomach' was used negatively, as in 'no stomach for ...'). It is perhaps more factually accurate to call it 'wind', or quality/quantity of airflow. This capacity is vital, especially in the racehorse. If 'oxygen in and carbon dioxide out' is compromised so too is performance, even with a 'good heart' and 'strong gut'

- possibly, pre-purchase veterinary examination

- structural and functional 'health'; whatever man's use of the horse through some 6,000 years, he has, consciously or not, analytically or 'through his breeches' benefited from the inherited structures and functionings imposed on Eohippus and its successors by the evolutionary survival requirements of its predecessors. Collectively these eventually made Equus and especially E. caballus, what it is – a suitable animal to ride and drive athletically.

Man, in his 'dominion over the horse' and his responsibility for it, procured means of transport which, by selective breeding, management and training, has been made even more useful – to become perhaps an elite athlete.

Whatever one's philosophy, and however one sees this investment for whatever return in the horse's potential, these structural and functional aspects of the species which made it 'one jump ahead' of extinction could, and often did, become a series of 'Achilles heels', or weak links, when man, in his enthusiasm, overstressed and so strained the horse's structure and functioning.

Herein lies the need for care and skill in managing, training and using the horse which, whatever its genetic background, remains an individual in response to feeding, handling and riding – an individual out of a common stock, built for a basic locomotor ability.

The domesticated athletic horse has no option but to remain a unit of structure and functioning in the compromising situation somewhere between the wild and the artificially elite. The further towards the latter, the greater the hazards.

During the rest period, the horsemaster will have paid particular attention to the state of the

- hooves *vis à vis*
  - ground condition, and the need to
  - trim accordingly
- skin and the coat, relative to seasonal influences, ectoparasites and protective clothing
- body condition, relative to the grazing and the need for supplementary feeding, and have checked on
- worming and vaccination programme dates

- recovery from previous dis-ease(s), and awareness of
- intercurrent dis-ease

During the last week of rest he will have arranged farrier attention (better to delay hind shoeing if several horses are together) and before and afterwards checked in-hand action on the hard.

The duration and the time of year for a rest period will vary with the discipline involved. The horsemaster will have managed the horse accordingly and will have aimed for a return to work as determined by the future dates within that competitive discipline. In general, an 8 week programme of fittening is the minimum. During the later weeks lower level work within the discipline will be practicable and advisable.

At the end of the rest period the horse will come up having been accustomed to a steady trickle diet based on grass; in good to fat 'soft' condition; unused to tack, grooming, and restrictions in its environment and activity.

It is the management of the necessary changes which requires skill, understanding and patience. Careful change especially from grass to conserved grass and then to concentrates, with possibly cereal straw bedding from the start, are essential to

- prevent digestive disorders and the risk of impaction
- prepare for the metabolic stresses of high energy feeding which will eventually be required
- balance the slow work induced loss of fat with the desired overall condition *vis à vis* the development of muscle

The basic *dietary change* should be made over 10 days. Concentrate feeding, unless as a carrier for prescribed supplements and/or as a 'sop' to the stabled horse which, from experience, will expect such a feed, is unlikely to be nutritionally necessary for 3 to 4 weeks. A convalescent mix is ideal if manger feeds are essential during this time.

Daily access to grazing will be part of the change-over programme, both for digestion and for relaxation and free activity. Beware of using lush pasture grass or exercise paddocks from which faeces have not been routinely cleared.

Coincidental with the husbandry changes from rest to work, the horsemaster must see to the immediate aspects of horse care in a more critical manner, i.e.

- state of skin, coat and general condition
- shoeing

- dentistry
- vaccinations

all with veterinary input if necessary

- veterinary inspection, especially if a dis-order was previously present
- recording of the vital parameters and body weight

and to plan ahead for the ultimate discipline targets

- the intermediate competition dates suitable for training within the overall fittening programme
- the advance ordering and/storing of fodder and forage
- when to clip
- the final check on
  - tack
  - clothing
  - transport
  - competition entries
- future preventative therapies

Stage 1 – Management Changes

Leisure horses do not have a 'close season' but between 'clock changes' the opportunity to ride is minimal unless good illuminated surfaces are available. Most such horses can live out throughout the year with the usual protection against cold, and supplements against poor grass in the winter – and care against excessively good grass (and flies) in the summer. Holidays for them are usually when the owner is away. They can be ridden from winter grass, but

- ponies and horses with a heavy coat should have no sweating work and no serious grooming, just over saddle and girth lightly
- other horses, if clipped out and NZ rugged, can do work commensurate with fitness – but must get dry and warm before being re-rugged and put out afterwards

Forward planning is not so critical for the non or lower competition horse. Feed changes are just as important, although an abrupt change from grass to stable is unlikely.

Stage 2 – Conditioning

Dependent on previous use, recent history and proposed future use, conditioning takes 4 weeks on average.

The aims are to accustom the horse to

- stabling
- handling
- routine controlled life
- feeding and feedstuffs – changeover
- grooming and strapping etc.
- tack and clothing (check saddle fit and again in 4–6 weeks)
- being ridden to 'harden' the connective tissues, stimulate all the systems and, importantly, to reduce unnecessary body fat

1. 'Hardening' the Connective Tissues

Whilst this slow work does not put all tissues to full stretch, the limited but controlled stress of stretch, compression and concussion on

- hoof horn
- interlocking laminae
- ligaments
- cartilage
- synovium
- tendons
- bone
- skin

does start to progressively condition all these tissues and in particular the collagen on which all are built, as well as the primary formative cells.

It is a necessary process to minimise the risk of overstress trauma in the coming faster work, either on hard or on extra soft surfaces.

Horses which have run free, at rest, on hard plains, prairies, steppes, etc. are already conditioned in the first respect. When put to work they are unlikely to 'meet' harder surfaces. They are not usually in initial overfat condition. Further but limited conditioning and subsequent fittening refine them for carrying a weight and for doing so faster and for longer periods.

Those such as in the UK and Ireland resting on usually wet (soft to firm, occasionally hard) pastures may spend much of their competition season 'going on the soft'. When the weather improves the horse is suddenly required to carry weight swiftly on hard going to which he has not been previously conditioned, and *it is then that some types of overstress will be more likely.* When and where possible some hard surface work, even if only road walking must be done.

Balance and action on soft going will come with practice.

The skin's outer layers of epidermis form its 'soft' surface. Although it is composed of dead cell layers the deeper most recently formed ones can be stressed into having denser, more compact keratin which acts as a greater protection to the 'live' deeper layer, or dermis, with its profuse capillary blood supply, hair follicles, sweat and sebaceous glands infolded into its depth, as well as the sensory nerve endings.

Damage occurs in two ways

- **pressure** with some friction, as from the saddle. The friction breaks the hairs, but more importantly the pressure causes interference with the flow of blood and intercellular fluid. As a consequence, blood serum and sometimes whole blood is pressurised to leak towards the surface and to lift the epidermal layer into a blister or gall. The swelling, and the possible eventual raw surface, is the source of pain. Secondary infection to cause a septic dermatitis may follow in the opened area

- **strong friction** with some pressure as from the girth. The affected area, as can be understood, is more elongated. Hairs are more widely broken and the epidermal surface is partly rubbed away. Blisters are less common in this site, but rawness predominates. The secondary infection is very often that of ringworm spores

- **friction only**, as over the neck from the rub of the reins. Usually slower in developing and often not until after clipping; also a site for ringworm

Prevention

- groom areas thoroughly to stimulate and tone
- tack up just sufficiently securely to keep saddle in place
- leave in box for 2 hours on first day
- tighten one hole more in each of the next 3 days and exercise without a rider for 15 minutes gradually increasing to 30 minutes
- thereafter for the next week tack up, leave just secure for half an hour before initial warming up in hand, and later tighten for riding on day 4 as further described

The bars of the mouth, covered with gum epidermis, are not so readily or easily abraded but leaving bridled as above for other tack will slowly condition them and the skin at the lip commissures. Later sores are another matter – rider/horse problem.

Hoof horn grows from the 'quick' of the coronet. It is a specialised skin composed of many quill-like tubules in the wall and flat layers on sole and frog. Pressure and friction problems do not arise in early conditioning as with skin, but the strength of the wall tubules does respond to footfall concussion and so strengthens as a result, even in the shod foot.

The **sole**, though 'off' the hard road, does indirectly benefit from the exercise. It takes surprisingly little concussion to trigger the response, after early conditioning, 10 minutes of trotting on the hard per day and, of course, plenty of walking. Conversely, too much and too severe, as from excessive and fast trotting on the hard, will over-concuss or jar with a damaging effect on the vascular supply and subsequently on the deeper tissues and the coffin joint.

The **frog** responds in a like manner.

Tendons and ligaments – there is no *direct* evidence of concussive or compression benefits from walking and trotting, but the increasing limb movements do stretch them and this, in itself, is beneficial to the 'tone' of the intrinsic cell and surrounding collagen matrix. Conversely, jarring can occur when work is done on the hard for too long and/or at too great a speed. Later fitting work will further 'train' these tissues to withstand slight overstretch on too soft, slippery and/or holding surfaces as well as against hard surface vibratory jarring.

Cartilage – a complex protein/carbohydrate material, acts as a shock absorber and as a lubricated frictionless joint surface. It does so by absorbing and ejecting the water of the joint oil or synovia. Being made to work, progressively its vitality and effectiveness are improved.

There is definite evidence that **bone**, especially in the limbs, responds to concussion, compression and torque. Extra bone is strategically laid down on the lining of the marrow cavity to give critical strength. It is thought that the basic bone becomes denser and stronger, in geometrical design and physiological integrity, by 10 minutes trotting per day on the hard; it does *not* become harder as is often thought. Increased trotting time on softer surfaces is necessary in the last week of conditioning. The gait at the walk and trot need not be above a working level.

2. Improving Suppleness
By making the horse walk then trot more 'out' as the days pass, joint movement range increases. The horse gets a spring in its step from the build-up of kinetic energy in tendons and ligaments as, e.g., the fetlock 'lets down' at weightbearing after the trot's suspension.

It stretches ligaments, and through the tendons, the muscles.

3. Stimulating the Controls of Movement and Metabolism
- the neuro-muscular system
- the hormonal system
- the enzymes

In practice, this stage is one of slow, progressively longer exercise. 'Long, slow work'.

Progressive regulated increases in levels of stress are effected, and to these the horse responds by improving in early fitness.

In addition to the above three aims the horse also begins to
- tone-up **muscles**, particularly the abdominals
- activate more powerful and faster **heart action**
- improve the general **circulation** by stimulating greater capillary bed involvement in the muscles
- improve **gaseous exchange** and open up quiescent alveolar areas
- 'burn off' **fat**

Fat stores in the resting, well-fed horse are laid down in specific subcutaneous areas and between muscle groups – resulting in the rounded, over-conditioned animal. They are also built up within the body cavities and especially within the abdomen, in the mesentery and the omentum, around the kidneys and particularly in the parietal ventral peritoneum – the inner belly. Through lack of intensive collected work, the resting horse also uses the abdominal muscles less – they sag under the weight of the fat and relatively larger amount of gut content.

Conditioning and appropriate feeding will slowly burn up the excess fat, thus reducing the abdominal weight. Conditioning will begin, and correct Stage 3 fitting with collection will develop the abdominal muscles. The horse will lose its grass belly and coincidentally become fit for asymmetric gaits which require flexion of the lumbar sacral articulation which is the dynamic responsibility of these muscles.

At the start of Stage 1 and thereafter, the following should be considered on a day-to-day basis
- the appearance, behaviour and general condition of the horse
- as work increases there is a greater need to check

- action in hand and under saddle, at walk and trot, over some 30 metres on a flat, hard surface and when turning in both directions, and

- the 'look and feel' of the limbs – compare with yesterday!

With practice, these observations will become almost automatic. To miss anything mild, especially in the limbs and action, risks more serious complications if work is done. This routine should be followed throughout a programme, especially for the high-performance animal.

A planned Stage 2 work programme might be as follows (remembering to check all contact areas after untacking each and every day, and sponge sweat off saddle and girth areas even though overall washing down is not yet necessary)

Week 1

Beginning after early conditioning to tack, *daily periods at grass*. In-hand loosening up and post-tacking passive stretches each day before work as now described

Day 1   15 mins walk on hard surfaces
Day 2   15 mins walk
Day 3   15 mins walk, but now 'in tack' which could have been fitted for an hour before work started, still in hand
Day 4   15 mins walk, still in hand, then 15 mins ridden (or led off another horse)
Day 5   30 mins ridden under saddle
Day 6   30 mins ridden under saddle
Day 7   30 mins ridden under saddle (no need for a day off yet)

A vigorous strapping every day is good practice.

The mornings of days 4, 5 and 6, provided the horse seems to have settled in, would be an ideal time to get the resting 'vital' signs measurements. If a horse is still unsettled, temperament-wise, this can be left for one or two weeks. These are

First – respiratory rate at rest

Second – heart rate (pulse) at rest

Third – temperature at rest, am & pm

The sequence is important. Any handling or undue noise will accelerate respiratory rate and heart rate. Quietly looking over stable door first will permit a respiratory count – at rest.

Haltering the horse next will cause a slight, short-lasting pulse rise: 'gentle' for 2 or 3 minutes, and it should be back to resting rate, ready to count. Then, with help and with care, take temperature. Do for three days: strike an average. Record.

These figures form a baseline for future comparisons. A routine blood test would give a further database, but this is not economically justified for any but high-performance horses.

At the end of the first week decide when and 'how' to clip.

Week 2

Day 1   40 mins ridden work, on hard surface on flat at walk
Day 2   40 mins ridden work, on hard surface on flat at walk
Day 3   40 mins ridden work, on hard surface on flat at walk
Day 4   40 mins ridden work, on hard surface on flat at walk including, in middle, 5 mins trot
Day 5   45 mins as on Day 4
Day 6   45 mins as on Day 5
Day 7   45 mins as on Day 6

Week 3

On firm grass or school surface.
Day 1   60 mins walk + 5 mins trot (mid-walk)
Day 2   60 mins walk + 5 mins trot (mid-walk)
Day 3   60 mins walk + 5 mins trot (mid-walk)
Day 4   60 mins walk + 5 mins trot + 2 x 5 mins trot at 20 mins & 40 mins after start (1 trot on hard, level surface if practicable)
Day 5   60 mins walk + 5 mins trot + 2 x 5 mins trot at 20 mins & 40 mins after start (1 trot on hard, level surface if practicable)
Day 6   60 mins walk + 5 mins trot + 2 x 5 mins trot at 20 mins & 40 mins after start (1 trot on hard, 1 trot uphill on firm surface, 1 on hard level surface if practicable)
Day 7   possibly a day off, if horse (or rider) seems in need of it. If so, then lead out to graze twice for 20 mins or turn out for *longer than on working days*

Week 4

Where possible use grass or prepared surface. More overall collection.

Day 1   80 mins ridden walk, including 2 x 5 mins trot (one uphill)

Day 2   80 mins ridden walk including 2 x 5 mins trot (one uphill)

Day 3   80 mins ridden walk including 2 x 5 mins trot (one uphill)

Day 4   80 mins and 2 x 10 mins, one uphill on soft to firm surface

Day 5   80 mins and 2 x 10 mins, one uphill on soft to firm surface

Day 6   80 mins and 2 x 10 mins, each uphill on soft to firm surface (use across hill as well). Walk down hill at this stage. A short trot on hard is still required

Day 7   day off: as for Week 3 Day 7, above

NB: When trotting up hills, adjust length to time so that you **trot to the top**. Do not trot downhill yet.

At the end of the first 4 weeks of conditioning work the decision as to moving on to Stage 3 or staying with Stage 2 is made on the ultimate degree of fitness required. A longer period in Stage 2 can pay dividends later.

It is a progressive programme and, as mentioned earlier, there is no clear demarcation.

Week 5

(If still on 'conditioning'.)

Day 1   2 hrs work – 40 mins walk on hard, 10 mins medium trot on soft, 40 mins walk on soft, 10 mins medium trot on soft. 5 mins trot on hard. Use hills for trotting wherever possible and across hills, both directions

Day 2   2 hrs work – 40 mins walk on hard, 10 mins medium trot on soft, 40 mins walk on soft. 10 mins medium trot on soft, 5 mins trot on hard. Use hills for trotting wherever possible and across hills, both directions

Day 3   2 hrs work – 30 mins walk on hard, 10 mins trot on soft, 10 mins **canter**, 5 mins trot on soft, 20 mins walk on soft or hard

Day 4   2 hrs – as for day 3 (add 5 mins to each trot or intersperse extra periods)

Day 5   2 hrs – as for day 4 (add 5 mins to each trot or intersperse extra periods; exchange 5 mins trotting on flat to cavalletti work, walk and trot

in the school or on soft to firm grass

Day 6   as for Day 4

Day 7   as for Week 3

The last trot and walk periods will in effect become the warming down time.

When the faster, asymmetric gait is introduced there is a need for more care

- pre-tacking
- correct tacking and techniques
- loosening up

Before the loosening-up work begins

- briskly groom or strap the fore and hindquarter muscle masses. Lightly strap or massage loin muscles. (See also techniques for passive stretches given below)
- in hand, turn horse quickly but carefully twice in both directions in box, bringing head and neck well round and getting him to cross hind legs over
- tack up, girth firm enough to hold saddle then for
- 'loosening up'
- bring out, walk both ways once in 10m circle. Push back several steps
- tighten girth as for mounting
- lift and extend each foreleg to pull skin under girth
    - flex each shoulder and pull back on extended fore leg
    - flex each hind leg high and lift slightly outwards then extend backwards (know your horse!)
- the carrot test is worthwhile, especially for older horses: tempt the horse to turn head and neck towards the chest wall, left and right, and then encourage head and neck down to eat the carrot at floor level; progress to between fore hooves. Spinal reflex stimulations will also help loosen up the back
- mount from 'leg up' or block
- ride off to warm up area

Cold-backed horses may need extra care.

Warm Up

Roughly 20 mins on loose rein, gradually collecting

- stimulates neuro-muscular and hormonal controls
- stimulates cardio-vascular system, capillary bed

opening and splenic emptying – the autonomic response to release extra red blood cells into the circulation

• stimulates respiration
• gives opportunity to check action under saddle and
• to adjust tack, especially the girth

Warm Down

15–20 mins slow trot into walk, onto loose rein

• to clear waste products from muscle cells etc.
• to continue heat regulation
• to continue limb circulation and lymph return flow
• to give opportunity to check heart and respiratory rates
• to check action at trot

After the warm-down, during recovery and dependent on fitness, the respiratory rate may continue faster than expected. Heat and humidity will influence this as will other factors within the horse itself.

Theoretically, the warming down should have the horse return home dry and breathing quietly, i.e. the oxygen debt will have been repaid. However, the opportunity should be taken to monitor the return of pulse and respiratory rates to resting normal even at these early stages of fittening. The limbs and feet should be inspected, as also the tack pressure areas. *Water may be offered once rates are halfway down or lower and half quantity of hard feed and succulents after the drink. Hay may be given after another hour.*

Later

In addition to usual stable routine check limbs for evidence of mild strain filling of cannon areas round sides and back. Give horse a good firm grooming or light strapping.

Next Day

Routine daily inspection. If a rest day, 20 mins in hand walk, and/or turn out for 2 x 20 mins grazing during the day. *Cut down feed to half that day.*

Week 6

As for Week 5, but more collection (flatwork) in all gaits

• increased trotting on soft, and add undulating terrain
• fast work on 3rd and 6th day (rest day on 7th, see above)

• increase these to 2 x 10 mins sessions
• increase hill work by 15%

Week 7

As for 6th week

• make certain to do 'the miles', and at least 5 mph at walk
• increase cantering to 1 x 10 mins and 1 x 15 mins
• increase hill work by another 5%

Week 8

As for 7th week. At end of the day's fast work, measure heart rate and respiratory rate and again when back at the stables.

The pre- and novice eventer will not require much faster work before the first event, but should have progressed to cantering over a course distance, but outside the time required after 6–7 weeks of Stage 2. In other words the last 2–3 weeks become, in fact, specific fittening work.

Cross-country and show jumping can be practised, in school with prepared fences – on days 1, 2, 4 and 5 or dressage movements as relevant. These activities will engage the propulsive muscles.

A crucial point for deciding on starting cantering work is, 'has the body weight dropped?' The assessment of this will relate to

• subjective appearance of
  • being thinner
  • muscle groups more clearly demarcated
• objectively measured by reduction in girth diameter
• feel of ribs, as if covered by skin and a thin layer of velvet
• lifting of belly floor

The cardio-vascular system to some extent, and the limbs even more so, could be over-stressed if asked to 'support' an overweight horse. Moreover, the heat control mechanism can be overtaxed.

A body-fat reduction, especially subcutaneous, causes condition score changes. The coincidental muscle development will further amend these. This is particularly important in the saddle area. Corrective re-flocking may be necessary at the end of the conditioning stage. Later when back, wither and shoulder muscles are well developed some further alterations should be considered.

By this time the cardio-vascular system will have been correctly progressively stressed as well as the locomotor muscular system. So too the respiratory system's gaseous exchange ability. To all intents and purposes the respiratory system cannot be trained. Synchronising breathing to symmetric gaits will be practised within **balanced** action.

The thermo-regulatory mechanism will have been activated and even at this point most horses should return to stables dry. Sweat at initial fast work is often soapy and dries scummy. It is also salty to the taste. **With fittening it flows clear, dries clean and loses the salt taste.**

In leisure horses which have not really been at rest but were put to Stage 2 in preparation for competitive work these weeks could be compressed

cantering could start in **Week 3** on good flat soft going or in a school (be careful of unbalanced horse on corners or circles) for 5 mins on 3rd day and again on 6th day as part of walking time: thus walk, trot, canter, trot, walk

Week 4 – 5 mins on 3rd day, and 10 mins on 6th day

At all times when cantering is done give time to warm up and down and cool off. Be more aware of leg interferences, injuries and early signs of overstress afterwards.

In the second month this type of horse could be given a 'jolly'. Use more undulating land with hills and different 'goings'. Small ditches can be negotiated as well as fallen trees (or poles and cavaletti in a school). Cantering uphill and across will give added benefit, twice weekly for 2 x 10 mins. Flatwork can be incorporated on days when faster work is not.

By this time fitness can be assessed and then a decision regarding the next stage can be taken. If 'weight' is to be carried at a competition it should be progressively carried in training.

Some Observations

There is a marked difference in the required levels of fitness between a Derby horse, an intermediate eventer and an RDA pony. The graduations up or down the athletic ladder do overlap, however.

A racehorse on the flat is trained to go a certain distance under a declared weight. Maximum anaerobic power cannot be increased by training, only 'reached' by careful training throughout and ultimate practice. It is rarely carried out during training, but short 'bursts' – 300 to 600m cantering at 200–250m/min progressively – in a balanced state are intermittently asked for; three-quarter speed in training usually suffices. The gallop ability is there to be asked for, as a rule, when required in a race or speed competition.

An eventer up to three-day event does not need maximum power (speed) but does have to be schooled in the skills necessary to successfully manage the cross-country and show-jumping difficulties set by the course designers and to finish within a certain time, without the stimulus of 'racing' against others. It should be able to go a little further than the competition will require but at a slower speed in this training. A full gallop is rarely required.

Both types must recover **in due course**, to go again. It is not a once-a-year, let alone a once-in-a-lifetime happening.

The RDA pony has to be biddable, quiet and 'understanding' in a school. In many situations it is also used for able riders and does, in fact, enjoy a 'jolly' provided it is without detriment to its prime use. Doing work keeps him fit, but must not encourage galloping!

The leisure horse, the novice eventer, the Grade C Jumper or lower, doing possibly 2 hours medium work a day, should be doing a daily mileage at walk and trot of around 15 (90 per week) and is fittening and strengthening as it works at its school work and other skills as well. Jumping, as has been said, is strength anaerobic work: strength comes from practice, not fittening. In practising, progressively, the explosive anaerobic power should build up.

Cantering must play a part in general fittening and vitality, but **galloping is not only unnecessary for most types but decidedly risky to the horse,** however much fun it might be to the rider!

The key to fitness is progressive work. When a certain distance in a certain time has been done without undue tiredness and certainly without exhaustion (fatigue), it can be said that the horse has responded to the stress and is now ready to be carefully stressed further.

The 'slower' type, and competition, horses keep themselves fit – for weeks on end – by working. They will remain plump, well covered, but underneath that their muscles should be developing. Only time will slim them down to some extent and, of course, no 'sentimental' feeding!

Days off are not essential, but if it so pleases the rider then do so but **reduce hard feed**, even rich roughage, **on** *that day, the night before and the morning after*. Such horses should be turned out to grass or, at least, put into a large yard for free if limited exercise. If the break is more than 4 days, go easy with faster work on first day back.

If longer rides are contemplated then do so instead of faster or more intensive exercising days, and slightly cut down the work on days either side. Step up the feed appropriately on the day of the longer ride. The duration of the ride could be split into two periods with a reasonable rest between, e.g. a circular 'picnic' ride of some 20 to 30 miles of walk, trot and canter, could have an hour's lunch break, provided sensible arrangements are made for stabling or grazing the horse during that time. In reasonable conditions of 'weather and going' the 30 miles could be completed in a round journey of 5 to 6 hours actual riding.

Stage 3 – Fittening

At all levels of fitness, 'fast' work days should be restricted to **2 per week**, especially for this advanced stage.

Pre-requisites

- rider – fit, well balanced mentally and physically, of more than average ability
- management – horse and stable
  - able to forecast potential of horse
  - knowledgeable about
    - feeding
    - grooming
    - hoof care
    - selection, fit and care of tack
    - transport
- on a day-to-day basis
  - able to know 'all is well'
  - quick to know 'all is not well'
  - what to do
  - able to monitor progress
    - subjective assessment
    - objective/scientific further assessment
  - good working knowledge of the disciplines involved and the effects of the variables which might occur, e.g.
    - weather
    - 'going'
    - terrain

- hazards
- technicalities
- and the requirements of the competition or event concerned, e.g.
  - weight to be carried
  - distance
  - time limits
  - difficulty factors

Performance Ability

- is structural and functional related
- can only be as good as weakest part of these
- is very dependent on management as well as riding
- improves by training and practising
  - a healthy horse can be got fit – within its genetic potential
  - an unhealthy horse cannot be got fully fit
  - but a conditioned, chronic unsound horse can be got relatively fit – consider COPD and laryngeal paresis

From grass rest to medium fitness or lower grade work will take 6 to 8 weeks, i.e. some 2 weeks into this stage in some cases. From grass rest to elite fitness and ability, 12 to 1 weeks. This is all relative to

- age
- previous fitness and training
- starting point – length of rest
- previous feeding – weight
  - in-between competitive work

Horses, in comparison to human athletes, lose conditioning and fitness slowly.

As a rough guide

- if off all work, the fitness reached goes after 4 weeks. If doing only slow walking, work after 6 weeks
- if off **all** work full, conditioning also goes after 6 weeks but, if less than 6 weeks, only 4 days road work (walk mins, trot 10 mins) will stimulate connective tissue responses and fitness returns with faster work after 2 weeks or so

The hoped-for performance requires an economical actio dependent upon

- balance
- obedience
- speed
- endurance or stamina
- pace
- strength
- skill – agility
- spirit – ability
- durability – part constitution, part fittening related

Most performance horses (except racing) up to three-day eventers mainly work aerobically; explosive work will involve anaerobic effort, as in jumping, and in advanced dressage, short distance and galloping if required. Horses have a greater intrinsic anaerobic potential than man.

Training increases aerobic and lactate threshold so delaying the need for anaerobic work. Practice increases strength – do it, repeat it.

Long, **fast** work up to submaximal speed and endurance may over-stress each time, with high risk of strain. Long, **low** work does not, but does develop heart and circulation; all gaseous exchange systems seem to benefit coincidentally.

Regulated or interval training for 'speed and endurance' stresses with minimal risk of strain. Strength equates with speed, which equates with muscle bulk, so as in humans, endurance helps speed improvement, but not *vice versa*. Endurance athletes do not want the weight of bulk, so speed work is not for them. In horses this is not yet proved, but is thought to be so.

Some differences are, e.g. a 14 hh Welsh pony will carry 200 kg (14 stone) shepherd at the walk, for hours in a day; but trot for 100 yards uphill, and it will be exhausted.

An endurance horse will complete 100 miles at average speed of 8 mph – walk, much trotting, some cantering. Gallop on, and it will be lucky to do a marathon distance without disaster.

A Grade A jumping track of under 2 minutes is quite possible for a strength-practised, up to end of Stage 2 conditioned horse. Ask it to do so for more than 5 minutes and fatigue will set in, unless there is a 5 to 10 minute break in jumping.

An intermediate, fit eventer will easily do a cross-country course in up to 10% slower than the set time; but push on for 10% faster, and fatigue will set in, in most cases.

Complicate a three-day-eventer's round with high temperature and humidity along with the roads and tracks and steeplechase, then heat exhaustion becomes a risk unless the rider slows down *considerably* and thermo-regulation is well managed.

In 4 or more weeks of the combined **Stages 3** and **4**, several targets are in sight
- increased muscle development, giving
  - increased power, through
    - improved energy conversion
    - recruitment of fast twitch fibres, and
      - the training of these for high oxidative metabolism for better oxygen utilisation
- enlargement of skeletal muscle capillary 'bed'
- increased strength and rate of heart muscle contraction, giving greater blood volume flow
- increased red blood cell size and efficiency, with increased haemoglobin content
- more efficient oxygen transport and gaseous exchange
- raised lactate threshold
- improved fat metabolism, to augment glucose use
- improved neuromuscular coordination and 'eye in', for balance and agility and accuracy
- increased adrenal cortex activity, other hormonal and enzyme action, all for improved performance, as well as
  - 'relaxation' without loss of motivation

and specific targets reached
- psychological familiarity
- improved thermo-regulation, so that there is
  - longer fatigue-free aerobic activity at faster speeds
  - faster heart and respiratory recovery rates
  - better anaerobic strength

Feeding will have been increased from about the beginning of the second week of Stage 2, but even now should always be 'behind' work being done. *Giving more on a few days before in anticipation of a hard day or a competition is not only a waste of money but can be detrimental:* if nothing else, it 'overheats' the horse. More the night before and during that day is sensible. Equally important is cutting down all hard feed on day off: not merely cutting out one ingredient.

Stage 3, including skill training, stage 4, can take 2 months, especially when Interval Training (IT – see below) is used, but generally one will suffice. It is a matter of long slow and then short fast continuous or intermittent, progressively faster work outs. Lower grade competitive work on the flat or over show jumps, and such as hunter trials and the Swedish 'Fartlek', are all possibilities – they give excitement and break the monotony!

The following suggestions are just that. Regularity in the training programme is what matters.

Interval or intermittent training (IT) refers to what is done on any one day. It is repeated twice weekly and, all going well, stepped up in intensity each week. Some horses 'recover' more quickly than others, but periods between should not be less than 3 days. (Competition days count as IT).

The aim of IT is to stress the systems without risking fatigue and subsequent injury. The horse is permitted a *partial* rest to trot or to walk after fast stage, when the heart is still well above rest rate and all the exhaust products are not completely cleared from the blood and lungs. It is then made to go faster again. In the later weeks he may go 3 or even 4 times and progressively for longer, faster work with shorter intervals. One must also do one to two hours slow work, walking (and some trotting, preferably uphill) to maintain a *total* mileage of approximately 60 per week for 2 more weeks, (the fit horse especially, and a horse in lower grade competitions but working up to its final target, can get by with less 'road' work, and it certainly should not be trotted on the hard for more than 5 minutes) with jumping, grid or flat work on the 3 other days, IT on 3rd and 6th and a rest on the 7th.

In addition to earlier suggestions for pre-work management it is beneficial to groom briskly and/or strap and repeat this after recovery on return to stable. Continue during Stage 4.

Week 1

Loosening, passive movements each work day as described.

Day 1 warm up, 20 mins at walk on hard or soft
warm up, 10 mins at trot on soft
school for 40 mins, at trot on soft school for 10 mins at canter
warm-down 20 mins, at trot and walk on hard or soft

Day 2 as above, but use school jumping and/or flatwork for the canter

Day 3 as above, but replace schooling or jumping with IT

Days 4 & 5
as for Day 1 and Day 2

Day 6 as for Day 3

Day 7 rest, but hand walk and graze 2 x 20 mins, or turn out to grass for longer than on work days

NB: **Never trot for more than 5 mins on the hard.** It not necessary to do any hard road work above walk aft end of Stage 2. It may be counter-productive.

Week 2

Day 1 as for Week 1, above
Day 2 as for Week 1, above
Day 3 IT
Day 4 as for Week 1, above
Day 5 as for Week 1, above
Day 6 as for Week 1, above
Day 7 as for Week 1, above

Week 3

Day 1 as for Week, 1 but replace canter with a countr 'jolly'
Day 2 as for Week, 1 but replace canter with a countr 'jolly'
Day 3 IT instead of canter
Day 4 as for Week 1, but replace schooling and 'jolly' with show jumping/dressage competition
Day 5 as for Week 1, but replace schooling and 'jolly' with show jumping/dressage competition
Day 6 as for Day 3
Day 7 as for Day 3

In the 3rd week and thereafter, weekly mileage can reduced to 40 miles walking.

Week 4

Day 1 as for Week 1, but on 'jolly' use increasing hill
Day 2 as for Week 1, but on 'jolly' use increasing hill
Day 3 IT instead of schooling – do dressage betwe fast periods
Day 4 as for Week 1, but increase trotting by 15 min
Day 5 as for Week 1, but increase trotting by 15 min
Day 6 IT. At slower periods during breaks in fast wo do dressage at walk and trot
Day 7 as for Week 1

The IT canter speeds, and on 'jolly', should never exce 300 metres per minute to keep within aerobic exerc levels.

The 'jolly' is really a good hack across known country where small ditches, fallen trees and other suitable objects can be jumped. Slow loping canters as well as the walking and trotting needed for the day's mileage can be done. *Uphill and across hill work is essential.*

In the 4th week and thereafter, an increase in this intensity can be made – hunter trials, sponsored rides, etc. so that times, speed, distance and 'country' can be varied. It is similar to the Swedish 'Fartlek'.

Beware severe weather changes, and marked changes in 'going'. Remember the weight to be carried in the competition.

Interval training sessions should only be undertaken with the help of experienced instructors or trainers.

An example to fit into the four or more weeks of Stages 3 and 4 might be

Week 1   canter 5 mins, walk 5 mins, canter 5 mins, warm down

Week 2   canter 6 mins, walk 5 mins, canter 6 mins, warm down

Week 3   canter 4 mins, trot 3 mins, canter 5 mins, trot 3 mins, canter 5 mins, warm down

Week 4   canter 6 mins, trot 3 mins, canter 6 mins, trot 3 mins, canter 6, warm down

Week 5   canter 7 mins, trot 4 mins, canter 7 mins, trot 4 mins, canter 2 mins, warm down

Each session is done on Days 3 and 6. The heart and respiratory rates are checked at the end of each IT total session. An old but useful alternative to IT is to train the horse to go for **longer** than that of the actual competition but at a **slower** speed required; and to go **faster** than **maximum estimated speed** required over a **shorter** distance. Extra monitoring for after-effects is required.

In fatter or laggardly horses, the first 2 weeks of Stage 3 IT can be three sessions of trot at less than 240 metres per minute, with 2 walks of 3 minutes. Thereafter, progressively as judged necessary.

From Week 3, introduce cantering 2 x 2 mins at less than 300 metres per minute, with 'break' of 2 minutes trotting.

From Week 4, 3 x 2 mins at 300 metres per minute, with 2-minute trotting breaks.

From Week 5, 3 x 3 mins at 300 metres per minute, with 2-minute trotting breaks.

Extra weeks may be required, but with only minor increases, if at all, in speed and repetition. See also 'pipe openers', below.

Short distances at over 600 metres per minute (Thoroughbred gallop) is anaerobic practice for sprint speed. *In all but flat sprinters, gallop practising to generic maximum is not required.* Some flat sprint trainers consider that this is not only unnecessary but is also risky to joints, bones, ligaments and tendons.

A programme should be individually designed.

Some gait speeds to produce a heart rate are

- medium walk   to reach 80 bpm
- trot   at 240 m per minute to reach 120 bpm
- canter   at 300 m per minute to reach 160 bpm

        at 360 m per minute to reach 200 bpm (this could be into anaerobic work)

Whatever the gait, the heart rate must be at the above on first attempt during the relevant Stage, in order to 'stress' the heart. In practice, by the time the rider has dismounted to take the reading they will have dropped to approximately 60, 80, 85, or 90 bpm.

On-board heart monitors will, of course, be more accurate for maximum work heart rates. Whilst getting to these rates is important, *it is the recovery rate which matters.* A rider's reading, after dismounting, should be between top reading and known resting normal, in 10 to 15 minutes.

However, before dismounting, read the rate when the horse is pulled up at the end of the last stretch of fast work, then ask it to 'go on' again for a short distance. If it does so willingly, immediately stop. If it does not, i.e. 'it drops the bit', investigate fatigue factors soon afterwards.

Heart respiration readings are of most use after the **first** (increased) fast or total IT work each week. Provided you do it at same time, it may be easier to give a 5 min trot before stopping and/or dismounting. In all situations the horse must be warmed down slowly thereafter; take temperature then.

The heart muscle can be specifically trained by short (one minute) bursts of speed, 'pipe openers', at around 300+ metres per minute plus. The warming up of walk, trot and canter, the burst, and canter/trot/walk is usually done on the day before a competition, or once weekly. In more advanced training, two half spells of fast work are intervalled by 2 minutes trotting. It lessens risks of leg injuries, as fatigue is less likely. This is a form of IT.

It must be realised that the suggested programmes for all

the stages are just that, suggestions. The time factors in Stage 2 are more precise out of necessity, but in Stages 3 and especially Stage 4 the trainer must use her own judgement for the individual animal. In IT the repetitions, the duration of hard work, to the interval of slower work between, the time, speed (and so the distance) are all variable; it is the principle of IT that matters.

Clinical Assessment of Fitness

By the Rider

- reached set objectives
- recognised horse's desire to go on
- first, heart rate and respiratory rate readings, as above

By the Trainer

- monitored physiological factors at 15 and 30 minutes after fast work
- inspected other parameters of 'all is well'

In more detail, that the horse

In the box	– is settled, excretes normally, eats and drinks well. All systems are normal
At exercise	– ready, willing and able
At measured work	– targets reached. Heart and respiratory rates normal. Respiratory noise normal
After work	– resting recovery rates normal. Thermo-regulation satisfactory. Temperature returns to normal inside 30 minutes
Next day	– action assessed in hand, or under saddle if necessary, is satisfactory
Weight	– as required, no loss of condition.
Results	– hindsight!

The leisure, low grade competition horse will, as previously emphasised, continue to fitten as it is used. Assessment in these situations is the subjective 'feel'

- does it do the work?
- does it want to do more that day, and go again tomorrow?
- does it hold its weight and bloom?
- as well as other A B C signs

As the intensity of work increases then extra, more objective, parameters are required.

Both rider and trainer should 'know the horse' and be able to record that, especially in competitions, it is doing the distance, in the time, with ease over terrain and obstacles, retaining enthusiasm, and meeting the requirements suggested above. Most importantly that there are no signs of leg 'reactions', and certainly no lameness.

Beware during fitness assessment (which is usually twice weekly after 'fast' sessions, or once after step up day)

- a *heart rate greater than expected* – this usually suggests pain. Check action, check tack zones, check mouth
- a *heart rate that is slower to recover* – suspect incipient metabolic upset. Check urine (being passed? colour?), check action behind, and check quarter and loin muscle for stiffness and pain (setfast?)
- a *respiratory rate greater than expected* – suspect intercurrent infection, and check for cough, nasal discharge, off food
- a *respiratory rate slower to recover* – suspect incipient metabolic upset

or it could be that progress was too quick for this horse. *If any disorder is perceived, seek advice.* If all seems normal next day, reduce next IT to previous lower level and start again from there.

If any of the four are 'wrong', *always take temperature*

- temperature higher than 39°C (102.5°F), monitor again at 15 then 30 minutes. If temperature higher than these for more than 30 minutes, *get the vet.*

After fast work and/or jumping carefully check in-hand action at walk and trot, later that day and on the next day before work. Feel legs regularly.

Exertion not Exhaustion

The competitor requires good *exertion* from the horse and should accept this in return for success, or at least completion without injury but with a degree of tiredness which wears off quickly.

Fatigue

Can develop at any stage of training. It is the inability to maintain a given exercise of predetermined intensity (speed, duration, difficulty). It is usually associated with increased work, longer duration, rise in ambient temperaure and humidity, illness or pain, and is caused by

- neuromuscular impairment
- energy production impairment
- limitations of fuel supply

Thus in high intensity work, i.e. greater than 400 metres per minute, or in slower work in adverse weather condi-ions, there is a rise in lactate level and a fall in pH in muscle cells.

In prolonged sub-maximal work, i.e. less than 400 m/m, here can be dehydration – excessive sweat loss, electrolyte imbalance, upset thermo-regulation – and, where there is depletion of glycogen, oxygen debt, and unavailability of free fatty acids.

There can, of course, be a combination of these. All lead to

- reduced circulation
- reduced perfusion of heart, brain and kidneys (the vital organs), especially if electrolyte or thermo-regulation are involved

Recovery is usually quick but **pain** or general discomfort is often evident. It is a matter of 'too far, too fast, too soon' in a particular stage of work. It is often associated with over-(wrong) feeding and under-working in days or even weeks previously.

If intercurrent problems, especially of respiratory and/or digestive systems, are present they may predispose to

- over-stress – strain
- metabolic upset

and low grade locomotor pain may also do so.

Recognition of Fatigue

During work the rider becomes aware

- horse drops bit
- needs encouragement
- does not respond
- drops head and neck
- breathes more noisily
- starts brushing fences
- changes leads and/or disunites
- changes rhythm 4 x to 3 x if gallop has been engaged
- begins to 'interfere'
- begins to stumble
- alters stride, length and rate to minimise weight-bearing and to ease muscles

At finish

- horse becomes imbalanced on slowing down, changes leads often repeatedly – weakness in fatigued postural muscles
- goes (too) quickly into trot, which causes overstress on the braking system

Afterwards

- there is prolonged oxygen debt repayment time
- a staggering gait and 'drooping'
- slow jugular and gum refill times
- skin-fold delay
- may go into exhaustion and/or heat stress syndrome

During work, and especially in a competition, the fatigued horse may

- fall and stay down
- injure itself before, and when falling
- get up unless injury prevents this
- strain ('break down') limb structures, without falling

Exhaustion

Being down and winded is a form, usually triggered by the tired horse falling at an obstacle

- the horse may collapse on the course
  - stay down
  - get up, but be weak or ataxic
  - keep falling down
- or collapse afterwards, as above
  - show a series of system upsets
  - die

These two extremes of work overstress should not happen.

Remember: any competition can be unexpectedly complicated by temperature/humidity increases, 'going' changes, or sudden adverse weather (e.g. driving rain just before or during an event), as well as by course builders' plans being more technical than trained for.

Heat Exhaustion

Prolonged sweating with excess loss of water and electrolyte, leading to

- failure of further sweating
- exhaustion

- loss of appetite *and thirst* (this last possibly associated with excessively low blood sodium lost in sweat)
- no urine passed
- temperature rise to 40.6°C (105°F) or higher
- increased respiratory and heart rates, with irregularities in heart rhythm, 'thumps'
- rhabdomyolysis (ER)or setfast
- colic (decreased intestinal motility)
- panting
- rigors
- alkalosis, with a fall in chlorine and a rise in potassium in the blood, as judged by lab examination of a blood sample – retrospective findings
- loss of anal tone
- coma
- death

Beware of competing when the sum of the temperature (expressed in °F) and the humidity (as a %) is greater than 150, especially if humidity accounts for more than half of the sum – *risk is high*. If greater than 180 – *don't compete.*

With or without these atmospheric complications, fatigue and exhaustion can become a greater risk, especially in endurance riding if hills and valleys are integrated with the distance. Not only do they require greater physical effort but humidity and temperature are often higher in narrow valleys.

There is also possible overstress associated with long-distance air transport. Horses can lose up to 30 kilos in body weight through sweat loss – more than they would in an elite competition. Seven days recovery may be required after a 9-hour flight.

MISTAKES IN MANAGEMENT

Mistakes may well handicap the fittening programme
- incorrect feedstuffs
  - mineral imbalances
  - too 'rich' cereals, especially high in glucose sources
  - too little fibre
  - mouldy material
- incorrect feeding
  - irregular times

- too much in manger, with long intervals between
  - rapid changes
- injudicious times for worming/vaccinating
- missed acquired conformational defects – incorrect trimming and shoeing, and
- ill-fitting tack (condition changes *vis à vis* saddle)
- changes in rider/trainer techniques: unsettled performance stress
- inconsiderate transporting – stress, dehydration
- failure to appreciate changes in weather, terrain, predisposing to
  - fluid imbalances
  - thermo-regulatory imbalances in and after competing
- failure to appreciate slight 'hiccoughs' in training schedule
- failure to appreciate possibility of contact virus infections at events, and need to monitor temperature of horse for next 7 days. *Elite athletes should have their temperature taken twice daily all through fit period and work*

Problems Associated with Training and Using

- locomotor over-stress, possibly leading to lameness
  - strain
  - hyper concussion – jarring
  - hyper compression
  - hyper extension of fast action joints, e.g. knee and fetlock
- metabolic over-stress
  - tying up, rhabdomyolysis (ER), with or without electrolyte imbalances as judged by lab tests
- minor loss of appetite and changes in thirst leading to low grade dehydration/electrolyte deficits
- gastric ulcers – stress induced as in young athletes
- respiratory dis-ease
  - viral
  - bacterial
  - fungal
  - allergic
  - 'bleeding'
- viral effect on cardio-vascular musculature and its neuro-control

- slower returns to resting pulse rate, possible arrythmias

temperament changes

- over the top – loss of interest
  - become stale
- been frightened
- been hurt: sub-clinical trauma will show up in fibrinogen increase in a blood sample. In poor performance syndromes investigations, which include blood sample analyses, it is now appreciated that an elevated fibrinogen level is of greater diagnostic and prognostic value than measuring haemoglobin levels. If fibrinogen is up *do not compete or hard exercise*
- transport defects' influence, heat stress, exhaustion from induced extra balancing requirements

Where such dis-ease situations arise, veterinary help is required for

clinical check-up and essential treatment

associated, 'aids to diagnoses' laboratory investigations, comparison with earlier database

further techniques

- radiography
- ultrasonography
- scintigraphy
- endoscopy and, in some more obscure cases
- electrocardiography
- muscle biopsy
- pulmonary function tests
- biodynamic assessments of locomotion (but only for elite horses!)

Heat Stress

Muscular activity catabolises stored energy into biochemical power (25%) and into heat (75%). The heat is primarily stored; the body can accept a rise up to 40C° (104F), but higher than this necessitates action to lose heat from the core temperature by **thermo-regulation**, a form of homeostasis.

Only man and horse exercise or work sufficiently vigorously to require thermo-regulated sweating; in most other animals hyperthermia is an environmental issue.

The mechanisms for losing or transferring heat away from the vital organs and the other systems are

Radiation – the movement of heat from one object to another not in direct physical contact, e.g. large wave radiation from a horse into the atmosphere around it; short wave, as from the sun onto a body surface in the path of its solar rays

Convection – as when cooler air moves over the surface of a warmer object such as a horse's skin when there is an outward transfer of heat. Humidity has no effect on this. If the air movement is increased by a wind (or the horse moves at speed) the convection becomes 'forced' – the wind chill factor. The air can be artificially blown, as by a fan for controlling cooling in rest areas

Conduction – heat transfer between two surfaces of different temperature but in direct contact with one another, e.g. from working muscle to in-contact body tissue such as blood flowing through them. The blood in turn loses heat to other tissues such as the skin where it is lost by radiation, convection and, when necessary, by evaporation

Evaporation – from moisture either in exhaled air or on the skin surface following the secretion of sweat onto it. Evaporation, in the horse, is the main form of excess heat loss, especially in warm weather which reduces the convection route.

Excessively hot weather, especially if accompanied by high humidity (the atmosphere can take on less, and more slowly, evaporated moisture), reduces further convection and limits radiation. Heat is dissipated more slowly and body temperature rises more quickly.

Biological methods can be augmented by

- dowsing down with ice-cold water, which increases conduction and supplies more in-contact water for evaporation and 'scraping off' as later described
- reducing solar radiation by keeping the horse in the shade in rest periods
- walking the horse (in the shade), to mimic increased air movement
- using fans, to the same end during breaks in and/or after high-intensity work

Exercise-induced body core temperature rise up to 40°C (104°F) is beneficial for continuing work. The mild hyperthermia of warming-up work (which protects against environmental cold) enhances enzymatic metabolism to give better force output of

- skeletal muscle
- cardiac muscle
  - increased oxygen delivery
  - overall better performance or exercise capacity

If heat rise continues, due to excessive work in excessive heat or failure of heat loss mechanisms, there will be unwanted effects, disorders of

- central nerve system functioning with ataxia and disorientation
- muscle metabolism, skeletal and cardiac, when
  - enzymes which are heat-labile fail to function at high temperatures
  - other hormonal-neural dysfunctions are decreased, leading to
    - dehydration and electrolyte loss
- sweat gland exhaustion with general
  - illness, and finally
    - death

Compared to man, the horse has a relatively less effective body surface area from which to radiate heat. It not only heats up to a greater extent but does so more quickly. It must compensate by a better sweating potential, and this it does.

However, even this inherited ability can be hazarded by work and 'weather'. Any horse at any competitive discipline, at any level, in any country, can suffer heat (over-) stress; even ponies at gymkhanas. A hot environment is one where the ambient temperature is above 26°C (80°F).

Cooling

Cold-water cooling is a satisfactory method if it is applied correctly. It can cool down hot horses rapidly, immediately after becoming hyperthermic, thereby speeding overall recovery and so reducing the risk of heat (over-) stress and coincidentally making their return to competitive fitness not only more likely but without the need for overlong recuperation. There is no evidence of any unwanted side-effects such as ER to the method advised.

This method depends upon augmenting convection and evaporation. The equipment required is

- very large buckets
- large blocks of ice
- cold water supplies, either from hose or (insulated) tanks
- two ordinary buckets, or supplement tubs
- three assistants
  - one to hold
  - one working on each side of the horse
- a shady spot in which to work
- fans, if feasible

Begin immediately after the work stage is finished, whilst taking the temperature. Liberally apply ice-cold water to *all parts* of the body, *including the quarters* where the bulk of the muscles are. *Do not* scrape excess water after each application, but carry on cooling for 20 to 30 seconds, then walk the horse around for 20–30 seconds. Continue this sequence; walking promotes vital circulation to muscles, to carry away by-products but especially it pushes air over the skin for cooling by convection and evaporation.

Check temperature at intervals, e.g. after a walk period but while still wetting. It should fall by about 1°C (2°F) in 10 minutes. Let the horse drink cool water (12 gulps at a time) with a choice of one supply with electrolytes at any competition breaks, and let it do so twice if it wishes or there is time available at 5 minute intervals. Internal heat loss is helped by conduction. *Do not* put ice in the drinking water. Stop cooling when, or if, the temperature is less than 38–39°C (100.4–102.2°F) and/or when the quarter skin remains cool after a walking period, if the respiration rate is less than 30 and/or if the horse shivers when put on a light rug.

Do not put ice into the horse's rectum – false temperature readings may result. *Do not* concentrate ice on focal parts of the body, or apply towels (which will soon dry out and act as a heat retainer).

Limit application of grease if overheating is present in the 10 min box. It will insulate skin where it is applied, and so minimise heat loss during the cross-country phase. *Do not* let the horse stand still for lengthy periods until well cooled down, obviously normally, and looking for grazing.

Feed hay and hard feed up to 4 hours *before* work starts. Leave water in stable until 15–30 minutes before leading away. Remember to always warm up before and where possible warm down, but *controlled cooling when necessary is paramount*.

Offer increased amounts of water as the horse eats, giving preference for plain or for electrolyte added as shown by the horse.

The End of the Season

When the competitive season is over it is not just a matter of removing shoes and turning out to grass.

'Let down' means slowly reducing hard feed and of changing grass for hay, etc. over 7 to 10 days, before roughing off. Continue to see the horse trot up, on hard, each day during this time. Critically inspect for low-grade sub-acute injury. Use professional and *specialist techniques* if necessary. Critically evaluate state of feet and need for remedially shoeing, for one set at least.

Rehabilitation

In convalescence, it is important to minimise residual pain and obviate a recrudescence of pain during this time by free movement – exuberant or uncontrolled – too much, too soon.

In rehabilitation, free movement out at grass or loose in school, remains a hazard which, in terms of limb morbidities, is best avoided.

Management of the memory of pain is important. It will require time, patience and perhaps re-exposure to the particular circumstances for a regaining of confidence. It is important to

minimise the 'mental' effects of the memory of the original pain

- the apprehension that a certain action will hurt (again)

Allow time to recover from this fear by

- progressive re-exposure to
    - regain confidence

controlled exercise on natural and on contrived artificial surfaces.

This applies primarily to ground surfaces and eventually to

articular movements on natural or usual surfaces

articular movements over 'obstacles' as met in the course of the discipline requirements

Rehabilitation is often slower than physical recovery. During post-acute and sub-acute inflammation or immediate recovery time, many of the proprioceptor sensations will become out of tune especially if box or yard rest is totally involved. Short-period, progressive, under-control locomotion will allow more extended activity and the 'feel' of the ground whatever that surface is at that time.

When work restarts, all the various external inputs, and the associated or relevant proprioceptor inputs of faster movement on variable surfaces have to be re-learnt and slowly retuned.

This re-learning process is stimulated by

Day 1   3 minutes each rein at walk. Increase by one minute each day, up to 15 minutes each way. Exercise at ridden walk or in hand, twice daily, over different natural, widely separated, safe surfaces, from

- firm to softish to hard (smooth, as on roads) on the level, then
- uphill and downhill (graduated at first), as well as
- across, on both 'reins', then after two weeks or so progress to

Day 14   twice daily walking in hand (and one to two weeks thereafter trotting in hand) on six or so different surfaces (see below), again on the level and each about 6 metres (18 feet) long, whereby the horse 'feels' the marked changes in the surface, and so retunes its proprioceptive memory of these. Increase from 3 minutes by 1 minute each day until 15 minutes is achieved

The surfaces will vary from firm to soft, hard, water over hard, stony, muddy, as examples of what eventual use might encounter, but in a controlled fashion. It is essential to encourage the horse to look where it is going, and where it is placing its feet.

The redevelopment of the locomotor system

- the originally traumatised area
- the secondarily affected areas, e.g. muscle atrophy

may well require complementary support, such as

- judicious analgesia
- physical (manual and electronic) therapy
    - other disciplines

NUTRITION

INTRODUCTION

As described in Chapter 1, EVOLUTION, the horse prehistorically was a scansorial (i.e. able to stand on its hind legs to feed) browser. Presently, it is a

- cursorial (i.e. with legs evolved for running) grazer – with browsing instincts – for saplings!
- herbivore
- trickle feeder

The indigenous sub-types of horse which developed from Equus 'learned' to live off what grasses grew in its nomadic territory. It had become structured to do so in terms of

- prehension
- mastication and salivation

and functionally adapted to the required

- trickle feeding – little and often over most of 24 hours
- the prolonged, up to 70 hours, fermentative digestion in the large bowel, necessary for the high cellulose content of the predominant coarse grasses, with the constant production, absorption and metabolism of the derived **volatile fatty acids**, the precursors of glucose and so of the energy necessary for living and breeding. This included locomotive output in order to ingest sufficient and to do so safely – a maintenance-plus diet
- the nutritive value of such grasses was seasonally variable but it *usually* supported the cursorial grazer to meet its genetically programmed
  - growth rates
  - maturation
  - ultimate size (height) and relative body mass
- the horse, in starts and stops, adjusted to these in terms of

- climate
- soil structure
- the quantity and the quality of the growing grasses

Compare the Mountain and Moorland pony with a heavy cold-blooded horse. The morphological difference reflects the plant varieties that best grew in moorland and mountain as well as the adjacent terrains on which the ponies moved – compared with the more nutritious pastures of lowland countries.

The different digestive powers and **metabolic** capabilities between the pony and the horse must still be borne in mind in present-day management, not only with regard to feeding but also to drugs given.

Man, in prehistoric days, could survive over winter on hunted meat, berries and fruit which grew or remained 'on the branch' well into winter. Times became more difficult when 'game' became scarce. Farming man 'invented' ways of

- selecting certain grasses with particularly generous seed heads which he gathered and stored as 'meal'
- preserving grass cut at its 'height', for winter feeding of stock including horses no doubt coralled for overnight safety, i.e. herded
- increasing the cereal grasses, i.e. becoming an arable farmer, thereby being able to share the harvested and stored grain with his breeding stock, horses and others

without knowing just why, but well aware that what grazing maintained a horse in the summer was, in winter insufficient for its needs, especially if it worked and particularly if the climate was colder.

It became necessary to supplement the declining stores

he standard 'maintenance' ration with one suitable for
production'. Experience taught him that

hay was not as nutritious as grass – the horse needed
more and soon reached a level of satiated appetite but
still nutritionally short

grain had its energy value *concentrated* into a more
compact or denser volume, and could satisfactorily
supplement the maintenance to give the extra energy
for production or work

t was many hundreds of years before the astute observa-
ions by the early farmer could be described and explained
s 'essential nutrients' in terms of quality and quantity,
eflecting

energy (as available from solubles)

fibre, of which the cellulose was a vital energy potential

protein

lipid (oil)

minerals, especially calcium and phosphorus

trace elements

vitamins, along with

water

vere all fully understood.

Continuing experience established that grass supplied two
istinct but integrated requirements

roughage – the total fibre, which

- required mastication, which thereby
  - stimulated salivation
- acted as stimulus to gut motility, and
  - a significant part of which was cellulose,
    fermentable by micro-organismic activity in the
    hind gut to produce
    - energy precursors, the volatile fatty acids
    - vitamins
  - the remainder was lignin, which was not
    fermented but passed on through as 'bulk'

solubles, intracellular and in the sap, were compound
sugars which with protein, minerals, trace elements,
and vitamins, were enzymatically digested in the small
intestine having been prepared to some extent
previously in the stomach, and which were programmed
for absorption from the small gut. Some did pass
through into the lower intestine but, if in excess, were
detrimental

It is to this fundamental structural and functioning digestion which evolved to cope with the roughage of indigenous pastures, that man must tailor his domesticated
feeding regimes and especially so to supply supplementary
forms of soluble, concentrated energy for work superimposed on top of 'living' requirements.

Plants

Anchored to a small area of soil by their root system are

- a reflection of that soil's minerals
- able to concentrate (**anabolise**) energy via the sun's rays
  on the chlorophyl (**photosynthesis**) in their leaf
  system, and store them in the
  - stem
  - leaf
  - fruit, and in some species in
  - tuber
  - root

for their own use in growth and the formation of their seed
which is the main reserve store of starch to feed the seed's
embryo as it eventually germinates in the soil into which it
had fallen.

Animals

In particular, herbivores are free to roam, to seek out and
to consume what they instinctively require for nourishment in stem, leaf, seed (and tuber and root where these
two exist and are available). They **catabolise** this stored
energy in the plant's cells, the sap and the seed, and use
the freed energy for their living via their digestive and
metabolic systems.

Man

Can alter the soil's mineral and moisture content by
agricultural techniques, especially the application of
fertilisers and/or control, and/or alter his animal's grazing
environment as well as that herbage which is harvested
and fed as straw, hay and cereal seed, thereby amending –
for good or for ill – his animal's metabolism for living, as
well as for growing, breeding, working and keeping warm
in winter time.

Nevertheless 'all flesh is grass'; the animal's living and
production (work by the horse) reflect the nutritive value
of what grows from the soil.

The Plant Embryo

Encased in the **seed**, it is stimulated to germinate in the
soil when that naturally warms, but stays moist, in the

spring

- the germination puts down
  - a root system into the soil
  - a stem and leaf system above the soil into the atmosphere
- the energy from this primary growth is from the
  - starch nourishment in the seed, helped by the
  - associated vitamins, especially the B group and E
- the early root absorbs the inorganic
  - mineral salts usually common to most soils
  - trace elements indigenous to that soil
  - other elements which will influence the formation of the future amino acids, e.g. nitrogen and sulphur
  - water

These travel upwards in the form of watery sap, to surround and to enter the cellular structure of the plant's immature component parts – not unlike the extravascular fluid of an animal but without the pumping action of a heart. The salts are now in an ionised state as electrolytes.

The leaf system produces chlorophyl, which incidentally gives the green colour to the plant. This chemical is sensitive to the sun's ultra violet rays and produces energy to replace the rapidly used energy of the concentrated starch in the seed. During daylight hours, by the process known as **photosynthesis**, the action of the sun's rays on the clorophyl first causes water in the leaves to be split into oxygen (which is released *to the atmosphere*) and hydrogen; the hydrogen is combined with carbon dioxide (*from the atmosphere*) to form

- carbohydrates – known as **solubles**
- cellulose and lignin – **insolubles**
- **lipids** (oils)
- **amino acids** (the forerunners of protein) some of which utilise sulphur as well as nitrogen

all of which are **nutrients**, 'the staff of life', and

- **ionised minerals** and **trace elements** also as **salts** and
- **vitamins** – the micro nutrients which are *essential* for life

This metabolism is **anabolic**, it *stores* energy.

As a plant grows, the ratios between the macro-nutrients change. During active stem growth the cells are rich in solubles. As the stem matures and stops much of its growth, its role changes to become a structural conduction system for the predominant carbohydrates, cellulose and lignin. The protein content lessens as does the moisture content. Similar changes follow in the leaves but because of their required metabolic functioning they remain softer between a network of cellulose scaffolding; within which there remains a soluble-rich sap.

With increasing maturity the predominant store of concentrated energy moves towards the flower and eventually into the seed. The leaves are now richer in cellulose but still sappy, whereas the stem becomes more straw-like. This progression is important in deciding when to cut grass to make hay. If before flowering, the stem will still have some solubles in the sap and cellulose in the framework of the cells available as a source of energy from the bacterial fermentative digestion in the animal into volatile fatty acids.

This distinguishes hay from the straw of cereal crops plentiful in indigestible lignin with nearly all the starch concentrated in the multiheaded seeds or grains of whatever 'corn' has been grown. It is then that cereals are harvested; except for oat straw, others are often no better

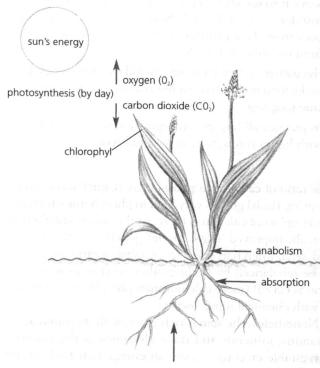

sun's energy

photosynthesis (by day)

oxygen (O_2)

carbon dioxide (CO_2)

chlorophyl

anabolism

absorption

water as a transporter of
minerals – major (Ca, P, Mg, K, Na, Cl, S, N) and
minor 'trace elements' (I_2, Fe, C, Co, Se, Mn, Mb, Sn)

'Nature' at work.

han bulk roughage or for bedding. The oat straw retains a
orthwhile proportion of cellulose, the others variably.

Growing grasses, as in permanent pasture where there
re several species each maturing at different times,
rovides a longer spell of nutritious grazing and a better
mple of hay in terms of bulk and of cellulose but
latively less soluble 'sugars'.

Ley hay is the richest but, as it is just one (or, at the
ost, two) species, getting economic bulk without risking
ver-maturity is difficult. Moreover, horses prefer variety,
pecially Timothy and some of the fescues. Their relative
ftness compared with the hardness of all rye grasses is
ot the disadvantage regarding mastication, salivation and
timate bulk once thought. (Man likes to think that a
oisy chew on rye hay must be more satisfying for the
orse! He anthropomorphises!)

Grass to be cut for hay presents difficult decisions, not
ast of all the problems of weather

let it grow to obtain maximum crop of stem and leaf

but cut it before flowering, and certainly before seeding
when much of the 'goodness' will have left the stem
and the leaf

leave it to seeding, and most of these will drop off to be
lost during the making. Whilst grass seed is relatively
poor in seed concentration, it has taken much away
from the stem and the leaf

the gathered stem (now straw) and the dying-back leaf
make for a harder hay – a less nutritious long fibre, a
true roughage

in practice all hay and all vegetation rich in cellulose
with lignin is **roughage** in feedstuff terms

he ratio of **calcium to phosphorus (Ca:P)** also changes.
owing (lush) grass is very high in phosphorus which also
cks up' what calcium is there, so the feed is unbalanced.
reals, improved 'grass' species grown as corn for grain
d seed, when harvested are of a similar ratio; these have
be rebalanced by feeding other substances where the
io is Ca>:P (more calcium than phosphorus) as in hay,
with chemical supplements.

Nonetheless the starch-rich grain, with its amino acids,
amins, minerals and trace elements, is the valuable
rvestable crop to become an energy rich feedstuff for
n and his animals.

Plants have a wide inter-species variation when their
nstituents are analysed either as growing or as harvested.
Despite this, agriculturalists have narrowed the range of
rbage and plants suitable for stock feeding by grazing or

by 'hand' feeding of the harvested forms such as

- grass meal
- silage
- haylage
- hay
- straw
- cereal grains
- others

Generally speaking, they are the sources of the major
nutrients for

- energy
- fibre
- protein
- minerals (ash)
- other micro nutrients

and are subgrouped as:

- roughage – hay and straw, seed husk, etc.
- concentrates – cereal grains

and on harvesting are recognised as having the ratios
shown in the table overleaf

The agriculturalist (who will examine several bales out of
a single field's yield, for the presence of weeds and other
noxious plants, especially ragwort) can estimate a hay's
nutritive value by randomly selecting a pull from the bale;
this should

- be greenish/yellow, and not brown or even darker
- smell sweet, neither malty nor musty
- be free from dust when shaken (a high clover content
  in bales more than 6 months old will release dust-like
  material from the disintegrating dried leaf)
- have a good proportion of intact leaf content
- have limited flower presence and little or no seed heads

The interpretation of these will be more accurate if he
knows

- if it is from permanent grassland, i.e. meadow hay
  which will have a wide variety of grasses not all
  maturing at the same time, or if it is seed hay (a 1–3
  year ley)
- age when cut – ideally no more than 8 weeks from the
  time growth started or regrowth if a second cut, i.e.
  before seed has developed and with limited flower
  formation

Chart of Percentage Composition of Plant Foodstuffs – and the Horse

	PLANTS			HORSE (less gut content)
	Grass	Hay	Corn	
Water	72	15	14	60
Protein	3	1	10	17
'Fat'	1	–	3	17
Carbohydrates	22	83 high in cellulose; low in solubles	70 high in solubles; low in cellulose	1
Minerals	2	1	1	5

- how long it took to 'make', and the weather during that time
- what fertiliser applications have been used

These facts will enable him to estimate the approximate

- energy value
- protein value
- fibre content
- calcium and phosphorus contents and ratios

The amateur owner/horsemaster should be able to inspect with regard to colour, smell, dustiness, and flower and seed content. If a more exact analysis is required, representative samples will be required for laboratory examination. This can be done via a food compounder or supplier.

Feeding

The advantages and disadvantages of feeding silage rather than hay are a matter for veterinary discussion. Haylages have several advantages as an intermediate conserve

- any moulds present but unseen are of much reduced risk, as the spores are unlikely to proliferate in the bag and those that do are mainly attached to the fibre – they will be harmlessly swallowed and **not inhaled**

- the producer, from analysis, will know the
  - dry matter (DM) content and protein percentage
  - the fibre percentage
  - possibly the mineral content

Thus the feed value and respiratory disease prevention factor are almost guaranteed, subject especially to the feeding practices being carefully followed.

Poor, badly made and stored hay is deficient in the vitamin A precursor Retinol and in the folates.

It is rare, and often inadvisable, for the private owner at all but the larger commercial stables or studs to buy 'straight' grains for home mixing of rations. This can more safely and, in the long run, more economical supplied by the corn merchant, who will

- compound the straights – including oil-rich cereals
- supplement with the necessary minerals and vitamins
- regulate the protein % level to **prevent unnecessary uneconomic excess**

and mill and/or heat-treat and bag them as flakes, cubes nuts or coarse mixes, to suit the

- energy requirements of different disciplines, and to
- balance the 'home' roughages – and these can be

analysed for more accurate rationing – to give a total feed best suited for the purpose for which that horse is kept

The compounder will advise:
- how much for the weight of horse, usually in terms of light, medium and heavy work
- how much roughage

and the eventual ratio of these as work intensity changes.

All the horsemaster needs to know is
- **how heavy** is the horse and is it basically a pony or is it a horse (height), and what is the dominant blood if it is a cross, and
- is it at the right **condition** for the
    - work
    - climate
- will this horse's temperament alter the feed levels required – from experience but this too can be evaluated with professional help
- is
    - condition being maintained
    - appetite retained
    - the horse still 'fresh and keen' and able, and does he
    - maintain these during the period of top work
        - at peak, as in racing
        - over time, in slower athleticism
- and **what are the rules of feeding** to these ends

A compounder can very accurately suggest that a
- a 500kg hunter will require xkg of a specified concentrate mix; and, if that is micronised, will only require ykg
- and zkg of good hay to supply long fibre roughage as well as an estimated energy input

He may suggest that, in the light of the horse's history
- excitability
- proneness to ER

and subject to veterinary advice for the latter, that oats, for example, are not incorporated in the feed but that oil can be substituted slowly and up to say 100ml (3.4fl oz) per day.

A very important reason for purchasing compounded feedstuffs is that they are balanced in terms of protein percentage (which need never be high, except for lactating mares, foals and young flat racehorses), and especially supplemented with vitamins and minerals to balance the analysis of these two ingredients in the hay, so that daily requirements of such micro-nutrients are covered.

It can been seen therefore that a feeding chart can be drawn up which tells the owner, e.g. that for a 15hh Thoroughbred horse weighing 450kg and in fair to good condition but fit, with a 24-hour ration calculated on the basis of DM feedstuffs equal to 2.5% of its bodyweight, an ideal total daily intake will be 11.25kg+ (25lb+). From experience and also by scientific statistical findings, a guide for the proportion of roughage to concentrate in this ration is determined.

Always feed by weight or 'weighed' known volume.

Water

The body fluids, and in particular the ever present water, act as a
- lubricant (as in synovia), and generally as a hydroelastic shock absorber, e.g. in connective tissue and cerebro-spinal fluid
- solvent to form hydrates
- ionising medium

Water has a
- high specific heat
- high surface tension
- high dielectric constant, and can
    - hydrolyse protein, fat and starch
- active role in all metabolic processes
- integral function for sound and sight as the fluid component of the respective sense organs

It is **the transport medium** within the three compartments of the body tissues
- intravascular – blood
- intercellular fluid – cytoplasm
- extracellular fluid – lymph

and in the digestive tract.

It must never be overlooked.

Minerals

From the plethora of advertisements for mineral supplements, horse owners could be led to believe that the science of mineral feeding was well understood. The cynics might interpret it otherwise and they would be nearer the mark. There is still much to learn.

Some important known features

- the important minerals are **calcium** (Ca) and **phosphorus** (P), which work together primarily but not only in bone structure and in metabolism generally
  - the digestion, the absorption and the metabolism of other minerals and the trace elements are 'controlled' by these two major elements' presence and ratios
- particularly with regard to calcium and phosphorus, there is a relatively wide range between an excess and a deficiency which could *endanger the life* of the adult horse. Miller's disease is such an extreme example – nutritional secondary hyperparathyroidism (NSH), where the mineral input is basically all phosphorus with little or no calcium. The feeding of bran as almost the entire diet meant the near total absence of Ca and a high intake of P

Most mineral disorders are associated with *imbalanced* ratios. Ca:P is a common example.

- work in human nutrition and in stock feeding has pinpointed certain metabolic disorders related to deficits (and occasionally excesses) of trace elements in the feedstuffs. Corrections by selection of nutrients and by appropriate supplementation are possible

Nutritional Secondary Hyperparathyroidism (NSH)

A metabolic dis-ease from feeding an incorrect ratio of calcium to phosphorus in the diet of natural or compounded feedstuffs. It is more likely to affect young stock and to show more quickly when they graze young, lush, improved pastures or are being fed concentrates when the phosphorus content is usually higher than calcium. It is made more probable if there is a vitamin D deficit and if the grazing contains oxalate-rich species. This 'chelates' or 'locks up' the calcium, thus compounding the problem.

The consequence is an attempt by nature to maintain calcium homeostasis in the blood by extracting calcium from the bone into the bloodstream. This is effected by positive feedback to the parathyroid glands which secret excess parathyroid hormone (PTH). A bone dystrophy, a osteoporosis, eventually develops with a relative increas of PTH in the bloodstream as well as a rising Ca level. Th osseous change is quicker in the young growing anima with its greater metabolic rate.

Other hormones such as renal calcitriol come into pla which, whilst naturally curative initially, will eventually, the diet is not corrected, result in fibrous (soft bone dystrophy, hypocalcaemia and renal failure.

Early diagnosis is difficult clinically, but is based on

- radiography to show bone changes – osteoporosis
- the dietary history
- the suspicious clinical signs
- serum analysis for the concentration of parathyroid hormone
- serum and urine tests for fractional excretion of excess phosphorus

Signs

- stiff gait
- shifting leg lameness
  - joint pain – the cartilage loses security on the epiphyseal bone
  - periostitis – from tearing of ligaments at origin and insertion ends, and tendons at their insertion off the weakened bone
  - micro-fractures – focal periosteal avulsion fracture
    - eventual spontaneous fractures on long bones
- a classical skull bone softening; the fibrous material occupies more space than the original bone, hence
  - 'big head' as in miller's (bran) disease
  - loss of dental security, pain on eating and masticating
    - weight loss
  - vertebral compression fractures
    - weakness
    - paresis

Treatment

Correct the Ca:P ration with veterinary and fee compounder's help. Increase calcium with alfalfa, e.

aiming for Ca:P of 4:1 until x-rays are normal. Reduce exercise to decrease bone metabolic loss of calcium.

Prevention

Monitor diet: beware a wrong Ca:P ratio, even a one day sudden switch to an all bran (medicinal/laxative) diet can upset the digestion.

Scientific investigation at the time, of a long established nutritional imbalance such as the extreme example of miller's disease, was not possible; mill stones are now more sophisticatedly driven than by a single horse power, but clinical appraisal did pave the way for an understanding of other similar but much less drastic imbalances related to Ca and P, such as

- bone dystrophy (DOD) in the immature horse
- electrolyte imbalances with other associated elements, such as potassium in the adult athlete, related to
    - fatigue syndrome in endurance horses
    - poor performance syndrome in the elite athletic horse

The levels of these two important minerals in feedstuffs varies

- cereals are deficient in calcium and rich in phosphorus
- grass has changing levels
    - low calcium in lush growing young crops, with high phosphorus
    - gradually changing to excess calcium to phosphorus, in grass ready for cutting or allowed to flower as a seed crop for harvesting
- hay reflects this; it is still richer in calcium than phosphorus **but often low in both** after losses during 'making and gathering'. So too is old pasture at the end of the growing season; they are poor sources of total minerals and trace elements

Generally speaking, good hay balances cereal concentrates' mineral ratios when the amounts fed are not lower than 50:50. It is important when feeding young stock and athletic animals and brood mares that the analyses are known **and corrected** to give what is thought to be a correct intake of total minerals, but **always more calcium than phosphorus**, certainly never less than 2:1 in the adult and never less than 4:1 in youngstock and performers.

Supplements

To correct natural or man-made imbalances of

- minerals
- trace elements
- (electrolytes)

as extra to those that are present in all feedstuffs in varying proportions. Some, like copper, calcium, phosphorus and magnesium can be stored in the body tissues such as bone, but this does not exonerate the horsemaster from maintaining a balanced daily input. Sodium, chlorine and potassium cannot be stored; they are serum electrolytes, and any excess fed is quickly excreted, but must be present in the animal on an on-going basis especially when hard exercise and sweat loss is anticipated.

They are necessary substances normally found in feedstuffs to varying percentages in varying nutrients, but which are deemed to be occasionally insufficient for

- that horse
- doing that work
- on a certain ration

They are supplied as straight inorganic minerals or, better, as organic 'salts'.

It may require more of a substance than a particular ration supplies; more to augment what that horse can utilise (metabolise) and more than the 'average' horse requires.

This may be proven by a range of

- analyses
    - metabolic tests
- diagnosed disorders

examples of which are

- electrolyte related ER
- nutritional secondary hyperparathyroidism

in which appropriate supplementation may

- cure a dis-ease

which is clinically apparent in one horse though not in others of the same age, type and use and **on the same basic ration**. They may be used preventatively in a horse (or horses) known to be susceptible.

A supplement can enhance the digestive and metabolic value of a ration by increasing the utilisation of oxygen by the systems to minimise the effect of exercise or to delay fatigue, e.g. dimethylglycine. It is usually added to a group exposed to the same exercise stress.

Conversely, a ration may be deficient in a

- trace element(s)
- mineral(s)
- vitamin(s)

whereby a significant number of similarly kept animals exhibit disorders known to be typical of the deficiency; they respond to the appropriate supplementation.

A straight deficiency of a major nutrient type whereby all the horses relative to the work expected are deficient in

- energy, or
- protein, or
- fibre

such is a true **mal-nutrition** which is corrected by upping the percentage of the deficient nutrient by a better

- ration formulation, or an improved
- quality/quantity input of the deficient nutrient

An **additive** is the feeding of a substance which, *per se*, has *no nutritive value* but which improves the

- palatability
- preservation
- digestibility of

an otherwise satisfactory, on analysis and by trial, ration.

Substances which have a medicinal value usually give the description '**medicated**' to the feedstuff which is then a vehicle for the oral prophylaxis or therapy against a particular disorder. Such supplements when added are called **Non Normal Nutrients**. They are known to alter the functioning of one or more physiological systems of the body for the better – or for the worse

- to enhance its action – to make the horse go faster, further and for longer duration than it has been genetically programmed to do
- to reduce its action – to slow it down
- to block painful nerve signals from the system to the central nervous system and thereby mask locomotor disturbances. This allows the horse to run better than it would (could) have done without the additive, i.e. bring it back to its pain-free genetic capability. (In competition circumstances these are said to be 'dopings'.)

All will culpably alter the forecasting of the horse's athleticism under 'rules and conditions'.

Fat *per se* is not normally found in equine rations vegetable oil is. It is known that a horse can be trained to utilise extra oil (or fat) for aerobic functioning.

Practical Applications of Nutrition Knowledge

Domestication of any herbivorous animal aims to

- prolong active life
- increase performance and fertility
- establish durability by feeding a ration of sufficient
    - coarse fibre (roughage)
    - energy concentration, including lipids
    - protein
    - micro nutrients (vitamins and minerals) which at the same time meets the average 'appetite' of DM for that horse

The need to observe the rules of feeding have been discussed. Attention elsewhere in this book has been drawn to

- maximum weight of concentrates in any one feed, and so the need for repeat feeds at regular intervals
- the danger of sudden changes in feedstuffs, and the use of contaminated or mouldy feedstuffs

It is fortuitous that the adult usually obtains sufficient crude digestible protein for living and up to hard (but not fast) work from the bulk foodstuffs. The immature horse, the brood mare and the elite athlete will require a protein supplement at critical times.

Unnecessary supplementary protein will not *per se* upset digestion and general metabolism: it will be another source of energy, an expensive source, but also *a strain on kidney functioning*.

The rations must blend with the horse's needs of its gut micro-organisms on the one hand; and on the other the induced ratio of blood cells to plasma, as to produce a hyper-concentration of cells and a relative deficiency of fluid. This is one reason for an athletic horse, on higher protein in its necessarily rich energy rations 'going over the top' too soon during full fitness, thus shortening the duration of peak performance. Care must be taken to recognise the premonitory signs when the horse becomes 'picky'. A let down in total feed intake and longer daily access to grazing is called for over 2 to 3 days with a gradual return.

Mistakes in feeding the bovine in which the dairy cow, especially, does require supplementary protein input commensurate with milk output (and meat production to a lesser extent in the beef animal), are easy to detect, explain and monitor

- litres of milk, of certain
  - butter fat
  - solids (not fat) per kilo of food fed
    - relative to fertility
  - fattening rates, and levels in kilos per kilo fed

In a milking herd or a beef unit, in well run establishments, the aim is to have little variation in not only genotype but also in phenotype, i.e. level base lines with reasonable equality in response to known feed levels, whereby the ratios and the actual total of

- energy
- fibre
- protein
- micro nutrients

could be accurately estimated and fed according to a tight ration. Any failure in a group could be investigated by

- clinical examination for dis-ease, including physical impediments such as lameness
- laboratory investigation
  - haematology
  - metabolic profile
  - liver and intestine functioning tests
  - urinary percentage clearance tests for minerals (electrolytes)
  - intercurrent sub-clinical dis-ease
- nutrient analyses

on the understanding that individual temperament was of little importance.

The horse is a sufficiently **different** herbivore to make production evaluations much less a reflection of functioning, since athletic production is not an exactly quantifiable parameter. The Thoroughbred can trace back genotypically but is more varied in actual on-going breeding. Phenotypically, many Thoroughbreds 'look' what they are but subtle differences in metabolism can be important performance wise. This is often relative to what, how and when they are fed.

Most importantly, the horse, whether pure bred or cross, is **always an individual**, particularly in

- keenness
- temperament and constitution
  - hormonal influences
  - feedstuff utilisation
  - response to day-to-day changes in environment (as a competitive athlete, these changes are often marked)

Moreover, it may have been bred for work in various disciplines requiring varied

- speed
- stamina
- agility

These, if nothing else, involve changes in locomotor muscle metabolism as well as what is best described as 'psychological attitude'.

Feeding errors of a minor nature make little difference to the adult horse but they could produce subtle disorders as part of Poor Performance Syndrome. The **quality** of the protein fed is important. It is essential to provide what are called **essential amino acids**, the building blocks of proteins.

Deficiency in **methionine, lysine** and **zinc** could be reflected in poor hoof and skin quality and would require supplementation with distillers grains and linseed meal in small quantities or as straight specific biochemicals.

Different breeds reach full maturity at different times, i.e. finish growth of the dorsal thoracic vertebral spines' cartilage caps to give the ultimate 'height at the withers', some as early as 6 years old, others not until 7 or even 8 years old. This variation may increase with cross-breds, especially with the introduction of hot blood lines into warm or even cold bloods and vice-versa.

This one parameter of height is genetically fixed; unless severe malnutrition is involved, a horse will reach its predetermined height – eventually – regardless of minor malnutrition.

Thoroughbreds are genetically programmed to mature early (as determined by the time of closure of the growth plates in the distal limb long bones); there is a significant implication in this *vis à vis* flat racing of 2 year olds and must be carefully fed to safely match the ratio requirements, especially of Ca and P.

It is also recognised, especially in Thoroughbreds and their close crosses, that energy feeding to effect rapid growth in weanlings can lead to asymmetries of relative growth between bone and muscle, and so associated limb deformities, the so-called 'contracted tendons syndrome'.

Racing on the flat is arguably the only reasonably accurate yardstick for proving a ration fed to a horse trained to 'go' a certain distance in a certain time. However, many factors can upset this 'on the day'

- sub-clinical viraemia
- certain bacterial infections paradoxically known as 'the Virus'
- temperament, as already emphasised
- 'wrong going' for a particular horse
- jockey error
- interference by other runners

Even so, the difference in time between first and last past the post is often so small that it is insignificant in estimating the performance (production) value of any one diet at any one time. This, in National Hunt racing, is even less helpful.

In endurance riding, the other extreme of stamina athleticism, some significant extrapolations can be made, e.g. rations with and without oil (fat), as judged by

- able to finish *and fit to continue*
- how close to a winning forecast time event or race
- not finishing
    - developing metabolic dis-orders during and after an event

being indicative of fatigue or 'running out of energy' in the absence of suspected or proven

- intercurrent dis-ease
- low grade lameness
- unexpected – untrained for – weather/terrain
- rider (un)fitness

Despite the breeding of

- close-bred lines or families with reasonably close
- matching conformation, and an
- athletic potential

there can be on-going different responses to

- feeding, as that determines 'condition'
- muscle development response related to training

possibly related to the effects of the individual constitution

- a good doer
- a bad doer
- a 'goer'
- a 'lazy devil', laid-back temperament

It is only by the horsemaster *taking all these into consideration* for tailoring the feeding amounts, ratios and times, that full use of feedstuffs can be attained.

It is accepted that in performance horse keeping, the cost of feeding is not high in the list of economic priorities but it is an important factor. It is more cost-concerning in the less athletic animal, particularly in regard to maintaining

- health and durability, e.g. in riding schools
- condition and physical ability, where other variable costs are low and fixed costs relatively so

Over-feeding and under-using are often justifiable criticisms of the private owner/horsemaster.

In any equine discipline success will depend upon the horse being at the **correct fitness** and the **right weight**. There is nothing to be gained, in fact much to be lost, by having a horse carry dead weight in the form of excess fat. Outwintering is another matter.

Show condition often means 'too well covered' which tells the judge nothing other than the horse is a good converter of food to body fat, but it also masks accurate assessment of skeletal conformation which is a basic parameter for physical performance potential.

The 'fighting fit', slimmed-down horse will reveal inter-muscle group demarcation and development *per se*; a fat animal will infill these marks and 'lard' over the muscle groups.

Fat must not be confused with inherited and developed muscle bulk: nor can fat be changed into muscle.

It is quite a skill to balance condition and weight; it is important that it is attempted, especially in the more athletic uses. Weight (static mass) can be measured; it will vary relative to condition (subcutaneous fat and muscle development) in any one horse.

When fittening begins the horse will have a certain weight which should be measured or estimated. It will also carry a certain percentage of this body weight as subcutaneous fat. The aim is to

- work the horse to
    - develop muscle bulk
    - burn off unwanted fat, and to
- feed it in such a manner as to maintain the required

- condition appearance, which is the relative
  - skeletal conformation which is unalterable
  - the muscle development gained at the time of near fitness to work without fatigue
  - the amount of subcutaneous fat thought to be ideal for that horse doing that discipline without it carrying unnecessary dead weight

There are no hard and fast measurements. It depends upon the trainer's skill, reflecting

past performance, against

present 'appearance' and training tests

Condition Score as a Guide

The evidence of subcutaneous fat, *especially* on the body areas used naturally for storing fat against times of need

seasonal malnutrition

excessive cold

seen at rest must be amended by

corrective feeding

progressive work

produce the ideal working condition

sub-cutaneous fat around the girth (along the heart line) the least likely to be in excess. Conversely, with weight loss it is the most readily measurable for 'a loss of subcutaneous fat' and *vice versa* for weight gain – a simple, easily accessible diameter measurement. In practice it is the measure of rise or fall that is important, not the actual estimated mass at any one time.

The horse *spends* energy as

maintenance for living – 'M-energy'

productive for working – 'P-energy'

eats and drinks to live. Its daily intake is limited to approximately 2.5% bodyweight of dry matter (erroneously called 'appetite'). When P-energy demands an increase more must be obtained from concentrates; the roughage consequently must be decreased, but **never to less than 20% of total intake** by weight and preferably 5–40% in the non-racing Thoroughbred.

Thoroughbred feeding, especially for young sprinters is a specialised and different matter.

the horsemaster must know what amount of feed, in terms

of energy and other constituents, which is necessary daily to

- reach an optimal static weight (mass x 0)
- body score for a particular job, and to
- maintain them there or thereabouts

The bovine digestive system has its 'fermentation vats' at the *anterior* end, the equine at the **posterior** in the form of the enlarged colon and the caecum. The horse is less able to withstand

- exposure to lush grazing, as distinct from the breed's indigenous grazing, e.g the moorland pony to bovine fattening grasslands which offer inadvisable intakes of solubles (starch) which do not have the requisite physiological time for enzymatic digestion in the horse's stomach and the small intestine before being 'washed' into the microbial fermentation processes of the large intestine, the caecum. It is the microbe which becomes dis-ordered with a strong potential for ill-effects
- sudden changes in diet, as from grass to hay

An increase in production output for the bovine requires a pro rata increase in energy **and** protein input. The horse's increase – an athletic output – does not require anything like the increase in input of protein but certainly does require a progressive input of energy sources. Herein lies the important difference in the two species.

A horse cannot be fed to go faster than its genetic token ability, but if its inherent ability of speed and stamina are invoked it needs to eat appropriately to fuel these functional outputs. It can be trained to

- more quickly and more efficiently metabolise its fat reserves, for aerobic muscle functioning
- more quickly induce type II high oxidative muscle fibres to become more efficiently aerobic in action
- become more efficient in
  - cardio-vascular output
  - gaseous exchange availability both pulmonary and systemically

to meet the manifold increase in metabolism required for high performance

  - delaying muscular fatigue

If underfed it will fuel its muscles 'off its back' by burning up fat (and muscle) for energy; it will lose condition.

The daily feed intake is **usually** always sufficiently available for maintenance and light work from summer grazing or hay and some concentrates in winter time. Some horses (ponies) relative to the type of grazing may have to walk (nomadic instinct) over considerable distances to find sufficient bulk. Even then, there is no guarantee that that amount of ingesta will supply all, or all of some, of the **essential** nutrients after digestion and metabolisation.

It will, however, be oblivious to any nutrient deficit, and be

- content in grazing, and
- eating and masticating

If and when an overall energy deficit arises, it will automatically 'call up' fat reserves. The related loss of condition in unprotected (uncovered) animals at grass in winter time will invoke heat retention tactics, and the horse

- seeks shelter
- huddles, and
- shivers – it is now 'aware' of its state

When the body core temperature can no longer be maintained, emaciation will follow – i.e. no subcutaneous fat is left for metabolism. There is, meanwhile, a protein (flesh) burn to augment heat but this is of limited use; weakness and death will follow.

The basic deficit is starvation. The 'sharp end' is hypothermia and the slowing down, and indeed cessation, of enzymatic functioning throughout all body cells.

CHAPTER
40 CARE OF THE OLDER HORSE

INTRODUCTION

The ages of the horse, relative to those of man, are approximately

5 horse	= 20 man
10 horse	= 40 man
15 horse	= 50 man
20 horse	= 60 man
25 horse	= 70 man
30 horse	= 80 man
35 horse	= 90 man

Hayes' *Veterinary Notes for Horse Owners*, quoting from *Smith's Veterinary Physiology*, lists horses living to an age ranging from 'Ladias' at 23 to Paerol at 36 years. The Guinness Book of Records has recorded a pony of 54 (France) and a horse, of Cleveland x Eastern blood, living to 62 (1760–1822).

There is little evidence that the horse's expectation of life has increased in the same way as man's, for whom better housing, contagious disease control (especially tuberculosis), and better incomes for better food, have all played vital roles.

Little work has been published as to longevity *vis à vis* occupation, but in general the quick-maturing breeds, e.g. the Thoroughbred, should have a shorter lifespan than the cold blood, and the slower-maturing purebreds such as the Arab.

In all breeds it is recognised that the more natural the life, the longer it is lived: the pony, hard-worked from grass, will outlive the stabled hunter. The brood animal will outlive one in work, apart from the hazards of breeding.

Work occupational hazards do of course shorten life, but mainly because the injuries and acquired defects shorten useful *economic* life – and only a minority of people believe in fully pensioning off a 'finished' hunter or chaser as distinct from using it as a nanny/companion.

Consequences of Ageing

Ageing brings with it
- a stretching or slackening – a 'tiring' of the
  - postural ligaments in the stay suspensory apparatus
    - going over at the knee, especially in the one-time athletic horse
    - a breaking back of the pastern/hoof axis
    - a sinking of the fetlock, especially in the hind limbs, along with weakness of the
  - supportive structures of the thoraco lumbar spine, leading to a
    - hollowing or sway back outline, especially in the brood mare, and to changing support pressure, with
  - hoof wall failures
    - distortion of the angle of the vulva, permitting entrapment of faeces and ascending infection of the vagina
- loss of some areas of fat deposition
  - the more hollow supra-orbital cavities
- variable disorders of the teeth
- deterioration in the quality of skin and coat
  - greater susceptibility to rain scald, and other dermatophilus disorders

Signs of old age.

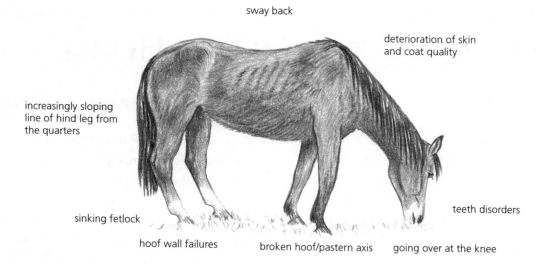

sway back

deterioration of skin and coat quality

increasingly sloping line of hind leg from the quarters

teeth disorders

sinking fetlock

hoof wall failures

broken hoof/pastern axis

going over at the knee

- diminished immunity, especially to secondary bacterial (and fungal) invaders of primary viral infections and to existing pulmonary allergies
- a susceptibility to the development of pituitary tumours, with the consequence of Cushingoid syndrome leading *inter alia* to
  - hirsutism
  - laminitis
  - diminished renal functioning

Overall there is a progressive deterioration in
- locomotor activity
  - weight carrying (and saddle fitting difficulty)
- degenerative joint dis-ease
- metabolism
  - liver function
  - stress control
  - weight loss – often multifactoral

There is little confirmable evidence of geriatric hearing difficulties.

Vision does deteriorate
- degenerative lens opacities (cataracts)
- changes in the vitreous body, with increased 'floaters' in it and liquefaction of its substance

- haemorrhages into both the aqueous and the vitreous chambers

All affect visual acuity for 'defence' against distant moving objects, but even these debilities do not markedly interfere with the old horse getting about in a known environment.

An increased incidence of ocular adnexal neoplasia does not help; they must be an irritating annoyance exacerbated by the attention of flies attracted to the associated discharges and the secondary excess tear formation.

Olfactory sensitivity is difficult to assess, but the continuing ability to feel what is presented to eat – via lip sensory endings and the tactile hairs – would seem to compensate along with gustatory sensibility.

The molar disorders, and any consequential caries and purulent gingivitis, will of course deaden this sense of **taste**, but most old horses will continue to be hungry and to prehend food even when the incisors and the molars,

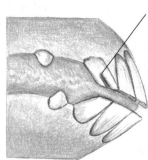

Galvayne's groove showing age of approx. 25 years; will 'grow' out entirely by approx. age 30

The angled teeth of an old horse.

especially, are causing increasing difficulty.

Horses do not die from an 'old' **heart**. The ageing of cardiac muscle and the possible interference with cardiac 'nerve' conduction associated with distortion of the ventricles and with earlier athletic hypertrophy or right side heart dilation from prolonged OPD and its pulmonary arterial obstruction, leaves this heart more susceptible to

- viral myositis
- myocardial malnutrition, and the effect of
- *sudden* exercise can lead to sudden failure

The equine failing heart usually gives warning with the horse, when ridden, slowing to a halt, slightly rearing, before stumbling and going down, usually with a loud whinnying.

The causes of human heart failure are not common in the horse but in a working geriatric horse an annual check-up is advisable.

The fatal rupture of one or other of the major arteries is more often seen in the younger (teenage) athletic horse. Those horses which make it to pensionable age rarely meet such stresses. The possible association of folic acid deficiency and thrombosis, as seen in the distal aorta in man and suspected in the horse with aortic-iliac thrombosis should not occur whilst grass is being eaten. There are pathogenic explanations other than old age.

The **respiratory system** is more susceptible, possibly because of

- recurrent viral inflammation
- secondary bacterial invasions
  - chronic bronchitis/bronchiolitis
- persisting allergic disorder of the bronchioles, as in COPD and ageing emphysema

but their usual 'pensioned off to grass' environment reduces their incidence. However, a new infection and invasion and/or an *acute* allergic exacerbation when fed dry hay, may well prove too much with consequent

- deterioration in gaseous exchange
- hypertension on the cardio-vascular system
  - liver and renal failure
  - CNS disturbance

Parasitism is important

- ageing deterioration of existing anti-helminth immunity

- exposure to permanent pasture grazing, with risk of heavy small redworm invasion
- possible thrombo-embolic colic, from large redworm larvae

less attention having been paid to routine worming, pasture hygiene and supplementary nutrition.

Lymphoid and lympho-sarcomatous **tumours** can occur in the body cavities, with

- destruction of gut wall integrity
  - protein-losing enteropathy
  - loss of absorption power
  - diarrhoea
- strangulation of the bowel by the pedicle of a tumour mass
- tumour masses in the
  - spleen (lowering immunity)
  - bone marrow (anaemia)
  - lungs (reduced gaseous exchange)

Melanomata, in themselves, are not usually worrying but

- intra-abdominally they are a further hazard to obstruction of the gut
- externally, especially in the perineum, they attract callophorine flies, the subsequent 'strike' predisposing to secondary infection and self-mutilation

Nutritional Deficits

- not sufficient nutrients in grazing offered
- difficulty in mastication
- gut wall problems as mentioned above

will lead to malnutrition, as will

- overall shortage – less than 2.5% body-weight intake per 24 hours, because of bare and/or 'poached' pastures
- specific deficiencies in vitamins and minerals and amino acids
- reduced digestion of protein, phosphorus and fibre
  - associated with chronic lower intestine mucosal damage

Most of the above are not primary geriatric digestive disorders but are relevant to geriatrics.

All these must receive attention if loss of condition and

increasing susceptibility to systemic and locomotor disease is to be avoided, as well as preventing hypothermia in the wet and cold of winter when there is a marked loss of body fat following malnutrition.

Horses can grow old gracefully, but are they happy if no longer suitable for work, such as

- gentle hacking – for a year or two longer, perhaps
- as a companion/nanny for young stock

As a lone animal they may be neglected.

The Old Mare

It is axiomatic that nature will control the likelihood of an old mare being hazarded by 'just one more foal', but if nature fails, the risks to a heavily pregnant old mare are

- debilitating abortion, with secondary
  - metritis
  - pneumonia
  - laminitis
- a difficult full-term foaling, and recumbency leading to
  - pneumonia
  - retained placenta
    - endotoxaemia
    - laminitis

and even the later stages of pregnancy overloading her weakened back and dropped hind fetlocks, with the ongoing risk of

- recumbency, or .
- laminitis, leading to
  - inability to get about and eventual
  - recumbency from postural weakness

Management of the Older Horse

An owner who for whatever reason wishes to maintain an equine pensioner **must**

- see to its teeth at the start
  - thereafter twice yearly
    - and be guided by the veterinary surgeon as to welfare considerations
- have the *feet attended to at least every six weeks*, and consider the need for advised special shoeing
  - pick them out each day, *even at grass*

- pay particular attention to
  - supplementary feeding
  - winter care and hypothermia risk
    - strict awareness of
      - mud fever
      - rain scald
      - fly strike, sweet itch and skin tumours
      - other injuries, lameness and systemic illnesses
    - Cushingoid syndrome

When the decision is reached to 'call it a day' – better sooner than later – then the method of euthanasia can be discussed with a veterinary surgeon, disposal likewise, but *you owe it to the horse to be there and to 'hold its hand'*

Cushing's Disease

This can be described as a mixed neoplastic/metabolic disease. The disease is called 'Cushingoid' or simply 'Equine Cushing's'. The name is taken from that used in human hyperadrenocorticism (HAC), in which a disorder of the adrenal glands produces a pathological excess of the hormone **adrenocortisol**.

It affects the older pony and cob, is less common in the hunter and less still in Thoroughbreds. An animal is susceptible between 12 and 34 years of age; and it is more common in geldings.

It is slow to develop, the coat changes, i.e. retained curly hair in patches being most diagnostic. Untreated, it is chronic up to 2 years. With treatment, a response should be seen in 6 weeks for the prognosis to be acceptable for longer treatment.

Oral ulcers are a common lesion.

Reference to CHAPTER 10, THE ENDOCRINE SYSTEM shows that the anterior pituitary gland (the adrenohypophysis) secretes a controlling hormone, adreno-corticotrophin hormone (ACTH) in response to information fed to it via the blood. When enough adrenocortisol is available, the negative feedback mechanism switches off the anterior pituitary gland, and so reduces the ACTH levels.

A main function of the adrenal hormone is the metabolism of glucose into the bloodstream. An excess of this glucose, **hyperglycaemia**, is a **transient** physiological response from

- adrenalin-induced glycogenesis

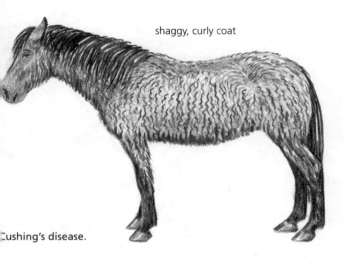

shaggy, curly coat

Cushing's disease.

- carbohydrate intake increase – dietary change
- insulin resistance brought about by, for example
  - stress, including strenuous exercise
  - pregnancy
  - obesity
- external factors
  - administration of corticosteroids
  - other drugs such as xylazine

All these are most marked in ponies and pony crosses which are genetically less sensitive to insulin activity. There is rarely sufficiently high or prolonged blood sugar level to cross the renal threshold to produce glycosuria – sugar in the urine.

Pathological causes such as adrenalin gland tumours are very rare in the horse.

However, persistent, pathological hyperglycaemia, as determined from blood tests, is the result of *uncontrolled* ACTH production. The most likely cause in the horse is a functional pituitary tumour. A *chronic* high glucose abnormality is relatively uncommon in the horse, and when it is diagnosed it is usually the result of HAC.

Repeat blood samples are necessary to differentiate the two types, but in practice the chronic form is suspected by the patient's history and slowly developing clinical signs and, from urine testing, an accompanying glycosuria.

HAC and functioning pituitary tumour is then strongly suspected.

The persistent form is not regulated by insulin as in human diabetes mellitus. This, and the associated pancreatic deficit, is extremely rare in the horse. Human secondary diabetes due to insulin blockage simulates HAC in the horse, and here a primary disorder must exist, namely the pituitary tumour. This can only be confirmed on autopsy or by computerised tomography, which is more or less impracticable in the horse.

The persistent hyperglycaemia affects the kidneys, leading to glycosuria, and these two cause polyuria and polydipsia – increased urinary output and excessive thirst, referred to as PUPD.

The tumour, an adenoma in the anterior of the three parts of the pituitary gland, causes an excess of cortisol, opiomelanocortin (POMC) peptide, in excess of the normal ACTH levels from the healthy gland.

The clinical signs of this failure to respond to negative feedback control are

- polyuria   in 76% of cases
- polydipsia   in 76% of cases
- weight loss   in 88% of cases
- hirsutism (retained coat)   in 94% of cases
- laminitis (corticosteroid toxicity)   in 82% of cases
- sweating   in 59% of cases
- neurological deficits   in 6% of cases
- supra orbital fat increase   in 12% of cases
- immunosuppression   in 50% of cases
- hyperglycaemia – lab tests   in 90% of cases
- hyperglycosuria – lab tests   in 80% of cases

There is no absolute cure, but good nursing and the *continuous* use of veterinary advised specific therapy can create an improved quality of life, even light work, but frequently the outcome is disappointing.

Repeated clipping of the excess coat is advisable, especially in hot weather. A slightly higher protein compound can be helpful, e.g. stud cubes 500g to 1kg (1–2lb) daily.

INDEX

Page numbers in **bold** type refer to illustrations

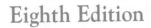

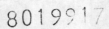

Eighth Edition

Clinical Nursing Skills

Basic to Advanced Skills

Sandra F. SMITH

President, National Nursing Review; Los Altos, California

Donna J. DUELL

Consultant to Deans and Directors of Nursing; California

Barbara C. MARTIN

Professor of Nursing, The University of Tulsa; Tulsa, Oklahoma

Pearson

Boston Columbus Indianapolis New York San Francisco Upper Saddle River
Amsterdam Cape Town Dubai London Madrid Milan Munich Paris Montreal Toronto
Delhi Mexico City Sao Paulo Sydney Hong Kong Seoul Singapore Taipei Tokyo

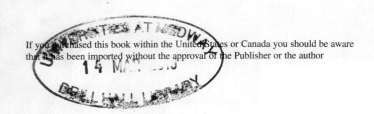
Notice: Care has been taken to confirm the accuracy of the information presented in this book. The authors, editors, and the publisher, however, cannot accept any responsibility for errors or omissions or for consequences from application of the information in this book and make no warranty, express or implied, with respect to its contents.

The authors and the publisher have exerted every effort to ensure that drug selections and dosages set forth in this text are in accord with current recommendations and practice at time of publication. However, in view of ongoing research, changes in government regulations, and the constant flow of information relating to drug therapy and drug reactions, the reader is urged to check the package inserts of all drugs for any change in indications of dosage and for added warnings and precautions. This is particularly important when the recommended agent is a new and/or infrequently employed drug.

The authors and publisher disclaim all responsibility for any liability, loss, injury, or damage incurred as a consequence, directly or indirectly, of the use and application of any of the contents of this volume.

Publisher: Julie Levin Alexander
Publisher's Assistant: Regina Bruno
Senior Acquisitions Editor: Kelly Trakalo
Assistant Editor: Lauren Sweeney
Development Editor: Karen Hoxeng
Managing Production Editor: Patrick Walsh
Production Liaison: Yagnesh Jani
Production Editor: Tracy Duff, PreMedia Global
Manufacturing Manager: Ilene Sanford
Manager, Design Development: John Christiana
Interior and Cover Design: Laura Gardner
Director of Marketing: David Gesell
Art Director: Jodi Notowitz
Marketing Manager: Phoenix Harvey
Marketing Specialist: Michael Sirinides
Media Product Manager: Travis Moses—Westphal
Media Project Managers: Rachel Collett / Leslie Brado
Composition: PreMediaGlobal
Printer/Binder: RR Donnelley/Von Hoffman
Cover Printer: Lehigh-Phoenix Color
Cover photos: Ronald May, Celina Burkhart, Rick Brady

Credits and acknowledgments borrowed from other sources and reproduced, with permission, in this textbook appear on appropriate page within text.

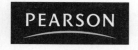

10 9 8 7 6 5 4 3 2 1

ISBN 13: 978-0-13-268360-9
ISBN 10:   0-13-268360-1